Translational Neuroscience:

Applications in Psychiatry, Neurology,
and Neurodevelopmental Disorders

Translational Neuroscience:

Applications in Psychiatry, Neurology,
and Neurodevelopmental Disorders

Edited by

James E. Barrett
Professor and Chair of Pharmacology and Physiology and Director of the Drug Discovery and Development Program at Drexel University College of Medicine, Philadelphia, PA, USA

Joseph T. Coyle
Eben S. Draper Chair of Psychiatry and Neuroscience at McLean Hospital, Harvard Medical School, Belmont, MA, USA

Michael Williams
Adjunct Professor of Pharmacology and Physiology, Faculty of the Drug Discovery and Development Program at Drexel University College of Medicine, Philadelphia, PA, USA

CAMBRIDGE UNIVERSITY PRESS

CAMBRIDGE UNIVERSITY PRESS
Cambridge, New York, Melbourne, Madrid, Cape Town,
Singapore, São Paulo, Delhi, Mexico City

Cambridge University Press
The Edinburgh Building, Cambridge CB2 8RU, UK

Published in the United States of America by
Cambridge University Press, New York

www.cambridge.org
Information on this title: www.cambridge.org/9780521519762

© Cambridge University Press 2012

This publication is in copyright. Subject to statutory exception
and to the provisions of relevant collective licensing agreements,
no reproduction of any part may take place without
the written permission of Cambridge University Press.

First published 2012

Printed in the United Kingdom at the University Press, Cambridge

A catalog record for this publication is available from the British Library

Library of Congress Cataloging-in-Publication data

Translational neuroscience: applications in psychiatry, neurology, and neurodevelopmental disorders / edited by James E. Barrett, Joseph T. Coyle, Michael Williams.
    p. ; cm.
    Includes bibliographical references and index.
    ISBN 978-0-521-51976-2 (Hardback)
    I. Barrett, James E. II. Coyle, Joseph T. III. Williams, Michael
    [DNLM: 1. Nervous System Diseases. 2. Drug Discovery.
3. Mental Disorders. 4. Neurosciences–methods. 5. Translational Research–methods. WL 140]
    616.8–dc23

2011043658

ISBN 978-0-521-51976-2 Hardback

Cambridge University Press has no responsibility for the persistence or accuracy of URLs for external or third-party internet websites referred to in this publication, and does not guarantee that any content on such websites is, or will remain, accurate or appropriate.

Every effort has been made in preparing this book to provide accurate and up-to-date information which is in accord with accepted standards and practice at the time of publication. Although case histories are drawn from actual cases, every effort has been made to disguise the identities of the individuals involved. Nevertheless, the authors, editors and publishers can make no warranties that the information contained herein is totally free from error, not least because clinical standards are constantly changing through research and regulation. The authors, editors and publishers therefore disclaim all liability for direct or consequential damages resulting from the use of material contained in this book. Readers are strongly advised to pay careful attention to information provided by the manufacturer of any drugs or equipment that they plan to use.

Contents

List of contributors vi
Preface ix
Acknowledgments xi

1 **The discovery and development of drugs to treat psychiatric disorders: Historical perspective** 1
Michael Williams and James E. Barrett

2 **Translational approaches to the treatment of anxiety disorders** 14
Charles F. Gillespie, Tamara Weiss, and Kerry J. Ressler

3 **Mood disorders** 27
Jorge A. Quiroz, Guang Chen, Wayne C. Drevets, Ioline D. Henter, and Husseini K. Manji

4 **Schizophrenia** 80
Darrick T. Balu and Donald C. Goff

5 **Addictive disorders** 107
Charles P. O'Brien

6 **Section summary and perspectives: Translational medicine in psychiatry** 118
Joseph T. Coyle

7 **Historical perspectives on the discovery and development of drugs to treat neurological disorders** 129
Michael Williams and Joseph T. Coyle

8 **Alzheimer's disease** 149
Donald L. Price, Alena V. Savonenko, Tong Li, and Philip C. Wong

9 **Pain therapeutics** 168
Anthony W. Bannon

10 **Multiple sclerosis** 178
Alfred W. Sandrock, Jr and Richard A. Rudick

11 **Parkinson's disease** 197
Jiang-Fan Chen

12 **Amyotrophic lateral sclerosis** 214
Nicholas J. Maragakis

13 **Epilepsy** 228
Maciej Gasior and Frank Wiegand

14 **Section summary and perspectives: Translational medicine in neurology** 253
James E. Barrett and Joseph T. Coyle

15 **Historical perspectives on the use of therapeutic agents to treat neurodevelopmental disorders** 261
Kimberly A. Stigler, Craig A. Erickson, David J. Posey, and Christopher J. McDougle

16 **Autism spectrum disorders** 273
Timothy P.L. Roberts, Michael Gandal, Steven J. Siegel, Paulo Vianney-Rodrigues, and John P. Welsh

17 **Attention deficit hyperactivity disorder** 303
Craig W. Berridge, David M. Devilbiss, Robert C. Spencer, Brooke E. Schmeichel, and Amy F.T. Arnsten

18 **Epigenetic mechanisms in central nervous system disorders** 321
Swati Gupta, Ryley Parrish, and Farah D. Lubin

19 **Section summary and perspectives: Neurodevelopmental disorders and regulation of epigenetic changes** 334
James E. Barrett and Joseph T. Coyle

20 **Promises and challenges of translational research in neuropsychiatry** 339
David L. Braff

Index 359
The color plate section can be found between pp. 148 and 149.

Contributors

Amy F.T. Arnsten
Department of Neurobiology, Yale University School of Medicine, New Haven, CT

Darrick T. Balu
Harvard Medical School, Belmont, MA

Anthony W. Bannon
Abbott Laboratories, Abbott Park, IL

James E. Barrett
Drexel University College of Medicine, Philadelphia, PA

Craig W. Berridge
Department of Psychology, University of Wisconsin, Madison, WI

David L. Braff
University of California San Diego School of Medicine, Department of Psychiatry, La Jolla, CA

Jiang-Fan Chen
Department of Neurology and Pharmacology, Boston University School of Medicine, Boston, MA

Guang Chen
Johnson & Johnson Pharmaceutical Research and Development, San Diego, CA

Joseph T. Coyle
Harvard Medical School, Boston, MA

David M. Devilbiss
Department of Psychology, University of Wisconsin, Madison, WI

Wayne C. Drevets
Laureate Institute for Brain Research and Department of Psychiatry, Oklahoma University College of Medicine, Tulsa, OK

Craig A. Erickson
Department of Psychiatry, Section of Child & Adolescent Psychiatry, Indiana University School of Medicine and the Christian Sarkine Autism Treatment Center, James Whitcomb Riley Hospital for Children, Indianapolis, IN

Michael Gandal
Department of Bioengineering and Department of Psychiatry, University of Pennsylvania, PA

Maciej Gasior
Discovery Medicine, Neuroscience, Bistol-Myers Squibb, Princeton, NJ

Charles F. Gillespie
Department of Psychiatry and Behavioral Sciences, Emory University School of Medicine, Atlanta, GA

Donald C. Goff
Massachusetts General Hospital, Boston, MA

Swati Gupta
The Evelyn F. McKnight Brain Institute, Department of Neurobiology, University of Alabama at Birmingham, Birmingham, AL

Ioline D. Henter
National Institute of Mental Health, National Institutes of Health, Bethesda, MD

Tong Li
Johns Hopkins University School of Medicine, Baltimore, MD

Farah D. Lubin
The Evelyn F. McKnight Brain Institute, Department of Neurobiology, University of Alabama at Birmingham, Birmingham, AL

List of contributors

Christopher J. McDougle
Lurie Center for Autism, Harvard University, Boston, MA

Husseini K. Manji
Johnson & Johnson Pharmaceutical Research and Development, Titusville, NJ

Nicholas J. Maragakis
Johns Hopkins University, Baltimore, MD

Charles P. O'Brien
Department of Psychiatry, University of Pennsylvania, Philadelphia, PA

Ryley Parrish
The Evelyn F. McKnight Brain Institute, Department of Neurobiology, University of Alabama at Birmingham, Birmingham, AL

David J. Posey
Department of Psychiatry, Section of Child & Adolescent Psychiatry, Indiana University School of Medicine and the Christian Sarkine Autism Treatment Center, James Whitcomb Riley Hospital for Children, Indianapolis, IN

Donald L. Price
Division of Neuropathology Alzheimer's Disease Research Center, Johns Hopkins University School of Medicine, Baltimore, MD

Jorge A. Quiroz
Pharma Research & Early Development, Neuroscience, Hoffmann-La Roche, Nutley, NJ

Kerry J. Ressler
Department of Psychiatry and Behavioral Sciences, Emory University School of Medicine, Atlanta, GA, Yerkes National Primate Research Center, Atlanta, GA and Howard Hughes Medical Institute

Timothy P.L. Roberts
Department of Radiology, University of Pennsylvania and Children's Hospital of Philadelphia, Philadelphia, PA

Richard A. Rudick
Mellen Center for Multiple Sclerosis Treatment and Research, Neurological Institute, Cleveland Clinic, Cleveland, OH

Alfred W. Sandrock, Jr
Neurology Research and Development, Biogen Idec, Inc., Cambridge, MA and Department of Neurology, Massachusetts General Hospital, Harvard Medical School, Boston, MA

Alena V. Savonenko
Departments of Pathology, Neurology and Division of Neuropathology, Johns Hopkins University School of Medicine, Baltimore, MD

Brooke E. Schmeichel
Department of Psychology, University of Wisconsin, Madison, WI

Steven J. Siegel
Department of Psychiatry, Translational Research Laboratory, University of Pennsylvania, Philadelphia, PA

Robert C. Spencer
Department of Psychology, University of Wisconsin, Madison, WI

Kimberly A. Stigler
Department of Psychiatry, Section of Child & Adolescent Psychiatry, Indiana University School of Medicine and the Christian Sarkine Autism Treatment Center, James Whitcomb Riley Hospital for Children, Indianapolis, IN

Paulo Vianney-Rodrigues
Department of Otorhinolaryngology, University of Pennsylvania, Philadelphia, PA

John P. Welsh
Center for Integrative Brain Research, Department of Pediatrics, Seattle Children's Research Institute, Seattle, WA

Tamara Weiss
Department of Psychiatry and Behavioral Sciences, Emory University School of Medicine, Atlanta, GA

Frank Wiegand
Johnson & Johnson Pharmaceutical Services LLC, Raritan, NJ

Michael Williams
Faculty of the Drug Discovery and Development Program at Drexel University College of Medicine, Philadelphia, PA

Philip C. Wong
Departments of Pathology and Neuroscience, Johns Hopkins University School of Medicine, Baltimore, MD

Preface

Translational medicine has emerged as a dominant theme within the context of the biomedical sciences. It has been somewhat difficult to define translational medicine as a formal discipline because, at the present time, there are no commonly accepted techniques or procedures that specifically delineate the methodological approaches or the conceptual framework within which the discipline is to evolve. In its most elemental form, translational medicine represents an effort to bridge the bidirectional gap between basic preclinical research and clinical studies in order to expedite the development of safe and effective therapeutics – the frequently articulated "bench to bedside" perspective. In a broader sense, translational medicine incorporates areas such as biomarker development, pharmacogenomics, clinical pharmacology, and clinical trial methodology to name just a few disciplines that have either embraced, or offer potential applications that can be applied to, translational research. Although the term translational medicine is relatively recent, the effort to bridge the divide between basic and clinical research is not new, having a clear precedent in the Congressional authorization to establish the National Institutes of Health Clinical Center in 1944. A substantial impetus for the recent emphasis to form a translational science initiative was based on the current paucity of new drugs, despite a considerable explosion of new technologies, insights into the molecular biology of new targets and mechanisms, and the discovery of new genetic pathways involved in various diseases. This lack of new drugs is all the more striking when one considers that research and development expenditures within the pharmaceutical industry have increased substantially over the past several years without a concomitant increase in the approval of new chemical entities and with many compounds failing in the later stages of development. No single factor is responsible for this outcome nor does a single solution or prescription address the many issues that are involved in the lengthy, exceedingly difficult process of drug discovery and development.

Multiple initiatives within the Federal Government that were launched by the creation of the "NIH Roadmap" in 2003, as well as those within academic research centers and the pharmaceutical industry, have emphasized the concept of translational medicine in an effort to address these many issues. These efforts have spawned the creation of approximately 60 Clinical and Translational Science Centers and the formation of the National Center for Advancing Translational Sciences. These efforts have prompted a nearly constant reexamination of drug discovery and development processes. It is too early to assess the impact of these and other initiatives because the drug discovery and development process is exceptionally complex, takes several years, and has numerous regulatory steps that are immutable in terms of timing and duration (e.g., toxicology studies). The transformational potential of these many efforts remains to be determined but, without question, the many concepts surrounding translational medicine have generated considerable activity and an appropriate as well as continuing evaluation of how to more effectively translate fundamental discoveries in basic science into clinical application. In these efforts to establish and apply translational research, it will be crucial not to neglect the need for continued support of basic research. Those activities, being the wellspring of new directions, provide essential insight into pathophysiological mechanisms and are therefore fundamental in translating basic research findings into new therapeutic benefits.

The dearth of novel therapeutics that has so frequently been raised as a critical issue is particularly true in the neurosciences where many of the current drugs used to treat neuropsychiatric and neurological disorders are derivatives of those discovered initially in the 1950s. It has been stated often that animal models of these disorders are poorly predictive of clinical efficacy, that psychiatric disorders in particular have overlapping phenotypes and show considerable comorbidity, making diagnosis and treatment difficult, and that there are no reliable or distinct biomarkers available. Furthermore, our understanding of the pathophysiology of both psychiatric and neurological disorders remains limited at the present time, thereby thwarting the development of more effective therapeutics. Although all of these factors are more or less true, it is also evident that basic and clinical neuroscience has made considerable progress in recent years in identifying new biological targets, molecular pathways, and potential points of therapeutic intervention that offer promising avenues and hope for patients suffering from these disorders, many of which are at this point intractable. Recently, it has also been recognized that some disorders have not been fully characterized from a phenotypic perspective. For example, treatments for schizophrenia need to address the currently neglected cognitive impairments and negative symptoms in addition to the positive symptoms, which are targeted by existing antipsychotics. As such, an effort to capture these exciting advances and couple them to developments emerging in translational and experimental medicine in a comprehensive text is timely and essential to facilitate progress in neuroscience and in the delivery of new medications to patients.

Translational Neuroscience: Applications in Psychiatry, Neurology, and Neurodevelopmental Disorders was conceived to provide a comprehensive disorder-focused perspective of this evolving discipline for individuals in academia, government, and industry. The text is divided into three major sections, focused separately on (i) psychiatric disorders such as anxiety, depression, and schizophrenia; (ii) neurological disorders such as Alzheimer's disease, pain, and Parkinson's disease; and (iii) neurodevelopmental disorders such as autism and fragile X syndrome. The authors of each chapter are experts in their field and represent a blend of individuals from academia and the pharmaceutical industry. It is our hope that the chapters that follow not only summarize the current status of research and clinical science in the respective therapeutic areas but also open new perspectives and spur translational initiatives in each of these critical areas of unmet medical need that will help to advance the scientific framework and approaches to translational neuroscience.

James E. Barrett
Joseph T. Coyle
Michael Williams

Acknowledgments

JEB thanks Maura Barrett for her support and patience throughout the editing of this book.

JTC thanks Genevieve Coyle and MW thanks Holly Williams for their support.

The editors thank all the authors for their contributions and commitment to this volume and also thank Pamela Fried for her diligent and professional assistance in the handling of manuscripts.

Chapter 1

The discovery and development of drugs to treat psychiatric disorders: Historical perspective

Michael Williams and James E. Barrett

Drugs to treat psychiatric disorders have added immeasurably to societal well-being, providing many patients with the ability to function adequately and productively under serious and often life-threatening psychiatric disorders. The initial discovery of drugs for the treatment of depression and schizophrenia was made over 50 years ago and was based on clinical observations of drugs used for indications other than depression and schizophrenia (Klein 2008; Preskorn 2010a). The mechanisms of these drugs were unknown at the time their efficacy in these disorders was established; however, the subsequent identification of these mechanisms was then used to define the mechanistic causality of the disease state. A historical perspective of these developments serves to underline and highlight a number of important aspects that have had a significant impact on the emergence of drug treatments for psychiatric disorders and is intended to provide focus for the chapters that follow as part of a current translational context.

First, there was and continues to be limited understanding of the molecular causality of psychiatric disorders, which are usually polygenomic, multifactorial, and complex (Enna and Williams 2009). This situation continues to exist despite the availability of effective drugs and represents a significant challenge in moving pharmacological treatment forward into new therapeutics. Second, the presumed mechanism of action of these drugs and their efficacy in treating disorders like schizophrenia, depression, and anxiety not only served to define these conditions biochemically but also provided the basis for the development of a variety of animal models (Day et al. 2008; Markou et al. 2009; Millan 2008; Spedding et al. 2005; van der Greef and McBurney 2005). Despite the proliferation of such models, both wild-type and transgenic, marked disconnects remain between putative animal models of human diseases and the human disease state itself (Nestler and Hyman 2010). Finally, because of historical precedents, the clinical trial paradigm continues to operate in a very opportunistic clinical mode with the expectation that any preclinical data are far from an absolute in terms of predicting what may happen in the clinic.

Psychiatric disorders are frequently treated with drugs that have diverse and often complex mechanisms of action that engage multiple targets. Conversely, different psychiatric disorders are often treated with the same agent, tending to confuse the disease/disorder cause-and-effect paradigm in addition to posing questions regarding diagnostic sensitivity. The paucity of new and improved psychoactive drugs has led to a renewed focus on hierarchical brain networks, neuronal plasticity, and signaling processes (Akil et al. 2010) as well as to the renewed interrogation of the predictive value of animal models in defining both psychiatric disorder causality and current translational approaches to psychiatric drug discovery. As many pharmaceutical companies appear to be abandoning their efforts in neuropsychiatric disorders (Miller 2010a; Nierenberg 2010; Nutt and Goodwin 2011; Stovall 2011), there is a pressing need to develop more in-depth information on the pathophysiological mechanisms contributing to these disorders and to develop innovative and alternative strategies for drug discovery and development.

Historical background

Although the origins of mood-altering substances like alcohol, nicotine, mescaline, and cocaine stretch back to antiquity, the utility for the CNS of other compounds like chloral hydrate, barbital, phenytoin, and epinephrine was only established in the late

Translational Neuroscience, ed. James E. Barrett, Joseph T. Coyle and Michael Williams. Published by Cambridge University Press. © Cambridge University Press 2012.

nineteenth and early twentieth centuries (Preskorn 2010a, 2010b). The "golden" age of psychopharmacology (Barrett 2002; Klein 2008) dates back to the late 1940s with the use of lithium urate for the treatment of mania (Cade 1949). The latter is widely considered a serendipitous discovery that was based on the ability of lithium to reverse urea toxicity in guinea pigs, the latter being a toxic agent present in the urine of manic patients. Lithium was in fact in use as a psychoactive drug in the late nineteenth century. At that time, excess uric acid had been linked to depression and mania. Because lithium could dissolve uric acid crystals, it had been used to treat mania in the 1870s but was abandoned as a therapeutic agent by 1900 due to the discrediting of the uric acid diathesis theory (Mitchell and Hadzi-Pavlovic 2000). Thus Cade more properly "rediscovered" the utility of lithium. This event was followed in the 1950s by the discovery of chlorpromazine (Ban 2007) and reserpine (Barsa and Kline 1955) for the treatment of schizophrenia, the monoamine oxidase (MAO) inhibitor, iproniazid, for the treatment of depression (Crane 1956; Zeller et al. 1952), and the benzodiazepine (BZ), chlordiazepoxide, for the treatment of anxiety (Sternbach 1979). These discoveries had a major impact in defining the neuropharmacology of the CNS (Jacobsen 1986) and were further aided by the emergence of the discipline of neurochemistry, which focused on the study of enzymes and receptors in the brain (Feldberg 1963; Foley 2007; McIlwain 1958). These discoveries also heralded an effort to develop appropriate animal behavior models in which these compounds could be assayed and which could serve as the basis for the discovery of new drugs (McArthur and Borsini 2008). In short, the identification of drugs to treat major psychiatric disorders launched the fields of biological psychiatry, behavioral pharmacology, and neuropsychopharmacology and had a profound impact not only on individuals suffering from these disorders and on the care and hospitalization of patients but also on the emergence of entirely new disciplines.

Neurochemical studies in cell homogenates, in situ, and in brain slices (McIlwain 1963) coupled with electrophysiological approaches (Llinas 1988) provided a facile means to measure the functional effects of transmitters on cell and tissue function and on metabolism and receptor signaling in relatively intact brain systems and provided the necessary context for the development of receptor binding assays (Snyder 2008). These created a new, target-based interface between small-molecule-based medicinal chemistry strategies and biological testing to advance the process of drug discovery via the rapid development of structure–activity relationships (SARs) for new chemical entities (NCEs) directed toward putative disease targets.

Shortly after its validation, the technique of radioligand binding was used to identify the first *drug* receptor, that for the BZ, diazepam (Braestrup and Squires 1978; Mohler and Okada 1977), the endogenous ligand for which, despite many interesting candidates, has still to be confirmed. With the ability to measure receptor interactions at a binding site as distinct from a functional tissue or whole animal response, a rapid, iterative strategy then became possible where the potency and the SAR of compounds or new chemical entities (NCEs) could be determined in vitro using small quantities (~ 1–2 mg) of newly synthesized NCEs. This process contrasted with the need for the 0.5 to 1 g or greater quantities that had been necessary to study compound effects in intact tissues and animals. In time, this process went through various iterations that further transformed the CNS drug discovery process and eventually led to industrial-level, high-throughput screening assays (Macarron et al. 2011) and combinatorial/parallel synthesis chemistry that could screen millions of compounds in the space of a week. The result was the generation of more data within a month than previously had been generated in several decades. These advances also unfortunately tended to replace the intellectual component of the research endeavor with a more technically biased, metrics-driven approach (Kubinyi 2003; Williams 2011).

Second-generation psychoactive agents

The astute observations in the clinical setting that led to the first generation of psychoactive drugs also created the putative framework for the potential discovery of new generations of psychotropic agents. Thus, by identifying the mechanistic attributes of clinically efficacious agents, a better understanding of the molecular causality of the disease could, theoretically, also be achieved. Newly identified targets could then be interrogated using the new tools of receptor binding and functional neurochemistry to identify second-generation compounds for evaluation in animal models that, theoretically, would be more selective in their actions and thus have improved efficacy, safety, and pharmacokinetic properties. A large number of second-generation compounds have been identified using this approach, some of which are now in clinical use. It is, however, the subject of considerable debate as to whether these NCEs represent clinical improvements over the agents initially discovered, especially in the case of the second-generation or atypical antipsychotics. The National Institute of Mental Health-sponsored CATIE (Clinical Antipsychotic Trials of Intervention Effectiveness) (McEvoy et al. 2006; Stroup et al. 2006) and National Health Service-sponsored CUtLASS (Cost Utility of the Latest Antipsychotic Drugs in Schizophrenia Study) (Jones et al. 2006) clinical trials, part of a comparative effectiveness research initiative, have led to the highly controversial (Insel 2010; Lewis and Lieberman 2008; Meltzer and Bobo 2006) conclusion that there are few major differences in the clinical effectiveness and safety of first- and second-generation antipsychotics.

Antipsychotics

The search for newer antipsychotics has been ongoing for the better part of the past 60 years. It has resulted in many thousands of compounds that have iterations on the receptor-binding properties of the seminal antipsychotics, haloperidol and chlorpromazine. These efforts have been largely based on the dopamine (DA) hyperfunction hypothesis of schizophrenia (Carlsson and Lindqvist 1963) that was substantiated by the finding that the binding of antipsychotics to brain DA receptors correlated with clinical potency (Creese et al. 1976). The additional finding that the presence of 5-HT$_{2A}$ antagonist activity improved the negative symptoms of the disease supported a role for 5-HT in the treatment of schizophrenia, as had been previously suggested by phenotypic similarities between LSD-induced hallucinations and schizophrenic psychosis (Meltzer 1999). This approach helped redefine the characteristics thought to be necessary in a second-generation antipsychotic agent (Kuroki et al. 2008; Marino et al. 2008) as did the discovery of the dibenzodiazepine antipsychotic, clozapine (Crilly 2007). The latter drug is generally considered the prototypic "second-generation" or atypical antipsychotic agent (see Chapter 4, this volume). Identified as a D$_2$ receptor antagonist with broad-spectrum efficacy in schizophrenia, clozapine was found to be effective in patients with treatment-resistant refractory schizophrenia. It also had a reduced incidence of extrapyramidal symptom liability (Bagnall et al. 2003; Wahlbeck et al. 2000) and could be used for longer periods prior to patient discontinuation compared with other antipsychotics. The positive attributes of clozapine were, however, limited by a high incidence of potentially fatal agranulocytosis that led to the compound being withdrawn in 1975. Following a subsequent trial in patients with treatment-resistant schizophrenia where it was found to be superior to first-generation compounds, clozapine was reintroduced in 1990 with labeling for continuous monitoring for blood dyscrasias in patients with nonresponsive positive symptoms.

Given its demonstrated superior therapeutic profile, considerable efforts have been directed toward identifying "clozapine-like" NCEs that have the improved antipsychotic efficacy but lack the risk of agranulocytosis. The search for "the mechanism of action" of clozapine was driven by the possibility that this drug might interact with a target that would provide insights into the mechanisms underlying its superior efficacy and side-effect profile and, by default, also provide a better understanding of the mechanistic nuances of schizophrenia. However, with the discovery of each new CNS receptor, the receptor-binding profile of clozapine – its "molecular fingerprint" – was similarly expanded, serving to emphasize the polypharmic profile of this unique antipsychotic drug. Clozapine appears to possess a classical privileged pharmacophore (Evans et al. 1988), making it truly a "magic shotgun"-like compound (Roth et al. 2004) and thus extremely challenging to replicate in an SAR-focused medicinal chemistry effort (Marino et al. 2008). The discovery and approval of another second-generation, atypical antipsychotic, aripiprazole (Shapiro et al. 2003), a partial agonist at the DA D$_2$ receptor, also focused attention on partial agonism/antagonism as an approach to what has been termed "third-generation" DA-based antipsychotics (Mailman and Murthy 2010).

The findings that psychotomimetics like phencyclidine and ketamine, antagonists of the N-methyl-D-aspartate (NMDA) subtype of the glutamate receptor, could mimic the positive, negative, and cognitive symptoms of schizophrenia (Javitt and Zukin 1991) has led to an alternative mechanistic hypothesis for the etiology of schizophrenia, namely that of glutamate hypofunction (Coyle et al. 2003; Jentsch and

Roth 1999; Kantrowitz and Javitt 2010; Millan 2005). NMDA receptor antagonists have been shown to exacerbate symptoms in patients with schizophrenia (Lahti et al. 1995) and trigger the re-emergence of symptoms in stable patients (Javitt and Zukin 1991). NMDA receptor co-agonists, including glycine, D-serine, and D-cycloserine, while having some beneficial effects in the treatment of schizophrenia (Heresco-Levy et al. 2005), have failed to show robust activity in subsequent trials (Buchanan et al. 2007). Inhibitors of the glycine transporter type 1 (GlyT1), e.g., sarcosine (Lane et al. 2006) and RG1678, that increase endogenous glycine have shown efficacy as an add-on therapy to antipsychotic agents. However, sarcosine and more potent GlyT1 inhibitors, e.g., ALX-5407, can produce hypoactivity/motor impairment and respiratory distress (Perry et al. 2008), an apparent function of compound residence time (Kopec et al. 2010), which has led to questions regarding the validity of GlyT1 inhibition as an approach to reversing NMDA hypofunction in schizophrenia. Endogenous sarcosine production may, however, be amenable to modulation using PPARα agonists including clofibrate and gemfibrozil (McBurney 2009), suggesting another mechanism for the NMDA receptor co-agonist approach.

Treatment of schizophrenic patients with LY404039, a group 2/3 metabotropic glutamate receptor agonist prodrug, resulted in significant improvements in both the positive and negative symptoms of schizophrenia compared with placebo without causing prolactin elevation, extrapyramidal symptoms, or weight gain (Patil et al. 2007). However, these initial results await further confirmatory studies. Positive allosteric modulators of the mGluR2 receptor, e.g., LY487379 (Galici et al. 2005), and the mGluR5 receptor, e.g. VU0360172 (Rodriguez et al. 2010), represent additional approaches to potentiating the effects of glutamate.

Genome-wide association studies in populations of patients with schizophrenia have identified more than 30 disease-associated genes (Marino et al. 2008) that include neuregulin, reelin, *DTNBP*, *RGS4*, *DISC1*, *CMYA5*, and the alpha 7 *NNR*, the role(s) of which in disease causality has yet to be established in the context of the existing dopamine/glutamate hyper/hypofunction hypotheses. The most recent gene association for schizophrenia, *CMYA5* (cardiomyopathy associated 5 gene or *myospryn*), was identified in 20 independent samples involving more than 33 000 participants (Chen et al. 2011). *Myospryn* binds to dysbindin (Benson et al. 2004), the protein product of the *DTNBP1* (dystrobrevin binding protein 1) gene, a major schizophrenia susceptibility factor (Kendler 2004). Like other genome-wide association studies candidate genes, the function of *myospryn* in schizophrenia is unclear. Its reported association with left ventricular hypertrophy (Nakagami et al. 2007) questions a specific role in the etiology of schizophrenia.

Anxiolytics

Since the 1960s, many NCEs have been identified that interact with the BZ receptor. The majority were iterations on the basic BZ pharmacophore, itself a privileged pharmacophore (Evans et al. 1988). Other ligands were identified by screening chemical libraries using radioligand binding assays, e.g., β-carbolines. The characterization of such compounds has become increasingly nuanced with the cloning and identification of the component α, β, and γ subunits of this pentameric ligand gated-ion channel receptor (Olsen and Sieghart 2009). The discovery of partial agonists that act at various subunit-containing complexes has been an active research area focused on the possibility to differentially and selectively modulate the many different effects of benzodiazepines that include anxiolytic, sedative, anticonvulsant, and cognitive activities (Rudolph and Möhler 2006). Unfortunately, the translational path from an "atypical" BZ ligand with superior anxiolytic efficacy and reduced side effects in various animal models of anxiety to an efficacious new drug remains a major challenge and has, thus far, been elusive (D'Hulst et al. 2009; see Chapter 2). Unlike the antipsychotic field, the clinical shortcomings of anxiolytics, while inherently present, are less of an issue in driving research efforts in the area.

Antidepressants

Following the discovery of the MAO inhibitor, iproniazid, as an antidepressant (Crane 1956), newer antidepressants were also discovered, one of which was the tricyclic antidepressant (TCA) imipramine, a product of medicinal chemistry efforts at CIBA-Geigy to develop a successor to the antipsychotic, chlorpromazine (Maxwell and Eckhardt 1990; Pletscher 1991). Since TCAs enhance extrasynaptic levels of the monoamines, 5-HT and norepinephrine (NE), by blocking the transporters for NE and 5-HT (SERT), this led to the biogenic amine hypothesis that depression was the result of a chronic decrease in the extrasynaptic levels of these monoamines (Schildkraut et al. 1965). As with the antipsychotics, the original TCA imipramine was joined by second- and third-generation compounds including desipramine, amitriptyline, and clomipramine. Due to a multitude of direct receptor interactions including serotonergic, muscarinic, histaminic, and α-adrenergic, the TCAs have multiple side effects that include sedation, orthostatic hypotension, and dry mouth that can limit their clinical use (Lieberman 2003). One of the TCAs, clomipramine, unlike imipramine, desipramine, and amitriptyline, proved to be more selective in its effects on 5-HT uptake than on NE uptake and led to the evolution of the 5-HT hypothesis of depression (Coppen 1967) and to the development of the selective serotonin reuptake inhibitors (SSRIs) that include fluoxetine (Wong et al. 2005), sertraline, and citalopram. The SSRIs have been highly successful drugs for the treatment of depression and led to various iterations on the TCAs that include the serotonin-norepinephrine reuptake inhibitors (SNRIs, e.g., venlaflaxine and duloxetine), the norepinephrine-dopamine reuptake inhibitors (NDRIs, e.g., buproprion), the selective serotonin reuptake enhancers (e.g., tianeptine), and the norepinephrine-dopamine disinhibitors (e.g., agomelatine) (de Bodinat et al. 2010) that, in antagonizing the 5-HT$_{2C}$ receptor, can modulate NE and DA release. A UK meta-analysis of antidepressant treatment (Baldwin et al. 2011) concluded that fluoxetine and sertraline appeared to have some advantages over other monoamine-based drug treatments and that duloxetine and escitalopram might be superior to venlafaxine and paroxetine.

The triple reuptake inhibitors that block the reuptake of all three monoamines, NE, DA, and 5-HT, such as DOV 21,947 and NS-2359/GSK-37247, while effective in animal models of depression, have failed to date to show robust clinical efficacy in depression. JZAD-IV-22 (Caldarone et al. 2010) is a newer triple reuptake inhibitor, the preclinical data for which suggest it may lack some of the side effects seen with other members of this class of potential antidepressants.

The search for new classes of antidepressants that are distinct from those acting via monoamines had, until recently, limited success. A major challenge was that the majority of antidepressants, in addition to various side effects related to their effects on monoamine function (Lieberman 2003), all have a delayed onset to action. This delay is of concern in that depressed patients do not undergo any beneficial effects from their medication for some 2–6 weeks or more after treatment is initiated, leading to rapid treatment dropouts (Pigott et al. 2010) and to suicide.

A major breakthrough in time to onset was the recent finding, albeit still controversial, that the NMDA receptor antagonist, ketamine, can rapidly (within 2 h) attenuate depression in patients, an effect that lasted up to a week (Zarate et al. 2006). These findings were extended (Diazgranados et al. 2010) to subjects with treatment-resistant bipolar depression in whom antidepressant effects were observed as soon as 40 minutes after they received ketamine (0.5 mg/kg). The use of ketamine is limited by the potential for the development of symptoms of mania, the necessity for its intravenous administration, and the short-lived nature of its antidepressant effects. Additional research in preclinical models showed that the rapid antidepressant effects of ketamine could be associated with increases in synaptic signaling proteins and synapse formation in the prefrontal cortex mediated via the mTOR pathway (Li et al. 2010). In these studies, the antidepressant actions of ketamine were mimicked to a degree by the NR2B antagonist, Ro25-6981, suggesting that a glutamate-associated brain mTOR pathway may represent a novel target for the development of improved antidepressant agents, provided that the psychotomimetic effects of ketamine can be "tuned out" in NCEs. This latter task was the major challenge in developing effective therapeutic treatments for ischemic stroke based on the glutamate excitotoxicity hypothesis and eventually proved to be insurmountable based on the pharmacodynamic properties of the pharmacophores evaluated (Hall 2007; Pangalos et al. 2007).

After some 60 years of research based almost exclusively on the monoamine hypothesis, the ketamine/glutamate approach to NMDA function may represent the first of several paradigm shifts in antidepressant research that may result in new medications for depression with the potential for a more rapid onset. The latter include growth factors, specifically BDNF (Chen et al. 2010), that affect neuronal survival and synaptic plasticity; the central melatonin system, where agomelatine produces its antidepressant effects in addition to its 5HT$_{2C}$ antagonist activities (de Bodinot et al. 2010); various members of the phosphodiesterase family (Halene and Siegel 2007); the 5-HT$_7$ receptor (Sarkisyan et al. 2010); neuropeptide receptor antagonists (e.g., CRF-1 and NK receptors); protein kinases as reflected in the mTOR findings discussed above (Li *et al.* 2010); protein phosphatases, e.g., MAPK kinase phosphatase-1 (Duric *et al.* 2010); GSK-3 inhibitors (Li and Jope 2010); and *bcl-2* proteins (Mathew *et al.* 2008). The finding that an endogenous microRNA, miR-16, complimentary to the 3'-untranslated region of SERT mRNA, mediates the effects of the SSRI fluoxetine on SERT expression via a pathway involving GSK-3 beta and *Wnt* (Baudry *et al.* 2010) further reinforces a potential role for GSK-3 in depression. Additionally, in line with an involvement of a glutamate axis in mood disorders as evidenced by the effects of the NR2B antagonist, Ro25-6981 in the mTOR model (Li *et al.* 2010), the PPARγ agonist rosiglitazone has been reported to have antidepressant-like actions (Eissa *et al.* 2009).

The translational research paradigm in CNS drug discovery

The key challenge in the search for a new generation of improved psychoactive drugs has focused on: (1) enhanced validation of the animal models used to characterize NCEs as bona fide models of the human disease and the use of these models to effectively translate NCEs to the human disease state (Day *et al.* 2008; Markou *et al.* 2009; Millan 2008; Nestler and Hyman 2010; Spedding *et al.* 2005; van der Greef and McBurney 2005); (2) ensuring that NCEs intended to produce their effects in the CNS actually reach their site of action at sufficient concentrations to produce efficacy (Frank and Hargreaves 2003; Sakoğlu *et al.* 2011); and (3) robust biomarkers for disease diagnosis and the assessment of disease progression and drug effects on progression (Flood *et al.* 2011; Ryten *et al.* 2009). As noted, efforts in CNS translational research have been confounded by (1) a focus on target-based approaches (Enna and Williams 2009; Lindner 2007; Sams-Dodd 2005) to the almost complete exclusion of more systems-based approaches to CNS function that include neuronal circuitry, signaling pathways, and database integration and interrogation (Akil *et al.* 2010; Haber and Rauch 2009; van der Greef and McBurney 2005); (2) shortcomings in the predictive value of animal models (Day *et al.* 2008; Markou *et al.* 2009; McArthur and Borsini 2008; Nestler and Hyman 2010; Pangalos *et al.* 2007) together with concerns related to the intrinsic pathophysiology of these models as they relate to the chronic nature of the majority of human CNS disease states (Spedding *et al.* 2005); and (3) by a lack of systematic effort in translational approaches to CNS disorders (Dawson *et al.* 2011; Wang *et al.* 2008; Williams and Enna 2011). The latter is also related to the issues surrounding patient diagnosis and the heterogeneous, overlapping nature of psychiatric disorders (Hyman 2010), clinical trial design, and analysis. The multifactorial causality of CNS diseases, genetic, developmental, and epigenetic, may be considered to be in marked contrast to the current "targephilic" (Enna and Williams 2009) approach that dominates current CNS drug discovery in both academia and industry (Conn and Roth 2008) and may also be considered as an impediment to the effective translation of preclinical findings to the clinic setting.

The translational research paradigm is generally viewed as a series of multidisciplinary steps that transition an optimized NCE from the preclinical setting to a phase II proof-of-concept outcome, the latter of which is a logical extension of the original research hypothesis (Duyk 2003; LoRusso 2009; Wehling 2009). For psychotropic drugs, this process generally involves the examination of uniquely selective and potent NCEs in animal models to predict potential human efficacy and dosing and ideally involves a bidirectional flow of data from the clinic to the research laboratory and vice versa (Sung *et al.* 2003). Despite the obvious logic in such an approach and the ample historical evidence that a close interface between preclinical scientists and clinicians can greatly facilitate clinical design paradigms, the translational interface in the CNS space has been described as an "unbridged gap" (Klein 2008) or a "valley of death" (Brady *et al.* 2009) that is greatly in need of reinvention to ensure that heuristically promising new approaches to the treatment of CNS disease states are not dismissed after evaluation of a single compound (Bloom 2009). The "unbridged gap" reflects the dependence on a history of clinical serendipity where NCEs had already made their way into the clinic, eliminating any requirement for a translational focus but instead requiring the funding of multiple trials in different CNS disorders to identify a match between the molecular, pharmacodynamic, and pharmacokinetic properties of the NCE and the human disease state. The "valley of death" refers to the chasm where drugs have failed during the transition from preclinical evaluation to clinical validation. More effective translational approaches are clearly needed that include a deeper understanding of the pathophysiology, a more reliable early predictors of clinical relevance, and the development of suitable biomarkers, to name just a few.

Animal models of human diseases

As noted, the majority of current preclinical animal models of CNS disease states reflect models in which drugs known to effectively treat CNS diseases have provided robust phenotypic signals (Day *et al.* 2008; Markou *et al.* 2009; McArthur and Borsini 2008; Nestler and Hyman 2010; Pangalos *et al.* 2007; Spedding *et al.* 2005). The use of these models, to a major extent, limits any additional hypothesis testing to the mechanistic approach to the disease state that underlies the mechanism of action(s), known or unknown, for the drugs used to define the model. A major cause of NCE attrition in the clinic occurs as the result of false positives from the present generation of animal assays or from the appearance of side effects that were not and could not be detected preclinically.

Although there has been considerable interest in the potential utility of transgenic models (Cryan and Holmes 2005; Zambrowicz and Sands 2003), few if any transgenic models fully recapitulate the disease symptoms. The use of gene ablation or gene knockins still reduces the experimental paradigm to the evaluation of the behavioral phenotype of the animal in the presence (wild-type), absence (knockout), or overexpression (knockin) of the proposed disease target. Although transgenic models have value in target identification and validation, they may contribute confounds, e.g., unknown and unknowable systems and target redundancies and abnormal CNS development, that can further complicate data interpretation.

Among the several recent reviews and monographs on the adequacy and current status of animal models of CNS diseases, Nestler and Hyman (2010) provide a challenge to the CNS research community to provide more rigor and insight – "clearly stated rationales and sober discussions of validity" – into the use and development of animal models for drug discovery rather than being "phenomenological." The authors take issue with the use of transgenic models with generic modifications that are not highly penetrant, that are dependent on rare or familial genetic mutations, or that focus on genes that have been associated with more than one CNS disease phenotype.

More recently, for schizophrenia, it has been suggested (Ibrahim and Tamminga 2011) that animal models should focus on individual components of the disease complex rather than model the disease as a single entity. This *component symptom complex* approach focuses on individual models for psychosis, cognitive dysfunction, and negative symptoms. Newer models reflecting the cognitive and negative symptom domains are under development (Neill *et al.* 2010). The potential difficulty here is that cognitive dysfunction in schizophrenia may be different than that in dementia or in other disorders, requiring a careful delineation and deeper understanding of the pathophysiological underpinnings of the phenotype that, on the surface, might appear to be similar.

Concerns related to animal model validity are not unique to the CNS area; numerous NCEs displaying target efficacy and safety (to the extent tested or testable) in animal models for multiple human disease states have failed in the clinic (Hackam and Redelmeier 2006), a result attributed to poor preclinical methods (Hackam 2007; Perel *et al.* 2007). These include a lack of blinding, randomization, and adequate powering/size of experiments; failure to conduct full dose–response curves; an "optimization bias" that can result in only positive data being reported (Lindner 2007; Pigott *et al.* 2010); genetic homogeneity in animals that contrasts with the heterogeneity present in the human population; and the absence of the chronic features of the human disease state in animals.

The CNS clinical translation disconnect?

Added to the concerns regarding the use of animal models in predicting clinical efficacy are concerns related to the clinical trials. Those for depression have undergone extensive post hoc assessment (Blier 2008; Kirsch 2009; Kramer 2005; Leventhal and Martell 2005; Pigott *et al.* 2010) and remain highly controversial, with major concerns regarding the contribution of placebo responses to reported efficacy (Klein 2008). A meta-analysis of data from 47 clinical trials covering the six most widely prescribed antidepressants approved between 1987 and 1999, fluoxetine, paroxetine, sertraline, venlafaxine, nefazodone, and citalopram, concluded that approximately 80% of the efficacy ascribed to an antidepressant was also seen in placebo controls, leading to the widely disseminated view that four out of six clinical trials for now-approved antidepressants failed to meet their stated end points. A subsequent analysis of fluoxetine, paroxetine, venlafaxine, and nefazodone (Kirsch *et al.* 2008) established that baseline severity was critical for antidepressant-related responses, with decreased responses to placebo rather than drug effects being responsible for positive clinical outcomes. Additional concerns, generic to most clinical trials, were that the patients recruited into clinical trials were not representative of the average depressed patient treated in practice (Fleischhaker and Goodwin 2009; Wisniewski *et al.* 2009) and the selective reporting of data in the literature (Eyding *et al.* 2010; Mathew and Charney 2009; Pigott *et al.* 2010; Turner and Rosenthal 2008; Turner *et al.* 2008). Thus, published data from 37 of 74 antidepressant trials registered with the FDA indicated that 94% of these trials yielded positive results. However, an analysis of the full 74 trials showed that only 51% of these were actually positive, indicating that the data selected for publication provided an overly optimistic view of compound efficacy. Additional analyses (Pigott *et al.* 2010) of published trials that included the STAR*D (Sequenced Treatment Alternatives to Relieve Depression) trial (Wisniewski *et al.* 2009) concluded that current antidepressant drugs were only "marginally efficacious" with "effectiveness ... probably even lower than ... reported ... with an apparent progressively increasing dropout rate across each study phase." The placebo effect issue in clinical trials for psychiatric medications, especially antidepressants, remains controversial (Silberman 2009), not only in terms of those compounds approved but also from the ability to effectively translate an NCE to an NDA approval. An additional factor that is of concern is the confounding of outcomes by the underreporting of negative trial results (Eyding *et al.* 2010; Mathew and Charney 2009; Pigott *et al.* 2010; Ramsey and Scoggins 2008; Turner *et al.* 2008).

Questioning the value of the *Diagnostic and Statistical Manual of Mental Disorders*

An additional challenge in developing new approaches to and treatments of mental disorders has been increasing concerns as to the intrinsic value of the *Diagnostic and Statistical Manual of Mental Disorders* (DSM) in defining psychiatric disorders and their diagnosis (Hyman 2010; Insel 2010). DSM diagnosis is based on the phenomenology of symptoms rather than objective causes. As a result, the DSM has been viewed as "hampering research" (Miller 2010*b*) and as being "arbitrary or hazy" (Hyman 2010) in the "targephilic"-based research environment that reflects current approaches to drug discovery (Enna and Williams 2009; Sams-Dodd 2005). The National Institute of Mental Health has recently undertaken a new initiative to classify psychiatric disorders in the context of Research Domain Criteria (RDoC) that are based on a neural circuitry approach (Insel *et al.* 2010) that involves five distinct domains: negative emotionality, positive emotionality, cognitive processes, social processes, and arousal/regulatory symptoms, with the expectation that this will provide greater clarity and differentiation for psychiatric disorders.

Conclusions

Arguably, the learning curve for CNS research over the past two decades that has relied so heavily on discrete drug targets and gene associations has come full circle as it again focuses on the unique complexity of the brain rather than treating it as an organ indistinguishable in composition and complexity and function from the heart or liver (Akil *et al.* 2010). Additional facets of this shift include a focus on database development and mining for specific CNS drug classes (Geerts 2009), information processing networks (Bassett *et al.* 2010), and a re-emergence of observational CNS pharmacology (the "pharmacometric screen" (Enna and Williams 2009) as embodied in both the classical Irwin test (Irwin 1968) and more recent automated versions (Kafkafi *et al.* 2009; Tecott and Nestler 2004).

With the productivity void in new CNS drugs after more than half a century of effort and the abandonment of efforts in pharma in the area of neuropsychiatric disorders (Miller 2010*a*; Nierenberg 2010; Stovall 2011), the position of a "the best we can do" approach, given the complex challenges of CNS function, is now giving way to a long-needed paradigm shift based on valid concerns. These concerns include animal models, diagnosis of psychiatric disorders, and the challenges of clinical trial design and analysis that can no longer be ignored. In addition to the controversial comparative effectiveness initiatives, other federally funded activities are designed to bridge the translational gap. These projects are presently in the area of schizophrenia (Brady *et al.* 2009) and include MATRICS (Measurement and Treatment Research to

Improve Cognition in Schizophrenia) (Marder and Fenton 2004) to delineate guidelines for the approval of NCEs to treat the cognitive aspects of schizophrenia; NCDDDGs (National Cooperative Drug Discovery and Development Groups) (Brady et al. 2009), and RDoC (Insel et al. 2010), major science-based initiatives that will hopefully aid in driving CNS research forward in more productive directions. Against the potential backdrop of a new world of CNS drug discovery, it is noteworthy that the present challenges are in many respects reminiscent of those faced by neuroscientists and psychiatrists over half a century ago. *Plus ça change, plus c'est la même chose.*

Given the complexity of CNS disease states and the equally complex path from concept to approval of NCEs in the CNS area, one can only be amazed that the discoveries made over 60 years ago as a result of clinical serendipity have proven to be so useful to so many patients. For translational neuroscience initiatives to be truly informative and *transformational* will require a concerted, data-driven effort toward a better understanding of the fundamental pathophysiological mechanisms in CNS disease causality that is directed by basic research and coupled in real time to clinical science and the drug discovery and development process.

References

Akil H, Brenner S, Kandel E et al. 2010. The future of psychiatric research: genomes and neural circuits. *Science* **327**:1580–1581.

Bagnall AM, Jones L, Ginnelly R et al. 2003. A systematic review of atypical antipsychotic drugs in schizophrenia. *Health Technol Assess* **7**:1–193.

Baldwin D, Woods R, Lawson R, Taylor D. 2011. Efficacy of drug treatments for generalised anxiety disorder: systematic review and meta-analysis. *Br Med J* **342**:d1199.

Ban TA. 2007. Fifty years chlorpromazine: a historical perspective. *Neuropsychiatr Dis Treat* **3**:495–500.

Barrett JE. 2002. The emergence of behavioral pharmacology. *Mol Interv* **2**:470–475.

Barsa JA, Kline NS. 1955. Reserpine in the treatment of psychotics with convulsive disorders. *Arch Neurol Psychiatry* **74**:31–35.

Bassett D, Greenfield D, Meyer-Lindenberg A et al. 2010. Efficient physical embedding of topologically complex information processing networks in brains and computer circuits. *PLoS Comput Biol* **6**:e10000748.

Baudry A, Mouillet-Richard S, Scneider B, Launay J-M, Kellermann O. 2010. MiR-16 targets the serotonin transporter: a new facet for adaptive responses to antidepressants. *Science* **329**:1537–1541.

Benson MA, Tinsley CL, Blake DJ. 2004. Myospryn is a novel binding partner for dysbindin in muscle. *J Biol Chem* **279**:10450–10458.

Blier P. 2008. Do antidepressants really work? *J Psychiat Neurosci* **33**:89–90.

Bloom FE. 2009. Commentary: Physician-scientist's frustrations fester. *Neuropsychopharmacology* **34**:1–5.

Brady LS, Winsky L, Goodman W, Oliveri ME, Stover E. 2009. NIMH initiatives to facilitate collaborations between industry, academia and government for the discovery and clinical testing of novel models and drugs for psychiatric disorders. *Neuropsychopharmacology* **34**:229–243.

Braestrup C, Squires RF. 1978. Brain specific benzodiazepine receptors. *Br J Psychiatry* **133**:249–260.

Buchanan RW, Javitt DC, Marder SR et al. 2007. The Cognitive and Negative Symptoms in Schizophrenia Trial (CONSIST): the efficacy of glutamatergic agents for negative symptoms and cognitive impairments. *Am J Psychiatry* **164**:1593–1602.

Cade JF. 1949. Lithium salts in the treatment of psychotic excitement. *Med J Aust* **2**:349–352.

Caldarone BJ, Paterson NE, Zhou J et al. 2010. The novel triple reuptake inhibitor, JZAD-IV-22, exhibits an antidepressant pharmacological profile without locomotor stimulant or sensitization properties. *J Pharmacol Exp Ther* **335**:762–770.

Carlsson A, Lindqvist M. 1963. Effect of chlorpromazine and haloperidol on formation of 3-methoxytyramine and normetanephrine in mouse brain. *Acta Pharmacol Toxicol (Copenh)* **20**:140–144.

Chen G, Twyman R, Manji HK. 2010. p11 and gene therapy for severe psychiatric disorders: a practical goal? *Sci Transl Med* **2**:54ps51.

Chen X, Lee G, Maher BS et al. 2011. GWA study data mining and independent replication identify cardiomyopathy-associated 5 (*CMYA5*) as a risk gene for schizophrenia. *Mol Psychiatry* **16**:1117–1129. Sep 14. [Epub ahead of print] doi:10.1038/mp.2010.96.

Conn PJ, Roth BL. 2008. Opportunities and challenges of psychiatric drug discovery: roles for scientists in academic, industry, and government settings. *Neuropsychopharmacology* **33**:2048–2060.

Coppen A. 1967. The biochemistry of affective disorders. *Br J Psychiatry* **113**:1237–1264.

Coyle JT, Tsai G, Goff D. 2003. Converging evidence of NMDA receptor hypofunction in the pathophysiology of schizophrenia. *Ann N Y Acad Sci* **1003**:318–327.

Crane GE. 1956. The psychiatric side-effects of iproniazid. *Am J Psychiatry* **112**:494–501.

Creese I, Burt DR, Snyder SH. 1976. Dopamine receptor binding predicts clinical and pharmacological potencies of antischizophrenic drugs. *Science* **192**:481–483.

Crilly J. 2007. The history of clozapine and its emergence in the US market: a review and analysis. *Hist Psychiatry* **18**:39–60.

Cryan JF, Holmes A. 2005. The ascent of mouse: advances in modelling human depression and anxiety. *Nat Rev Drug Discov* **4**:775–790.

Dawson GR, Craig KJ, Dourish CT. 2011. Validation of experimental medicine methods in psychiatry: the P1vital approach and experience. *Biochem Pharmacol* **81**:1435–1441.

Day M, Balci F, Wan HI, Fox GB, Rutkowski JL, Feuerstein G. 2008. Cognitive endpoints as disease biomarkers: optimizing the congruency of preclinical models to the clinic. *Curr Opin Investig Drugs* **9**:696–707.

de Bodinat C, Guardiola-Lemaitre B, Mocaer E et al. 2010. Agomelatine, the first melatonergic antidepressant: discovery, characterization and development. *Nat Rev Drug Discov* **9**:628–642.

D'Hulst C, Atack JR, Kooy RF. 2009. The complexity of the GABA$_A$ receptor shapes unique pharmacological profiles. *Drug Discov Today* **14**:866–875.

Diazgranados N, Ibrahim L, Brutsche NE et al. 2010. A randomized add-on trial of an N-methyl-D-aspartate antagonist in treatment-resistant bipolar depression. *Arch Gen Psychiatry* **67**:793–802.

Duric V, Banasr M, Licznerski P et al. 2010. A negative regulator of MAP kinase causes depressive behavior. *Nat Med* **16**:1328–1332.

Duyk G. 2003. Attrition and translation. *Science* **302**:603–605.

Eissa A, Amany A, Al-Rasheed NM, Al-Rasheed NM. 2009. Antidepressant-like effects of rosiglitazone, a PPAR[gamma] agonist, in the rat forced swim and mouse tail suspension tests. *Behav Pharmacol* **20**:635–642.

Enna SJ, Williams M. 2009. Challenges in the search for drugs to treat central nervous system disorders. *J Pharmacol Exp Ther* **329**:404–411.

Evans BE, Rittle KE, Bock MG et al. 1988. Methods for drug discovery: development of potent, selective, orally effective cholecystokinin antagonists. *J Med Chem* **31**:2235–2246.

Eyding D, Lelgemann M, Grouven U et al. 2010. Reboxetine for acute treatment of major depression: systematic review and meta-analysis of published and unpublished placebo and selective serotonin reuptake inhibitor controlled trials. *Br Med J* **341**:c4737.

Feldberg W. 1963. *A Pharmacological Approach to the Brain from Its Inner and Outer Surface*. Baltimore, MD: Williams and Wilkins.

Fleischhaker WW, Goodwin GM. 2009. Effectiveness as an outcome measure for treatment trials in psychiatry. *World Psychiatry* **8**:23–27.

Flood DG, Marek GM, Williams M. 2011. Developing predictive CSF biomarkers – a challenge critical to success in Alzheimer's disease and neuropsychiatric translational medicine. *Biochem Pharmacol* **81**:1422–1434.

Foley P. 2007. Succi nervorum: a brief history of neurochemistry. *J Neural Transm Suppl* **72**:5–15.

Frank R, Hargreaves R. 2003. Clinical biomarkers in drug discovery and development. *Nat Rev Drug Discov* **2**:566–580.

Galici R, Echemendia NG, Rodriguez AL, Conn PJ. 2005. A selective allosteric potentiator of metabotropic glutamate (mGlu) 2 receptors has effects similar to an orthosteric mGlu2/3 receptor agonist in mouse models predictive of antipsychotic activity. *J Pharmacol Exp Ther* **315**:1181–1187.

Geerts H. 2009. Of mice and men: bridging the translational disconnect in CNS drug discovery. *CNS Drugs* **23**:915–926.

Haber SN, Rauch SL. 2009. Neurocircuitry: a window into the networks underlying neuropsychiatric disease. *Neuropsychopharmacology* **35**:1–3.

Hackam DG. 2007. Translating animal research into clinical benefit. *Br Med J* **334**:163–164.

Hackam DG, Redelmeier DA. 2006. Translation of research evidence from animals to humans. *J Am Med Assoc* **296**:1731–1732.

Halene TB, Siegel SJ. 2007. PDE inhibitors in psychiatry – future options for dementia, depression and schizophrenia? *Drug Discov Today* **12**:870–878.

Hall ED. 2007. Stroke/traumatic brain and spinal cord injury. In *Comprehensive Medicinal Chemistry II, Vol. 6*. Taylor JB, Triggle DJ, eds. Oxford: Elsevier, pp. 253–277.

Heresco-Levy U, Javitt DC, Ebstein R et al. 2005. D-serine efficacy as add-on pharmacotherapy to risperidone and olanzapine for treatment-refractory schizophrenia. *Biol Psychiatry* **57**:577–585.

Hyman SE. 2010. The diagnosis of mental disorders: the problem of reification. *Annu Rev Clin Psychol* **6**:155–179.

Ibrahim HM, Tamminga CA. 2011. Schizophrenia: treatment targets beyond monoamine systems. *Annu Rev Pharmacol Toxicol* **51**:189–209.

Insel T, Cuthbert B, Garvey M et al. 2010. Research domain criteria (RDoC): toward a new classification framework for research on mental disorders. *Am J Psychiatry* **167**:748–751.

Insel TR. 2010. Disruptive insights in psychiatry: transforming a clinical discipline. *J Clin Invest* **119**:700–705.

Irwin S. 1968. Comprehensive observational assessment: 1a. A systematic, quantitative procedure for assessing the behavioural and physiologic state of the mouse. *Psychopharmacologia* **13**:222–257.

Jacobsen E. 1986. The early history of psychotherapeutic drugs. *Psychopharmacology (Berl)* **89**:138–144.

Javitt DC, Zukin SR. 1991. Recent advances in the phencyclidine model of schizophrenia. *Am J Psychiatry* **148**:1301–1308.

Jentsch JJ, Roth RH. 1999. The neuropsychopharmacology of phencyclidine: from NMDA receptor hypofunction to the dopamine hypothesis of schizophrenia. *Neuropsychopharmacology* **20**:201–225.

Jones PB, Barnes TR, Davies L et al. 2006. Randomized controlled trial of the effect on quality of life of second- vs first-generation antipsychotic drugs in schizophrenia: Cost Utility of the Latest Antipsychotic Drugs in Schizophrenia Study (CUtLASS 1). *Arch Gen Psychiatry* **63**:1079–1087.

Kafkafi N, Yekutieli D, Elmer GI. 2009. A data mining approach to in vivo classification of psychopharmacological drugs. *Neuropsychopharmacology* **34**:607–623.

Kantrowitz JT, Javitt DC. 2010. N-methyl-d-aspartate (NMDA) receptor dysfunction or dysregulation: the final common pathway on the road to schizophrenia? *Brain Res Bull* **83**:108–121.

Kendler KS. 2004. Schizophrenia genetics and dysbindin: a corner turned? *Am J Psychaitry* **161**:1533–1536.

Kirsch I. 2009. *The Emperor's New Drugs: Exploding the Antidepressant Myth*. London: The Bodley Head.

Kirsch I, Deacon BJ, Huedo-Medina TB et al. 2008. Initial severity and antidepressant benefits: a meta-analysis of data submitted to the Food and Drug Administration. *PLoS Medicine* **5**:e45.

Klein DF. 2008. The loss of serendipity in psychopharmacology. *J Am Med Assoc* **299**:1063–1065.

Kopec K, Flood DG, Gasior M et al. 2010. Glycine transporter (GlyT1) inhibitors with reduced residence time increase prepulse inhibition without inducing hyperlocomotion in DBA/2 mice. *Biochem Pharmacol* **80**:1407–1417.

Kramer PD. 2005. *Against Depression*. New York, NY: Viking.

Kubinyi H. 2003. Drug research: myths, hype and reality. *Nat Rev Drug Discov* **2**:665–668.

Kuroki T, Nagao N, Nakahara T. 2008. Neuropharmacology of second-generation antipsychotic drugs: a validity of the serotonin-dopamine hypothesis. *Prog Brain Res* **172**:199–212.

Lahti AC, Koffel B, LaPorte D, Tamminga CA. 1995. Subanesthetic doses of ketamine stimulate psychosis in schizophrenia. *Neuropsychopharmacology* **13**:9–19.

Lane H, Huang C, Wu P et al. 2006. Glycine transporter I inhibitor, N-methylglycine (sarcosine), added to clozapine for the treatment of schizophrenia. *Biol Psychiatry* **60**:645–649.

Leventhal AM, Martell CR. 2005. *The Myth of Depression as Disease: Limitations and Alternatives to Drug Treatment*. Santa Barbara, CA: Praeger.

Lewis S, Lieberman J. 2008. CATIE and CUtLASS: can we handle the truth? *Br J Psychiatry* **192**:161–163.

Li N, Lee B, Liu R-J et al. 2010. mTOR-dependent synapse formation underlies the rapid antidepressant effects of NMDA antagonists. *Science* **329**:959–964.

Li X, Jope RS. 2010. Is glycogen synthase kinase-3 a central modulator in mood regulation? *Neuropsychopharmacology* **35**:2143–2154.

Lieberman III, JA. 2003. History of the use of antidepressants in primary care. *J Clin Psychiatry* **5** (Suppl. 7):6–10.

Lindner M. 2007. Clinical attrition due to biased preclinical assessments of potential efficacy. *Pharmacol Ther* **115**:148–175.

Llinas RR. 1988. The intrinsic electrophysiological properties of mammalian neurons: insights into central nervous system function. *Science* **242**:1654–1664.

LoRusso PM. 2009. Phase 0 clinical trials: an answer to drug development stagnation? *J Clin Oncol* **27**:2586–2588.

Macarron R, Banks MN, Bojanic D et al. 2011. Impact of high throughput screening in biomedical research. *Nat Rev Drug Discov* **10**:188–195.

Mailman RB, Murthy V. 2010. Third generation antipsychotic drugs: partial agonism or receptor functional selectivity? *Curr Pharm Design* **16**:488–501.

Marder SR, Fenton W. 2004. Measurement and Treatment Research to Improve Cognition in Schizophrenia: NIMH MATRICS initiative to support the development of agents for improving cognition in schizophrenia. *Schizophr Res* **72**:5–9.

Markou A, Chiamulera C, Geyer MA, Tricklebank M, Steckler T. 2009. Removing obstacles in neuroscience drug discovery: the future path for animal models. *Neuropsychopharmacology* **34**:74–89.

Marino MJ, Knutsen LJS, Williams M. 2008. Emerging opportunities for antipsychotic drug discovery in the postgenomic era. *J Med Chem* **51**:1077–1107.

Mathew SJ, Charney DS. 2009. Publication bias and the efficacy of antidepressants. *Am J Psychiatry* **166**:140–145.

Mathew SJ, Manji HK, Charney DS. 2008. Novel drugs and therapeutic targets for severe mood disorders. *Neuropsychopharmacology* **33**:2080–2092.

Maxwell RA, Eckhardt SB. 1990. *Drug Discovery: A Casebook and Analysis.* Clifton, NJ: Humana, pp. 133–141.

McArthur RA, Borsini F. 2008. *Animal and Translational Models for CNS Drug Discovery, Vol. 1. Psychiatric Disorders.* Burlington, MA: Academic Press.

McBurney RN. 2009. Methods of increasing sarcosine levels for treating schizophrenia. PCT patent application, publication number WO/2009/039266.

McEvoy JP, Lieberman JA, Stroup TS et al. 2006. Effectiveness of clozapine versus olanzapine, quetiapine, and risperidone in patients with chronic schizophrenia who did not respond to prior atypical antipsychotic treatment. *Am J Psychiatry* **163**:600–610.

McIlwain H. 1958. Neurochemistry and therapeutic endeavor. *Arch Neurol Psychiatry* **80**:292–297.

McIlwain H. 1963. *Chemical Exploration of the Brain.* New York, NY: Elsevier.

Meltzer HY. 1999. The role of serotonin in antipsychotic drug action. *Neuropsychopharmacology* **21**:106S–115S.

Meltzer HY, Bobo WV. 2006. Interpreting the efficacy findings in the CATIE study: what clinicians should know. *CNS Spectr* **11**:14–24.

Millan MJ. 2005. N-methyl-D-aspartate receptors as a target for improved antipsychotic agents: novel insights and clinical perspectives. *Psychopharmacology (Berl)* **179**:30–53.

Millan MJ. 2008. The discovery and development of pharmacotherapy for psychiatric disorders: A critical survey of animal and translational models and perspectives for their improvement. In *Animal and Translational Models for CNS Drug Discovery, Vol. 1.* McArthur RA, Borsini F, eds. Burlington, MA: Academic Press. pp. 1–57.

Miller G. 2010a. Is pharma running out of brainy ideas? *Science* **329**:502–504.

Miller G. 2010b. Beyond DSM – seeking a brain-based classification of mental illness. *Science* **327**:1437.

Mitchell PB, Hadzi-Pavlovic D. 2000. Lithium treatment for bipolar disorder. *Bull WHO* **78**:515–517.

Mohler H, Okada T. 1977. Benzodiazepine receptor: demonstration in the central nervous system. *Science* **198**:849–851.

Nakagami H, Kikuchi Y, Katsuya T et al. 2007. Gene polymorphism of myospryn (cardiomyopathy-associated 5) is associated with left ventricular wall thickness in patients with hypertension. *Hypertens Res* **30**:1239–1246.

Neill JC, Barnes S, Cook S et al. 2010. Animal models of cognitive dysfunction and negative symptoms of schizophrenia: focus on NMDA receptor antagonism. *Pharmacol Ther* **128**:419–432.

Nestler EJ, Hyman SE. 2010. Animal models of neuropsychiatric disorders. *Nat Neurosci* **13**:1161–1179.

Nierenberg AA. 2010. The perfect storm: CNS drug development in trouble. *CNS Spectr* **15**:282–283.

Nutt DJ, Goodwin G. 2011. ECNP Summit on the future of CNS drug research in Europe 2011. *Eur Neuropsychopharmacol* **21**:495–499.

Olsen RW, Sieghart W. 2009. $GABA_A$ receptors: subtypes provide diversity of function and pharmacology. *Neuropharmacology* **56**:141–148.

Pangalos MN, Schecter LE, Hurko O. 2007. Drug development for CNS disorders: strategies for balancing risk and reducing attrition. *Nat Rev Drug Discov* **6**:521–532.

Patil ST, Zhang L, Martenyi F et al. 2007. Activation of mGlu2/3 receptors as a new approach to treat schizophrenia: a randomized phase 2 clinical trial. *Nat Med* **13**:1102–1107.

Perel P, Roberts E, Sena E et al. 2007. Comparison of treatment effects between animal experiments and clinical trials: systematic review. *Br Med J* **334**:197–202.

Perry KW, Falcone JF, Fell MJ et al. 2008. Neurochemical and behavioral profiling of the selective GlyT1 inhibitors ALX5407 and LY2365109 indicate a preferential action in caudal vs. cortical brain areas. *Neuropharmacology* **55**:743–754.

Pigott HE, Leventhal AM, Alter GS et al. 2010. Efficacy and effectiveness of antidepressants: current status of research. *Psychother Psychosom* **79**:267–279.

Pletscher A. 1991. The discovery of antidepressants: a winding path. *Cell Mol Life Sci* **47**:4–8.

Preskorn SH. 2010a. CNS drug development. Part I: The early period of CNS drugs. *J Psychiatr Res* **16**:334–339.

Preskorn SH. 2010b. CNS drug development. Part II: Advances from the 1960s to the 1990s. *J Psychiatr Res* **16**:413–415.

Ramsey S, Scoggins J. 2008. Commentary: practicing on the tip of the information iceberg? Evidence of underpublication or registered clinical trials in oncology. *Oncologist* **13**:925–929.

Rodriguez AL, Grier MD, Jones CK et al. 2010. Discovery of novel allosteric modulators of metabotropic glutamate receptor subtype 5 reveals chemical and functional diversity and in vivo activity in rat behavioral models of anxiolytic and antipsychotic activity. *Mol Pharmacol* **78**:1105–1123.

Roth BL, Sheffler DG, Kroeze WK. 2004. Magic shotguns versus magic bullets: selectively non-selective drugs for mood disorders and schizophrenia. *Nat Rev Drug Discov* **3**:353–359.

Rudolph U, Möhler H. 2006. GABA-based therapeutic approaches: GABA$_A$ receptor subtype functions. *Curr Opin Pharmacol* **6**:18–23.

Ryten M, Trabzuni D, Hardy J. 2009. Genotypic analysis of gene expression in the dissection of the aetiology of complex neurological and psychiatric diseases. *Brief Funct Genomic Proteomic* **8**:194–198.

Sakoğlu Ü, Upadhyay J, Chin C-L et al. 2011. Paradigm shift in translational neuroimaging of CNS disorders. *Biochem Pharmacol* **81**:1374–1387.

Sams-Dodd F. 2005. Target-based drug discovery: is something wrong? *Drug Discov Today* **10**:139–147.

Sarkisyan G, Roberts AJ, Hedlund PB. 2010. The 5-HT$_7$ receptor as a mediator and modulator of antidepressant-like behavior. *Behav Brain Res* **209**:99–108.

Schildkraut JJ, Klerman GL, Hammond R et al. 1965. Excretion of 3-methoxy-mandelic acid (VMA) in depressed patients treated with antidepressant drugs. *J Psychiatric Res* **2**:257–266.

Shapiro DA, Renock S, Arrington E et al. 2003. Aripiprazole, a novel atypical antipsychotic drug with a unique and robust pharmacology. *Neuropsychopharmacology* **28**:1400–1411.

Silberman S. 2009. Placebos are getting more effective. Drugmakers are desperate to know why. [article written August 24, 2009.] *Wired* September 17. Available at: http://www.wired.com/medtech/drugs/magazine/17-09/ff_placebo_effect?currentPage=all. Accessed July 27, 2011.

Snyder SH. 2008. *Science and Psychiatry. Groundbreaking Discoveries in Molecular Neuroscience.* Washington, DC: American Psychiatric Press, pp. 439–455.

Spedding MT, Jay T, Costa E, Silva Jl, Perret L. 2005. A pathophysiological paradigm for the therapy of psychiatric disease. *Nat Rev Drug Discov* **4**:467–476.

Sternbach LH. 1979. The benzodiazepine story. *J Med Chem* **22**:1–7.

Stovall S. 2011. R&D cuts curb brain-drug pipeline. *Wall St Journal* March 27, 2011. Available at: http://online.wsj.com/article/SB10001424052748704474804576222463927753954.html. Accessed July 27, 2011.

Stroup TS, Lieberman JA, McEvoy JP et al. 2006. Effectiveness of olanzapine, quetiapine, risperidone, and ziprasidone in patients with chronic schizophrenia following discontinuation of a previous atypical antipsychotic. *Am J Psychiatry* **163**:611–622.

Sung NS, Crowley WF Jr, Genel M et al. 2003. Central challenges facing the national clinical research enterprise. *J Am Med Assoc* **289**:1278–1287.

Tecott LJ, Nestler EJ. 2004. Neurobehavioral assessment in the information age. *Nat Neurosci* **7**:462–466.

Turner EH, Matthews AM, Linardatos E, Tell RA, Rosenthal R. 2008. Selective publication of antidepressant trials and its influence on apparent efficacy. *N Engl J Med* **358**:252–260.

Turner EH, Rosenthal R. 2008. Efficacy of antidepressants. *Br Med J* **336**:516–517.

Van der Greef J, McBurney RN. 2005. Rescuing drug discovery: in vivo systems pathology and systems pharmacology. *Nat Rev Drug Discov* **4**:961–967.

Wahlbeck K, Cheine M, Essali MA. 2000. Clozapine versus typical neuroleptic medication for schizophrenia. *Cochrane Database Syst Rev* CD000059.

Wang PS, Heinssen R, Oliveri M, Wagner A, Goofman W. 2008. Bridging bench and practice: translational research for schizophrenia and other psychotic disorders. *Neuropsychopharmacology* **34**:204–212.

Wehling M. 2009. Assessing the translatability of drug projects: what needs to be scored to predict success? *Nat Rev Drug Discov* **8**:541–546.

Wisniewski SR, Rush AJ, Nierenberg AA et al. 2009. Can phase III trial results of antidepressant medications be generalized to clinical practice? A STAR*D report. *Am J Psychiatry* **166**:599–607.

Williams M. 2011. Productivity shortfalls in drug discovery: contributions from qualitative, consensus-dependent, technology-driven preclinical science? *J Pharmacol Exp Ther* **329**:404–411.

Williams M, Enna SJ. 2011. Prospects for neurodegenerative and psychiatric disorder drug discovery. *Exp Opin Drug Discov* **6**:1–7.

Wong DT, Perry KW, Bymaster FP. 2005. The discovery of fluoxetine hydrochloride (Prozac). *Nat Rev Drug Discov* **4**:764–774.

Zambrowicz BP, Sands AT. 2003. Knockouts model the 100 best-selling drugs – will they model the next 100? *Nat Rev Drug Discov* **2**:38–51.

Zarate Jr, CA, Singh JB, Carlson PJ et al. 2006. A randomized trial of an N-methyl-D-aspartate antagonist in treatment-resistant major depression. *Arch Gen Psychiatry* **63**:856–864.

Zeller EA, Barsky J, Fouts JR, Kirchheimer WF, Van Orden LS. 1952. Influence of isonicotinic acid hydrazide (1NH) and 1-*iso*nicotinyl-2-*iso*propyl hydrazine (IIH) on bacterial and mammalian enzymes. *Experientia* **8**:349–350.

Chapter 2

Translational approaches to the treatment of anxiety disorders

Charles F. Gillespie, Tamara Weiss, and Kerry J. Ressler

Fear is a basic emotion that facilitates adaptation to threat in the environment. This adaptation comes in the form of anxiety, which may be thought of as an emotional state linked to a cognitive association that relates the experience of fear to events, their outcome, and their meaning (Izard 1992). Anxiety disorders are characterized by the presence of maladaptive anxiety or fear and are the most common type of psychiatric disorder with a lifetime prevalence of over 28% (Garakani et al. 2006; Kessler et al. 2005). A subset of anxiety disorders including posttraumatic stress disorder (PTSD), panic disorder, social anxiety disorder, and specific phobias appear to be based, in part, on associative learning that occurs in conjunction with a fear-provoking experience, or the mental representation of such a real or imagined experience, that triggers excessive fear and is managed primarily by inappropriate avoidance.

Preclinical research examining the biological basis of fear learning, emotional memory regulation, and the expression of fear has, in conjunction with clinical research in patients with anxiety disorders, fostered the progressive development of a biologically grounded understanding of the pathophysiology of fear-related anxiety disorders and suggested points of biological intervention that may yield novel treatments for these diseases. As outlined in Fig. 2.1, fear-related disorders, such as PTSD, do not develop immediately at the time of the trauma or stressful event, nor do they only develop when symptoms become apparent. Rather, the risk for a dysregulated fear response, overconsolidation of the fear memory, increased sensitization, and impaired fear recovery are all part of a timeline of progression of the disorder. By understanding the neurobiology of risk and resilience and how the neurobiology of memory formation and regulation affects fear-related disorders, it is hoped that new approaches to prevention, recovery, and treatment will be produced. We review evidence of the following tenets:

1. Fear-based anxiety disorders are responsive to behavioral therapy, which facilitates new emotional learning to compete with or inhibit the aversive memories, and the emotional learning process may be enhanced by select pharmacologic agents.
2. The initial consolidation of a fear memory may be disrupted before the "overlearning" of a traumatic experience occurs and subsequent anxiety disorder develops.
3. Preclinical research with laboratory animals suggests that already-formed memories become labile when reactivated, and consequently, may be susceptible to a disruption in the same way that consolidation of new memories is vulnerable to interference.

Translationally informed treatment of anxiety disorders

The neurobiology of fear

The prevailing model of the pathogenesis of fear-related anxiety disorders is based on the acquisition of fear-related memories through associative learning and reinforcement of this fear association through persistent avoidance (reviewed in Mineka and Oehlberg 2008). Insight into the etiology of anxiety disorders in humans has been acquired, in part, from preclinical research examining fear learning in rodents. In classical fear conditioning paradigms in rodents an initially neutral conditioned stimulus (CS), such as a tone, is paired with an aversive unconditioned stimulus (UCS), such as a foot shock. This pairing elicits a collection of behavioral and physio-

---

Translational Neuroscience, ed. James E. Barrett, Joseph T. Coyle and Michael Williams. Published by Cambridge University Press. © Cambridge University Press 2012.

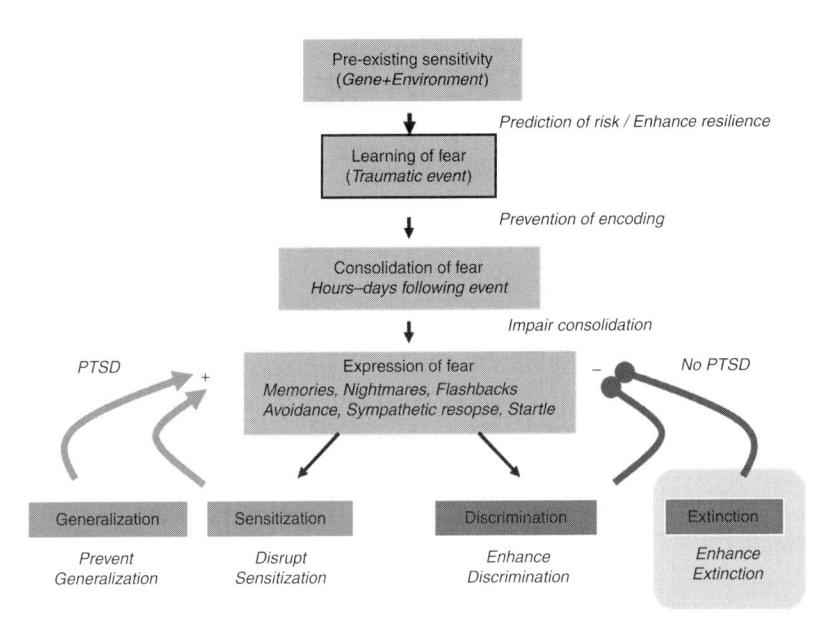

Figure 2.1. The developmental progression of fear-related disorders, such as posttraumatic stress disorder (PTSD). The strength and regulation of fearful memories are affected by numerous factors both before and after the traumatic or fearful event occurs. Genetic heritability comprises up to about 40% of the risk for stress-related disorders, such as depression, panic disorder, and PTSD, and early childhood abuse is a strong risk factor for all mood and anxiety disorders. Further understanding of the roles of genes and environment may allow enhanced prediction of risk and enhancement of resilience in vulnerable populations. Memories are not permanent at the time of the trauma, and psychological and pharmacological approaches to prevent the initial encoding of the trauma are under study. Additionally, memories then undergo a period of consolidation in which they shift from a labile state to a more permanent state. Impairing the consolidation (or even reconsolidation) would be an alternative way of preventing the sequelae of long-term trauma memories. The expression of traumatic memories, which can be the source of many symptoms in fear-related disorders, is diminished by the process of extinction, whereby repeated therapeutic exposures to the fear-related cues reduce or inhibit the fear memories over time. In contrast, some evidence suggests that, in those who develop PTSD and other pathological conditions, a combination of avoidance of sufficient exposure with intrusive and uncontrollable memories leads to sensitization of the fear response. Enhancing discrimination and extinction of fear memories is key to recovery in the psychotherapeutic approaches to treating PTSD and other fear-related disorders such as panic disorder and social phobia. Reprinted with permission from the *American Journal of Psychiatry*, Vol. 167, Jovanovic T, Ressler KJ. How the neurocircuitry and genetics of fear inhibition may inform our understanding of PTSD, pp. 648–662. (Copyright © 2010). American Psychiatric Association.

logical responses, known as the conditioned response (CR). After the CS-UCS pairing is made, the CS is able to elicit the CR in the absence of the UCS. In addition, the environmental context in which the initial conditioning occurred will also be able to elicit the CR. The CR serves as an observable and quantifiable representation of the emotional memory that was established. Decades of work have demonstrated that a hard-wired fear response serves as the basis of this CR. The clinical symptoms of a panic attack, which occur in all of the fear-related disorders (panic disorder, specific phobia, social phobia, acute stress disorder, and PTSD) result in the same series of fear response reflexes that have been shown to occur with activation of the central nucleus of the amygdala (Fig. 2.2). Thus, an understanding of what leads to differential activation of this hard-wired neural reflex is a critical question both for understanding the pathological acquisition of fear responding and the inability to normally inhibit fear in a safe situation.

The inhibition of learned fear, a process known as extinction, has been studied extensively in laboratory animals as well as in humans and is a form of "active" learning as opposed to simply a form of unlearning or forgetting a conditioned association (reviewed in Myers and Davis 2002). During extinction training, the CS (such as a previously learned fear trigger for a patient with an anxiety disorder) is repeatedly presented in the absence of the fear-inducing UCS, leading to inhibition of the previously conditioned fear response to the otherwise neutral CS. Considered in operational terms, extinction may thus be defined as "a reduction in the strength or probability of a conditioned fear response as a consequence of repeated presentation of the CS in the absence of the UCS" (Rothbaum and Davis 2003).

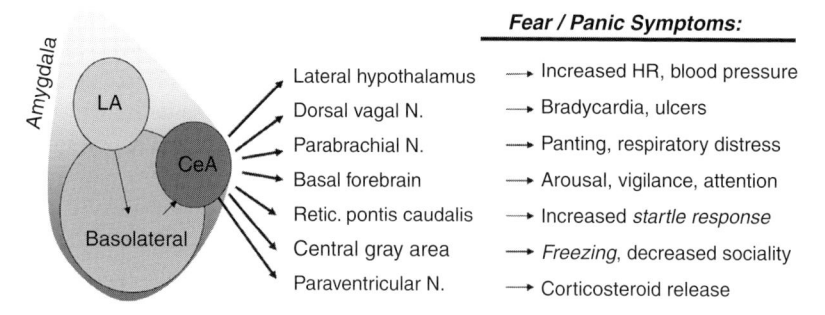

Figure 2.2. The neural circuitry of the fear response. The symptoms that underlie the syndrome of a panic attack closely align with the hard-wired conditioned responses that are downstream of central amygdala (CeA) activation. The amygdala is composed of numerous subnuclei, but the lateral amygdala (LA), basolateral amygdala (BLA), and CeA appear to be most important in the emotion of fear. The LA and BLA receive input from a large array of sensory and associative areas and are thought to be critical for the synaptic plasticity events underlying conditioned associations. When these areas activate the CeA, then a variety of downstream events occur (Davis, 1992). The CeA is connected with numerous hypothalamic and brainstem areas that lead to essentially reflexive behavioral fear responses, which include the majority of the DSM–IV definitions for the symptoms occurring with a panic attack. Note that the acoustic startle reflex and the freezing response are two of the most common measures of fear response in animal models. HR, heart rate; N, nerve.

Pharmacological enhancement of extinction-based treatment

Clinically, the principles of extinction learning form much of the foundation for the most effective behavioral therapies for fear-related anxiety disorders (reviewed in Abramowitz 2006; Norton and Price 2007; Rothbaum and Schwartz 2002) though gaps in efficacy remain (Brown and Barlow 1995; Clark et al. 1994; Margraf et al. 1993). In practice, this situation involves progressively graded exposure to the feared object or event in the absence of any actual harm – a process that is analogous to a rodent's exposure to a fear-related CS without repeated pairing of the aversive UCS in extinction training. The environmental context of therapeutic exposure may be *imaginal* in nature wherein the patient reads or listens to a narrative of the feared event or *in vivo* wherein the patient is directly exposed to the feared stimulus. Of note, some of the most well-controlled and novel behavioral exposure therapy techniques have involved virtual reality approaches. In these paradigms the patient is exposed, via a computerized virtual environment, often wearing three-dimensional head goggles, with surround sound, for a full-immersion event (Rothbaum et al. 1997). Virtual reality exposure therapy has been shown to be efficacious for PTSD (Difede et al. 2007; Gerardi et al. 2008), social phobia (Wallach et al. 2009), and specific phobia (Ressler et al. 2004; Rothbaum et al. 2000). Furthermore, stimulus control and reproducibility make it an excellent research tool for examining the mechanisms of exposure therapy.

A large body of literature derived from preclinical studies using animal models as well as clinical research with human subjects has deepened our understanding of the neurobiology of fear conditioning and extinction (reviewed in Myers and Davis 2007; Rodrigues et al. 2009; Sehlmeyer et al. 2009). In particular, the excitatory amino acid neurotransmitter, glutamate, acting on the N-methyl-D-aspartic acid (NMDA) receptor has been found to play a pivotal role in the acquisition and extinction of fear learning (Gillespie and Ressler, 2005). Infusion of NMDA receptor antagonists into the rat amygdala blocks the acquisition (Miserendino et al. 1990) as well as the extinction (Falls et al. 1992) of conditioned fear whereas peripheral or central infusion of the partial NMDA receptor agonist, d-cycloserine (DCS), facilitates the extinction of conditioned fear in rats. Importantly, DCS does not reduce fear in rats in the absence of extinction training; this finding suggests that the effects of DCS are not related to anxiolysis but rather are directed toward the facilitation of new learning (described and reviewed in Myers and Davis 2007; Vervliet 2008).

The site of DCS action is the strychnine-insensitive glycine recognition site of the NMDA receptor complex (Hood et al. 1989; Monahan et al. 1989), which, when bound by either endogenous glycine or D-serine or by exogenous DCS, facilitates the activity of previously silent NMDA synapses (Gomperts et al. 1998). Because DCS is a partial agonist, the effects of DCS on NMDA receptor function are complex and are contingent on synaptic glycine concentrations

(Emmett et al. 1991; Hood et al. 1989; Watson et al. 1990). DCS administration under conditions of high full agonist concentration (in which binding sites are saturated by endogenous glycine or D-serine) reduces NMDA receptor activity, presumably as a consequence of competitive displacement of the endogenous agonists by DCS and the lower intrinsic efficacy of DCS compared to glycine/D-serine. Conversely, administration of DCS under conditions of low synaptic glycine and minimal agonist occupancy of glycine binding sites results in enhanced NMDA receptor activity relative to baseline, because DCS occupies otherwise empty glycine sites. The modulating effects of DCS on NMDA receptor activity may thus promote neuroplasticity as well as interference with the reconsolidation (see below) of fear memories resulting in increased effectiveness of extinction training (reviewed in Krystal 2007; Vervliet 2008).

Previous attempts to combine symptom-directed pharmacotherapy with behavior therapy to obtain treatment synergy have not generally been successful (Foa et al. 2002; Otto 2002). Occasionally, combined treatments have even worsened clinical outcomes (Barlow et al. 2000; Marks et al. 1993). One explanation for this potentially paradoxical effect, at least for some of the benzodiazepine trials combined with therapy, is that the gains made in psychotherapy may be encoded in a state-dependent manner that does not transfer to an internal state after the benzodiazepine washout period. Regardless of the mechanism of lack of synergy, extinction-based therapies for anxiety may be an exception to this trend insofar as the role of the medication is to specifically enhance the process of extinction rather than to separately target symptom clusters. The qualitative similarity between extinction training in rodents and exposure therapy for anxiety disorders in humans in conjunction with the prior safe use of DCS as an adjunctive antibiotic in the treatment of tuberculosis in humans (Heifets 1994) made it an attractive candidate compound to examine for utility in augmenting the effectiveness of extinction-based behavior therapies for anxiety disorders.

Six studies evaluating the use of DCS combined with exposure therapy on the extinction of fear in clinical populations with anxiety disorders have been published to date (review and meta-analysis by Norberg et al. 2008). DCS combined with exposure therapy has been shown to be effective in the treatment of fear of heights (Ressler et al. 2004) and social anxiety disorder (Guastella et al. 2008; Hofmann et al. 2006).

In addition, two positive trials (Kushner et al. 2007; Wilhelm et al. 2008) and one negative trial (Storch et al. 2007) have been reported for the use of DCS combined with exposure and response-prevention therapy for obsessive-compulsive disorder. Methodological differences between the positive (Kushner et al. 2007; Wilhelm et al. 2008) and negative (Storch et al. 2007) obsessive-compulsive studies with respect to the dose of DCS, timing of DCS administration relative to the timing of the exposure treatment, and a floor effect induced by a high rate of response of all groups to the behavior therapy component may be responsible for the differences in outcomes observed in these studies (reviewed in Rothbaum 2008).

The effect of DCS on extinction in healthy human subjects has been evaluated in a small series of studies as well (reviewed in Grillon 2009; Vervliet 2008). In contrast to the effectiveness of DCS combined with exposure therapy in the treatment of anxiety in clinical populations, DCS combined with exposure has not been effective in the extinction of subclinical fear of spiders (Guastella et al. 2007a) or laboratory-conditioned fear (Guastella et al. 2007b; Kalisch et al. 2009) as well as nonemotional memory in normal human research subjects (Otto et al. 2009). The reasons for the discordant results observed between clinical and nonclinical populations with respect to DCS effects on the extinction of fear are unclear. It has, however, recently been proposed (Grillon 2009) that dual, threat-responsive neural systems exist in humans that are differentially engaged by the lower-intensity laboratory fear-conditioning protocols compared with the high-intensity environmental exposures that result in anxiety disorders. In such a model, the phylogenetically older threat response system common to rodents and primates geared to rapid and robust response to threat may be the system primarily responsive to DCS augmentation of extinction and the system responsible for fear-related anxiety disorders. Conversely, a higher order threat response system, not responsive to DCS, common only to primates, may be the system engaged by laboratory-based fear conditioning or low-intensity fear. Another explanation is the possibility that, at least in some of the nonclinical studies, the subjects may all have had relatively rapid emotional learning and thus have been subject to a floor effect in the decrease in their fear response, so that any additional added effect of DCS might not be appreciated.

Finally, a recent meta-analysis (Norberg et al. 2008) using data extracted from over 40 preclinical and clinical manuscripts from 1998 to 2007 examined the effect of DCS augmentation of extinction protocols in rodents as well as in human clinical and nonclinical populations. Collectively, the results indicate that DCS enhances fear extinction/exposure therapy in both animals and anxiety-disordered humans with moderate effect sizes. Timing and magnitude of DCS dose were also identified as important variables with efficacy maximized when DCS is administered a limited number of times and immediately before or after extinction training or exposure therapy. Because the effects of DCS seem to decrease over repeated sessions, the major contribution of DCS to exposure-based therapy might be to increase its speed or efficiency. In summary, DCS continues to be promising as an agent for pharmacological enhancement of psychotherapy and may guide translational research toward future potential agents that effectively enhance behavioral therapy.

Disruption of traumatic memory consolidation

Within the general class of anxiety disorders, PTSD is unique in the sense that the precipitating traumatic event may provide the opportunity for acute intervention before the onset of symptoms and before memories have been consolidated. Thus, in some cases, it may be possible to mitigate the development of disease. However, in much the same way that the surgical and medical management of patients with life-threatening physical trauma during the so-called golden hour following injury is fraught with both peril and opportunity so is the acute treatment of patients following psychologically traumatic experiences. Evidence-based practice of the acute management of patients following exposure to psychological trauma is limited. Several psychological interventions have been investigated for use in acutely trauma-exposed individuals and found to be either minimally effective or in some cases harmful (review in Mansdorf 2008; review and meta-analysis in Roberts *et al.* 2009). However, as our understanding of the neurobiology of memory has evolved, researchers have identified novel pharmacological interventions targeting the disruption or attenuation of the aversive component of traumatic emotional memory.

Consolidation is the process whereby a short-term memory is transformed into a long-term memory. A large body of preclinical research (reviewed in Dudai 2004; McGaugh 2000; Rodrigues *et al.* 2004) indicates that during the period of consolidation, short-term memories are labile and subject to disruption by a wide variety of interventions. The central implication of this finding is that, following trauma exposure in human patients, it may be possible selectively to disrupt the consolidation of the new fear memories that are in the process of being formed while retaining declarative memory for the traumatic event (Pitman and Delahanty 2005). This may be possible, given that the encoding of memory is a parallel, distributed process whereby declarative/explicit memory systems involving hippocampal–cortical pathways encode the "what, when, and where" of an event while parallel, amygdala–cortical pathways encode the emotional salience of the memory. Ideally, with such treatments, it may be possible to block the overconsolidation of the aversive emotional components of a memory while preserving the declarative aspects of the memory.

In theory, such a practice would not render the patient fully amnestic but could potentially prevent PTSD or reduce the intensity of symptoms. However, the inherent value placed on all components of experience, both positive and negative, as they help define our uniqueness as individuals, has prompted a variety of ethical questions with respect to potential interventions that have selective emotional amnesia as clinical end points in the treatment of fear memories in acutely traumatized patients (reviewed in Levy and Clarke 2008).

Much of what is presently understood about the process of consolidation as it applies to the psychobiology of fear is derived from preclinical studies with rodents using the inhibitory avoidance paradigm (reviewed in McGaugh 2000). In avoidance learning paradigms, an animal, typically a rodent, is placed in a box with two compartments. On stepping from one compartment into the adjacent compartment, the animal receives a mild foot shock. After completion of this training, the animal then avoids spending time in the compartment in which it was shocked, even if it receives no more reinforcing shocks (McGaugh and Cahill 1997). The basolateral amygdala plays a critical role in the consolidation of fear memory (reviewed in McGaugh 2004) as observed in inhibitory avoidance (Parent and McGaugh 1994) as well as classical fear conditioning paradigms (Vazdarjanova and McGaugh 1999). Concurrent activation of the endogenous fight or flight adrenergic (Ferry *et al.* 1999a, 1999b, 1999c; reviewed in Ferry and McGaugh 2000) and of glucocorticoid (Quirarte *et al.* 1997;

Roozendaal and McGaugh 1997) responses to fear-evoking events during inhibitory avoidance training appears to be a critical step in the post-event strengthening of these memories within the basolateral amygdala. Consolidation of fear memories is additionally influenced by a wide variety of other neurotransmitter systems (reviewed in McGaugh and Roozendaal 2009) including dopamine (Guarraci *et al.* 2000) and glutamate-NMDA pathways (Shimizu *et al.* 2000). In multiple preclinical studies, propranolol, a commonly used β-adrenergic antagonist, and glucocorticoids have been found to alter consolidation of newly formed fear memories, especially in inhibitory avoidance paradigms. Translational studies in humans based on these approaches are reviewed below.

Propranolol

Propranolol is a β-adrenergic receptor antagonist that is commonly used to treat hypertension. The use of propranolol to treat individuals with posttraumatic stress symptoms was initially described in a case series of physically and sexually abused children with severe symptoms of agitation. Administration of propranolol reduced agitation but, following discontinuation of propranolol, these symptoms promptly returned, indicating that the effects of propranolol were limited to symptom reduction (Famularo *et al.* 1988). However, preclinical research on the role of adrenergic receptors in the consolidation of emotional memory prompted further investigation into the use of propranolol to interfere with fear acquisition. Studies in healthy human subjects (Cahill *et al.* 1994) and rodents (Cahill *et al.* 2000) later demonstrated the capacity of propranolol to attenuate emotional memory. A subsequent case report (Taylor and Cahill 2002) describing the reduction of posttraumatic stress symptoms in a patient with PTSD following new traumatic exposure suggested the potential clinical application of propranolol as an emotional memory modulating agent in the acute treatment of patients following trauma exposure.

At present, four studies have examined the use of propranolol in the treatment of patients following acute exposure to a traumatic event (McGhee *et al.* 2009; Pitman *et al.* 2002; Stein *et al.* 2007; Vaiva *et al.* 2003). Pitman and colleagues (2002) examined subjects who presented to an emergency room immediately following a traumatic event (primarily motor vehicle accidents). In this study, patients were randomized to receive either propranolol or placebo, orally four times daily for 10 days, followed by a taper period. The first dose of medicine was administered, on average, 4 hours after the traumatic event occurred. One month following the trauma, PTSD symptom measures trended lower in the 11 completers that received propranolol compared with the 20 completers who did not. In addition, when exposed to script-driven mental imagery of the trauma approximately 3 months after the trauma, a significant number of those who took placebo had ongoing physiological symptoms of PTSD whereas none of the subjects taking propranolol experienced such symptoms.

Vaiva and colleagues (2003) performed an open-label evaluation in which 19 subjects were recruited from hospital emergency departments, 11 of whom took propranolol three times daily beginning 2 to 20 hours after the trauma for 7 days followed by a taper period. Two months post-trauma, levels of PTSD symptoms were significantly different in the patients treated with propranolol.

More recently, Stein and colleagues (2007) performed a randomized, double-blind, placebo-controlled trial comparing 14 days of the β-blocker propranolol (n = 17), the anticonvulsant gabapentin (n = 14), or placebo (n = 17) administered within 48 hours of injury to patients admitted to a surgical trauma center. Assessments of posttraumatic stress and depressive symptoms were performed at 1, 4, and 8 months following initial injury, and neither propranolol nor gabapentin showed a significant benefit over placebo on depressive or posttraumatic stress symptoms.

Finally, McGhee and colleagues (2009) conducted a retrospective study examining the relationship between PTSD prevalence and propranolol administration during burn treatment in soldiers injured in Operation Iraqi Freedom and Operation Enduring Freedom. Propranolol was not administered systematically in this study and was given at the discretion of the treating physician. Variables considered in the analysis included receipt of propranolol as a categorical variable, number of surgeries, anesthetic/analgesic regimen, amount of surface area burned, and injury severity score collected from patients charts. PTSD was assessed using the PTSD Checklist-Military. Thirty-one soldiers received propranolol and 34 soldiers matched on the above variables did not. No significant difference was observed in the prevalence of PTSD between patients receiving propranolol and those who did not. Thus the data on whether propranolol prevents consolidation of emotional trauma memories in humans remain unclear. In the studies discussed above, it is possible that propranolol (given hours to days following the trauma) may not have been given sufficiently early following the trauma (e.g., in the animal studies, it is usually given minutes following fear learning) to disrupt the early critical period of emotional memory consolidation.

Glucocorticoids

An alternative consolidation-blockade approach to the use of propranolol involves the administration of glucocorticoids to trauma-exposed patients. The rationale for this approach is based on the findings in some studies that lower post-trauma cortisol levels predict subsequent risk for PTSD (Yehuda 2001; Yehuda et al. 1995, 2004). Additionally, a large body of data (reviewed in de Quervain et al. 2009) indicates that glucocorticoids promote emotional memory consolidation and impair memory retrieval. Together, these findings suggest that administration of stress doses of glucocorticoids following trauma exposure may interrupt the cycle of retrieval, re-experiencing, and reconsolidation by impairing memory retrieval. Thus, this process may attenuate the intensity of aversive emotional memories. Interestingly, glucocorticoid-induced memory retrieval deficits may be reduced by concurrent administration of propranolol (de Quervain et al. 2007). The initial findings of clinical research conducted in patients hospitalized for septic shock in intensive care units support the hypothesis that administration of glucocorticoids during the time of trauma exposure reduces the intensity of posttraumatic stress symptoms (reviewed in Schelling et al. 2006). Schelling and colleagues (1999) conducted a small pilot study and found that exogenously administered stress doses of cortisol reduced the development of subsequent posttraumatic stress symptoms in medical-surgical patients following septic shock. This finding was subsequently replicated by a large randomized, double-blind, placebo-controlled study in patients with septic shock (Schelling et al. 2001). It was further extended to patients undergoing cardiothoracic surgery (Schelling et al. 2004; Weis et al. 2006). Further, Aerni and colleagues (2004) reported that repeated administration of low-dose cortisol to patients with PTSD reduced PTSD symptoms.

Collectively, the work on the use of medications that interfere with emotional memory consolidation remains in its early stages but carries the potential of true disease prevention. Interpretation of the outcome of the preceding studies is limited by methodological differences between studies and small sample size across studies. As our understanding of the mechanisms of fear consolidation becomes more sophisticated, we remain hopeful that it will lead to direct translational interventions that may eventually prevent the development of trauma-related disorders in acutely traumatized subjects.

Disruption of traumatic memory reconsolidation

Similar to what occurred with consolidation, work over the last several years has examined the hypothesis that memories remain labile and susceptible to new associations following reactivation (Nader et al. 2000; Przybyslawski and Sara 1997; Przybyslawski et al. 1999). In a fascinating series of studies, it was shown that reactivated memories are sensitive to pharmacological disruption (reviewed in Nader and Hardt 2009). Most of this work has been based on the early findings that local infusion of protein synthesis inhibitors into discrete brain regions in rodents appears to prevent the reconsolidation of the memory after it is made labile again through reactivation. In the initial recent study examining this process, Nader et al. (2000) showed that consolidated fear memories, when reactivated during retrieval, return to a labile state in which infusion of anisomycin, a protein synthesis inhibitor, shortly after memory reactivation produces amnesia on later tests. The same treatment with anisomycin, in the absence of memory reactivation, left memory intact. Consistent with a time-limited role for protein synthesis production in consolidation, delay of the infusion until 6 hours after memory reactivation produced no amnesia. The authors argue that these data show that consolidated fear memories, when reactivated, return to a labile state that requires *de novo* protein synthesis for reconsolidation.

Protein synthesis inhibitors generally do not easily cross the blood–brain barrier and can be toxic; thus, they are unlikely to be used in translational studies in humans. However, a few studies have suggested that other, more benign drugs, given acutely during recall of fear memories in animals, may also act to reduce later memory expression, possibly through inhibiting reconsolidation mechanisms. For example, in recent years, the earliest demonstration of blockade of reconsolidation was shown with NMDA antagonists by Sara and colleagues (Przybyslawski and Sara 1997). This group also demonstrated that the β-adrenergic antagonist, timolol, prevented reconsolidation (Przybyslawski *et al.* 1999; Roullet and Sara 1998). This finding was later replicated by LeDoux and colleagues using propranolol (Debiec and Ledoux 2004). Interestingly, this study found that propranolol impaired reconsolidation but not the initial consolidation of Pavlovian fear conditioning, which is in contrast with the effects of propranolol on consolidation of inhibitory avoidance learning as discussed previously. This difference in the animal models may have to do with the different neural circuits involved in cued fear conditioning, as performed by Ledoux's group, and inhibitory avoidance learning, as performed by McGaugh's group.

Eisenberg and Dudai (2004) suggested that reconsolidation effects are found following newly learned memories but not following remotely acquired memories. The lack of a reported finding in humans using propranolol to block reconsolidation has been curious, because the initial report in animals appeared almost a decade ago. Given the relative experimental ease and safety of such an experiment, one possibility is that the propranolol human pilot studies that intended to block consolidation following trauma in the emergency room (above) were actually not targeting consolidation but were instead targeting the early reactivation and thus reconsolidation processes in the days and weeks after the trauma occurred. Together, these data suggest that treatment with a β-adrenergic antagonist in the weeks following initial trauma exposure might be effective in preventing PTSD, possibly through impairing reconsolidation and sensitization processes early, but that disrupting the remote memories from chronic PTSD may not be possible using reconsolidation impairing approaches. If that turns out to be the case, we can hope the mechanisms discussed above to enhance extinction of fear may be optimal in such situations.

Translational trials of glucocorticoids and propranolol in reconsolidation

Glucocorticoids have also been examined with respect to reconsolidation. Cai and colleagues (2006) examined the role of post-reactivation glucocorticoids on fear memory. They found that when glucocorticoids were administered immediately after reactivation of a contextual fear memory, subsequent recall was significantly diminished. Additional experiments support the interpretation that glucocorticoids not only decrease fear memory retrieval but also augment consolidation of fear memory extinction rather than decrease reconsolidation. These findings provide a rodent model for a potential treatment of established acquired anxiety disorders in humans, as suggested by others (Aerni *et al.* 2004; Schelling *et al.* 2004), based on a mechanism of enhanced extinction. More recently, Soravia and colleagues (2006) reported that glucocorticoid administration was effective in the reduction of fear symptoms in a cohort of patients with social phobia and an additional cohort of patients with spider phobia.

Studies with propranolol have yielded both positive and negative findings in human trials of reconsolidation impairment. Brunet and colleagues (2008) tested the effect of propranolol given after the retrieval of memories of past traumatic events. Subjects with chronic PTSD described their traumatic event during a script preparation session and then received a 1-day dose of propranolol (n = 9) or placebo (n = 10), randomized and double-blind. A week later, they engaged in script-driven mental imagery of their traumatic event. Physiological (but not necessarily subjective emotional) responses were significantly smaller in the subjects who had received post-reactivation propranolol. Similarly, Kindt *et al.* (2009) reported that administration of propranolol before memory reactivation in humans erased the behavioral expression of a learned preclinical fear memory 24 hours later and apparently prevented the return of this conditioned fear. Note that these approaches have been used in negative trials as well. Tollenaar and colleagues (2009) tested the effects of propranolol on physiological responding to emotional memories in 79 healthy young men. After preparing a script of a negative disturbing memory, participants were instructed to imagine this event 1 week later after ingestion of 35 mg cortisol, 80 mg propranolol, or a placebo. Physiological responding to the script-driven imagery was recorded during this reactivation as well as a week later after drug washout. The authors found that emotionality of the memories was reduced over time but that it was not affected by either cortisol or propranolol treatment during memory reactivation. The authors concluded that whereas healthy men do respond psychophysiologically to personal emotional scripts, the effects of cortisol and propranolol on physiological responses to emotional memories might be specific to clinical groups characterized by emotional hyper-responsiveness as observed clinically in patients with PTSD.

Combined extinction–reconsolidation approaches

It has become increasingly clear that the minutes to hours following fear memory consolidation as well as reconsolidation may provide for a particularly labile period in memory formation. Myers *et al.* (2006) reasoned that extinction initiated shortly following fear acquisition preferentially engages depotentiation or unlearning, whereas extinction initiated after longer delays recruits a different mechanism. They found, consistent with an inhibitory learning mechanism of extinction, that rats extinguished 24 hours to 72 hours following acquisition exhibited reinstatement, renewal, and spontaneous recovery (the classic measures of fear memory "savings" as exhibited following extinction). In contrast, and consistent with an erasure mechanism, rats extinguished 10 minutes to 1 hour after acquisition exhibited little or no reinstatement, renewal, or spontaneous recovery. These data support a model in which different neural mechanisms are recruited depending on the temporal delay of fear extinction.

More recently, an exciting development was reported by Monfils and colleagues (2009). The authors used a behavioral design in which a fear memory in rats is destabilized and reinterpreted as safe by presenting an isolated retrieval trial before an extinction session. Essentially, they found that if they provided an extinction session at short periods of time for a single reactivation session, the rats no longer exhibited reinstatement, renewal, or spontaneous recovery, suggesting that this protocol led to either profound extinction or erasure or the previously trained fearful memory. This procedure thus appears to permanently attenuate the fear memory without the use of drugs. This approach is now being tried in several ongoing human preclinical and clinical trials (D. Schiller and M. Monfils, personal communication) and offers a potentially exciting new approach to mechanisms of fear treatment with exposure therapy.

Conclusions

Considered collectively, the novel approaches we have described are examples of the translation of preclinical research data examining the biology of fear learning and emotional memory into new treatments for fear-related anxiety disorders. The anxiety disorders, particular disorders of fear dysregulation, appear to be some of the most low-hanging fruit in psychiatry. The neurobiological circuits mediating fear have been well worked out over several decades, and the approaches to understanding the molecular neurobiology of synaptic plasticity and learning are at the forefront of neuroscience. Together, these burgeoning scientific areas hope to bring new, rationally designed, translational approaches to some of the most devastating psychiatric disorders.

This chapter has examined the use of DCS as well as potentially other new approaches that enhance emotional learning when combined with exposure therapy. In addition, memory reactivation, combined with mechanisms of reconsolidation blockade, provides for another novel and potentially powerful approach to reduce the intensity of maladaptive fear memories. Enhancing the extinction, or inhibition, and disrupting the reconsolidation of previously existing traumatic and fearful memories together open up new avenues for providing a long-term cure for patients with emotional disorders. Finally, clinically directed interference with initial memory consolidation through the use of β-blockers or glucocorticoids following acute trauma exposure could prevent or attenuate the formation of traumatic emotional memory and reduce risk of PTSD.

Decades of research on the temporal nature of memory acquisition, consolidation, expression, and extinction combined with an increased understanding of the molecular mechanisms of memory formation are now leading to new approaches that together offer exciting promise for the field of psychiatry for those it serves.

Acknowledgments

This work was primarily supported by National Institutes of Mental Health MH082256 to CFG & MH071537 to KJR, and the Burroughs Wellcome Fund.

Financial disclosures

No commercial sponsors or commercial relationships are related to the current work. All additional past and present financial ties of the investigators are disclosed herein. Dr. Gillespie has received funding from APIRE/Wyeth, the National Alliance for

Research on Schizophrenia and Depression (NARSAD), the National Institute on Drug Abuse (NIDA), and the National Institute of Mental Health (NIMH). Dr. Ressler has received awards and/or funding support related to other studies from Lundbeck Inc., Burroughs Wellcome Foundation, Pfizer, NARSAD, NIMH, and NIDA and is a cofounder of Extinction Pharmaceuticals. None of the above funding agencies had any role in the review or approval of the manuscript.

References

Abramowitz JS. 2006. The psychological treatment of obsessive-compulsive disorder. *Can J Psychiatry* **51**:407–416.

Aerni A, Traber R, Hock C et al. 2004. Low-dose cortisol for symptoms of posttraumatic stress disorder. *Am J Psychiatry* **161**:1488–1490.

Barlow DH, Gorman JM, Shear MK, Woods SW. 2000. Cognitive-behavioral therapy, imipramine, or their combination for panic disorder: a randomized controlled trial. *J Am Med Assoc* **283**:2529–2536.

Brown TA, Barlow DH. 1995. Long-term outcome in cognitive-behavioral treatment of panic disorder: clinical predictors and alternative strategies for assessment. *J Consult Clin Psychol* **63**:754–765.

Brunet A, Orr SP, Tremblay J et al. 2008. Effect of post-retrieval propranolol on psychophysiologic responding during subsequent script-driven traumatic imagery in post-traumatic stress disorder. *J Psychiatr Res* **42**:503–506.

Cahill L, Pham CA, Setlow B. 2000. Impaired memory consolidation in rats produced with beta-adrenergic blockade. *Neurobiol Learn Mem* **74**:259–266.

Cahill L, Prins B, Weber M, McGaugh JL. 1994. Beta-adrenergic activation and memory for emotional events. *Nature* **371**:702–704.

Cai WH, Blundell J, Han J, Greene RW, Powell CM. 2006. Postreactivation glucocorticoids impair recall of established fear memory. *J Neurosci* **26**:9560–9566.

Clark DM, Salkovskis PM, Hackmann A et al. 1994. A comparison of cognitive therapy, applied relaxation and imipramine in the treatment of panic disorder. *Br J Psychiatry* **164**:759–769.

Davis M. 1992. The role of the amygdala in fear and anxiety. *Annu Rev Neurosci* **15**:353–375.

de Quervain DJ, Aerni A, Roozendaal B. 2007. Preventive effect of beta-adrenoceptor blockade on glucocorticoid-induced memory retrieval deficits. *Am J Psychiatry* **164**:967–969.

de Quervain DJ, Aerni A, Schelling G, Roozendaal B. 2009. Glucocorticoids and the regulation of memory in health and disease. *Front Neuroendocrinol* **30**:358–370.

Debiec J, Ledoux JE. 2004. Disruption of reconsolidation but not consolidation of auditory fear conditioning by noradrenergic blockade in the amygdala. *Neuroscience* **129**:267–272.

Difede J, Cukor J, Jayasinghe N et al. Virtual reality exposure therapy for the treatment of posttraumatic stress disorder following September 11, 2001. *J Clin Psychiatry* **68**:1639–1647.

Dudai Y. 2004. The neurobiology of consolidations, or, how stable is the engram? *Annu Rev Psychology* **55**:51–86.

Eisenberg M, Dudai Y. 2004. Reconsolidation of fresh, remote, and extinguished fear memory in Medaka: old fears don't die. *Eur J Neurosci* **20**:3397–3403.

Emmett MR, Mick SJ, Cler JA et al. 1991. Actions of D-cycloserine at the N-methyl-D-aspartate-associated glycine receptor site in vivo. *Neuropharmacology* **30**:1167–1171.

Falls WA, Miserendino MJ, Davis M. 1992. Extinction of fear-potentiated startle: blockade by infusion of an NMDA antagonist into the amygdala. *J Neurosci* **12**:854–863.

Famularo R, Kinscherff R, Fenton T. 1988. Propranolol treatment for childhood posttraumatic stress disorder, acute type. A pilot study. *Am J Dis Child* **142**:1244–1247.

Ferry B, McGaugh JL. 2000. Role of amygdala norepinephrine in mediating stress hormone regulation of memory storage. *Acta Pharmacol Sin* **21**:481–493.

Ferry B, Roozendaal B, McGaugh JL. 1999a. Basolateral amygdala noradrenergic influences on memory storage are mediated by an interaction between beta- and alpha1-adrenoceptors. *J Neurosci* **19**:5119–5123.

Ferry B, Roozendaal B, McGaugh JL. 1999b. Involvement of alpha1-adrenoceptors in the basolateral amygdala in modulation of memory storage. *Eur J Pharmacology* **372**:9–16.

Ferry B, Roozendaal B, McGaugh JL. 1999c. Role of norepinephrine in mediating stress hormone regulation of long-term memory storage: a critical involvement of the amygdala. *Biol Psychiatry* **46**:1140–1152.

Foa E, Franklin ME, Moser J. 2002. Context in the clinic: how well do cognitive-behavioral therapies and medications work in combination? *Biol Psychiatry* **52**:987–997.

Garakani A, Mathew SJ, Charney DS. 2006. Neurobiology of anxiety disorders and implications for treatment. *Mt Sinai J Med* **73**:941–949.

Gerardi M, Rothbaum BO, Ressler K, Heekin M, Rizzo A. 2008. Virtual reality exposure therapy using a virtual Iraq: case report. *J Trauma Stress* **21**:209–213.

Gillespie CF, Ressler KJ. 2005. Emotional learning and glutamate: translational perspectives. *CNS Spectrums* **10**:831–839.

Gomperts SN, Rao A, Craig AM, Malenka RC, Nicoll RA. 1998. Postsynaptically silent synapses in single neuron cultures. *Neuron* **21**:1443–1451.

Grillon C. 2009. D-cycloserine facilitation of fear extinction and exposure-based therapy might rely on lower-level, automatic mechanisms. *Biol Psychiatry* **66**:636–641.

Guarraci FA, Frohardt RJ, Falls WA, Kapp BS. 2000. The effects of intra-amygdaloid infusions of a D2 dopamine receptor antagonist on Pavlovian fear conditioning. *Behav Neurosci* **114**:647–651.

Guastella AJ, Dadds MR, Lovibond PF, Mitchell P, Richardson R. 2007a. A randomized controlled trial of the effect of D-cycloserine on exposure therapy for spider fear. *J Psychiatr Res* **41**:466–471.

Guastella AJ, Lovibond PF, Dadds MR, Mitchell P, Richardson R. 2007b. A randomized controlled trial of the effect of D-cycloserine on extinction and fear conditioning in humans. *Behav Res Ther* **45**:663–672.

Guastella AJ, Richardson R, Lovibond PF et al. 2008. A randomized controlled trial of D-cycloserine enhancement of exposure therapy for social anxiety disorder. *Biol Psychiatry* **63**:544–549.

Heifets LB. 1994. Antimycobacterial drugs. *Sem Respir Infect* **9**:84–103.

Hofmann SG, Meuret AE, Smits JAJ et al. 2006. Augmentation of exposure therapy with D-cycloserine for social anxiety disorder. *Arch Gen Psychiatry* **63**:298–304.

Hood W, Compton R, Monahan J. 1989. D-cycloserine: a ligand for the N-methyl-D-aspartate coupled glycine receptor has partial agonist characteristics. *Neurosci Lett* **98**:91–95.

Izard CE. 1992. Basic emotions, relations among emotions, and emotion-cognition relations. *Psychol Rev* **99**:561–565.

Jovanovic T, Ressler KJ. 2010. How the neurocircuitry and genetics of fear inhibition may inform our understanding of PTSD. *Am J Psychiatry* **167**:648–662.

Kalisch R, Holt B, Petrovic P et al. 2010. The NMDA agonist D-cycloserine facilitates fear memory consolidation in humans. *Cereb Cortex* **19**:187–196.

Kessler RC, Chiu WT, Demler O, Merikangas KR, Walters EE. 2005. Prevalence, severity, and comorbidity of 12-month DSM-IV disorders in the National Comorbidity Survey Replication. *Arch Gen Psychiatry* **62**: 617–627.

Kindt M, Soeter M, Vervliet B. 2009. Beyond extinction: erasing human fear responses and preventing the return of fear. *Nat Neurosci* **12**:256–258.

Krystal JH. 2007. Neuroplasticity as a target for the pharmacotherapy of psychiatric disorders: new opportunities for synergy with psychotherapy. *Biol Psychiatry* **62**:833–834.

Kushner MG, Kim SW, Donahue C et al. 2007. D-cycloserine augmented exposure therapy for obsessive-compulsive disorder. *Biol Psychiatry* **62**:835–838.

Levy N, Clarke S. 2008. Neuroethics and psychiatry. *Curr Opin Psychiatry* **21**:568–571.

Mansdorf IJ. 2008. Psychological interventions following terrorist attacks. *Br Med Bull* **88**:7–22.

Margraf J, Barlow DH, Clark DM, Telch MJ. 1993. Psychological treatment of panic: work in progress on outcome, active ingredients, and follow-up. *Behav Res Therapy* **31**:1–8.

Marks I, Swinson R, Basoglu M et al., 1993. Alprazolam and exposure alone and combined in panic disorder with agoraphobia. A controlled study in London and Toronto. *Br J Psychiatry* **162**:776–787.

McGaugh JL. 2000. Memory – a century of consolidation. *Science* **287**:248–251.

McGaugh JL. 2004. The amygdala modulates the consolidation of memories of emotionally arousing experiences. *Annu Rev Neurosci* **27**:1–28.

McGaugh JL, Cahill L. 1997. Interaction of neuromodulatory systems in modulating memory storage. *Behav Brain Res* **83**:31–38.

McGaugh JL, Roozendaal B. 2009. Drug enhancement of memory consolidation: historical perspective and neurobiological implications. *Psychopharmacology* **202**:3–14.

McGhee LL, Maani CV, Garza TH et al. 2009. The effect of propranolol on posttraumatic stress disorder in burned service members. *J Burn Care Res* **30**:92–97.

Mineka S, Oehlberg K. 2008. The relevance of recent developments in classical conditioning to understanding the etiology and maintenance of anxiety disorders. *Acta Pychol (Amst)* **127**:567–580.

Miserendino MJD, Sananes CB, Melia KR, Davis M. 1990. Blocking of acquisition but not expression of conditioned fear-potentiated startle by NMDA antagonists in the amygdala. *Nature* **345**:716–718.

Monahan JB, Handelmann GE, Hood WF, Cordi AA. 1989. D-cycloserine, a positive modulator of the N-methyl-D-aspartate receptor, enhances performance of learning tasks in rats. *Pharmacol Biochem Behav* **34**:649–653.

Monfils MH, Cowansage KK, Klann E, LeDoux JE. 2009. Extinction-reconsolidation boundaries: key to persistent attenuation of fear memories. *Science* **324**: 951–955.

Myers KM, Davis M. 2002. Behavioral and neural analysis of extinction. *Neuron* **36**:567–584.

Myers KM, Davis M. 2007. Mechanisms of fear extinction. *Mol Psychiatry* **12**:120–150.

Myers KM, Ressler KJ, Davis M. 2006. Different mechanisms of fear extinction dependent on length of time since fear acquisition. *Learn Mem* **13**:216–223.

Nader K, Hardt O. 2009. A single standard for memory: the case for reconsolidation. *Nat Rev Neurosci* **10**:224–234.

Nader K, Schafe GE, Le Doux JE. 2000. Fear memories require protein synthesis in the amygdala for reconsolidation after retrieval. *Nature* **406**:722–726.

Norberg MM, Krystal JH, Tolin DF. 2008. A meta-analysis of D-cycloserine and the facilitation of fear extinction and exposure therapy. *Biol Psychiatry* **63**:1118–1126.

Norton PJ, Price EC. 2007. A meta-analytic review of adult cognitive-behavioral treatment outcome across the anxiety disorders. *J Nerv Ment Dis* **195**:521–531.

Otto M. 2002. Learning and "unlearning" fears: preparedness, neural pathways, and patients. *Biol Psychiatry* **52**:917–920.

Otto MW, Basden SL, McHugh RK et al. 2009. Effects of D-cycloserine administration on weekly nonemotional memory tasks in healthy participants. *Psychother Psychosom* **78**:49–54.

Parent MB, McGaugh JL. 1994. Posttraining infusion of lidocaine into the amygdala basolateral complex impairs retention of inhibitory avoidance training. *Brain Res* **661**:97–103.

Pitman RK, Delahanty DL. 2005. Conceptually driven pharmacologic approaches to acute trauma. *CNS Spectr* **10**:99–106.

Pitman RK, Sanders KM, Zusman RM et al. 2002. Pilot study of secondary prevention of posttraumatic stress disorder with propranolol. *Biol Psychiatry* **51**:189–192.

Przybyslawski J, Roullet P, Sara SJ. 1999. Attenuation of emotional and nonemotional memories after their reactivation: role of beta adrenergic receptors. *J Neurosci* **19**:6623–6628.

Przybyslawski J, Sara SJ. 1997. Reconsolidation of memory after its reactivation. *Behav Brain Res* **84**:241–246.

Quirarte GL, Roozendaal B, McGaugh JL. 1997. Glucocorticoid enhancement of memory storage involves noradrenergic activation in the basolateral amygdala. *Proc Nat Acad Sci USA* **94**:14048–14053.

Ressler KJ, Rothbaum BO, Tannenbaum L et al. 2004. Cognitive enhancers as adjuncts to psychotherapy: use of D-cycloserine in phobic individuals to facilitate extinction of fear. *Arch Gen Psychiatry* **61**:1136–1144.

Roberts NP, Kitchiner NJ, Kenardy J, Bisson JI. 2009. Systematic review and meta-analysis of multiple-session early interventions following traumatic events. *Am J Psychiatry* **166**:293–301.

Rodrigues SM, LeDoux JE, Sapolsky RM. 2009. The influence of stress hormones on fear circuitry. *Annu Rev Neurosci* **32**:289–313.

Rodrigues SM, Schafe GE, LeDoux JE. 2004. Molecular mechanisms underlying emotional learning and memory in the lateral amygdala. *Neuron* **44**:75–91.

Roozendaal B, McGaugh JL. 1997. Basolateral amygdala lesions block the memory-enhancing effect of glucocorticoid administration in the dorsal hippocampus of rats. *Eur J Neurosci* **9**:76–83.

Rothbaum BO. 2008. Critical parameters for D-cycloserine enhancement of cognitive behavioral therapy for obsessive-compulsive disorder. *Am J Psychiatry* **165**:293–296.

Rothbaum BO, Davis M. 2003. Applying learning principles to the treatment of post-trauma reactions. *Ann N Y Acad Sci* **1008**:112–121.

Rothbaum BO, Hodges L, Kooper R. 1997. Virtual reality exposure therapy. *J Psychother Pract Res* **6**:219–226.

Rothbaum BO, Hodges L, Smith S, Lee JH, Price L. 2000. A controlled study of virtual reality exposure therapy for the fear of flying. *J Consult Clin Psychol* **68**: 1020–1026.

Rothbaum BO, Schwartz AC. 2002. Exposure therapy for posttraumatic stress disorder. *Am J Psychotherapy* **56**:59–75.

Roullet P, Sara S. 1998. Consolidation of memory after its reactivation: involvement of beta noradrenergic receptors in the late phase. *Neural Plast* **6**:63–68.

Schelling G, Briegel J, Roozendaal B et al. 2001. The effect of stress doses of hydrocortisone during septic shock on posttraumatic stress disorder in survivors. *Biol Psychiatry* **50**:978–985.

Schelling G, Kilger E, Roozendaal B et al. 2004. Stress doses of hydrocortisone, traumatic memories, and symptoms of posttraumatic stress disorder in patients after cardiac surgery: a randomized study. *Biol Psychiatry* **55**:627–633.

Schelling G, Roozendaal B, Krauseneck T et al. 2006. Efficacy of hydrocortisone in preventing posttraumatic stress disorder following critical illness and major surgery. *Ann N Y Acad Sci* **1071**: 46–53.

Schelling G, Stoll C, Kapfhammer HP et al. 1999. The effect of stress doses of hydrocortisone during septic shock on posttraumatic stress disorder and health-related quality of life in survivors. *Crit Care Med* **27**:2678–2683.

Sehlmeyer C, Schoning S, Zwitserlood P et al. 2009. Human fear conditioning and extinction in neuroimaging: a systematic review. *PloS One* **4**: **e5865**.

Shimizu E, Tang YP, Rampon C, Tsien JZ. 2000. NMDA receptor-dependent synaptic reinforcement as a crucial process for memory consolidation. *Science* **290**: 1170–1174.

Soravia LM, Heinrichs M, Aerni A et al. 2006. Glucocorticoids reduce phobic fear in humans. *Proc Nat Acad Sci USA* **103**:5585–5590.

Stein MB, Kerridge C, Dimsdale JE, Hoyt DB. 2007. Pharmacotherapy to prevent PTSD: results from a randomized controlled proof-of-concept trial in physically injured patients. *J Trauma Stress* **20**:923–932.

Storch EA, Merlo LJ, Bengtson M et al. 2007. D-cycloserine does not enhance exposure-response prevention therapy in obsessive-compulsive disorder. *Int Clin Psychopharmacol* **22**:230–237.

Taylor F, Cahill L. 2002. Propranolol for reemergent posttraumatic stress disorder following an event of retraumatization: a case study. *J Trauma Stress* **15**: 433–437.

Tollenaar MS, Elzinga BM, Spinhoven P, Everaerd W. 2009. Psychophysiological responding to emotional memories in healthy young men after cortisol and propranolol administration. *Psychopharmacology (Berl)* **203**:793–803.

Vaiva G, Ducrocq F, Jezequel K et al. 2003. Immediate treatment with propranolol decreases posttraumatic stress disorder two months after trauma. *Biol Psychiatry* **54**:947–949.

Vazdarjanova A, McGaugh J. 1999. Basolateral amygdala is involved in modulating consolidation of memory for classical fear conditioning. *J Neurosci* **19**:6615–6622.

Vervliet B. 2008. Learning and memory in conditioned fear extinction: effects of D-cycloserine. *Acta Psychol (Amst)* **127**:601–613.

Wallach HS, Safir MP, Bar-Zvi M. 2009. Virtual reality cognitive behavior therapy for public speaking anxiety: a randomized clinical trial. *Behav Modif* **33**:314–338.

Watson GB, Bolanowski MA, Baganoff MP, Deppeler CL, Lanthorn TH. 1990. D-cycloserine acts as a partial agonist at the glycine modulatory site of the NMDA receptor expressed in *Xenopus* oocytes. *Brain Res* **510**:158–160.

Weis F, Kilger E, Roozendaal B et al. 2006. Stress doses of hydrocortisone reduce chronic stress symptoms and improve health-related quality of life in high-risk patients after cardiac surgery: a randomized study. *J Thorac Cardiovasc Surg* **131**:277–282.

Wilhelm S, Buhlmann U, Tolin DF et al. 2008. Augmentation of behavior therapy with D-cycloserine for obsessive-compulsive disorder. *Am J Psychiatry* **165**:335–341, quiz 409.

Yehuda R. 2001. Biology of posttraumatic stress disorder. *J Clin Psychiatry* **62**:41–46.

Yehuda R, Golier JA, Yang RK, Tischler L. 2004. Enhanced sensitivity to glucocorticoids in peripheral mononuclear leukocytes in posttraumatic stress disorder. *Biol Psychiatry* **55**:1110–1116.

Yehuda R, Kahana B, Binder-Brynes K et al. 1995. Low urinary cortisol excretion in Holocaust survivors with posttraumatic stress disorder. *Am J Psychiatry* **152**:982–986.

Chapter 3

Mood disorders

Jorge A. Quiroz, Guang Chen, Wayne C. Drevets, Ioline D. Henter, and Husseini K. Manji

Mood disorders – in particular major depressive disorder (MDD) and bipolar disorder (BPD) – are common, chronic, recurrent mental illnesses that affect the lives and functioning of millions of individuals worldwide and are a major public health concern. Indeed, the World Health Organization's (WHO) Global Burden of Disease projects that mood disorders will be the leading cause of disability worldwide within the next decade (Murray and Lopez 1996). A growing number of recent studies indicate that outcome is poor for many individuals with mood disorders. The illnesses are characterized by high rates of relapse, chronicity, lingering residual symptoms, subsyndromes, cognitive and functional impairment, psychosocial disability, and diminished well-being.

Furthermore, available therapeutic options for the treatment of mood disorders are often insufficient for effectively managing the acute episodes, relapses, cyclicity, and recurrences that are the hallmarks of these disorders or for restoring premorbid functioning (Insel and Scolnick 2006; Machado-Vieira et al. 2008). A sizeable proportion of patients fail to respond to or tolerate currently available treatments; indeed, it is particularly sobering to note that, with the exception of lithium, all available Food and Drug Administration (FDA)-approved treatments for BPD are either anticonvulsant or antipsychotic drugs originally developed to treat other conditions (Zarate and Manji 2008). In psychiatry, there is wide consensus that better treatments for mood disorders are urgently needed. "Better treatments" essentially means treatments that are more effective for more patients, that act faster, and that have fewer side effects. The inordinately high personal, familial, societal, and financial burden of these disorders underscores the urgent need to develop novel drugs to treat them.

Mood disorders are, obviously, extraordinarily complex diseases. Previously, neurobiological studies of mood disorders focused primarily on abnormalities of the monoaminergic neurotransmitter systems, on characterizing alterations of individual neurotransmitters in disease states, and on assessing response to mood stabilizer and antidepressant medications. The monoaminergic neuronal systems project extensively throughout the network of limbic, striatal, and prefrontal cortical neuronal circuits thought to support the behavioral and visceral manifestations of mood disorders (Drevets 2000). Studies of cerebrospinal fluid (CSF) chemistry, neuroendocrine responses to pharmacological challenge, and neuroreceptor and transporter binding sites have demonstrated a number of abnormalities in monoaminergic neurotransmitter and neuropeptide systems in mood disorders (Goodwin and Jamison 2007). Unfortunately, these observations did not greatly advance our understanding of the underlying biology of recurrent mood disorders, which must be able to explain the episodic and often profound mood disturbances that can become progressive over time. Severe mood disorders likely arise from the complex interaction of multiple susceptibility (and protective) genes and environmental factors. The phenotypic expression of the disorder includes not only mood disturbance but also a constellation of cognitive, motor, autonomic, endocrine, and sleep/wake abnormalities.

The last decade has been a truly remarkable one for biomedical research. The "molecular medicine revolution" has brought to bear the power of sophisticated cellular and molecular biological methods to tackle many of society's most devastating illnesses. Psychiatry, like much of the rest of medicine, has entered a new and exciting age characterized by current rapid advances and the future promise of genetics,

---

Translational Neuroscience, ed. James E. Barrett, Joseph T. Coyle and Michael Williams. Published by Cambridge University Press. © Cambridge University Press 2012.

molecular and cellular biology, and improving technologies. Whereas knowledge of the full human genetic sequence was a major step forward, many other advances of significant importance have aided our efforts to elucidate the pathophysiology of severe psychiatric illnesses. The development of a multitude of new methods for brain imaging, genetic and genomic analyses, molecular engineering of mutant animals, novel routes for drug delivery, and sophisticated cross-species behavioral assessments makes it possible to study psychiatric and neurological diseases and disorders at the physiological level. Thus, recent years have witnessed a more wide-ranging understanding of the neural circuits and the various mechanisms of synaptic and neural plasticity, the molecular mechanisms of receptor and post-receptor signaling, a finer understanding of the process by which genes code for specific functional proteins, and the identification of potential susceptibility and protective genes in many neuropsychiatric disorders that, in toto, reduce the complexity in gene-to-behavior pathways.

Our goals are twofold. First, we describe the recently identified molecular, cellular, and brain circuits thought to be responsible for the phenotypic behaviors that characterize mood disorders. It is becoming increasingly clear that these neurochemical and structurally related abnormalities are closely associated with abnormalities in cellular plasticity. We present these findings as well as the accompanying hypotheses that have markedly influenced the field. In all cases, we first present preclinical evidence and, whenever possible, discuss data from relevant clinical studies. Our second goal is to provide a thorough overview of the most recent neuroimaging findings in mood disorders, highlighting how the extant data implicate a network formed by the medial prefrontal cortex (PFC) and anatomically related areas of the striatum, thalamus, anterior temporal cortex, hippocampus, amygdala, hypothalamus, and brain stem in the pathophysiology of mood disorders. It is our hope that this chapter will provide readers with a way to make sense of the many novel findings presented, to extract integrated themes, and to draw insight from the data.

Novel leads from preclinical and clinical studies

It is clear that genetic factors play a major role in the etiology of mood disorders. Indeed, the strong familiality and heritability of mood disorders have long been some of the best clues to their etiology. However, although it is clear that we are on the verge of truly identifying susceptibility (and likely protective) genes for these disorders, it is also clear that there is no one-to-one relationship between genes and behavior, so that different combinations of genes – and the resultant changes in neurobiological expression – contribute to complex behaviors (normal or abnormal) (Hasler *et al.* 2006). It is also critically important to remember that gene polymorphisms are likely simply *associated* with mood disorders; that is, such genes are more likely to lend a higher probability for the subsequent development of mood disorders than invariably determine outcome. Obviously, genes never code for abnormal behaviors per se but rather code for proteins that make up cells, thereby forming circuits that in combination affect facets of both abnormal and normal behavior. These expanding and interconnected levels of interaction have, in part, made the study of psychiatric diseases so difficult. The next task of psychiatric genetic research is to study how and why variations in these genes impart a greater probability of developing mood disorders and then to direct therapeutic agents at the pathophysiological alterations (Gould and Manji 2004).

We are not yet at a point where we can focus on susceptibility genes to guide us in our search to fully elucidate the pathophysiology of these illnesses. Thus, our field has had to rely on more indirect strategies. As noted above, the monoaminergic neurotransmitter systems have heretofore received the greatest attention in neurobiological studies of these illnesses. Clinical studies over the past 40 years have attempted to uncover the biological factors mediating the pathophysiology of mood disorders using a variety of biochemical and neuroendocrine strategies. Assessments of CSF chemistry, neuroendocrine responses to pharmacological challenge, and neuroreceptor and transporter binding have, in fact, demonstrated a number of abnormalities of the serotonergic, noradrenergic, and other neurotransmitter and neuropeptide systems in mood disorders. It is also important to note that, whereas most antidepressants exert their initial effects by increasing the intrasynaptic levels of serotonin and/or norepinephrine, their clinical antidepressant effects are only observed after chronic (days to weeks) administration, suggesting that a cascade of downstream events is ultimately responsible for their therapeutic effects. These observations have led to the sense that, although dysfunction within the monoaminergic neurotransmitter systems is likely key to mediating some facets of the pathophysiology of mood disorders, such dysfunction likely represents the downstream effects of other, more primary abnormalities (Manji and Lenox 2000).

Despite these formidable obstacles, considerable progress has been made in our understanding of the underlying molecular and cellular basis of mood disorders in recent years. In particular, recent evidence demonstrates that impaired signaling pathways may play a role in the pathophysiology of mood disorders and that antidepressants and mood stabilizers exert major effects on signaling pathways that regulate synaptic and neural plasticity. These data have generated considerable excitement in the clinical neuroscience community and are reshaping views about the neurobiological underpinnings of these disorders (Duman 2002; Manji *et al.* 2001*b*; Nestler *et al.* 2002).

It is our contention that mood disorders arise from abnormalities in cellular plasticity, leading to aberrant information processing in synapses and circuits mediating affective, cognitive, motor, and neurovegetative function. Cellular signaling cascades form complex networks that allow the cell to receive, process, and respond to information (Bhalla and Iyengar 1999; Bourne and Nicoll 1993). These intracellular networks facilitate the integration of signals across multiple time scales and the generation of distinct outputs depending on input strength and duration, and regulate intricate feed-forward and feedback loops (Weng *et al.* 1999). These signaling cascades play a critical role as molecular switches subserving acute and long-term alterations in neuronal information processing. It is also becoming clear that observed neurochemical and structurally related abnormalities in mood disorders are closely associated with abnormalities in cellular plasticity, including the ability of neuronal and glial cells to resist or adapt to environmental stressors (cellular resilience), the ability of these cells to undergo remodeling of synaptic connections (synaptic plasticity), and their ability to undergo cell regeneration (neurogenesis) (Quiroz and Post 2009) (Fig. 3.1).

Translational research is essential for elucidating the neurobiology of mood disorders as well as for developing biomarkers and novel therapeutics to prevent mood disorders and rapidly relieve symptoms (Coyle and Duman 2003; Krishnan and Nestler 2008; Manji *et al.* 2001*a*). Indeed, preclinical translational studies have discovered a variety of molecular and cellular actions for antidepressants, electroconvulsive therapy (ECT), and the rapid-acting N-methyl-D-aspartate (NMDA) antagonist ketamine in brain regions involved in mood regulation. Some of these have been further evaluated at the behavioral level. The alterations induced by early life events, chronic unpredictable stress, and social defeat have also been studied in animal models, as have the effects of antidepressant treatments on some of these measures. The findings suggest intriguing leads for developing novel therapeutics and biomarkers for mood disorders.

We discuss some of these findings as well as the hypotheses that have markedly influenced the field. We begin by presenting preclinical evidence and, whenever possible, review data pertaining to relevant clinical studies.

Molecular targets of existing antidepressants and mood stabilizers: beyond the monoamine systems

The cyclic adenosine monophosphate pathway

Currently available antidepressants increase norepinephrine and serotonin levels in the synaptic cleft, which in turn stimulate G-protein-coupled receptors (Tanis and Duman 2007). Activation of Gs (stimulatory G-protein-coupled receptors) such as $5HT_{4,6,7}$ and beta adrenergic receptors increases adenylyl cyclase (AC) activity (Tanis and Duman 2007). AC converts adenosine triphosphate (ATP) to cAMP, a second messenger that in turn activates protein kinase A (PKA) (Cooper 2003; Pierre *et al.* 2009; Tanis and Duman 2007). PKA phosphorylates and alters the function of a variety of proteins including cAMP response element binding protein (CREB), a transcription factor (Cooper 2003; Pierre *et al.* 2009; Tanis and Duman 2007). cAMP accumulation can also result from activation of Gq/G11 coupled receptors such as $5HT_{1,5}$ and alpha-1 adrenergic receptors. This activation leads to increased phospholipase C activity, which hydrolyzes phosphatidylinositol 4,5-bisphosphate (PIP2) to inositol trisphosphate (IP3) together with diacylglycerol (DAG). IP3 triggers calcium release in the endoplasmic reticulum (ER) and calcium-enhanced calcium-dependent ACs (Cooper 2003; Pierre *et al.* 2009; Tanis and Duman 2007). AC subtypes can also be activated by the Gbg complex (Cooper 2003; Pierre *et al.* 2009; Tanis and Duman 2007).

In vivo activation of the cAMP pathway by antidepressants is largely supported by findings showing

Chapter 3: Mood disorders

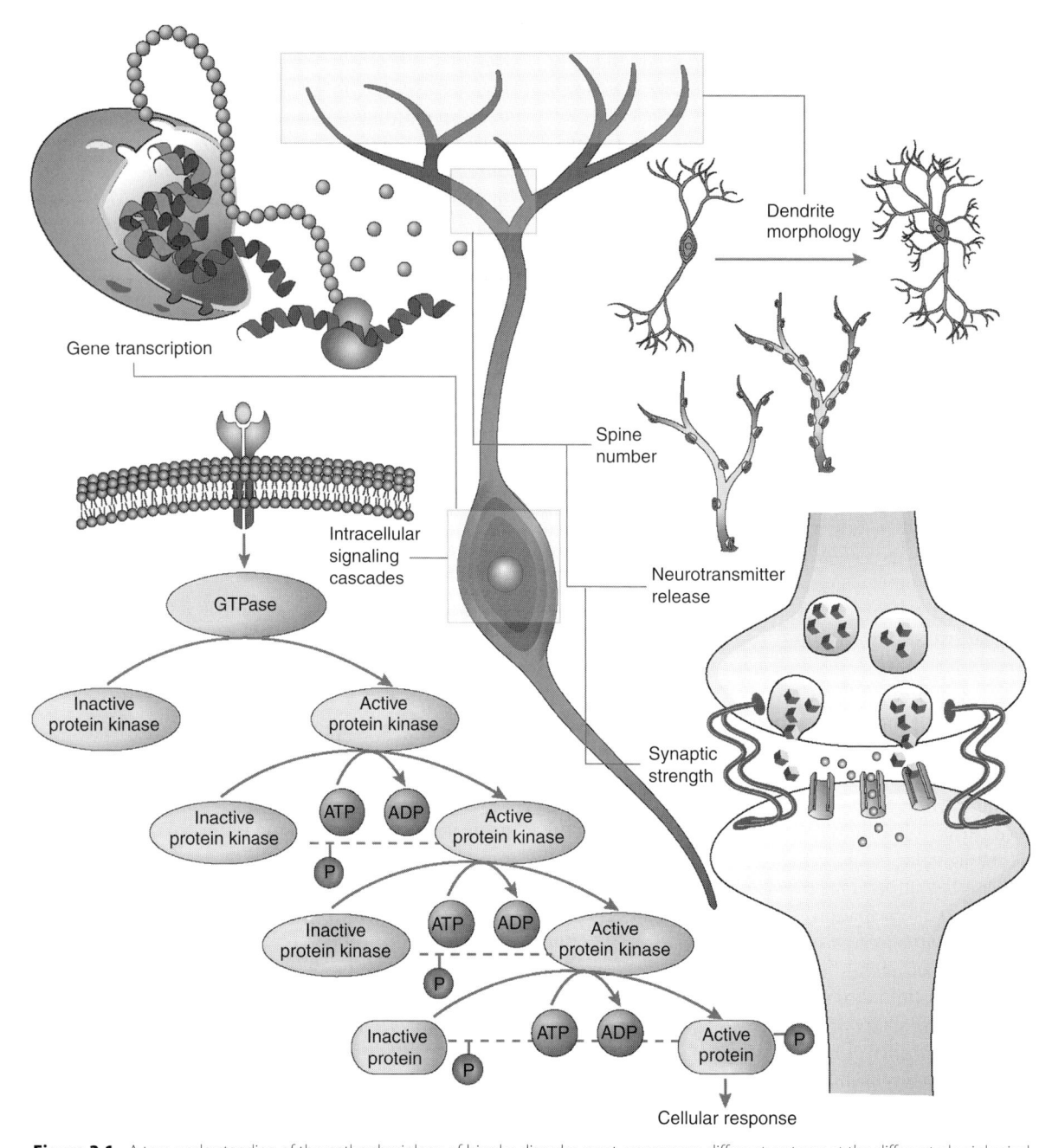

Figure 3.1. A true understanding of the pathophysiology of bipolar disorder must encompass different systems at the different physiological levels at which the disease manifests itself: molecular, cellular, and behavioral. Reprinted with permission from *Neuropsychopharmacology*, Vol. 33, Schloesser RJ, Huang J, Klein PS, Manji HK. Cellular plasticity cascades in the pathophysiology and treatment of bipolar disorder, pp. 110–133, copyright 2008. This figure is reproduced in color in the color plate section.

that antidepressant treatment increased protein phosphorylation at the PKA site and altered the function of these proteins. PKA is known to phosphorylate CREB, thus enhancing its transcriptional activity (Cooper 2003; Pierre *et al*. 2009; Tanis and Duman 2007). Acute and chronic treatment with fluoxetine increased the phosphorylation of DARPP-32 (dopamine- and cAMP-regulated phosphoprotein of M(r) 32,000) at serine 137, a PKA site (Svenningsson *et al*. 2002). Interestingly, antidepressant treatment also increased phosphorylation of alpha-amino-3-hydroxy-5-methyl-4-isoxazolepropionic acid (AMPA) receptor subunit GluR1, also at a PKA site (Svenningsson et al. 2002). Furthermore, GluR1 phosphorylation increased after treatment with imipramine, lamotrigine, riluzole, and tianeptine (Du et al. 2004, 2007; Svenningsson et al. 2007). A variety of kinases, including PKA, were found to phosphorylate glycogen synthase kinase 3 (GSK-3) alpha at ser-21 and GSK-3 beta at ser-9. Notably, this phosphorylation inactivated GSK-3 (Gould et al. 2007; Jope and Roh 2006), and studies have shown that imipramine, fluoxetine, atypical antipsychotics, and a combination of these treatments all increased GSK-3 phosphorylation at these sites (Li et al. 2007; Roh et al. 2005). In addition, treatment with a variety of antidepressants and with ECT increased CREB phosphorylation and CREB-mediated reporter gene expression in a region-specific manner (Nibuya et al. 1996; Thome et al. 2000). Several genes are known to be regulated by CREB and upregulated by antidepressant treatment and ECT, including brain-derived neurotrophic factor (BDNF), B-cell lymphoma 2 (Bcl-2), and cocaine- and amphetamine-regulated transcript (CART) (Duman 2009; Hunsberger et al. 2009b; Roh et al. 2009).

The forced swim and tail suspension tests are two common animal models of depression; reduced immobility in these tests is typically seen in response to a variety of antidepressants, as well as the NMDA antagonist ketamine and some mood stabilizers (Chen et al. 2010a). Forskolin, a known AC activator, as well as its derivative, reduced immobility in the forced swim test without locomotor activation (Maeda et al. 1997). This finding suggests that AC stimulation produced antidepressant-like effects. Ten AC subtypes have been identified (Cooper 2003; Pierre et al. 2009), and genetically mutant AC1, AC5, AC7, and AC8 mice have been studied in behavioral tests related to anxiety and depression. Male AC5 knockout (KO) mice were found to be hyperactive in the open field test, were less anxious-like in the elevated plus maze and light–dark tests, showed less immobility in the forced swim test, and spent less time with wild-type mice in two social interaction tests (Krishnan et al. 2008); the overall outcome was opposite to the hypothesis that stimulating AC5 would produce antidepressant-like effects. Female, but not male, AC7 heterozygous KO mice showed increased immobility in the forced swim and tail suspension tests (Hines et al. 2006). Male and female AC1/8 double KO (DKO) mice were hypoactive in the open field test, had reduced liquid consumption and sucrose preference in the sucrose preference test, and spent more time with wild-type mice in two social interaction tests (Krishnan et al. 2008). Male, but not female, AC1/8 DKO mice showed reduced immobility in the forced swim test (Krishnan et al. 2008). Taken together, it appears that with regard to regulating behaviors related to depression, the role of any particular AC, as well as its interaction with other factors such as gender and development, is complex. Further elucidation is needed before ACs can be selectively targeted as putative therapeutics for the treatment of mood disorders.

Few studies have investigated the behavioral effects of direct PKA stimulation. One brief report (Branski et al. 2008) noted that intracerebroventricular (ICV) injection of 8-bromo-cyclic adenosine monophosphate (8-Br-cAMP) and imipramine reduced immobility in the forced swim test. The effect of this membrane-permeable PKA activator could be blocked by Rp-cAMPS (Rp-adenosine 3' 5'cyclic monophosphorothioate), a PKA inhibitor. As noted previously, several animal models exist in which repeated or chronic, but not acute, treatment with antidepressants produces behavioral effects on measures related to the symptoms of depression. These models include the learned helplessness, chronic mild or unpredictable stress, and social defeat paradigms (Krishnan and Nestler 2008). It remains to be elucidated whether direct PKA activation can produce antidepressant-like effects in such paradigms.

Phosphodiesterase (PDE) breaks the phosphodiester bonds of cAMP and cyclic guanosine monophosphate (cGMP), and converts them to AMP and GMP (Zhang 2009). It has been proposed that PDE inhibition may in fact have antidepressant effects; the initial test of this hypothesis was conducted over half a century ago by Helmut Wachtel (Zhang 2009). Preclinical studies found that chronic administration of the PDE4 inhibitor rolipram had antidepressant-like behavioral effects on differential-reinforcement of low rate (DRL) behavior and in the forced swim test (O'Donnell and Frith 1999). Approximately 25 different variants of PDE4 exist, resulting from different splicing of four PDE4 genes (PDE4A-D) (Zhang 2009). Both PDE4B and PDE4D KO strains displayed reduced immobility in the forced swim test; the PDE4D KO strain also showed reduced immobility in the tail suspension test (Siuciak et al. 2008; Zhang et al. 2002, 2008). Despite their possible usefulness, the development of PDE4 inhibitors as antidepressants is further complicated by the fact that antidepressants increase the levels of some isoforms of PDE4; sleep deprivation also increases hippocampal PDE activity and PDE4A5 protein levels in rodents (Nibuya et al. 1996; Takahashi et al. 1999).

In humans, the putative antidepressant effects of PDE4 inhibitors were tested in both open (Zeller et al. 1984) and controlled clinical trials (Bertolino et al. 1988; Bobon et al. 1988; Fleischhacker et al. 1992; Hebenstreit et al. 1989), where they demonstrated antidepressant-like effects. Rolipram has shown some antidepressant efficacy in depressed patients (Hebenstreit et al. 1989; Scott et al. 1991), but its use has been limited due to its associated side effects of nausea and emesis. Since the publication of these clinical studies, no new evidence of the antidepressant effects of rolipram or other PDE inhibitors has been demonstrated. Only one clinical neuroimaging positron emission tomography (PET) study is currently ongoing using 11-C rolipram; to clarify the role of selective serotonin reuptake inhibitors (SSRIs) on PDE4 levels in patients with MDD (http://www.clinicaltrials.gov/ct2/show/NCT00369798?term=depression+PDE&rank=1).

Transcription factors: CREB and DeltaFosB

Treatment with different classes of antidepressants as well as ECT has been found to increase CREB mRNA and transcriptional targets of CREB and BDNF in selected brain regions (Nibuya et al. 1996; Shirayama et al. 2002; Thome et al. 2000); antidepressant treatment was subsequently found to increase temporal cortical CREB levels in the temporal cortex in patients with MDD (Dowlatshahi et al. 1998). The mood stabilizers lithium and valproate (VPA) increased CREB phosphorylation as well as BDNF and Bcl-2 expression in the frontal cortex and hippocampus (Einat et al. 2003), and the effects of these agents on CREB were found to be involved in upregulating Bcl-2 expression (Creson et al. 2009). Additional studies found that treatment with antidepressants increased CREB function and that local expression of CREB in the hippocampus produced antidepressant-like effects in the learned helplessness paradigm and forced swim test (Shirayama et al. 2002). These data are consistent with recent data showing that Bcl-2 and its family proteins modulate outcome in the same behavioral models (Maeng et al. 2008a).

However, it appears that CREB plays opposing roles in mediating outcome in various behavioral paradigms in a manipulation-specific manner that is also temporal- and brain region-dependent. Local expression of CREB in the nucleus accumbens (NAc) worsens escape deficits and, conversely, local expression of mutant CREB produces antidepressant-like effects (Newton et al. 2002). In addition, local expression of CREB in the basolateral amygdala before the inescapable shock paradigm also worsened escape deficits; however, local CREB expression after inescapable shock improved them (Wallace et al. 2004). Lastly, the social defeat and social isolation paradigms produced opposing phospho-CREB binding patterns in the NAc (Wallace et al. 2009). Thus, it appears that the best method for targeting CREB in a controlled, brain region-specific manner requires further research.

The transcription factor Delta FosB is a truncated splice variant of FosB (unlike the full length FosB protein), resulting in unusual stability and the accumulation of this transcription factor following repeated stimulation (Nestler et al. 1999). Chronic treatment with cocaine, amphetamine, antidepressants, antipsychotics, and ECT increased expression of DeltaFosB in specific brain regions (Chen et al. 1995, 1997; Hope et al. 1992, 1994; Nye and Nestler 1996). Notably, one documented effect of Delta FosB upregulation is increased levels of the NMDA receptor 1 (NMDAR1) glutamate receptor subunit NR1 in the frontal cortex after ECT (Hiroi et al. 1998). In rodents, Delta FosB overexpression in the NAc increases daily wheel running (a natural reward for rodents) (Werme et al. 2002). Long-term overexpression of Delta FosB in the brain increased the rewarding effects of cocaine (McClung and Nestler 2003). In addition, local overexpression of Delta FosB in the NAc enhanced the rewarding effects of morphine (Zachariou et al. 2006), facilitated food-reinforced instrumental performance and progressive ratio responding (Olausson et al. 2006), increased sucrose intake (Wallace et al. 2008), and promoted some sexual behaviors (Wallace et al. 2008). These data demonstrate that Delta FosB positively mediates natural and drug-associated reward mechanisms in rodents.

In the learned helplessness paradigm, some animals that receive inescapable food shocks develop escape deficits (Chen et al. 1997), and these increase Delta FosB expression in the ventrolateral periaqueductal gray

(PAG) (Berton et al. 2007). Interestingly, the strongest Delta FosB inductions were observed in animals that did not develop escape deficits. Local overexpression of Delta FosB in the ventrolateral PAG further reduced the escape deficits and inhibited the shock-induced release of substance P, whereas over-expression also reduced immobility in the forced swim test. These data show that Delta FosB is a positive modulator of the stress coping response (Berton et al. 2007). Overall, given its role in reward and stress coping, Delta FosB can be considered a potential target for developing novel antidepressants.

Protein kinase C inhibition in mania

Protein kinase C (PKC), a family of enzymes involved in the regulation of intracellular signaling regulation, plays an important role in the modulation of pre- and postsynaptic neurotransmission, including the regulation of neuronal excitability, synaptic plasticity, neurotransmitter release, and various forms of learning and memory. As occurs with other intraneuronal signaling pathways, several neurotransmitters may induce PKC activity. Changes in PKC signaling after treatment with lithium and VPA have been studied extensively (Chen et al. 1994; Friedman et al. 1993; Hahn and Friedman 1999; Manji et al. 1993; Manji and Lenox 1999; Young et al. 1999), and significant decreases have been noted in the membrane-associated PKC isozymes alpha and epsilon in brain regions of interest.

Tamoxifen, a relatively selective PKC inhibitor that crosses the blood–brain barrier, is available for human use. Based on the hypothesis that PKC inhibition may be relevant to the treatment of manic episodes, a single-blind clinical study conducted a decade ago confirmed that tamoxifen significantly decreased manic symptoms within a short period of time (3–7 days) in a small cohort of patients (Bebchuk et al. 2000). Two subsequent, double-blind, placebo-controlled studies recently confirmed those preliminary findings (Yildiz et al. 2008; Zarate et al. 2007), as did a third pilot study of hormone modulation in a subgroup of women with hypomanic and manic symptoms (Kulkarni et al. 2006). In the first study, 16 acutely manic or mixed patients with BPD, with or without psychotic features, received oral tamoxifen or placebo for 3 weeks. Tamoxifen was associated with significant antimanic effects, with efficacy observable as early as day 5 of treatment; response rates were 63% for tamoxifen and 13% for placebo (Zarate et al. 2007). Similar results were obtained from a larger study looking at 66 patients with mania (Yildiz et al. 2008). The antimanic effects of tamoxifen were not due to sedation, and no increased risk of depression was observed. Other studies have also confirmed the relevance of PKC inhibition in antimanic agents (Kulkarni et al. 2006). *In toto*, the evidence demonstrates that PKC inhibition is an effective and viable target for developing new antimanic agents to treat BPD.

Growth factors and neurotrophins

BDNF is a key neurotrophin involved in synaptic plasticity (Martinowich et al. 2007), particularly neuronal survival, neurogenesis, neuronal growth processes, and synaptogenesis in the central nervous system (CNS) and peripheral nervous system (Hunsberger et al. 2009b). BDNF has a high affinity for the tyrosine kinase B (TrkB) receptor (Martinowich et al. 2007) and binds to p75 (also known as low affinity nerve growth factor receptor or LNGFR) (Martinowich et al. 2007). Furthermore, genetic variants of BDNF have been linked to increased risk for schizophrenia and mood disorders (Martinowich et al. 2007).

Notably, chronic treatment with a variety of antidepressants and ECT was found to increase BDNF expression (Duman 2009; Hunsberger et al. 2009b; Nibuya et al. 1995, 1996), and chronic treatment with mood stabilizers similarly increased BDNF expression (Einat et al. 2003; Fukumoto et al. 2001; Hunsberger et al. 2009b). Several studies also found that behavioral stress lowered brain BDNF levels; for instance, social defeat stress suppressed BDNF III and IV transcript expression through epigenetic mechanisms (Tsankova et al. 2006). Imipramine treatment upregulated BDNF expression and increased histone acetylation within its promoter regions (Tsankova et al. 2006).

Results from a recent meta-analysis of human plasma BDNF levels were consistent with the notion that BDNF is reduced in individuals with depression (Sen et al. 2008). An elegant preclinical study further demonstrated that direct infusion of BDNF, but not nerve growth factor (NGF), into the dentate gyrus (DG) of the hippocampus produced antidepressant-like effects in the forced swim test and learned helplessness paradigms (Shirayama et al. 2002). Midbrain infusion of BDNF also appeared to prevent the development of escape deficits in the learned helplessness paradigm and reduced immobility in the forced swim test (Siuciak *et al.* 1997). Preliminary data further suggest that peripheral BDNF administration produced antidepressant-like effects in the forced swim test, the chronic unpredictable stress paradigm, and the novelty-induced hypophagia test of anxiety (Schmidt and Duman 2008).

As the evidence reviewed above suggests, BDNF is a promising target for the development of therapeutic agents to treat mood disorders; however, several issues require further consideration. For instance, sustained application of BDNF downregulates TrkB levels in cultured hippocampal neurons and brain regions around the infusion site (Frank *et al.* 1996, 1997). Studies also found that the behavioral regulatory role of BDNF is temporal- and brain region-specific; BDNF infusion into the ventral tegmental area (VTA) reduced latency to immobility in the forced swim test, an effect opposite to that seen with antidepressants (Eisch *et al.* 2003); and expression of a dominant-negative TrkB in the NAc produced antidepressant-like effects in the forced swim test (Eisch *et al.* 2003). Investigators created forebrain-inducible BDNF KO mice and found that early deletion of BDNF caused hyperactivity and impaired cue- and context-dependent conditioning in the fear conditioning paradigms (Monteggia *et al.* 2004); BDNF deletion in adults caused context-dependent fear conditioning. Interestingly, the deletion did not alter immobility in the forced swim test; however, the effects of desipramine on immobility were no longer significant in the KO mice. Other investigators found that BDNF over-expression in the forebrain caused anxiogenic-like effects, likely mediated through amygdalar spinogenesis, although the over-expressing mice displayed reduced immobility in the forced swim test (Govindarajan *et al.* 2006). Finally, it should be noted that the potential behavioral toxicity of brain regional BDNF overactivation requires further investigation.

From a clinical standpoint, only one experimental study was conducted in patients with amyotrophic lateral sclerosis (ALS) in an attempt to directly increase BDNF brain availability by intrathecal infusion (Ochs *et al.* 2000). This clinical study used recombinant methionyl human BDNF (mBDNF). Many side effects were noted, including sensory symptoms, paresthesias or a sense of warmth, sleep disturbance, dry mouth, agitation, and other behavioral effects. Although apparently well tolerated, the treatment was not effective, and no further studies have been reported. Current efforts are now focusing on pharmacological methods to increase BDNF expression due to the mounting evidence (described above) that neuroplasticity plays a major role in the pathophysiology of mood disorders.

With regard to other neurotrophins, studies using the gene expression profiling approach demonstrated that repeated ECT increased vascular endothelial growth factor (VEGF), VGF (non-acronymic), and neuritin expression as well as BDNF in the hippocampus (Newton *et al.* 2003). VEGF is a trophic factor that stimulates the growth of new blood vessels. VEGF binds to its receptors, which are also tyrosine kinase receptors, and induces receptor dimerization, transphosphorylation, and activation. A follow-up study showed that ECT, as well as fluoxetine and desipramine, upregulated VEGF protein levels in the hippocampus (Warner-Schmidt and Duman 2007). ICV infusion of VEGF reduced immobility in the forced swim test and attenuated escape deficits in the learned helplessness paradigms (Warner-Schmidt and Duman 2007). Infusion of VEGF receptor (Flk-1) inhibitor blocked the effects of antidepressants on hippocampal neurogenesis and their behavioral effects (Warner-Schmidt and Duman 2007). It is interesting to note that a preliminary study also showed that acute treatment with the NMDA receptor antagonist and antidepressant agent ketamine increased VEGF expression in the hippocampus (Li *et al.* 2009). Finally, a human genetic-imaging study revealed that two VEGF variants, single nucleotide polymorphism (SNP)-2 and SNP-3, influenced hippocampal volume in healthy individuals (Blumberg *et al.* 2008). Thus, VEGF and its signaling pathway in the hippocampus are clearly candidates for the development of novel therapeutics to treat mood disorders.

In the aforementioned gene expression profiling study, hippocampal expression of 33 genes, including VGF, was found to be altered during wheel running (Hunsberger *et al.* 2007). The VGF gene encodes a precursor protein that is cleaved to several polypeptides that play a role in energy homeostasis, metabolism, and synaptic plasticity. Both CREB activation and neurotrophins such as BDNF are known to induce VGF expression. Furthermore, microinjection of an active VGF fragment (AQEE-30 amino acids 588–617) into the lateral ventricles was found to reduce immobility in the forced swim and tail suspension tests and to reduce feeding latency in the novelty-induced hypophagia model of anxiety (Hunsberger et al. 2007). VGF KO mice showed the opposite outcome in behavioral tests (Hunsberger et al. 2007). Taken together, the data suggest that VGF may play a role in behavioral regulation related to antidepressant effects and depression. In addition to BDNF, VEGF and VGF, other trophic factors such as IGF-1 and FGF2 have also been implicated in the development of novel antidepressants (Duman 2009). Clinical evidence regarding the use of this strategy requires further development.

The Bcl-2 family proteins

Bcl-2 was the first of the antiapoptotic Bcl-2 family proteins to be discovered (Hunsberger et al. 2009b; Maeng et al. 2008a). It is expressed in the brain and modulates fundamental neural processes including neurogenesis, neuronal survival, and neuronal process growth and regeneration (Hunsberger et al. 2009b; Maeng et al. 2008a); it also regulates calcium signaling and plays a critical role in functional plasticity (Hunsberger et al. 2009b; Maeng et al. 2008a). In addition, Bcl-2 expression is involved in regulating mitochondrial function (Hunsberger et al. 2009b; Maeng et al. 2008a). The expression of the antiapoptotic Bcl-2 protein is also promoted by CREB phosphorylation, counterbalancing the potentially damaging consequences of stress-induced neuronal endangerment, particularly due to its role in regulating mitochondrial activity (Zarate et al. 2003) (Fig. 3.2).

An open-ended, genome-wide search revealed that chronic treatment with the mood stabilizers lithium and VPA upregulated Bcl-2 protein levels in various brain regions (Chen et al. 1999b). These effects were at least partly due to activation of the MAP kinase/ERK pathway by these mood stabilizers (Creson et al. 2009). Other studies have shown that antidepressant and ECT treatment also increased Bcl-2 expression (Hunsberger et al. 2009b). Interestingly, postmortem studies revealed that brain Bcl-2 levels were lower in the brains of individuals with mood disorders (Kim et al. 2010). Preclinical studies showed that Bcl-2 heterozygous mice exhibited more anxious-like behaviors during anxiety-related tests and were more prone to developing escape deficits in the learned helplessness paradigm (Chen et al. 2007). The mice also showed delayed recovery from escape deficits. Thus, Bcl-2 upregulation would have considerable utility in treating a variety of disorders associated with endogenous or acquired impairments of cellular resilience (Manji et al. 2003).

Bcl-2 associated athanogene (BAG-1) is a co-chaperone that potentiates Bcl-2 activity, modulates the function of intracellular signaling molecules, and mediates glucocorticoid receptor (GR) translocation and signaling (Maeng et al. 2008a). A microarray study demonstrated that chronic treatment with lithium and VPA upregulated BAG-1 expression and altered BAG-1 function, including GR trafficking to nuclei (Zhou et al. 2005). Mice with selective brain overexpression of BAG-1 showed less anxious-like behaviors in the elevated plus maze test and rapid spontaneous recovery from helplessness in the learned helplessness paradigm (Maeng et al. 2008a). BAG-1 heterozygous (HET) KO mice showed an increased tendency to become helpless in the learned helplessness paradigm (Maeng et al. 2008a). These data suggest that BAG-1 may regulate depressive lability and resilience.

Finally, stimulation of tumor necrosis factor (TNF) receptor-1 activates caspase-8 that, in turn, cleaves BH3 interacting domain death agonist (BID) to truncated BID (tBID), which antagonizes Bcl-2 and potentiates BAX/BAK, the proapoptotic members of the Bcl-2 family proteins. Recent preclinical studies found that a BID inhibitor reduced immobility in the forced swim and tail suspension tests and facilitated recovery from escape deficits in the learned helplessness paradigm (Malkesman et al. in press). In the absence (until recently) of a pharmacological means of increasing CNS Bcl-2 expression, all studies heretofore used transgenic mouse models or viral vector-mediated delivery of the Bcl-2 gene into the CNS. In these models, Bcl-2 overexpression prevented motor neuron death induced by facial nerve axotomy and sciatic nerve axotomy, saved retinal ganglion cells from axotomy-induced death, protected cells from the deleterious effects of MPTP or focal ischemia, and protected photoreceptor cells from two forms of inherited retinal degeneration; interestingly, neurons that survived ischemic lesions or traumatic brain injury in vivo showed upregulation of Bcl-2 (see Bonfanti et al. 1996; Chen et al. 1997; Lawrence et al. 1996; Merry and Korsmeyer 1997; Raghupathi et al. 1998; Sadoul 1998; Yang et al. 1998, and references therein).

Overexpression of Bcl-2 was also shown to prolong survival and attenuate motor neuron degeneration in a transgenic animal model of ALS (Kostic et al. 1997). Not only does Bcl-2 overexpression protect against apoptotic and necrotic cell death, it

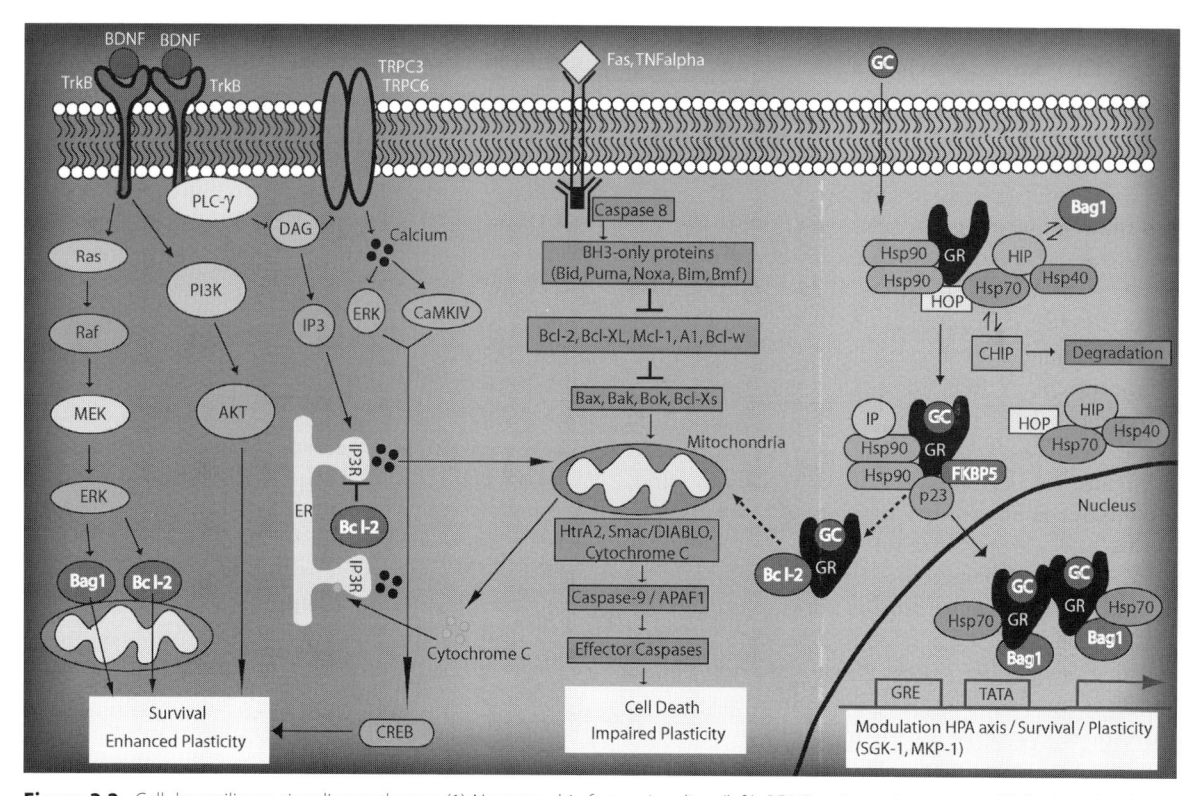

Figure 3.2. Cellular resiliency signaling pathways. (1) Neurotrophic factor signaling (left). BDNF activates its receptor, TrkB; phosphorylation can then activate either the ERK signaling cascade, PI3K, or PLC-γ. Ultimately, these independent pathways converge to enhance plasticity and cell survival. (2) Antiapoptotic signaling (center). Following activation of procaspases (e.g., caspase 8), proapoptotic factors are activated (BH3-only proteins), which in turn inhibit antiapoptotic proteins such as Bcl-2. This step enables proapoptotic members to form pores on the outer mitochondrial membrane, ultimately leading to the release of cytochrome C, activation of effector caspases (e.g., caspase 3) and, eventually, impaired plasticity and cell death. (3) GR signaling. Following a stress response, GCs are released and downregulate the HPA axis, eventually turning off the stress response. At the cellular level, GCs bind to their receptors, whereby different co-chaperones can modulate GR nuclear trafficking. FKBP5 and BAG-1 are two such co-chaperones that have opposing roles in either attenuating or enhancing GR nuclear trafficking, respectively. Once inside the nucleus, GRs bind to GREs and turn on downstream gene targets (e.g., SGK-1 and MKP-1), leading to enhanced survival and plasticity mechanisms. Alternatively, the GR can associate with Bcl-2 (dashed line) following acute doses of corticosterone. This complex translocates (dotted line) to the mitochondria to enhance survival, leading to enhanced cellular plasticity and resiliency. BDNF, brain-derived neurotrophic factor; CREB, cAMP response element binding protein; ERK, extracellular response kinase; GC, glucocorticoid; GR, glucocorticoid receptor; GRE, glucocorticoid response element; HPA, hypothalamic-pituitary-adrenal; TNF, tumor necrosis factor; TrkB, tyrosine kinase B. Reprinted from Brain Research, Vol. 1293, Hunsberger JG, Austin DR, Chen G, Manji HK. Cellular mechanisms underlying affective resiliency: the role of glucocorticoid receptor- and mitochondrially-mediated plasticity, pp. 76–84, copyright 2009, with permission from Elsevier. This figure is reproduced in color in the color plate section.

can also promote *regeneration* of axons in the mammalian CNS, leading to the intriguing postulate that Bcl-2 acts as a major regulatory switch for a genetic program that controls the *growth* of CNS axons (Chen *et al.* 1997). Because Bcl-2 was also shown to promote neurite sprouting, increasing CNS Bcl-2 levels may represent an effective therapeutic strategy for the treatment of many neurodegenerative diseases (Chen *et al.* 1997).

In view of its major effects on GSK-3 (reviewed below), Bcl-2, and BAG-1, it is not surprising that recent studies investigated lithium's potential neuroprotective effects in several preclinical paradigms, where it was found to have robust neuroprotective properties against a variety of insults (reviewed in Bachmann *et al.* 2005; Chuang and Priller 2006; Manji *et al.* 2000). Notably, lithium pretreatment protected cerebral and cerebellar neurons in primary culture from glutamate-induced, NMDA receptor-mediated apoptosis (reviewed in Chuang and Priller 2006). Excessive NMDA activation is likely involved in stress-induced hippocampal atrophy and has been implicated in the pathogenesis of a variety of neurodegenerative diseases such as stroke, Huntington's disease, ALS, spinal cord injury, traumatic brain injury (TBI), and cerebellar degeneration. In cultured neurons, lithium-induced neuroprotection against glutamate excitotoxicity occurred within the therapeutic concentration range of this drug and required 5 to 6 days pretreatment for maximal effects. Lithium also showed beneficial effects in a number of animal models of neurodegenerative diseases. For example, pre- or post-insult treatment with lithium suppressed cerebral ischemia-induced brain infarction, caspase-3 activation, and neurological deficits in rats. These neuroprotective effects were associated with induction of heat shock protein 70 and decreased expression of Bax (Ren et al. 2003; Xu et al. 2003). Several independent studies demonstrated that lithium has neuroprotective effects in animal and cellular models of Alzheimer's disease, Huntington's disease, Parkinson's disease, retinal degeneration, spinal cord injury, and HIV infection (reviewed in Chuang and Priller 2006).

Although the body of preclinical data demonstrating neurotrophic and neuroprotective effects of lithium is striking, considerable caution must be exercised in extrapolating to the clinical situation with humans. In view of lithium's robust effects on the levels of the cytoprotective protein Bcl-2 in the anterior cingulate, one study re-analyzed older data demonstrating ~ 40% reductions in subgenual PFC volumes in familial mood disorder subjects (Drevets 2001). Consistent with the neurotrophic/neuroprotective effects of lithium, they found that patients treated with chronic lithium or VPA exhibited subgenual PFC volumes that were significantly higher than those in non-lithium- or non-VPA-treated patients and not significantly different from those of controls. To investigate the potential neurotrophic effects of lithium in humans more definitively, one study used proton magnetic resonance spectroscopy (MRS) to demonstrate that treatment of patients with BPD with lithium for 4 weeks increased the level of N-acetyl aspartate (NAA), a marker of neuronal viability, in the cerebral cortex (Moore et al. 2000a). A follow-up volumetric magnetic resonance imaging (MRI) study demonstrated that 4 weeks of lithium treatment also significantly increased *total gray matter content* in the human brain (Moore et al. 2000b), suggesting the possibility of an increase in the volume of the neuropil (the moss-like layer composed of axonal and dendritic fibers that occupies much of the cortex gray matter volume). A subsequent study confirmed a similar increase in gray matter volume in response to lithium compared with the brains of untreated patients and healthy subjects (Sassi et al. 2002).

Another study of familial pediatric BPD revealed that subjects with BPD with past exposure to lithium or VPA tended to have greater amygdala gray matter volume than subjects with BPD without such exposure (Chang et al. 2005). One study compared the volume of the hippocampus, hippocampal head (Hh), and body/tail (Hbt) in three groups with no history of medication use before entry into the study: (a) a group of patients treated with lithium for 1 to 8 weeks and then scanned; (b) a group comprising patients who were unmedicated at the time of scan; and (c) a group of patients treated with either VPA or lamotrigine for 1 to 8 weeks. They observed a bilateral increase in hippocampal and Hh volumes in the lithium-treated group compared with the unmedicated group, an effect that was apparent even over a brief treatment period (Yucel et al. 2008) (Fig. 3.3).

Another study used high-resolution MRI and cortical pattern matching methods to map gray matter differences in 28 BPD patients, 20 of whom were lithium-treated, and 28 healthy controls (Bearden et al. 2007). Their results showed that gray matter density was significantly greater in diffuse cortical regions in patients with BPD than in healthy subjects; the differences were most pronounced in the bilateral cingulate and paralimbic cortices, which are areas used in attention, motivation, and emotion. In addition, the data revealed greater gray matter density in the right anterior cingulate in lithium-treated patients relative to the BPD subjects not taking lithium. The lithium-treated sample included subjects who had received lithium for varying amounts of time, and their dosages were not uniform. The lack of difference in gray matter density between the untreated patients and healthy controls, as well as the growing evidence that lithium exerts major effects on a number of cellular proteins and pathways (see above) known to regulate cell atrophy/death, lends support to the view that the gray matter enlargement is mediated through the trophic actions of lithium in the brain (Chuang and Manji 2007).

Clinical studies have been conducted with pramipexole, a D_2–D_3 agonist used to treat Parkinson's disease that also upregulates Bcl-2 in several brain areas (Kitamura et al. 1998; Takata et al. 2000; Zarate et al. 2004b). Interestingly, pramipexole induced an antidepressant response in individuals with Parkinson's disease and in open-label studies of individuals with treatment-resistant MDD (Lattanzi et al. 2002)

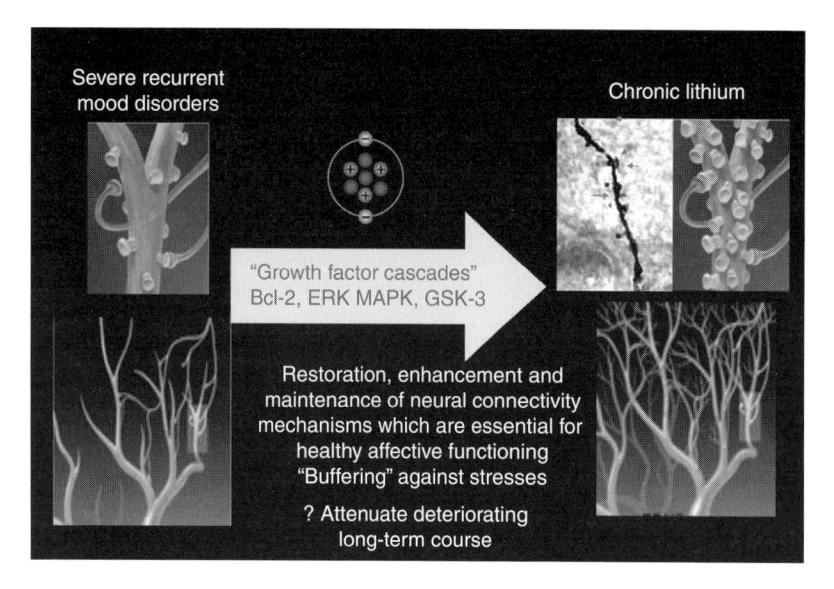

Figure 3.3. Potential impact of the neurotrophic effects of lithium. Many patients with severe mood disorders exhibit volumetric reductions in critical brain areas. However, the available data suggest that – in contrast to traditional neurodegenerative diseases like Alzheimer's disease – severe mood disorders are associated with regional atrophic changes rather than widespread degenerative changes. This figure depicts (left) the reduced neuronal branches and reductions in spine density. It is our contention that these structural impairments contribute to the neural circuitry abnormalities observed in patients (because the dendritic spines represent the processes on which one neuron synapses onto another, the atrophy of dendritic spines results in impaired synaptic connectivity). Lithium exerts major effects on a number of neurotrophic pathways, most notably via inhibition of GSK-3, activation of ERK MAP kinases, and upregulation of neurotrophic members of the Bcl-2 family. Lithium, via these cellular effects, is thought to reverse the illness-related atrophic changes, thereby restoring the synaptic and neural circuitry mediating affective, cognitive, motoric, and neurovegetative functions. These effects would also serve to "buffer" against stresses and likely play a role in attenuating long-term deterioration. GSK-3, glycogen synthase kinase 3. Adapted from *Neuron*, Vol. 34, Nestler EJ, Barrot M, DiLeone RJ, Eisch AJ, Gold SJ, Monteggia LM. Neurobiology of depression, pp. 13–25, copyright 2002, with permission from Elsevier. This figure is reproduced in color in the color plate section.

as well as in preliminary (Sporn *et al.* 2000) and randomized double-blind studies of individuals with bipolar depression (Goldberg *et al.* 2004; Zarate *et al.* 2004*b*). In a randomized, double-blind, placebo-controlled, add-on study, 21 depressed patients with BPD-II who were receiving adjunctive treatment with either lithium or VPA were treated for 6 weeks with pramipexole. Response, as assessed by a 50% decrease in ratings of depression severity, was observed in 60% of patients taking pramipexole and 9% taking placebo; no difference was observed in switch to mania, but the presence of mood stabilizers in these studies may have prevented such mood switches (Zarate *et al.* 2004*b*). A second, similarly designed study looked at 22 subjects with bipolar depression and found that 67% of 12 patients taking pramipexole and 20% of 10 taking placebo showed a clinical response (Goldberg *et al.* 2004). It is important to note that the dopaminergic agonistic effects of pramipexole may have also contributed to the observed response, because an antidepressant response has also been observed with other D_2 agents (piribedil and bromocriptine) (Post *et al.* 1978). Taken together, the neurochemical, postmortem human brain, preclinical behavioral, and clinical studies indicate that enhancing Bcl-2 function may be a worthwhile strategy for preventing and treating mood disorders.

Glycogen synthase kinase 3 (GSK-3) signaling cascade

GSK-3 is a multifunctional, highly active serine/threonine kinase that regulates diverse signaling pathways (e.g., the phosphoinositide 3-kinase [PI3K] pathway, the Wnt pathway, PKA, and PKC). GSK-3 (isoforms α and β) is a key regulator of glycogen synthesis, gene transcription, synaptic plasticity, apoptosis (cell death), cellular structure, and resilience (Jope 2003). GSK-3 is believed to regulate behavior by affecting β-catenin, glutamate receptors, circadian rhythms, and serotonergic neurotransmission (reviewed in Beaulieu *et al.* 2008). All of these have been implicated in the pathophysiology of severe mood disorders.

Studies have shown that lithium directly inhibits GSK-3 at therapeutically relevant concentrations in vitro (Klein and Melton 1996) as well as in vivo in diverse cell types, including cultured neurons and rodent brain (Gould *et al.* 2004a; Hedgepeth *et al.* 1997; Hong *et al.* 1997; Lovestone *et al.* 1999; Munoz-Montano *et al.* 1997; Noble *et al.* 2005; O'Brien *et al.* 2004; Stambolic *et al.* 1996). Many of the known effects of lithium can in fact be explained in terms of GSK-3 inhibition, including glycogen synthesis, early development (Klein and Melton 1996), neurogenesis, neuronal survival (Chalecka-Franaszek and Chuang 1999; Chuang 2004; Gould *et al.* 2006; Li *et al.* 2002), and behavior (Beaulieu *et al.* 2004; Gould *et al.* 2004a; Kaidanovich-Beilin *et al.* 2004; O'Brien *et al.* 2004). Lithium also induces neurotrophic and neuroprotective effects in rodents, partly due to GSK-3β inhibition (reviewed in Gould and Manji 2005). However, GSK-3 inhibition by lithium occurs at the higher end of its therapeutic range, raising some questions about whether this level of inhibition is sufficient to cause relevant biological effects. To address this issue, investigators proposed that secondary modes of inhibition might enhance direct GSK-3 inhibition (De Sarno *et al.* 2002). These modes would include inhibition of the phosphatase that dephosphorylates GSK-3 (which is itself regulated by GSK-3) (Zhang *et al.* 2003), activation of Akt through an unknown mechanism (Chalecka-Franaszek and Chuang 1999), and induction of N-terminal phosphorylation (Bhat *et al.* 2000; Chalecka-Franaszek and Chuang 1999; De Sarno *et al.* 2002; Hall *et al.* 2002; Lochhead *et al.* 2006; Noble *et al.* 2005; Roh *et al.* 2005; Song *et al.* 2002; Zhang *et al.* 2003). In support of this indirect mode of inhibition, evidence for increased N-terminal phosphorylation of GSK-3 in peripheral blood mononuclear cells has been reported in patients treated with lithium (Li *et al.* 2007) (Fig. 3.4).

Preclinical studies have demonstrated that mice over-expressing a constitutively active form of brain GSK-3β displayed increased locomotor activity and decreased habituation in the open field test. In contrast, and similar to the effects of lithium, pharmacological or genetic inhibition of GSK-3β significantly decreased dopamine-dependent locomotor hyperactivity and induced similar molecular changes (Beaulieu *et al.* 2008; O'Brien *et al.* 2004). Similarly, mice treated with VPA for 5 to 10 days displayed reduced immobility in the forced swim test (Semba *et al.* 1989) and reduced exploratory behavior without a concomitant reduction in locomotor activity or rearing (File and Aranko 1988; Rao *et al.* 1991). Lithium and VPA also attenuated amphetamine- and chlordiazepoxide-induced hyperlocomotion (Cao and Peng 1993; Murphy 1977). Pharmacological and genetic evidence supports the hypothesis that these behavioral effects could be mediated by direct or indirect inhibition of GSK-3. For instance, two structurally distinct GSK-3 inhibitors – AR-A014418 (Gould *et al.* 2004b) and the peptide L803-mts (Kaidanovich-Beilin *et al.* 2004) – reduced immobility in the forced swim test and attenuated amphetamine-induced hyperactivity. VPA was initially reported to inhibit GSK-3β activity in SH-SY5Y cells (Chen *et al.* 1999a; Chuang 2005), but these effects have not been confirmed in neuronal cells (Gurvich and Klein 2002). The anticonvulsant carbamazepine was also reported to be involved in signal transduction of cAMP second messenger systems, but no effect on Akt/GSK-3β has yet been reported (Gould *et al.* 2004b). Few studies have been carried out using other agents effective in mood disorders; however, results to date suggest that this signaling pathway is not affected by all mood stabilizers (Aubry *et al.* 2009; Li *et al.* 2002).

Taken together, extant findings suggest that this class of compounds has relevant antimanic and antidepressant effects. However, GSK-3β inhibition is associated with some limitations due to its involvement with diverse pathways that contain multiple substrates that may lead to side effects or toxicity (Rayasam *et al.* 2009). Presently, no blood–brain barrier-penetrant GSK-selective inhibitors have been clinically tested. Proof of principle studies with selective and safe GSK-3β inhibitors are needed to establish the potential safety and therapeutic relevance of this target in mood disorders.

p11: an unexpected target for depression

Studies have shown that p11, also known as S100A10, plays a critical role in behavioral regulation related to depression (Svenningsson *et al.* 2006). p11 increases cell surface localization of the 5-HT1B and 5-HT4 receptors (Warner-Schmidt *et al.* 2009) as well as several ion channels (Svenningsson *et al.* 2006; Warner-Schmidt *et al.* 2009). Its levels were decreased in the brain tissue of depressed patients and of animals that had achieved helplessness in the learned helplessness paradigm, and increased in the brain tissue of animals treated with antidepressants or

Chapter 3: Mood disorders

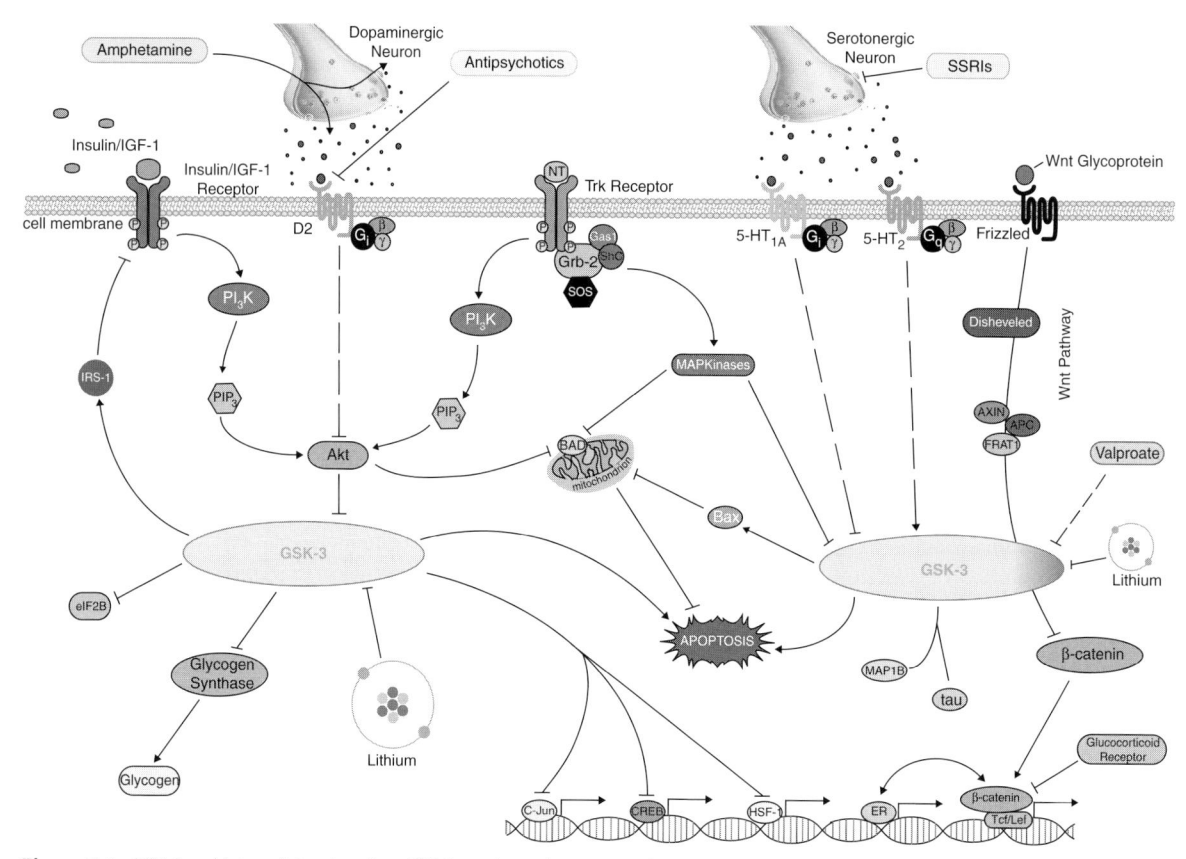

Figure 3.4. GSK-3 and intracellular signaling. GSK-3 regulates diverse signaling pathways in the cell. These pathways include insulin/IGF-1 signaling, neurotrophic factor signaling, and Wnt signaling. Insulin signaling through its Trk receptor activates PI3K-mediated signaling, resulting in GSK-3 inhibition. GSK-3 inhibition activates glycogen synthase and eIF2B while inhibiting IRS-1, an inhibitor of the insulin receptor. Insulin is generally thought to minimally affect central nervous system (CNS) neurons; however, IGF-1 interacting with its cognate receptor appears to have similar functions. NTs act through Trk receptors A, B, and C to activate PI3K and Akt and to inhibit GSK-3. Many effectors have been implicated in the neurotrophic effects of GSK-3 including transcription factors (e.g., HSF-1, C-Jun, and CREB) and BAX, a proapoptotic member of the Bcl-2 family. In the Wnt signaling pathway, secreted Wnt glycoproteins interact with the Frizzled family of receptors and, through disheveled-mediated signaling, inhibit GSK-3. Stability of this process requires the scaffolding proteins AXIN and APC. Normally active GSK-3 phosphorylates β-catenin, leading to its ubiquitin-dependent degradation. However, when GSK-3 is inhibited in the Wnt pathway, β-catenin is not degraded, allowing for its interaction with TCF to act as a transcription factor. β-catenin activity is modulated by the intracellular ER, which also affects transcription of an independent set of genes. As shown in the figure, medications used to treat mood disorders have both direct and indirect effects on GSK-3 and GSK-3-regulated cell signaling pathways, including the direct effects of lithium and indirect effects of antipsychotics, amphetamine, and SSRIs. These distinct pathways have convergent effects on cellular processes such as bioenergetics (energy metabolism), neuroplasticity, neurogenesis, resilience, and survival. Thus, lithium (and other medications) may act by enhancing these processes via GSK-3 inhibition. However, as detailed in the text, GSK-3 modulates a number of signaling pathways not shown in the figure. It remains to be determined which pathway(s) are most relevant to the actions of lithium in the treatment of bipolar disorder and major depressive disorder. G_i refers to G_i/G_o; G_q refers to G_q/G_{11}. APC, adenomatous polyposis coli; CREB, cyclic AMP response element binding protein; eIF2B, eukaryotic initiation factor 2B; ER, estrogen receptor; GSK-3, glycogen synthase kinase 3; HSF-1, heat shock factor-1; insulin-like growth factor 1; IRS-1, insulin receptor substrate-1; NT, neurotrophin; Tcf, T cell-specific transcription factor; Trk, tyrosine receptor kinase. Reprinted from Current Drug Targets, Vol. 7, Gould TD, Picchini AM, Einat H, Manji HK. Targeting glycogen synthase kinase-3 in the CNS: implications for the development of new treatments for mood disorders, pp. 1399–1409, copyright 2006, with permission from Bentham Science Publishers. This figure is reproduced in color in the color plate section.

ECT (Svenningsson et al. 2006). p11 KO mice displayed increased anxiety-like behaviors (thigmotaxis) in the open field test, increased immobility in the tail suspension test, and consumed less palatable 2% sucrose solution than their wild-type littermates (Svenningsson et al. 2006).

A recent study further investigated which brain region was critical to the action of p11 on behaviors related to depression. The investigators studied two regions – the anterior cingulate cortex (ACC) and the NAc – using adeno-associated virus (AAV) vectors delivered by siRNA for knockdown of endogenous p11 mRNA and p11 cDNA for p11 over-expression. Focal knockdown of p11 in the NAc increased immobility time in the tail suspension and forced swim tests in otherwise normal adult C57B1/6 mice. However, knockdown in the ACC had no effect on immobility measures. The investigators further demonstrated that AAV-mediated p11 focal expression in the NAc of p11 KO mice alleviated this increased immobility time in the tail suspension test; the same treatment had no significant effect on immobility time in wild-type mice. In addition, focal NAc p11 expression in p11 KO mice increased their consumption of 2% sucrose solution but not water. Lastly, significantly lower p11 protein levels were found in NAc tissue from depressed patients compared with controls. Taken together, these data demonstrate that p11 in the NAc modulates depression-related behaviors; the role of the ACC in mediating other mood and cognitive symptoms requires further investigation. As discussed, upregulation of BDNF is a common effect of diverse antidepressants as well as of ECT and mood stabilizers. Recent studies demonstrated that the effects of BDNF infusion into the lateral ventricle on immobility in both the tail suspension and forced swim tests were absent in p11 KO mice (discussed in Chen *et al.* 2010*b*). Furthermore, p11 is known to dramatically enhance tissue plasminogen activator (tPA) activity (Kim and Hajjar 2002). This finding is particularly notable because a large proportion of neuronal BDNF is secreted in the pro-form, which is subsequently converted to mBDNF by extracellular proteases such as plasmin or matrix metalloproteinases (discussed in Martinowich *et al.* 2007). tPA, an extracellular protease that converts the inactive zymogen plasminogen to plasmin, is of particular interest due to its ability, via plasmin activation, to convert proBDNF to mBDNF in the hippocampus; this conversion is required for late-phase, long-term potentiation (LTP) (discussed in Martinowich *et al.* 2007). Additional researchers are investigating the role of p11 in mood disorders and in novel treatments for mood disorders in monkeys and humans.

Neuroactive cytokines

Neuroactive cytokines are known to influence brain structural plasticity and function (Dantzer *et al.* 2008; Miller *et al.* 2009). Notably, short-term administration of proinflammatory cytokines in animals causes a series of behavioral changes known as "sickness behavior," including deficits in social and exploratory activities that echo the symptoms of depression (Dantzer *et al.* 2008; Miller *et al.* 2009). Antidepressant treatment decreased TNF-alpha expression in the brain (Nickola *et al.* 2001), whereas ICV microinfusion of TNF-alpha increased immobility. In contrast, the infusion of TNF-alpha antibodies reduced immobility in the forced swim test (Reynolds *et al.* 2004). A related study reported that TNF receptor-1 KO mice showed reduced immobility in the forced swim test without locomotor alterations in the home cage or open field tests and reduced memory in the fear conditioning paradigm (Simen *et al.* 2006). In addition, TNF receptor-2 KO mice showed reduced immobility in the first 5 minutes of a 15-minute forced swim test, and both KO strains demonstrated increased consumption of sucrose solution after water deprivation. Studies have also been conducted using IL-1β and interferon, and results suggest that these molecules similarly play a critical role in mediating stress response, fear conditioning, and anxiety, and are potential targets for treating depression (Duman 2009).

A recent, related exciting area of research is the regulation of glutamatergic system function and synaptic plasticity by neuroactive cytokines (reviewed in Khairova *et al.* 2009). Interestingly, multiple studies have shown that cytokines, notably IL-1 and TNF-alpha, modulate GluR1-containing AMPA receptor trafficking and surface expression. Recent evidence further supports the trafficking mechanism of this action; specifically, a pool of AMPA receptors that recycle in endosomes supplies the synapse with receptors in as little as 20 minutes after NMDA receptor-mediated stimuli that induced LTP (Lu *et al.* 2001; Park *et al.* 2004). This AMPA receptor exocytosis is mediated by the activation of TNFR1 through a PI3K-dependent pathway (Stellwagen *et al.* 2005). The newly expressed AMPA receptors had lower stoichiometric amounts of GluR2, making the receptors permeable to calcium ions. Similarly, an earlier study showed that long-term treatment (24–48 hours) of cultured hippocampal neurons with TNF-alpha increased calcium currents by ~30%, as measured by whole cell perforated patch-clamp recording (Furukawa and Mattson 1998).

These TNF-alpha-induced changes in AMPA receptor surface expression may have important implications for synaptic plasticity (Carroll *et al.* 2001). TNF-alpha appears to directly affect dendritic branching in cultured neurons (Neumann *et al.* 2002), probably through its TNFR2 receptor, which is known to transduce the trophic effect of TNF-alpha (Yang *et al.* 2002). This observation is supported by the results of an in vivo study showing that TNFR1 and TNFR2 KO mice had decreased arborization of the apical dendrites of the CA1 and CA3 regions and accelerated DG development (Golan *et al.* 2004). In addition to its involvement in hippocampal morphogenesis, TNF-alpha deficiency specifically improved the performance of affected mice on behavioral tasks related to spatial memory. Moreover, basal levels of TNF-alpha regulated BDNF and NGF levels during hippocampal development (Golan *et al.* 2004). Modulation of these factors governs granular cell migration in the DG and dendritic tree formation by pyramidal cells in regions CA1 and CA3.

In addition to the effects of TNF-alpha on LTP, TNF-alpha may be part of the core signaling pathway that homeostatically regulates neuronal synaptic strength. Indeed, prolonged inhibition of neuronal activity by tetrodotoxin triggers release of glial TNF-alpha, which then increases the membrane trafficking of AMPA receptors and consequently increases miniature excitatory postsynaptic currents in a compensatory manner (Stellwagen *et al.* 2005; Stellwagen and Malenka 2006). Together, these findings provide further evidence that TNF-alpha promotes activity-dependent changes at the level of the glutamatergic synapse and may thus play a crucial role in the molecular mechanisms of synaptic plasticity.

Notably, numerous proinflammatory cytokines have been reported to be elevated in patients suffering from MDD compared with nondepressed subjects or, in some cases, correlated with symptom severity (Dantzer *et al.* 2008; Miller *et al.* 2009). These include increased acute-phase proteins (C-reactive protein, alpha-1-acid glycoprotein, alpha-1-antichymotrypsin, haptoglobin), increased expression of chemokines and adhesion molecules (including human macrophage chemoattractant protein-1 [MCP-1], soluble intracellular adhesion molecule-1 [sICAM-1], and E-selectin), increased serum and/or plasma concentrations of interleukin (IL)-1β, IL-6, and TNF-alpha, both in peripheral blood and in the CNS (particularly in CSF); elevated levels of TNF-alpha and IL-6 have been noted most consistently. Recent studies also suggest that functional allelic variants of the genes for IL-1β and TNF-alpha increase the risk for depression and are associated with reduced responsiveness to antidepressant therapy (reviewed in Miller *et al.* 2009).

In connection with this evidence, an interesting clinical study investigated the effects of etanercept (a soluble TNF-alpha receptor that prevents TNF-alpha-mediated cellular response by competitively inhibiting the interaction of TNF-alpha with cell-surface receptors) on symptoms of depression and fatigue associated with psoriasis. In this clinical trial, 618 patients with moderate to severe psoriasis received double-blind treatment with placebo or intravenous infusion of 50 mg of twice-weekly etanercept. The primary efficacy end point was improvement of psoriasis, but secondary end points included the Hamilton Rating Scale for Depression (HAM-D), the Beck Depression Inventory (BDI), and the Functional Assessment of Chronic Illness Therapy Fatigue (FACIT-F) scale. A greater proportion of patients receiving etanercept had at least a 50% improvement on the HAM-D or BDI at week 12 compared with the placebo group; furthermore, patients treated with etanercept also had significant, clinically meaningful improvements in fatigue. In addition, improvements in depressive symptoms were less correlated with measures of skin clearance or joint pain (Tyring *et al.* 2006). Although the population studied did not have MDD, the results suggest that future studies exploring pharmacological interventions with anticytokine activity (particularly anti-TNF-alpha activity) are warranted, and that these might have a role in treating MDD. In fact, at least two ongoing studies are exploring this hypothesis. The first is of the P38a kinase inhibitor GW856553X, which inhibits the production of proinflammatory cytokines (details available at: http://www.clinicaltrials.gov/ct2/show/NCT00976560?term=cytokine+depression&rank=7), and the second is a study using infliximab (Remicade, an antibody anti-TNF-alpha) (details are available at: http://www.clinicaltrials.gov/ct2/show/NCT00463580?term=cytokine+depression&rank=8).

The glutamatergic system

Glutamate is the main excitatory synaptic neurotransmitter in the brain (Fig. 3.5). It mediates neurotransmission across excitatory synapses and modulates several physiological brain functions such as synaptic plasticity, learning, and memory (Bannerman *et al.* 1995; Collingridge 1994; Collingridge and Bliss 1995; Watkins and Collingridge 1994). Excessive

Chapter 3: Mood disorders

Physiological role in regulation of homeostatic plasticity

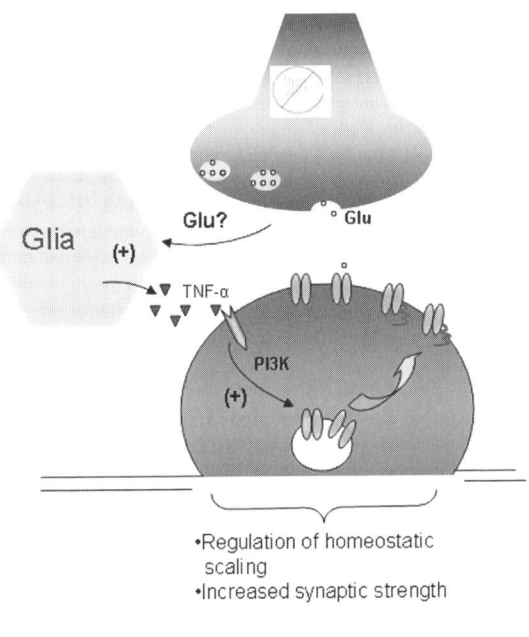

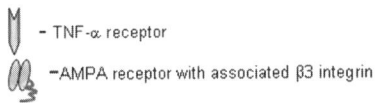

Pathophysiological role in regulation of synaptic plasticity in depression

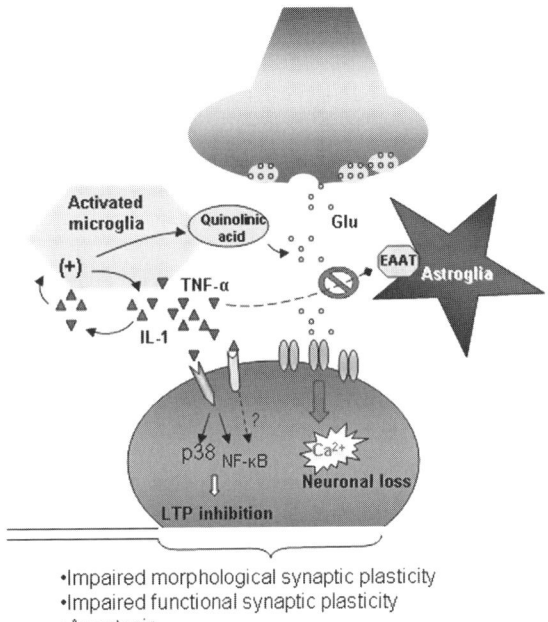

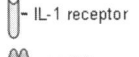

Figure 3.5. Dual role of proinflammatory cytokines in regulating synaptic plasticity. The diagram on the left depicts the critical role of constitutively expressed TNF-alpha in regulating homeostatic synaptic plasticity in the normal brain. Decreased neuronal activity and consequently reduced glutamate release from axons is sensed by glia, which trigger release of TNF-alpha. TNF-alpha activates neuronal TNF-alpha receptor type I (TNFR1), leading to activation of the phosphoinositide-3 kinase (PI3K) pathway and upregulation of the specific adhesion molecule-β3 integrin; this step in turn triggers AMPA receptor insertion to the membrane and increases synaptic strength. The diagram on the right depicts the various signaling cascades initiated by high pathophysiological levels of proinflammatory cytokines in the brain by activated microglia, which might underlie at least some aspects of the pathophysiology of depression. (1) TNF-alpha and IL-1 trigger production of quinolinic acid and release of glutamate by microglia; (2) TNF-alpha and IL-1 inhibit glutamate removal by astrocytes, leading to excess extracellular glutamate and neurotoxicity; (3) TNF-alpha acts via TNFR1 to upregulate membrane expression of calcium-permeable AMPA receptor subunits, thus leading to increased calcium influx and neuronal death; (4) TNFR1 activation coupled to activation of p38 and NF-κB pathways inhibits the early and late phases of LTP. These effects of pathophysiological levels of proinflammatory cytokines on synaptic plasticity at both morphological and functional levels might underlie the cognitive disturbances and memory impairments seen in patients with depression. AMPA, alpha-amino-3-hydroxy-5-methyl-4-isoxazolepropionic acid; Glu, glutamate; TNF, tumor necrosis factor. Reproduced from *International Journal of Neuropsychopharmacology*, Vol. 12, Khairova R, Machado-Vieira R, Du J, Manji HK. A potential role for pro-inflammatory cytokines in regulating synaptic plasticity in major depressive disorder, pp. 561–578, copyright 2009, with permission from Cambridge University Press. This figure is reproduced in color in the color plate section.

concentrations of glutamate are directly involved in the dysregulation of brain neuroplasticity and cellular resilience observed in patients with mood disorders (Sanacora *et al*. 2008). Emerging data also indicate that glutamate plays a critical role in both acute and long-term processes involved in the action of currently available mood stabilizers and antidepressants. Consequently, several glutamatergic modulators have been investigated in an attempt to regulate dysfunctional glutamatergic transmission. Pharmacological interventions targeting different components of this neurotransmitter system have been evaluated in patients with mood disorders (Zarate *et al*. 2002, 2006). Such interventions have alternately worked at the synaptic release level or by antagonizing NMDA receptors, modulating AMPA receptor activity, or modulating the function of metabotropic receptors (Fig. 3.6).

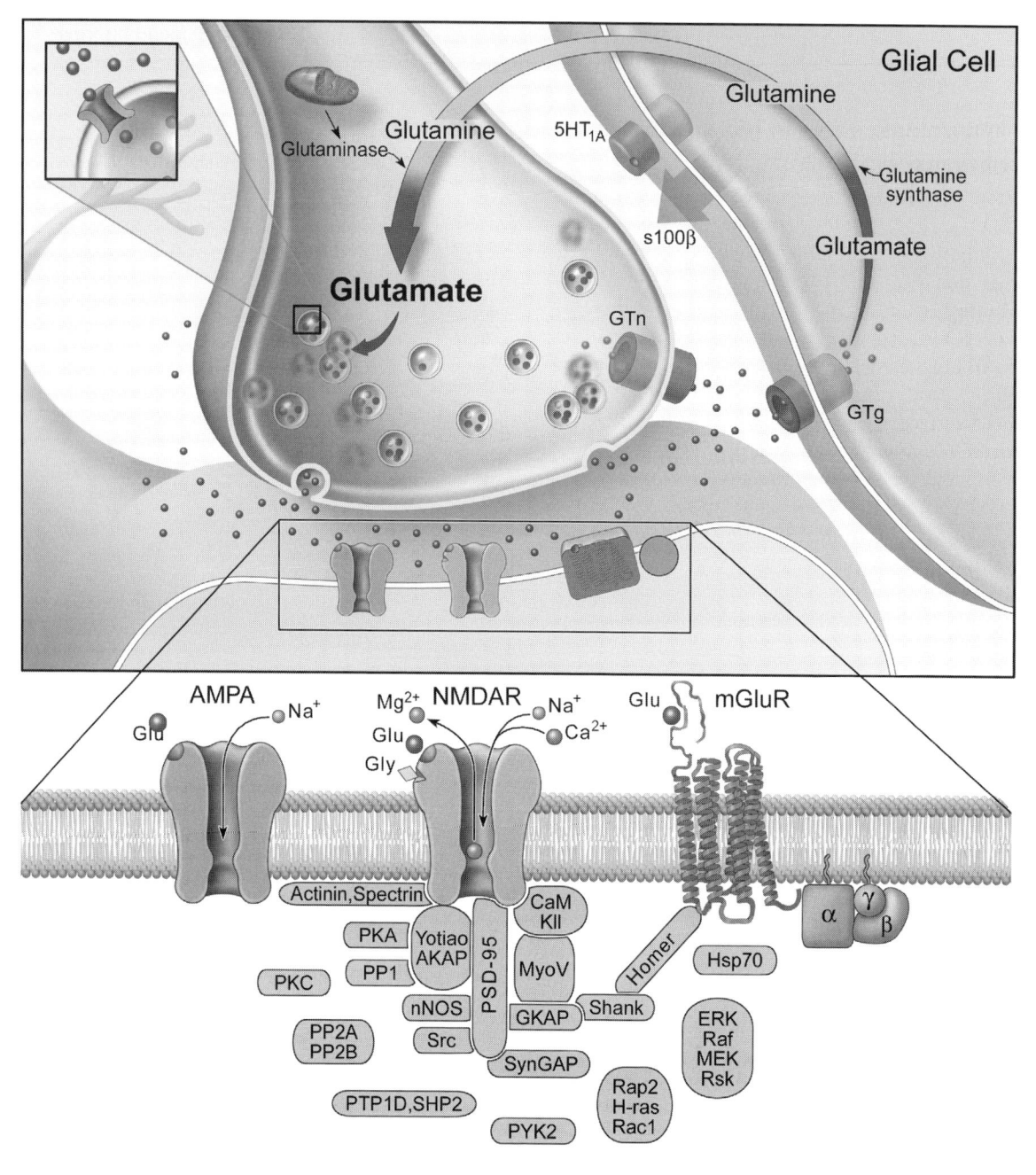

Receptor Subunit Types

Ionotropic			Metabotropic		
NMDA	AMPA	Kainate	Group I	Group II	Group III
NR1	GluR 1	GluR 5	mGlu 1 a-b-c-d	mGlu 2	mGlu 4 a-b
NR2 A-B-C-D	GluR 2	GluR 6	mGlu 5 a-b	mGlu 3	mGlu 6
NR3 A-B	GluR 3	GluR 7			mGlu 7 a-b
	GluR 4	KA 1			mGlu 8 a-b
		KA 2			

Figure 3.6. This figure depicts the various regulatory processes involved in glutamatergic neurotransmission. The biosynthetic pathway for glutamate involves synthesis from glucose and the transamination of a-ketoglutarate; however, a small proportion of glutamate is formed more directly from glutamine by glutamine synthetase. The latter is actually synthesized in glia and, via an active process (requiring ATP),

Agents that regulate glutamate release and AMPA receptor trafficking: riluzole

Riluzole (2-amino-6-trifluoromethoxybenzothiazole), an FDA-approved medication for the treatment of ALS, inhibits synaptic glutamate release. Preclinical studies demonstrated that lamotrigine and riluzole significantly enhanced the surface expression of GluR1 and GluR2 in a time- and dose-dependent manner in cultured hippocampal neurons; in contrast, the mood stabilizer and anticonvulsant VPA significantly reduced surface expression of GluR1 and GluR2 (Du et al. 2007). Concomitant with GluR1 and GluR2 changes, the peak value of depolarized membrane potential evoked by AMPA was significantly higher in lamotrigine- and riluzole-treated neurons, supporting the surface receptor changes. Phosphorylation of GluR1 at the PKA site (S845) was enhanced in both lamotrigine- and riluzole-treated hippocampal neurons but reduced in VPA-treated neurons. In addition, lamotrigine and riluzole, as well as the traditional antidepressant imipramine, increased GluR1 phosphorylation at GluR1 (S845) in the hippocampus after long-term treatment in vivo (Du et al. 2007).

Due to its mechanism of action, a series of hypothesis-driven clinical studies were conducted to explore the putative efficacy of riluzole in mood disorders. An initial open-label study was conducted in 19 patients with treatment-resistant MDD; significant improvements in depressive symptoms were observed over 6 weeks (Zarate et al. 2004a). This study was followed by an 8-week, open-label trial of riluzole in combination with lithium in 14 subjects with bipolar depression, which similarly reported that riluzole was associated with significant treatment effects (Zarate et al. 2005). Similar results were also obtained in a pilot study of 10 subjects with treatment-resistant MDD (Sanacora et al. 2007). Taken together, the findings suggest that riluzole may indeed have antidepressant efficacy; additional studies are ongoing. Recently, using a different strategy, researchers administered riluzole to maintain the antidepressant effects achieved by the NMDA antagonist ketamine (see below for a full discussion of ketamine's antidepressant effects). However, riluzole failed to prevent depressive relapses in the first month after treatment with ketamine (Mathew et al. 2010).

NMDA receptor antagonists

Three subgroups of glutamatergic receptor-ion channels have been identified on the basis of their pharmacological ability to bind different synthetic ligands: NMDA, AMPA, and kainate receptors. NMDA receptor antagonists have demonstrated antidepressant-like effects in diverse preclinical paradigms (Maeng and Zarate 2007; Moryl et al. 1993; Papp and Moryl 1993; Przegalinski et al. 1997; Trullas and Skolnick 1990; Zarate et al. 2002). The NMDA receptor antagonists dizocilpine (MK-801) and CGP 37849 showed antidepressant-like effects alone or in combination with standard antidepressants in several preclinical studies (Meloni et al. 1993; Padovan and Guimaraes 2004; Papp and Moryl 1993; Skolnick et al. 1992; Trullas

Figure 3.6. (cont.)
is transported to neurons where, in the mitochondria, glutaminase is able to convert this precursor to glutamate. Furthermore, in astrocytes, glutamine can undergo oxidation to yield a-ketoglutarate, which can also be transported to neurons and participate in glutamate synthesis. Glutamate is either metabolized or sequestered and stored in secretory vesicles by VGluTs. Glutamate can then be released by a calcium-dependent excitotoxic process. Once released from the presynaptic terminal, glutamate binds to numerous excitatory amino acid (EAA) receptors, including ionotropic receptors (e.g., NMDA and mGluRs). Presynaptic regulation of glutamate release occurs through mGluR$_2$ and mGluR$_3$, which subserve the function of autoreceptors; however, these receptors are also located on the postsynaptic element. Glutamate has its action terminated in the synapse by reuptake mechanisms using distinct glutamate transporters (labeled VGT in the figure) that exist on not only presynaptic nerve terminals but also astrocytes; indeed, current data suggest that astrocytic glutamate uptake may be more important for clearing excess glutamate, raising the possibility that astrocytic loss (as has been documented in mood disorders) may contribute to deleterious glutamate signaling, but more so by astrocytes. It is now known that a number of important intracellular proteins are able to alter the function of glutamate receptors (see figure). Also, growth factors such as glial-derived neurotrophic factor (GDNF) and S100b secreted from glia exert a tremendous influence on glutamatergic neurons and synapse formation. Notably, serotonin$_{1A}$ (5-HT$_{1A}$) receptors are regulated by antidepressant agents; this receptor is also able to modulate the release of S100b. Modified from Szabo et al. 2004. AKAP, A kinase anchoring protein; CaMKII, Ca^{2+}/calmodulin–dependent protein kinase II; ERK, extracellular response kinase; GKAP, guanylate kinase-associated protein; Glu, glutamate; Gly, glycine; GTg, glutamate transporter glial; GTn, glutamate transporter neuronal; Hsp70, heat shock protein 70; MEK, mitogen-activated protein kinase/ERK; mGluR, metabotropic glutamate receptor; MyoV, myosin V; NMDAR, NMDA receptor; nNOS, neuronal nitric oxide synthase; PKA, protein kinase A; PKC, protein kinase C; PP-1, PP-2A, PP-2B, protein phosphatases; RSK, ribosomal S6 kinase; SHP2, src homology 2 domain–containing tyrosine phosphatase; vGluTs, vesicle glutamate transporters. Reprinted from Szabo S, Gould TD, Manji HK. Neurotransmitters, receptors, signal transduction pathways and second messengers, pp. 3–52, *American Psychiatric Publishing Textbook of Psychopharmacology*, copyright © 2004, with permission from the American Psychiatric Association. This figure is reproduced in color in the color plate section.

and Skolnick 1990). D-cycloserine, an antibiotic used to treat tuberculosis, acts as a partial agonist on the glycine recognition site of the NMDA receptor. In preclinical studies, it was found to inhibit the hypermobility induced by methamphetamine but not that induced by apomorphine (Dall'Olio et al. 1994) and to decrease aggressiveness in the resident-intruder test (McAllister 1994). Clinical studies with D-cycloserine found no efficacy for treatment-resistant MDD (Heresco-Levy et al. 2006), although it is possible that the doses studied were too low. This agent is currently being tested for the treatment of bipolar depression.

Ketamine

Ketamine is a pharmacological agent that non-competitively antagonizes the postsynaptic NMDA ionotropic glutamatergic receptor by binding to a site within the open channel. Preclinical studies found that a single injection of ketamine had both antidepressant and anxiolytic effects in diverse paradigms, including acute and sustained effects on immobility in the forced swim test and reversed escape deficits in the learned helplessness paradigm (Aguado et al. 1994; Garcia et al. 2008; Maeng et al. 2008b; Mickley et al. 1998; Silvestre et al. 1997).

Clinically, an initial, small (n = 7), double-blind, placebo-controlled study found that ketamine had rapid, robust antidepressant effects in subjects with treatment-resistant MDD (Berman et al. 2000). These findings were subsequently confirmed in a randomized, double-blind, placebo-controlled study of patients with treatment-resistant MDD; patients receiving ketamine showed significant improvement in depressive symptoms compared with those receiving placebo. These effects began within 2 hours of intravenous ketamine administration and lasted for at least 1 week (Zarate et al. 2006). Notably, the magnitude of the effect was similar to that observed after weeks of treatment with currently available antidepressants, and the antidepressant response to a single infusion of ketamine was not associated with the dissociative symptoms usually induced by this agent. Ketamine also produced rapid, prolonged antidepressant effects in patients with bipolar depression (Berman et al. 2000; Diazgranados et al. 2010b; Zarate et al. 2006) and was further associated with rapid, beneficial effects on suicidal ideation in depressed patients (Diazgranados et al. 2010a; Price et al. 2009). One small, recent trial evaluated 10 patients who received repeated ketamine infusions – six infusions over 12 days (aan het Rot et al. 2010). Response criteria were met by nine patients after the first through sixth infusions, suggesting that repeated NMDA blocking is a feasible approach for treating acute, treatment-resistant MDD. Furthermore, recent studies that used ketamine as an experimental tool found that increased ACC activity in response to fearful faces (Salvadore et al. 2009) and positive family history of alcohol dependence (Phelps et al. 2009) both predicted initial antidepressant response to ketamine but that BDNF levels did not (Machado-Vieira et al. 2009). These research efforts are expected to generate insights into the mechanism by which NMDA antagonism is associated with rapid antidepressant response.

NR2B antagonists

Preclinical studies and clinical trials assessing the efficacy of more subtype-selective NMDA antagonists are underway to determine whether these antidepressant effects can occur safely without causing ketamine's psychomimetic side effects. The NR2B selective antagonist Ro-25 6981 mimicked ketamine's effects in the forced swim test (Maeng et al. 2008b), and a single injection of ketamine or Ro-25 6981 was similarly found to restore sucrose preference deficits in the chronic unpredictable stress model.

A randomized, placebo-controlled, clinical trial was conducted using the NR2B subunit-selective NMDA receptor antagonist, CP-101,606 (Preskorn et al. 2008). A single intravenous infusion of this agent produced a greater decrease of depressive symptoms than placebo. HAM-D response rates were 60% for the drug and 20% for the placebo. Interestingly, and as observed with ketamine, 78% of CP-101,606-treated responders maintained response status for at least 1 week after the infusion. The agent was safe and well tolerated and did not produce dissociative effects (Preskorn et al. 2008). Oral agents with this mechanism of action (MK-0657 and EVT-101) are now being investigated in a population of treatment-resistant patients (details available at: http://www.clinicaltrials.gov/ct2/show/NCT00472576?term=nr2b&rank=2; http://www.clinicaltrials.gov/ct2/show/NCT01128452?term=EVT-101&rank=1).

Modulation of AMPA receptor function

AMPA receptors are ionotropic receptors mediating the fast components of excitatory neurotransmission that play a major role in learning and memory.

Diverse classes of compounds regulate AMPA receptors by binding to allosteric sites and are termed AMPA receptor positive modulators or AMPA receptor potentiators (ARPs). ARPs modulate AMPA receptors indirectly by decreasing the receptor desensitization rate and/or deactivation in the presence of an agonist (e.g., AMPA and glutamate) (see Black 2005 for a review). In contrast to the receptor activation by agonists, ARPs decrease receptor desensitization and/or deactivation rates in the presence of an agonist (see Bleakman and Lodge 1998; Borges and Dingledine 1998 for review). Particular attention has focused on the role of a subclass of AMPA potentiators known as AMPAkines, which are small benzamide compounds that produce positive allosteric effects in the AMPA receptors. These compounds include benzoylpiperidines (e.g., CX-516), benzothiazides (e.g., cyclothiazide), pyrrolidones (piracetam, aniracetam), and birylpropylsulfonamides (e.g., LY392098). Consistent with the enhancement of AMPA receptor transmission, animal studies using the ARP LY451646 found that this compound reduced immobility time in the forced swim and tail suspension tests (Bai et al. 2001; Li et al. 2001). Treatment with the ARP LY392098 also produced antidepressant-like effects in the forced swim test and in an unpredictable chronic mild stress paradigm (Farley et al. 2010).

Animal studies have also demonstrated that treatment with antidepressants modulated both AMPA and NMDA receptors in the brain. GluR1 (an AMPA receptor subunit) can be phosphorylated by PKC at serine 831 and by PKA at serine 845, which is thought to increase the membrane insertion and function of GluR1. Chronic treatment with fluoxetine, imipramine, tianeptine, lamotrigine, and riluzole are all known to increase GluR1 phosphorylation (Du et al. 2004, 2007; Svenningsson et al. 2002, 2007). Both ketamine and lithium reduced GluR1 phosphorylation and immobility in the forced swim test, and AMPA receptor antagonists blocked both of these effects (Du et al. 2004; Gould et al. 2008; Maeng et al. 2008b). Thus, one hypothesis to explain the antidepressant actions of acute ketamine and chronic antidepressant treatment is that these may increase AMPA/NMDA activation (Maeng et al. 2008b), as ketamine is also known to increase glutamate release (Moghaddam et al. 1997).

It is also interesting to note that although alterations in GluR1 phosphorylation as an indicator of AMPA receptor functional change have been well documented, preliminary data do not support GluR1 phosphorylation per se as critical for antidepressant action. In GluR1 double phospho-mutant mice, an NR2B antagonist and imipramine, but not tianeptine, effectively decreased immobility time, whereas GluR1 KO mice showed the opposite effect in the forced swim test (Kiselyczyk et al. 2009). Thus, the involvement of selective AMPA receptor subunits in antidepressant action requires further elucidation.

As with other glutamatergic strategies discussed in this chapter, AMPAkines also possess antidepressant properties in animal models of depression (including models of inescapable stress, the forced-swim test, the tail-suspension test, induced immobility tests, the learned-helplessness paradigm, and chronic mild stress exposure (reviewed in Black 2005; Miu et al. 2001). One animal study showed that chronic treatment with the AMPAkines CX731, CX691, or CX516 produced fluoxetine-like effects in the submissive behavioral paradigm (Knapp et al. 2002). In another animal study, the AMPAkine Ampalex induced antidepressant effects in the first week of treatment, whereas fluoxetine showed similar effects only after 2 weeks of treatment (Knapp et al. 2002).

No clinical trials are currently being conducted with AMPAkines, because prior studies encountered safety concerns that prompted researchers to stop developing these compounds for use in humans. However, the potential impact in patients with depressive symptoms may still represent an exciting new avenue for the development of novel therapeutics.

Because ARPs appear to have antidepressant-like properties, it is possible that AMPA receptor antagonists could display antimanic effects. The first group of selective AMPA receptor antagonists to be characterized was the quinoxalinedione derivatives, such as 2,3-dioxo-6-nitro-1,2,3,4-tetrahydrobenzo[*f*]quinoxaline-7-sulfonamide, which acts at the AMPA receptor recognition site. In contrast, recent AMPA receptor antagonists, such as GYKI 52466, block AMPA receptors on the receptor-channel complex via an allosteric site (Donevan and Rogawski 1993). Talampanel (a GYKI 52466 analog [GYKI 53773; LY300164]) possesses anticonvulsant effects and appears to be well tolerated in clinical trials; sedation has been the only notable side effect (reviewed by Rogawski 2006). This agent is currently undergoing phase II clinical trials for the treatment of ALS. Other similar agents include the competitive AMPA receptor antagonist NS1209; in preclinical models, this agent appeared to have faster and more complete anticonvulsant effects than diazepam (Pitkanen et al. 2007). NS1209 showed good CNS bioavailability and was well tolerated in phase I/II clinical trials; it is currently being tested in patients with treatment-refractory epilepsy (reviewed in Nielsen et al. 1999; Rogawski 2006).

It is plausible that the putative antidepressant effects of ARPs are mediated through AMPA receptor trafficking (including receptor insertion, internalization, and delivery to synaptic sites), which plays a critical role in the activity-dependent regulation of synaptic strength as well as in various forms of neural and behavioral plasticity (Sanacora et al. 2008).

Targeting metabotropic glutamate receptors

The metabotropic glutamate receptors (mGluRs) comprise eight receptor subtypes (mGluR1 to GluR8) classified into three groups on the basis of their sequence homology, coupling to second messenger systems, and agonist selectivity. Group I mGluRs (mGluR1 and mGluR5) are coupled to the phospholipase C signal transduction pathway. Group II (mGluR2 and mGluR3) and group III (mGluR4 and mGluR6 to mGluR8) receptors are both coupled in an inhibitory manner to the adenylyl cyclase signal transduction pathway, which is generally involved in regulating the release of glutamate or other neurotransmitters such as gamma-aminobutyric acid (GABA), based on synaptic localization (Conn and Pin 1997).

mGluRs play a role in the early phases of memory formation and in the mechanisms of long-term depression (Riedel et al. 2003; Salinska and Stafiej 2003; Tan et al. 2003). Rapidly accumulating evidence supports the notion that the regulation of glutamatergic neurotransmission via mGluRs is linked to CNS-related disorders (Zarate et al. 2002) and to mood disorders in particular (Witkin et al. 2007; Zarate et al. 2002). In preclinical studies, group II mGluRs agonists (e.g., LY341495) dose-dependently decreased the immobility time of rodents in the forced swim and tail suspension tests (Chaki et al. 2003). Moreover, the group II mGluR antagonist MGS-0039 was effective in the learned helplessness model of depression (Yoshimizu et al. 2006) and increased cell proliferation in the adult mouse hippocampus (Yoshimizu and Chaki 2004). Interestingly, activation of AMPA receptors has been shown to be responsible at least in part for the antidepressant-like activity of group II

mGluR antagonists; the AMPA antagonist 2,3-dioxo-6-nitro-1,2,3,4-tetrahydrobenzo[f]quinoxaline-7-sulfonamide blocked the antidepressant-like activity of MGS-0039 in the tail suspension test in mice (Karasawa et al. 2005).

Clinically, compounds that antagonize the group I mGluR5 receptors are being investigated for several neurological and psychiatric indications; relevant to this discussion is RO4917523, which has already reached the clinical phase of development with exploratory efficacy endpoints in treatment-resistant MDD (details available at: (http://www.clinicaltrials.gov/ct2/show/NCT00809562?term=roche+depression&rank=1). This family of receptors is likely to provide several novel targets with antidepressant properties and remains an exciting development in translational research.

Long-term changes induced by early life events

Early life experiences, including maternal care, childhood traumatic events, and maltreatment (including verbal, physical, or sexual abuse) shape the trajectory of human psychology and behavior, with long-term impact on cognition and emotion (Feder et al. 2009; Lupien et al. 2009; Tsankova et al. 2007). Clinical studies have demonstrated that early life adverse events, alone or in combination with genetic variants such as SNPs of FKBP5, BDNF, or CRHR1, increase risk for psychiatric illnesses, especially depression and post-traumatic stress disorder (PTSD) (Binder et al. 2008; Gatt et al. 2009; Gillespie et al. 2009; Polanczyk et al. 2009). Several animal models have been developed that partially simulate this human phenomenon. Sustained alterations in the expression of GRs (McGowan et al. 2009; Weaver et al. 2004, 2005, 2007), arginine vasopressin (AVP) (Murgatroyd et al. 2009), and BDNF (Roth et al. 2009) were demonstrated in modeled animals.

Stress and the hypothalamic-pituitary-adrenal axis

Acute and chronic stress alters the function of the hypothalamic-pituitary-adrenal (HPA) axis. Animal data have consistently shown that behavioral stress alters HPA axis function; causes structural remodeling in the hippocampus, PFC, and amygdala; and induces deficits in behavioral tests for cognitive and emotional functioning. In turn, hippocampal GR activation is thought to be involved in the negative regulation of the HPA axis response to stress (Feder *et al.* 2009; Lupien *et al.* 2009; Tsankova *et al.* 2007). Notably, over-activity of the HPA axis in depression (both MDD and bipolar depression) has been reported repeatedly, as evidenced by the lack of dexamethasone suppression of plasma cortisol levels, increased adrenocorticotropic hormone (ACTH) response to corticotropin-releasing hormone (CRH) and altered responses to the combined dexamethasone/corticotropin release hormone challenge (Ising *et al.* 2007; Plotsky *et al.* 1998). In addition, early childhood psychosocial stress has also been associated with adult-onset MDD (Heim *et al.* 2001) and an adverse course for BPD (Brown *et al.* 2005; Garno *et al.* 2005; Leverich *et al.* 2002). Some human genetic studies also suggest that variants of the HPA axis components confer risk for depression (Claes 2009).

Attempts to modify HPA axis abnormalities in mood disorders, intervening at the axis at different levels and with diverse strategies, have been investigated over the last decade (reviewed in Quiroz *et al.* 2004); double-blind, placebo-controlled clinical studies have been reported using inhibitors of glucocorticoid synthesis (Malison *et al.* 1999; Wolkowitz *et al.* 1999), GR antagonists (Belanoff *et al.* 2001; Young *et al.* 2004), downregulation of the HPA axis with hydrocortisone (DeBattista *et al.* 2000), dehydroepiandrosterone utilization (Bloch *et al.* 1999; Wolkowitz *et al.* 1999), and CRF-1 antagonists (Zobel *et al.* 2000).

Glucocorticoid receptors and epigenetic modifications

Maternal nursing activities (including licking and grooming of pups and arched-back nursing in the first 10 postnatal days) have been associated with attenuated ACTH and corticosterone responses to restraint stress (20 minutes), increased sensitivity to the inhibitory effects of glucocorticoids on stress-induced HPA axis activation, and increased levels of hippocampal GRs (Liu *et al.* 1997, 2000). A series of studies laid out a plausible molecular and cellular mechanism for the phenomena known as epigenetic (re)programming of hippocampal GR gene expression and stress responses by maternal behavior (Weaver 2009; Zhang and Meaney 2010). Maternal licking and grooming and arched-back nursing elevate hippocampal serotonin (5-HT) turnover and stimulate the 5-HT7 receptor in offspring, thereby activating the expression of the transcription factor nerve growth factor-inducible protein-A (NGFI-A)

through phosphorylated-CREB (pCREB) activity. NGFI-A translocates to its cognate binding site on the GR exon 17 promoter and recruits CREB-binding protein (CBP, a histone acetylase transferase that increases acetylation of histones and accessibility to the DNA demethylase [MBD2]) to the site. DNA hypermethylation and histone deacetylation are the epigenetic processes underlying inactivation of the gene promoters. Thus, the actions of CBP stabilize GR promoter activation. A recent study showed that GR expression from a neuron-specific GR (NR3C1) promoter was lower in postmortem hippocampus obtained from suicide victims with a history of childhood abuse compared with suicide victims with no childhood abuse or controls (McGowan *et al.* 2009). The investigators also found cytosine methylation of an NR3C1 promoter. These data provide direct evidence to support the preclinical studies suggesting that maternal care and postnatal maltreatment alter hippocampal GR expression levels through epigenetic mechanisms.

In most situations, gene expression set by epigenetic controls is permanent (Sweatt 2009). However, one study (Weaver *et al.* 2006) showed that a hippocampal injection of the HDAC inhibitor trichostatin A (TSA) to the offspring of adult rats who had experienced low maternal nursery activity enhanced histone acetylation, facilitated demethylation, and increased activation of the GR exon 17 promoter. Conversely, l-methionine (MET), which inhibits DNA demethylation and increases DNA methylation, blocked NGFI-A binding and attenuated GR exon 17 promoter activity in offspring who had experienced high maternal nursery activities. That study also suggested that AVP might play a role in the long-term behavioral effects of early life stress (Murgatroyd *et al.* 2009). AVP is a pituitary-adrenocorticotropin released from the hypothalamus that stimulates the secretion of ACTH from the pituitary in response to stress. ACTH then enters blood circulation and stimulates the release of glucocorticoids from the adrenal gland. Maternal separation (3 hours daily for first 10 postnatal days) is known to cause baseline hypersecretion of corticosterones, hypersensitivity of the HPA axis to acute stress, and blunted response to dexamethasone-induced suppression in adult animals (Murgatroyd *et al.* 2009). A recent study found that maternal separation also caused memory deficits in the step-down avoidance learning test and increased immobility in the forced swim test (Murgatroyd *et al.* 2009). The sustained changes were associated with increased expression of AVP but not of CRH in the paraventricular nucleus (PVN). The researchers further demonstrated that the separation caused hypomethylation in the enhancer region of the AVP gene. The AVP V1b receptor antagonist SSR149415 reduced memory deficits and increased immobility in mice subjected to the early life stress associated with maternal separation. Thus, separation stress appears to produce stable upregulation of AVP expression through epigenetic mechanisms that in turn trigger neuroendocrine and behavioral alterations.

Although not strictly related to GR modifications, other interesting developments regarding the epigenetic modification of BDNF are worth mentioning. Alterations of BDNF in the brain, CSF, and plasma of individuals with depression have been reported (Duman 2009), supporting a putative role for BDNF in mood disorders. One study that investigated altered BDNF expression following exposure of rat neonates (postnatal 1–7, Long-Evans strain) to either a stressed, behaviorally abusive mother or a cross-foster caregiving mother found that, compared with those exposed to caregiving mothers, the adult rats previously exposed to abusive mothers had significantly lower levels of exon IX BDNF mRNA in the PFC (Roth *et al.* 2009). The females exposed to abusive mothers displayed increased self-grooming and rearing in the prepartum period, behaviors thought to be related to anxiety. In addition, these females displayed more abusive behaviors toward the neonates. DNA methylation is one of the epigenetic mechanisms underlying sustained inactivation of gene promoter. Further studies revealed that exposure to an abusive mother increased exon IX BDNF DNA methylations at postnatal day 8, day 30 (young), and day 90 (adult). Methylation of exon IV BDNF DNA was also increased in adult rats exposed to an abusive mother. Thus, early life adverse experiences caused long-term suppression of BDNF expression in the PFC through epigenetic mechanisms. Interestingly, the researchers also noted that the animals cared for by mothers exposed to an abusive mother in their early development developed exon IV BDNF hypermethylation in the hippocampus. A daily infusion of zebularine, a DNA methylation inhibitor, into the left third ventricle for 7 days normalized the increases in BDNF DNA methylation. These data raise the possibility that chemical intervention can interrupt the chain of events triggered by abusive maternal behaviors by stressed mothers in the first generation, early life stress and epigenetic alterations in the second generation, maternal behavior alterations in the second generation, and epigenetic alterations in the third generation.

Clinical studies of glucocorticoid receptors

Pharmacological antagonism of GRs has also been considered a therapeutic target in the treatment of mood disorders. Mifepristone (RU-486), a nonselective GR antagonist, was investigated in clinical trials for the treatment of MDD, including MDD with psychotic symptoms; though initially encouraging, results were not subsequently replicated (Belanoff *et al.* 2001, 2002; DeBattista *et al.* 2006; Flores *et al.* 2006; Murphy *et al.* 1993; Simpson *et al.* 2005). Mifepristone was further evaluated in a double-blind, crossover design, placebo-controlled trial of 1 week in individuals with BPD. Patients in the mifepristone group showed improved neurocognitive functioning (spatial working memory, verbal fluency, and spatial recognition memory); HAM-D, and Montgomery–Åsberg Depression Rating Scale (MADRS) scores were also significantly reduced compared with baseline (Young *et al.* 2004). These efficacy data require further confirmation and careful evaluation of the risk–benefit ratio due to the side effect profile associated with this target.

Treatment with glucocorticoid synthesis inhibitors (GSIs) such as ketoconazole and metyrapone appears to significantly improve depressive symptoms in clinical and preclinical studies (reviewed in Quiroz *et al.* 2004). In a double-blind, randomized, placebo-controlled trial, metyrapone was effective as an adjunctive treatment in depression, accelerating the onset of antidepressant action (Jahn *et al.* 2004). Ketoconazole (up to 800 mg/day) was given as an add-on therapy to six depressed patients with a diagnosis of treatment-resistant BPD (Brown *et al.* 2001); reduced depressive symptoms were observed in three patients who received a dose of at least 400 mg/day, with no development of manic symptoms. Ketoconazole also reduced cortisol levels in individuals with BPD and depression, but these preliminary results need replication (Brown *et al.* 2001). Furthermore, the toxicity risk and drug interactions associated with ketoconazole use rule out its possible continuous use in mood disorders.

CRF receptor antagonists

Many of the behavioral effects observed in animals after central administration of CRH mimic symptoms of depression in humans including behavioral despair, disrupted sleep patterns, and decreased food consumption. Stress also elicits this response and is reversed by a specific CRH receptor antagonist (Berridge and Dunn 1987). Antidepressants in vitro modulate GR mRNA expression, GR protein levels, and GR function (see Carvalho and Pariante 2008). Several classes of CRF-1 inhibitors have been identified (see Holmes et al. 2003; Saunders and Williams 2003 for a review). In preclinical studies, CRF-1 antagonists diminished CRF-induced ACTH release as well as CRF-induced cAMP production.

Oral administration to non-human primates of antalarmin, a pyrrolopyrimidine compound, significantly reduced CRF-stimulated ACTH release as well as the pituitary-adrenal, sympathetic, and adrenal medullary responses to stress. It also reversed stress-induced inhibition of exploratory and sexual behaviors (Habib et al. 2000). In mice, antalarmin and fluoxetine significantly improved measures of physical state, weight gain, and emotional response in the chronic stress model (Ducottet et al. 2003). This compound also decreased swim-stress-induced ACTH response, but showed no antidepressant-like effects in the forced swim test (Jutkiewicz et al. 2005). The CRF inhibitor CP-154,526 also had antidepressant-like properties in the learned helplessness paradigm. Like antalarmin, it had significant brain-barrier penetrability and decreased synthesis of CRF in the PVN (Mansbach et al. 1997; Seymour et al. 2003). Similarly, SSR125543A, a 2-aminothiazole derivative that displays a high affinity for human CRF-1 receptors, reversed chronic mild stress-induced suppression of neurogenesis, also improving depressive-like symptoms and reducing aggressive behavior in three different animal models (Alonso et al. 2004; Farrokhi et al. 2004; Griebel et al. 2002).

In an open-label clinical trial, the CRF-1 receptor antagonist R-121919 reduced anxiety and depressive symptoms in patients with MDD (Zobel et al. 2000), but further clinical development of the compound was discontinued because of elevated liver enzyme levels (Kunzel et al. 2003). However, in an extended data report, no serious side effects were noted in the hypothalamic-pituitary-gonadal system, the hypothalamic-pituitary-thyroid axis, the renin-angiotensin system, or in prolactin or vasopressin secretion, encouraging the development of CRF-1 antagonists as antidepressant medications (Kunzel et al. 2003). Two recent double-blind, placebo-controlled studies exploring the safety and efficacy of the CRF-1 antagonist CP-316,311 in treating MDD were conducted. One study was stopped for futility during an interim analysis; though safe and well tolerated in this study population, it failed to demonstrate efficacy (Binneman et al. 2008). A more recent report (unpublished data) of patients with MDD suggested that GSK561679, a CRF-1 antagonist, also failed to demonstrate a treatment effect in a phase II clinical trial compared with placebo.

Neurogenesis

Both human brain imaging and postmortem studies implicate volumetric reductions in prefrontal cortical and hippocampal regions associated with depression (Manji et al. 2001a) (see "Functional neuroanatomy, translational neuroimaging, and new therapeutic approaches" below for further details). Studies in animals showed that behavioral stress caused dendritic spine remodeling in prefrontal cortex hippocampus and blunted neurogenesis in the hippocampal DG (Lupien et al. 2009) and that antidepressant treatment enhanced hippocampal neurogenesis in adult animals (Malberg et al. 2000). Furthermore, treatment with mood stabilizers, ECT, and atypical antipsychotics enhanced hippocampal neurogenesis (Hunsberger et al. 2009b). Adult hippocampal neurogenesis is a multiple stage process. One study showed that fluoxetine enhanced only proliferation of progenitor cells (Encinas et al. 2006); another study found that antidepressants increased neuronal turnover in the DG (Sairanen et al. 2005) (Fig. 3.7).

Although the role of neurogenesis in the pathogenesis of depression and in the behavioral action of antidepressants has been studied, results to date are conflicting. A seminal animal study investigated the effects of suppressing neurogenesis through irradiation restricted to the hippocampus. The investigators found that restricted hippocampal irradiation blocked the behavioral effects of antidepressants on feeding activity in the novelty-suppressed feeding paradigm for anxiety and on coat condition and grooming activity after chronic unpredictable stress (Santarelli et al. 2003). However, later studies found that hippocampal irradiation did not block the chronic effects of fluoxetine in the forced swim test in BALB/cJ mice (Holick et al. 2008). Hippocampal irradiation also blocked the effects of fluoxetine treatment in mice treated with corticosterone; immobility was not

Chapter 3: Mood disorders

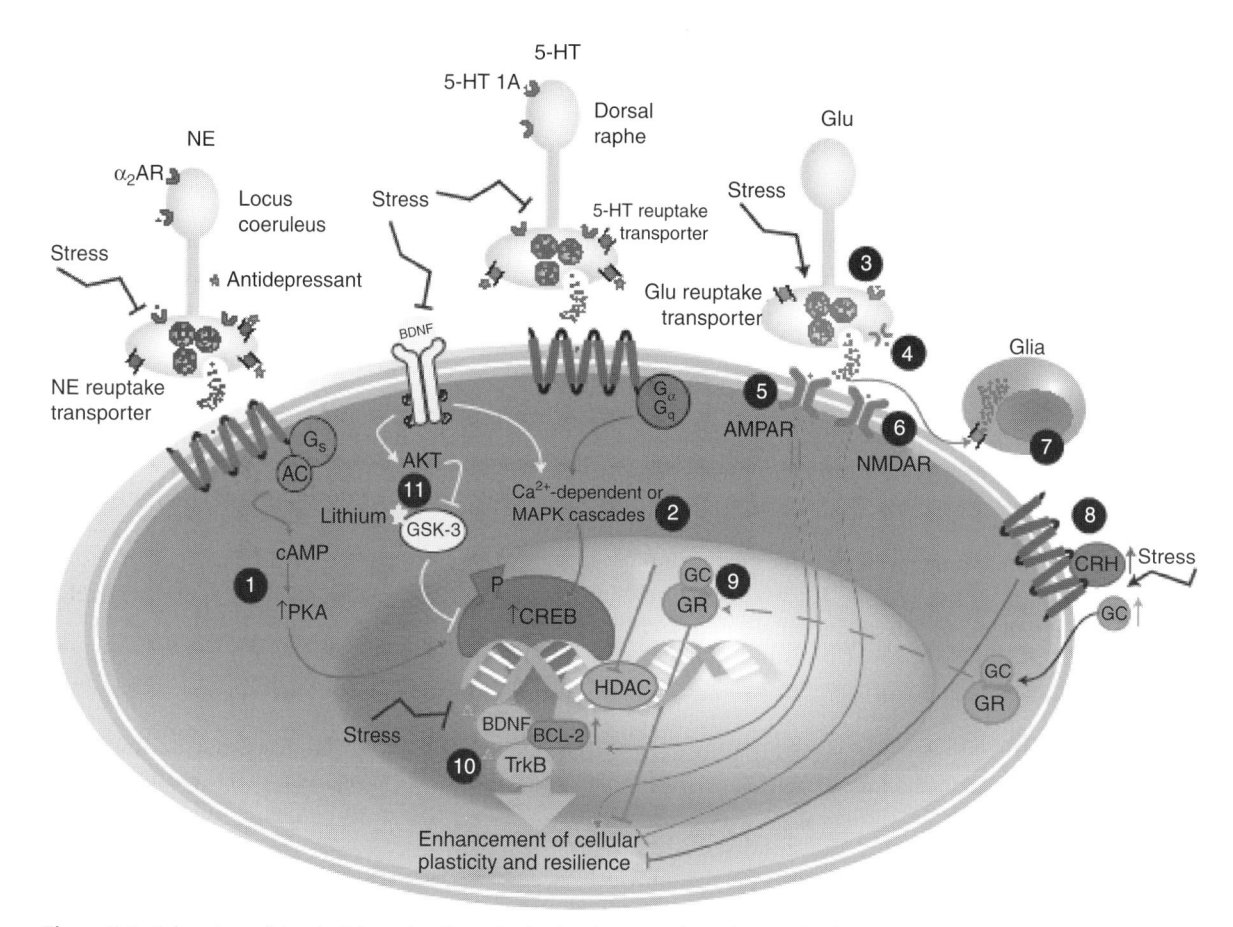

Figure 3.7. Enhancing cellular plasticity and resilience in the development of novel agents for the treatment of severe mood disorders. This figure depicts the multiple targets through which cellular plasticity and resilience may potentially be regulated in the treatment of severe mood disorders. Genetic/neurodevelopmental factors, repeated affective episodes (and likely elevations of glucocorticoids), and illness progression may all contribute to the impaired cellular resilience, volumetric reductions, and cell death and atrophy observed in mood disorders. Bcl-2 attenuates apoptosis by sequestering pro-forms of death-driving cysteine proteases (called caspases), by preventing the release of mitochondrial apoptogenic factors such as calcium, cytochrome c, and AIF into the cytoplasm, and by enhancing mitochondrial calcium uptake. Antidepressants regulate the expression of BDNF, and its receptor TrkB. Both TrkA and TrkB use the PI3K/Akt and ERK MAP kinase pathways to bring about their neurotrophic effects. The ERK MAP kinase cascade also increases the expression of Bcl-2 via its effects on CREB. (1) Phosphodiesterase inhibitors increase the levels of pCREB; (2) MAP kinase modulators increase Bcl-2 expression; (3) mGluR II/III agonists modulate the release of excessive levels of glutamate; (4) drugs such as lamotrigine and riluzole act on sodium channels to attenuate glutamate release; (5) AMPA potentiators upregulate the expression of BDNF; (6) NMDA antagonists such as ketamine enhance plasticity and cell survival; (7) novel drugs to enhance glial release of trophic factors and clear excessive glutamate may be useful for treating mood disorders; (8) CRH and (9) glucocorticoid antagonists attenuate the deleterious effects of hypercortisolemia, and CRH antagonists may exert other beneficial effects in the treatment of depression through non-HPA mechanisms; (10) agents that upregulate Bcl-2 (e.g., lithium, valproate, or pramipexole) could be useful in treating severe mood disorders as well as other disorders associated with atrophic changes; (11) GSK-3 inhibition may prevent apoptosis while also playing a role in synaptic plasticity. AIF, apoptosis-inducing factor; AMPA, alpha-amino-3-hydroxy-5-methyl-4-isoxazolepropionic acid; Bcl-2, B-cell lymphoma 2; BDNF, brain-derived neurotrophic factor; CREB, cAMP response element binding protein; CRH, corticotropin-releasing hormone; Glu, glutamate; HT, hydroxytryptophan; NE, norepinephrine; NMDA, N-methyl-D-aspartate; pCREB, phosphorylated-CREB. Reprinted from *Science Signaling STKE*, Issue 225, 2004. Charney DS, Manji HK. Life stress, genes, and depression: multiple pathways lead to increased risk and new opportunities for intervention, p. re5. This figure is reproduced in color in the color plate section.

affected by corticosterone, and the effects of fluoxetine on immobility were not affected by irradiation. Finally, in humans, a postmortem brain study found no evidence of altered hippocampal neural stem cell proliferation in individuals with mood disorders compared with controls (Reif *et al.* 2006).

Nestin is expressed by neural progenitor cells in both the subventricular zone (SVZ) and subgranular zone (SGZ) in the brain. Thymidine kinase (tk) converts ganciclovir (GCV) into a toxin that induces cell death. The expression of tk under the control of a nestin enhancer has been used to create transgenic mice in which neurogenesis can be stopped by administering GCV. In tk-expressing mice treated with GCV, chronic treatment with imipramine still reduces immobility in the tail suspension test (Singer et al. 2009). Methylazoxymethanol (MAM), an anticancer cytostatic agent, has also been used to prevent neurogenesis. Treatment with MAM alone was found to block neurogenesis (Bessa et al. 2009); furthermore, the chronic mild stress paradigm reduced neurogenesis, a change accompanied by reduced sucrose preference and increased immobility in the forced swim test. However, treatment with MAM did not block the recovery effects of antidepressants on chronic mild stress-induced sucrose preference and immobility deficits. Interestingly, MAM treatment alone increased latency to feed in the NSF test, whereas the effects of antidepressants on feeding were insignificant in MAM-treated animals. Whether or not neurogenesis is necessary for the effects of antidepressant medications requires further investigation.

Dendritic spine remodeling

The chronic restraint stress paradigm, which involves daily restraint for weeks, is a commonly used rodent stress paradigm. This paradigm causes lower body and thymus weights, spatial and working memory deficits, and anxious-like behaviors (Chen et al. 2009; Wood et al. 2004). These chronic restraint stress-induced changes correlated with brain region-specific dendritic spine remodeling (Chen et al. 2009; Mitra et al. 2005; Watanabe et al. 1992; Wood et al. 2004). Afterward, dendritic spine densities were reduced in subregions of the hippocampus and mPFC (Wood et al. 2004) and increased in the basolateral amygdala (Johnson et al. 2009; Mitra et al. 2005). Treatment with lithium or tianeptine prevented chronic restraint stress-induced neuronal structural remodeling (Johnson et al. 2009; Watanabe et al. 1992; Wood et al. 2004). It remains to be resolved whether chronic restraint stress-induced dendritic structure remodeling correlates with deficits in pleasure-seeking activity or reflects anhedonia, a core feature of depression.

The learned helplessness paradigm is frequently used to model depression and to assess antidepressant response. The escape deficits induced by the inescapable foot shock portion of the learned helplessness paradigm can also be reversed by a single injection of ketamine. In addition to escape deficits, the inescapable footshock also causes pleasure-seeking deficits as assessed by the female urine sniffing test. One recent study revealed that inescapable foot shocks reduced hippocampal synapses, a finding quantified using electron microscopic stereology (Hajszan et al. 2010). Another study found that in the chronic mild stress paradigm, stress-induced changes observed in sucrose preference and immobility correlated with reduced dendritic length and spine density in subregions of the middle PFC and hippocampus (Bessa et al. 2009). Notably, antidepressant treatment reversed these behaviors that correlated with structural reversals. Desipramine treatment for 5, but not for 1 or 3 days, improved the escape deficits and recovered the hippocampal synapse loss induced by the inescapable footshock (Hajszan et al. 2010). In summary, both the learned helplessness and chronic mild stress data clearly link the effects of stress and antidepressant treatment on dendritic remodeling and on behavioral alterations; however, whether these two correlated events are causally related requires further research.

Functional neuroanatomy, translational neuroimaging, and new therapeutic approaches
Neurocircuitry underlying the pathophysiology of mood disorders

The neurochemical abnormalities associated with mood disorders reviewed above putatively exert their pathophysiological effects to generate depressive and manic phenotypes by acting within the neural circuits that regulate emotional behavior and visceral function. The extant neuroimaging and neuropathological data particularly implicate a network formed by the mPFC and anatomically related areas of the striatum, thalamus, anterior temporal cortex, hippocampus, amygdala, hypothalamus, and brain stem in the pathophysiology of mood disorders. Many of the structures that form this extended medial prefrontal network contain abnormalities in gray matter volume, cell counts, synaptic markers, neurophysiological activity, receptor pharmacology, and/or gene expression in individuals with MDD and/or BPD. This network exerts forebrain control over emotional behavior, stress responses, and visceral functions mediated via the hypothalamus and brain stem. Dysfunction within these circuits may thus conceivably account for the disturbances in autonomic and

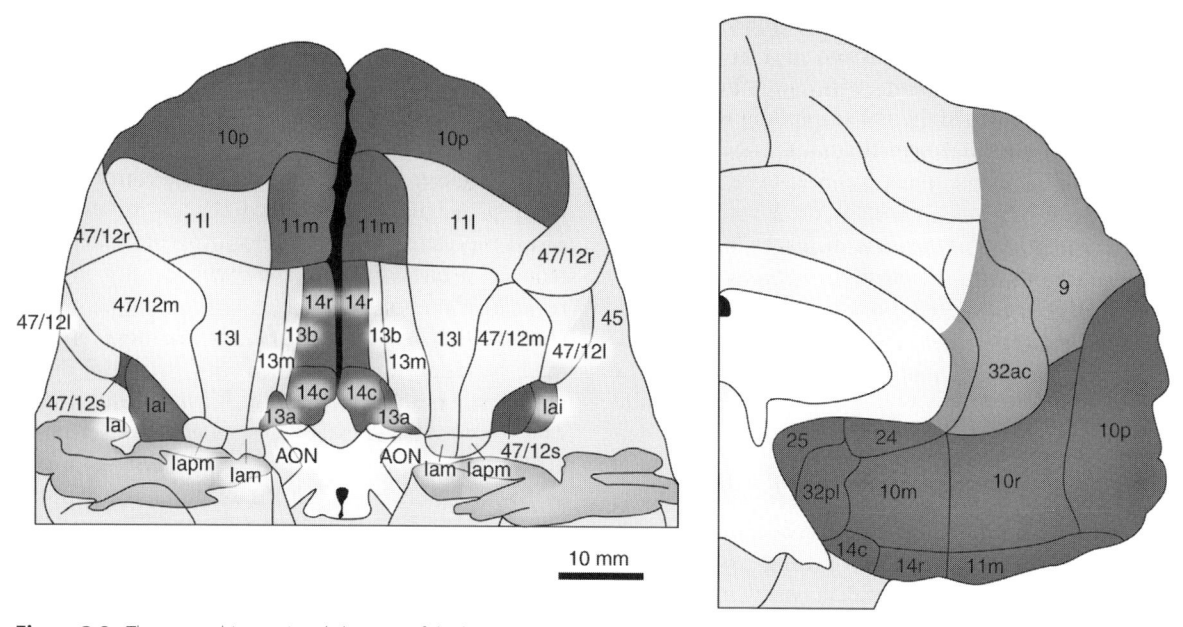

Figure 3.8. The cytoarchitectonic subdivisions of the human medial prefrontal (right) and orbital (left) cortex surfaces are distinguished here as being predominantly in the medial (red) and orbital (yellow) prefrontal networks. The orange areas are part of the dorsal prefrontal system. Modified from *Journal of Comparative Neurology*, Vol. 460, Ongur D, Ferry AT, Price JL. Architectonic subdivision of the human orbital and medial prefrontal cortex, pp. 425–449, copyright 2003, with permission from John Wiley and Sons. This figure is reproduced in color in the color plate section.

neuroendocrine function, mood, emotion–cognition interactions, and physiological and psychological responses to stress associated with mood disorders.

Convergent results from clinical studies conducted using neuroimaging and postmortem techniques further implicate these circuits as targets for antidepressant and mood-stabilizing agents. These data support the conclusions of the preclinical studies reviewed above that the effects of such agents on neuroplasticity and glutamatergic neurotransmission may underlie their therapeutic mechanisms in human mood disorders. In addition, the data obtained using neuroimaging and neuropathological techniques have converged with data in the literature regarding the circuits in which neurosurgical interventions ameliorate depression to guide the development of novel deep brain stimulation (DBS) approaches for treatment-refractory depression.

Networks involving the orbital and medial prefrontal cortex

Experiments in macaque monkeys extended previous work defining the cortical and subcortical circuits related to the orbitomedial PFC and defined two networks, referred to as the "orbital" and "medial" prefrontal networks. The areas within each network interconnect preferentially with other areas within the same network and form common connections with other parts of the cerebral cortex (Carmichael and Price 1996). Whereas structures within both the orbital and medial networks have shown abnormal hemodynamic responses during emotional, reward, and autobiographical memory studies in mood disorders, the medial network more specifically appears to contain reductions in gray matter and histopathological changes resembling those associated with rodent stress models (Price and Drevets 2010).

The PFC regions that characterize the medial network consist of areas on the ventromedial surface of the frontal lobe, rostral and ventral to the genu of the corpus callosum, areas along the medial edge of the orbital cortex, and a caudolateral orbital region at the rostral end of the anterior insula (Carmichael and Price 1996) (Fig. 3.8). The most prominent connections with the amygdala and other limbic areas also involve the medial rather than the orbital network (Carmichael and Price 1995; Kondo *et al.* 2005). In addition, the medial network forms connections with other cortical regions of the superior temporal, entorhinal, and parahippocampal cortices that have been implicated in functional and structural anatomical studies of mood disorders (reviewed in Price and Drevets 2010). Moreover, the medial network is primarily connected with the ACC and posterior cingulate cortex, whereas the orbital network connects primarily to the middle portion of the cingulate cortex (Miller *et al.* 2008). This network is also characterized by outputs to visceral control areas in the hypothalamus and PAG. None of the areas related to the medial network are directly related to a sensory modality. Instead, they together resemble the "default" system defined in functional neuroimaging studies as areas that are active in a resting state but decrease activity in some cognitive–behavioral tasks (Drevets and Raichle 1998; Grimm *et al.* 2009; Raichle *et al.* 2001). Thus, whereas the orbital network appears to subserve a sensory-related system, the medial network instead appears to constitute a system that modulates visceral function related to emotion, stress, reward, or other factors.

Although substantial outputs from the medial prefrontal network target the hypothalamus, the PAG, and other visceral control centers (An *et al.* 1998; Barbas *et al.* 2003; Freedman *et al.* 2000; Ongur *et al.* 1998a; Rempel-Clower and Barbas 1998), the cortex ventral to the corpus callosum genu (i.e., "subgenual") provides the heaviest projections, which terminate in both the medial and lateral hypothalamus and in both the dorsolateral and ventrolateral columns of the PAG. The fibers from the lateral part of the medial network (i.e., part of the agranular anterior insula and intrasulcal 47/12) are restricted to the lateral hypothalamus and ventrolateral PAG (An *et al.* 1998; Ongur *et al.* 1998a). Electrical stimulation of these medial network areas disturbs autonomic functions such as heart rate and respiration (Kaada 1960), and functional MRI studies show that activity in the medial PFC correlates with changes in autonomic activity (Critchley *et al.* 2000; Teves *et al.* 2004; Williams *et al.* 2000). Conversely, lesions of the medial PFC decrease parasympathetic autonomic regulation of heart rate but *increase* sympathetic autonomic, glucocorticoid, and behavioral responses to stressors or fear-conditioned stimuli in rats (Diorio *et al.* 1993; Frysztak and Neafsey 1994; Morgan and LeDoux 1995; Sullivan and Gratton 1999). In humans, lesions of the ventromedial PFC abolish the normal visceral response to emotive stimuli (Bechara *et al.* 2000; Damasio *et al.* 1990) and impair the ability to use emotional processing to guide social behavior. To account for such deficits, investigators proposed that the visceral reaction accompanying emotion serves as a warning or guide to decision-making and social behavior (Damasio 1994). In mood disorders, overactivation of this system may conceivably produce the chronic sense of "unease" that is a common component of depression, compatible with evidence that depression severity correlates positively with metabolism in ventromedial PFC regions during depressive episodes (e.g., Hasler *et al.* 2008; Osuch *et al.* 2000).

Within the lateral PFC, several areas are closely related to the medial and orbital prefrontal networks. Notably, the lateral PFC areas consistently implicated in studies of depression interconnect specifically with the medial prefrontal network. These regions include areas 9, 46d, and 10 at the frontal pole and area 45a. As with the medial network, these regions send efferent projections to the hypothalamus and PAG, positioning this lateral PFC system anatomically so that it also can modulate visceral functions.

The axonal projections sent by the amygdala, hippocampal subiculum, and the primary olfactory, entorhinal, perirhinal, and parahippocampal cortices to both the orbital and medial PFC (Carmichael and Price 1995; Carmichael *et al.* 1994; Kondo *et al.* 2005) and the mediodorsal thalamic nucleus – medial portion (MDm) (Russchen *et al.* 1985) are excitatory and probably glutamatergic. The MDm also receives GABAergic inputs from the ventral pallidum and rostral globus pallidus (Churchill *et al.* 1996; Kuroda and Price 1991a), which form part of the cortico-striato-pallido-thalamic loop involving the orbital and medial PFC. In the MDm, the GABAergic terminals of afferent pallidal fibers synapse on the same dendrites and often on the same dendritic spines as the excitatory terminals from the amygdala and other limbic structures (Kuroda and Price 1991b). These convergent but antagonistic inputs presumably interact to modulate reciprocal thalamo-cortical interactions between the orbital and medial PFC and MDm. Although limbic inputs predominate, the sustained thalamo-cortical and cortico-thalamic activities allow for continuing behavior patterns. When pallidal inputs become more prominent, ongoing patterns are interrupted, allowing a switch from one behavior to another. The affected "behaviors" would presumably include those associated with the orbital and medial PFC: mood, value assessment of objects, and stimulus–reward associations (Price and Drevets 2010). Thus, lesions of the ventral striatum and pallidum, MD, or the orbital and medial PFC can cause perseverative deficits in stimulus–reward reversal tasks in rats and monkeys, such that the animals have difficulty switching from previously rewarded, but now unrewarded, stimuli (Ferry *et al.* 2000*a*; Kazama and Bachevalier 2009; McBride and Slotnick 1997; Roberts *et al.* 1990). A similar deficit in mood disorders might be the persistence of a negative mood or mind-set beyond the resolution of traumatic or stressful events.

Within the striatum, the orbital and medial PFC projects principally to the rostral ventromedial striatum (Calzavara *et al.* 2007). The PFC regions involved in the medial network project to the NAc and the adjacent medial caudate nucleus (Ferry *et al.* 2000*b*). The amygdala input to the striatum coexists with the medial network. Notably, area 25 in the subgenual PFC projects specifically to the "shell" of the NAc, where dysfunction may particularly interfere with reward- or goal-directed behaviors.

Structural neuroimaging abnormalities in mood disorders

The neuroimaging abnormalities found in MDD and BPD converge with observations based on clinical manifestations of lesions or degenerative illnesses of the striatum and lesions of the orbital and medial PFC to implicate the limbic-cortico-striato-pallido-thalamic circuitry in the pathophysiology of mood disorders. Because the neurological disorders that involve this limbic cortico-striato-pallido-thalamic circuitry affect synaptic transmission in diverse ways, it appears that dysfunction that alters transmission in a variety of ways can produce the pathological emotional symptoms that manifest as MDD (Drevets *et al.* 2004*a*).

Patients with mood disorders show morphological or morphometric abnormalities in several cortical and limbic structures associated with the medial prefrontal network (Price and Drevets 2010). The prominence or presence of these abnormalities depends partly on clinical characteristics such as age of onset, capacity for developing psychosis or mania, and evidence of familial aggregation of illness. Depressed individuals who consistently show volumetric abnormalities within the medial prefrontal network exhibit early age of onset and presence of illness in first-degree relatives. In contrast, elderly individuals with late-onset depression or mania show nonspecific imaging correlates of cerebrovascular disease (reviewed in Drevets *et al.* 2004*a*). Similarly, individuals with MDD or BPD who have either delusions or late-life onset show nonspecific atrophy manifested by lateral ventricle enlargement. Nevertheless, such cases have been differentiated more specifically from relevant control groups on the basis of lesions or more prominent gray matter loss within the orbital and medial PFC (Coryell *et al.* 2005; MacFall *et al.* 2001).

The most prominent volumetric abnormalities reported in MDD and BPD have been reduced gray matter in the left subgenual ACC (i.e., BA 24 subgenual) and infralimbic cortex (i.e., BA 25) (Botteron *et al.* 2002; Coryell *et al.* 2005; Drevets *et al.* 1997; Hirayasu *et al.* 1999; Koo *et al.* 2008; Ongur *et al.* 1998*b*, 2003). The extant data suggest that this volumetric reduction exists early in the illness and in young adults at high familial risk for MDD (Boes *et al.* 2008; Botteron *et al.* 2002; Drevets *et al.* 2004*b*; Hirayasu *et al.* 1999) and shows progression in subjects with psychotic mood disorders (Koo *et al.* 2008). The deficit applies to males (Boes *et al.* 2008; Hastings *et al.* 2004) and females (Botteron *et al.* 2002), to psychotic MDD, to bipolar depression (Adler *et al.* 2007; Coryell *et al.* 2005; Hirayasu *et al.* 1999), and to bipolar-spectrum illness (Haznedar *et al.* 2005). In individuals with BPD, chronic lithium treatment was associated with increasing gray matter volume toward normal in treatment responders in the subgenual ACC and other PFC areas (Drevets *et al.* 2008; Moore *et al.* 2009); in contrast, reduced subgenual ACC volume persisted in individuals with MDD despite successful treatment with SSRIs (Drevets *et al.* 1997).

The abnormal reduction in subgenual ACC volume has been identified primarily in subjects with mood disorders characterized by familial aggregation (Hirayasu *et al.* 1999). Notably, studies showed that reduced volume of the right "perigenual" ACC (including both the subgenual ACC and the "pregenual" ACC situated anterior to the corpus callosum genu) was associated with increasing genetic risk for BPD based on the number of affected relatives (McDonald *et al.* 2004). Moreover, the left perigenual ACC volume was smaller in boys with subclinical depressive symptoms and correlated inversely with depressive symptoms in boys with a family history of depression (Boes *et al.* 2008). These data suggest that genetic vulnerability factors play a role in the pathogenesis of MDD. One finding relevant to this conclusion is that the short allele of the serotonin transporter promoter region length polymorphism (5HTT-PRL), which reportedly increases vulnerability for developing MDD within the context of stress (Caspi et al. 2003), was also associated with reduced subgenual ACC gray matter volume (Pezawas et al. 2005).

Gray matter is also reduced in parts of the orbitofrontal cortex (BA 11 and intrasulcal 47) in patients with MDD and BPD, in the ventrolateral PFC (BA 45), frontal polar/dorsal anterolateral PFC (BA 9, 10), parahippocampal gyrus, and temporopolar cortex in MDD, and in the posterior cingulate cortex and superior temporal gyrus in patients with BPD (Bowen et al. 1989; Drevets and Price 2005; Drevets et al. 2004a; Lyoo et al. 2004; Nugent et al. 2006; Rajkowska et al. 1999). Some studies also reported reduced hippocampal volume in MDD ranging in magnitude from 8% to 19%, although other studies did not replicate these differences (reviewed in Drevets et al. 2004a). One study reported that reduced hippocampal volume was limited to depressed women who suffered early-life trauma (Vythilingam et al. 2002), and others reported that hippocampal volume correlated inversely with time spent depressed (e.g., Sheline et al. 2003). The reduced hippocampal volume persisted despite prolonged symptom remission (Neumeister et al. 2005).

Amygdalar volume has been reported to be increased in some studies but decreased in others in individuals with depression relative to controls (reviewed in Drevets et al. 2004a). Nevertheless, higher resolution volumetric MRI data indicated that amygdalar volume is abnormally smaller in unmedicated individuals with BPD, but larger in patients with BPD receiving mood-stabilizing treatments that exert neurotrophic effects in experimental animals (Savitz et al. 2010). In the striatum, investigators found a smaller caudate nucleus volume in individuals with depression than in controls, consistent with a postmortem study (Baumann et al. 1999) that found that caudate and accumbens area volumes were decreased in both MDD and BPD samples relative to controls (Baumann et al. 1999; Krishnan et al. 1992). Nevertheless, other imaging studies reported inconsistent results in striatal or pallidal volumes between MDD subjects and controls (reviewed in Drevets et al. 2004a).

Finally, consistent with evidence that HPA axis function is elevated in some individuals with mood disorders, the pituitary and adrenal glands are enlarged in patients with MDD (Drevets et al. 2004a; Krishnan et al. 1991), probably reflecting elevated stimulation by CRH and ACTH. The findings of blunted ACTH responses to CRF in vivo, reduced CRF receptor density in the PFC, and increased corticotrophic cell size and mRNA levels in the pituitary in postmortem samples of individuals with mood disorders also indicate chronic activation of the HPA axis (Gold and Chrousos 2002; Lopez et al. 1992; Swaab et al. 2005).

Neurophysiological imaging studies of patients with mood disorders

Many regions in which structural abnormalities appear in people with mood disorders also have abnormalities of blood flow and glucose metabolism. Generally, the structures that form the medial prefrontal network show increased glucose metabolism in the depressed phase relative to the remitted phase of MDD – for instance, as manifested by longitudinal studies of depressed patients scanned before compared with after treatment (e.g., Drevets et al. 2002) and of remitted patients imaged before compared with during depressive relapse (e.g., Hasler et al. 2008; Neumeister et al. 2004). Nevertheless, the reduced gray matter volume in some structures appears sufficiently prominent to produce partial volume effects in functional brain images due to their low spatial resolution. For example, whereas some studies found that depressed subjects with MDD and BPD show metabolic activity that appears *reduced* in the subgenual ACC relative to controls (Drevets et al. 1997, 2002; Kegeles et al. 2003; Ketter et al. 2001; Kruger et al. 2003; Liotti et al. 2002; Pizzagalli et al. 2004), other studies reported increased metabolic activity in the subgenual ACC in primary (Bauer et al. 2005; Clark et al. 2006; Dunn et al. 2002; Kumano et al. 2006; Mah et al. 2007; Mayberg et al. 2005) or secondary depression (Inagaki et al. 2007). These apparently discrepant results may be explained by the inter-relationship between deficits in gray matter volume and physiological imaging data measured using low resolution PET, because correction of the metabolic data for partial volume averaging effect indicates that metabolism is actually *increased* in the subgenual ACC in the unmedicated depressed phase (Drevets and Price 2005).

Compatible with this conclusion, subgenual ACC metabolism (1) increases in remitted individuals with MDD during depressive relapse by either tryptophan depletion (Neumeister et al. 2004) or catecholamine depletion (Hasler et al. 2008); (2) decreases during successful treatment with antidepressants (Drevets et al. 1997, 2002; Holthoff et al. 2004; Mayberg et al. 2000) or DBS (Mayberg et al. 2005); (3) is positively correlated with the severity of depression in MDD (e.g., Osuch et al. 2000); (4) increases in healthy humans during experimentally induced sadness (George et al. 1995; Mayberg et al. 1999); (5) appears abnormally elevated in depressed subjects with BPD medicated chronically with lithium, in whom gray matter volume presumably has normalized, thus eliminating the partial volume effect associated with regional atrophy (Bauer et al. 2005; Drevets et al. 2008; Mah et al. 2007; Moore et al. 2009).

Hemodynamic activity increases in the perigenual ACC during a variety of emotional–behavioral tasks including sadness induction (George et al. 1995; Mayberg et al. 1999), exposure to traumatic reminders (reviewed in Rauch and Drevets 2008), selecting sad versus happy targets (Elliott et al. 2000), monitoring internal states (Gillath et al. 2005), and extinction learning (Phelps et al. 2004). In contrast, more dorsal regions of the pregenual ACC show physiological responses to more diverse types of emotional stimuli (Bush et al. 2000; Critchley et al. 2003; Drevets and Raichle 1998). Notably, *higher activity* in the pregenual ACC holds *positive prognostic significance* in MDD, because improvement during antidepressant treatment correlates with higher *pretreatment* pregenual ACC metabolism and electrophysiological activity (Mayberg et al. 1997; Pizzagalli et al. 2001; Wu et al. 1992).

Although the pattern of activity in the medial network is generally one of elevated metabolism in the depressed compared with the remitted phases, the relationship between activity and symptom severity differs in valence across structures, consistent with preclinical evidence that distinct medial PFC structures are involved in opposing processes with respect to emotional behavior (Vidal-Gonzalez et al. 2006). Regions where metabolic activity correlates *negatively* with depression severity in MDD include the left ventrolateral PFC/lateral OFC (approximately BA 45a and 47s, respectively) (Drevets et al. 2004a; Price and Drevets 2010), where increased activity during depressive episodes appears to reflect a compensatory response that modulates depressive symptoms. In contrast, regions where metabolism correlates *positively* with depression severity include the amygdala, subgenual ACC, and ventromedial frontal polar cortex (reviewed in Price and Drevets 2010). Metabolism and blood flow decrease in these regions during recovery associated with antidepressant drug treatment or with DBS of the subgenual ACC or anterior capsule (Drevets et al. 2002; Mayberg et al. 1999, 2005; Van Laere et al. 2006). Conversely, individuals with MDD who recovered and then experienced depressive relapse under experimental conditions involving catecholamine or serotonin depletion show increased metabolic activity in the subgenual ACC and ventromedial frontal polar cortex (Hasler et al. 2008; Neumeister et al. 2004). Left amygdala activity also increased during tryptophan depletion-induced relapse, but only in individuals with MDD who were homozygous for the long allele of the 5HTT-PRL polymorphism (Neumeister et al. 2006b). Evidence for additional clinical specificity comes from findings demonstrating that, under resting baseline conditions, elevated metabolic activity in the amygdala and other structures occurs predominantly in depressed subjects classified as having BPD, familial pure depressive disease (FPDD), or melancholic subtype and to subjects who show cortisol hypersecretion or responsiveness to total sleep deprivation (reviewed in Drevets 2001; Drevets et al. 2002).

Abnormal hemodynamic responses in the amygdala to specific types of emotional stimuli have been observed in a broader range of depressed subjects. In individuals with MDD, the amygdala shows exaggerated hemodynamic responses during exposure to sad words (Siegle et al. 2002), explicitly presented sad faces (Drevets et al. 2001; Fu et al. 2004), masked fearful faces (Sheline et al. 2001; Victor et al. 2010), and masked sad faces (Fu et al. 2004). Similar increases in amygdala activity in response to sad faces were observed in unmedicated-remitted subjects with MDD (Neumeister et al. 2006a; Victor et al. 2010), suggesting that this abnormality is trait-like in MDD. These data appear generally consistent with behavioral evidence that depressed patients manifest a mood-congruent processing bias in which stimulus processing is preferentially directed toward negative information (Elliott et al. 2000; Murphy et al. 1999; Murray et al. 1999).

Finally, in the depressed phases of MDD or BPD, metabolism in the accumbens, medial thalamus, and posterior cingulate cortex is abnormally elevated and hemodynamic responses to rewarding or emotional stimuli are altered (Drevets *et al.* 2002, 2004*a*). For example, in functional MRI studies, individuals with MDD show attenuated hemodynamic responses in the ventral striatum in reward-processing tasks and in the ventral striatum and posterior cingulate cortex in tasks involving negative feedback (e.g., Drevets 2007; Knutson *et al.* 2007; Taylor Tavares *et al.* 2008).

Neuropathological correlations with neuroimaging abnormalities

The structural imaging abnormalities observed in mood disorders discussed above are associated with histopathological abnormalities in postmortem studies of MDD and BPD: reduced gray matter volume thickness or wet weight in the subgenual ACC, posterior orbital cortex, and ventral striatum (Baumann *et al.* 1999; Bowen *et al.* 1989; Ongur *et al.* 1998*b*; Rajkowska *et al.* 1999) and greater decrements in volume following fixation (interpreted as indicating a neuropil deficit) in the hippocampus (Stockmeier *et al.* 2004) in MDD and BPD subjects relative to controls; reductions in glia, synapses or synaptic proteins, and neuronal size have also been noted in MDD and BPD samples (Cotter *et al.* 2001, 2002; Eastwood and Harrison 2000, 2001; Ongur *et al.* 1998*b*; Rajkowska *et al.* 1999; Uranova *et al.* 2004). Abnormal reductions in glial cell counts and density and glia-to-neuron ratios also extend to the pregenual ACC (Cotter *et al.* 2001), dorsal anterolateral PFC (BA 9) (Cotter *et al.* 2002; Uranova *et al.* 2004), and amygdala (Bowley *et al.* 2002; Hamidi *et al.* 2004) in MDD. Finally, the mean size of neurons was abnormally reduced in the dorsal anterolateral PFC (BA 9) in patients with MDD (Rajkowska *et al.* 1999), and the density of nonpyramidal neurons was decreased in the ACC and hippocampus in patients with BPD (Benes *et al.* 2001; Todtenkopf *et al.* 2005), and in the dorsal anterolateral PFC (BA 9) in those with MDD (Rajkowska *et al.* 2007). Reductions in synapses and synaptic proteins were evident in BPD subjects in the hippocampal subiculum/ventral CA1 region (Eastwood and Harrison 2000; Rosoklija *et al.* 2000), and the expression of multiple genes involved in axonal growth and synaptic function was reduced in MDD subjects in the middle temporal cortex (Aston *et al.* 2005).

The glial cell type implicated most consistently in mood disorders has been the oligodendrocyte (e.g., Hamidi *et al.* 2004; Uranova *et al.* 2004), including the satellite (perineuronal) oligodendrocytes (Uranova *et al.* 2001; Vostrikov *et al.* 2007). Perineuronal oligodendrocytes are immunohistochemically reactive for glutamine synthetase, suggesting that they function like astrocytes to take up synaptically released glutamate for conversion to glutamine and cycling back into neurons (D'Amelio *et al.* 1990). Reductions in astroglia or astroglial markers also have been observed in postmortem studies of individuals with mood disorders (Johnston-Wilson *et al.* 2000), although other studies found no abnormalities in the number of glial fibrillary acidic protein-stained cells or glial fibrillary acidic protein levels in individuals with MDD or BPD (Hamidi *et al.* 2004; Webster *et al.* 2001). These reductions in perineuronal oligodendroglia, and possibly also in astrocytes, suggest that clearance of intrasynaptic glutamate may be impaired in people with mood disorders because of the important role that these cells play in glutamate transport and cycling.

MRS measures of glutamate, glutamine, and GABA

MRS studies of individuals with MDD show reduced cerebral concentrations of GABA and a reduced "Glx" spectral peak, which reflect the combined concentrations of glutamate plus glutamine. These findings appear compatible with the postmortem observation of cellular reductions, because these spectra are overwhelmingly dominated by the intracellular pools of the associated neurotransmitters. Depressed individuals with MDD show abnormally reduced GABA levels in the dorsomedial/dorsal anterolateral PFC and occipital cortex (Hasler *et al.* 2007; Sanacora *et al.* 1999). Most of the GABA pool exists within GABAergic neurons, so the reduction in GABA in the dorsal anterolateral PFC is compatible with the reduction in GABAergic neurons found in this region (BA 9) in patients with MDD (Rajkowska *et al.* 2007). Depressed patients also show abnormally reduced Glx levels in the dorsomedial/dorsal anterolateral and ventromedial PFC (Hasler *et al.* 2007), compatible with the postmortem reductions in glial cells found in the same regions in individuals with MDD.

Relationship to rodent stress models

In regions that appear homologous to the areas where gray matter reductions are evident in depressed humans (i.e., medial PFC, hippocampus), in rodents, repeated stress results in dendritic atrophy and reduced oligoglial cell counts (Banasr and Duman 2007; Czeh et al. 2005; McEwen and Magarinos 2001; Radley et al. 2008; Wellman 2001). Dendritic atrophy would be reflected by a decrease in the volume of the neuropil that occupies most of the gray matter volume, leading to the hypothesis that a homologous process accounts for the reduced gray matter volume in hippocampal and PFC structures in patients with MDD and BPD (McEwen and Magarinos 2001). In rats, stress-induced dendritic atrophy in the medial PFC was associated with impaired extinction to fear-conditioned stimuli (Izquierdo et al. 2006), suggesting that this process can alter emotional behavior.

In contrast, in the basolateral amygdala (BLA), chronic unpredictable stress produced dendritic atrophy whereas chronic immobilization stress instead *increased* dendritic branching (Banasr and Duman 2007; Vyas et al. 2002, 2003). Moreover, repeated stress resulted in hyperexcitability in the BLA in rodents, a finding associated with exaggerated fear responses (Shekhar et al. 2005; Vyas et al. 2006). These findings suggest mechanisms that may contribute to pathological amygdala activity in depression.

The finding that reduced cortex volume or histopathological changes appear specifically in regions that show elevated glucose metabolism during depression raises the possibility that excitatory amino acid transmission plays a role in the neuropathology of mood disorders. Cerebral glucose metabolism largely reflects the energy requirements associated with glutamatergic transmission (Shulman et al. 2004). In agreement with the neuroimaging evidence of elevated activity in this circuit, postmortem studies of the NMDA receptor complex in suicide victims found that glutamatergic transmission was increased in the PFC antemortem in individuals with depression (Paul and Skolnick 2003). Because stress-induced dendritic remodeling depends on interactions between glucocorticoid hypersecretion and NMDA receptor stimulation, the elevated glutamatergic transmission within discrete anatomical circuits in patients with MDD and BPD also may explain the targeted nature of gray matter changes in those with mood disorders (e.g., affecting the left more than the right subgenual ACC) (Drevets and Price 2005; McEwen and Magarinos 2001; Shansky et al. 2009).

Implications of neurocircuitry-based models of depression for treatment mechanisms

The abnormalities of structure and function evident within the extended medial prefrontal network may impair this network's modulation of endocrine, autonomic, emotional, and behavioral responses to aversive and reward-related stimuli or to stressful and social contexts (Ongur et al. 2003), potentially accounting for the disturbances seen within these domains in mood disorders. Through potentially diverse mechanisms, antidepressant and mood-stabilizing treatments may exert their therapeutic actions by countering dysregulation within this network. For example, neurophysiological activity in the amygdala decreases in rats, monkeys, and humans during administration of antidepressant drugs from multiple pharmacological classes, vagal nerve stimulation, or DBS of the anterior capsule (Drevets et al. 2002; Fu et al. 2004; Gerber et al. 1983; Henry et al. 1998; Horovitz 1966; Sheline et al. 2001; Van Laere et al. 2006). In depressed humans, metabolism and blood flow also decrease in the subgenual ACC/ventromedial PFC in response to chronic treatment with antidepressant drugs, vagus nerve stimulation, or DBS of the subgenual ACC or anterior capsule (Conway et al. 2006; Drevets et al. 2002; Mayberg et al. 1999, 2005; Nahas et al. 2007; Van Laere et al. 2006). Preliminary reports further suggest that the abnormally elevated metabolism in the accumbens area in primary depression or in depression associated with obsessive-compulsive disorder is attenuated by chronic SSRI treatment or DBS of the anterior capsule (Drevets et al. 2006; Van Laere et al. 2006). Similarly, DBS applied via electrodes situated in the accumbens area/ventral internal capsule improves depressive symptoms in individuals with treatment-refractory MDD (Schlaepfer et al. 2008). Thus, a variety of treatments for depression, involving pharmacological, neurosurgical, or DBS methods, appear to suppress pathological activity within components of the extended medial prefrontal network (Drevets and Price 2005; Drevets et al. 2002; Mayberg et al. 2005; Van Laere et al. 2006).

Finally, as discussed previously, some mood-stabilizing and antidepressant drugs may exert therapeutic effects by enhancing the expression of neurotrophic factors that protect or restore medial network function from the effects of repeated stress (Manji et al. 2001a; Santarelli et al. 2003). For example, cognitive–behavioral strategies for managing depressive symptoms theoretically rely on enhancing the function of PFC systems that modulate limbic activity, thereby enhancing the normal role of cortico-limbic circuits in modulating emotional expression and experience (Siegle *et al.* 2006). The neuroplastic effects of mood-stabilizing and antidepressant treatments reviewed in this chapter may thus play a critical role in preserving or restoring the function of PFC projections that enable "top-down" modulation of emotional and visceromotor processing in individuals vulnerable to mood disorders.

Conclusions

We have provided an overview of some of the most fundamental aspects of recent translational research into the pathophysiology of mood disorders, focusing on preclinical, clinical, and neuroimaging findings. As noted in the Introduction, the pathophysiology of these disorders must account not only for profound changes in mood seen in these disorders but also for a constellation of neurovegetative features derived from dysfunction in limbic-related regions such as the hippocampus, hypothalamus, and brain stem. Notably, the highly integrated monoamine and prominent neuropeptide pathways are known to originate and project heavily within these regions of the brain; it is thus not surprising that abnormalities have been noted in their function across clinical studies. Whereas dysfunction within these neurotransmitter and neuropeptide systems is likely to play an important role in mediating some facets of illness pathophysiology, they likely represent the downstream effects of other, more primary abnormalities in cellular signaling. Thus, these illnesses can best be conceptualized as genetically influenced disorders of synapses and circuits rather than simply as deficits or excesses in individual neurotransmitters. Furthermore, many of these pathways play critical roles not only in synaptic (and therefore behavioral) plasticity but also in long-term atrophic processes. Abnormalities in cellular signaling that regulate diverse physiological functions also likely explain the tremendous comorbidity with a variety of medical conditions (notably cardiovascular disease, diabetes mellitus, obesity, and migraine) and substance abuse seen in individuals with mood disorders.

The abnormalities in cellular plasticity likely also represent the underpinnings of the impaired structural plasticity seen in morphometric studies of mood disorders. Many of these pathways play critical roles not only in "here and now" synaptic plasticity but also in long-term cell growth/atrophy and cell survival/cell death. For instance, the atrophic changes observed in multiple cell types (neurons and glia), as well as the reversibility of the changes with treatment, support a role for intracellular plasticity cascades. It is likely that the major defect is in the ability to regulate neuroplastic adaptations to perturbations (both physiological and pathophysiological) – an inability to handle "normal loads" (e.g., neurochemical, hormonal, stress-induced, pharmacologically induced) without failing or invoking compensatory adaptations that overshoot and predispose to oscillations. This allostatic load contributes to long-term disease progression (and potentially to cycle acceleration). Many of the same "plasticity regulators" also play a critical role in cell survival, cell death, and cellular resilience. These observations serve to explain the atrophic, and perhaps degenerative, aspect of the illness in some patients as well as the presence of signs normally associated with ischemic and hypoxic insults, such as white matter hyperintensities.

It is also becoming increasingly clear that, for many patients with refractory mood disorders, new drugs simply mimicking the "traditional" drugs that directly or indirectly alter biogenic amine levels and those that bind to their cell surface receptors may be of limited benefit. Such strategies implicitly assume that the target receptor(s) and downstream signal mediators are functionally intact and that altered synaptic activity will thus be transduced to modify the postsynaptic "throughput" of the system. However, the possible existence of abnormalities in intracellular signal transduction pathways suggests that, for patients refractory to conventional medications, improved therapeutics may only be obtained by directly targeting postreceptor sites. Recent discoveries concerning a variety of mechanisms involved in the formation and inactivation of second messengers offer the promise of developing novel pharmacological agents designed to target signal transduction pathways (Guo *et al.* 2000).

Although it would clearly be more complex than developing receptor-specific drugs, it may be possible to design novel agents to selectively affect second messenger systems, because they are heterogeneous at the molecular and cellular levels, are linked to receptors in a variety of ways, and are expressed in different stoichiometries in different cell types (Manji and Duman 2001). In addition, because signal transduction pathways display certain unique characteristics depending on their activity state, they offer built-in targets for relative specificity of action, depending on the "set-point" of the substrate. It is also notable that a variety of strategies to enhance neurotrophic factor signaling are currently under investigation. An increasing number of strategies are being investigated to develop small molecular switches for protein–protein interactions, which have the potential to regulate the activity of growth factors, MAP kinase cascades, and interactions between homo- and heterodimers of the Bcl-2 family of proteins (Guo *et al.* 2000).

Taken together, the evidence presented in this chapter advances our understanding of the pathophysiology of mood disorders and suggests that recent translational research holds much promise for developing improved therapeutics to treat these devastating illnesses and improve the lives of millions worldwide.

Disclosure/Conflict of interest: All authors report no potential conflict of interest related to this work. Dr. Drevets was supported by an unrestricted grant from the William K. Warren Foundation. Drs. Chen and Manji are full-time employees of Johnson and Johnson Pharmaceuticals Group. Dr. Quiroz is a full-time employee of Hoffman-LaRoche, Inc. Ms. Henter gratefully acknowledges the support of the Intramural Research Program of the National Institute of Mental Health, National Institutes of Health.

References

aan het Rot M, Collins KA, Murrough JW *et al.* 2010. Safety and efficacy of repeated-dose intravenous ketamine for treatment-resistant depression. *Biol Psychiatry* 67:139–145.

Adler CM, Delbello MP, Jarvis K *et al.* 2007. Voxel-based study of structural changes in first-episode patients with bipolar disorder. *Biol Psychiatry* 61:776–781.

Aguado L, San Antonio A, Perez L, del Valle R, Gomez J. 1994. Effects of the NMDA receptor antagonist ketamine on flavor memory: conditioned aversion, latent inhibition, and habituation of neophobia. *Behav Neural Biol* 61:271–281.

Alonso R, Griebel G, Pavone G *et al.* 2004. Blockade of CRF(1) or V(1b) receptors reverses stress-induced suppression of neurogenesis in a mouse model of depression. *Mol Psychiatry* 9:278–286, 224.

An X, Bandler R, Ongur D, Price JL. 1998. Prefrontal cortical projections to longitudinal columns in the midbrain periaqueductal gray in macaque monkeys. *J Comp Neurol* 401:455–479.

Aston C, Jiang L, Sokolov BP. 2005. Transcriptional profiling reveals evidence for signaling and oligodendroglial abnormalities in the temporal cortex from patients with major depressive disorder. *Mol Psychiatry* 10:309–322.

Aubry JM, Schwald M, Ballmann E, Karege F. 2009. Early effects of mood stabilizers on the Akt/GSK-3beta signaling pathway and on cell survival and proliferation. *Psychopharmacol (Berl)* 205:419–429.

Bachmann RF, Schloesser RJ, Gould TD, Manji HK. 2005. Mood stabilizers target cellular plasticity and resilience cascades: implications for the development of novel therapeutics. *Mol Neurobiol* 32:173–202.

Bai F, Li X, Clay M, Lindstrom T, Skolnick P. 2001. Intra- and interstrain differences in models of "behavioral despair". *Pharmacol Biochem Behav* 70:187–192.

Banasr M, Duman RS. 2007. Regulation of neurogenesis and gliogenesis by stress and antidepressant treatment. *CNS Neurol Disord Drug Targets* 6:311–320.

Bannerman DM, Good MA, Butcher SP, Ramsay M, Morris RG. 1995. Distinct components of spatial learning revealed by prior training and NMDA receptor blockade. *Nature* 378:182–186.

Barbas H, Saha S, Rempel-Clower N, Ghashghaei T. 2003. Serial pathways from primate prefrontal cortex to autonomic areas may influence emotional expression. *BMC Neurosci* 4:25.

Bauer M, London ED, Rasgon N *et al.* 2005. Supraphysiological doses of levothyroxine alter regional cerebral metabolism and improve mood in bipolar depression. *Mol Psychiatry* 10:456–469.

Baumann B, Danos P, Krell D *et al.* 1999. Reduced volume of limbic system-affiliated basal ganglia in mood disorders: preliminary data from a post mortem study. *J Neuropsych Clin Neurosci* 11:71–78.

Bearden CE, Thompson PM, Dalwani M *et al.* 2007. Greater cortical gray matter density in lithium-treated patients with bipolar disorder. *Biol Psychiatry* 62:7–16.

Beaulieu JM, Sotnikova TD, Yao WD *et al.* 2004. Lithium antagonizes dopamine-dependent behaviors mediated by an AKT/glycogen synthase kinase 3 signaling cascade. *Proc Natl Acad Sci USA* 101:5099–5104.

Beaulieu JM, Zhang X, Rodriguiz RM *et al.* 2008. Role of GSK3 beta in behavioral abnormalities induced by serotonin deficiency. *Proc Natl Acad Sci USA* 105:1333–1338.

Bebchuk JM, Arfken CL, Dolan-Manji S *et al.* 2000. A preliminary investigation of a protein kinase C inhibitor in the treatment of acute mania. *Arch Gen Psychiatry* **57**:95–97.

Bechara A, Damasio H, Damasio AR. 2000. Emotion, decision making and the orbitofrontal cortex. *Cereb Cortex* **10**:295–307.

Belanoff JK, Flores BH, Kalezhan M, Sund B, Schatzberg AF. 2001. Rapid reversal of psychotic depression using mifepristone. *J Clin Psychopharmacol* **21**:516–521.

Belanoff JK, Rothschild AJ, Cassidy F et al. 2002. An open label trial of C-1073 (mifepristone) for psychotic major depression. *Biol Psychiatry* **52**:386–392.

Benes FM, Vincent SL, Todtenkopf M. 2001. The density of pyramidal and nonpyramidal neurons in anterior cingulate cortex of schizophrenic and bipolar subjects. *Biol Psychiatry* **50**:395–406.

Berman RM, Cappiello A, Anand A et al. 2000. Antidepressant effects of ketamine in depressed patients. *Biol Psychiatry* **47**:351–354.

Berridge CW, Dunn AJ. 1987. A corticotropin-releasing factor antagonist reverses the stress-induced changes of exploratory behavior in mice. *Horm Behav* **21**:393–401.

Bertolino A, Crippa D, di Dio S et al. 1988. Rolipram versus imipramine in inpatients with major, "minor" or atypical depressive disorder: a double-blind double-dummy study aimed at testing a novel therapeutic approach. *Int Clin Psychopharmacol* **3**:245–253.

Berton O, Covington HE, 3rd, Ebner K et al. 2007. Induction of deltaFosB in the periaqueductal gray by stress promotes active coping responses. *Neuron* **55**:289–300.

Bessa JM, Ferreira D, Melo I et al. 2009. The mood-improving actions of antidepressants do not depend on neurogenesis but are associated with neuronal remodeling. *Mol Psychiatry* **14**:764–773, 739.

Bhalla US, Iyengar R. 1999. Emergent properties of networks of biological signaling pathways. *Science* **283**:381–387.

Bhat RV, Shanley J, Correll MP et al. 2000. Regulation and localization of tyrosine216 phosphorylation of glycogen synthase kinase-3beta in cellular and animal models of neuronal degeneration. *Proc Natl Acad Sci USA* **97**:11074–11079.

Binder EB, Bradley RG, Liu W et al. 2008. Association of FKBP5 polymorphisms and childhood abuse with risk of posttraumatic stress disorder symptoms in adults. *J Am Med Assoc* **299**:1291–1305.

Binneman B, Fletner D, Kolluri S et al. 2008. A 6-week randomized, placebo-controlled trial of CP-316,311 (a selective CRH1 antagonist) in the treatment of major depression. *Am J Psychiatry* **165**:617–620.

Black MD. 2005. Therapeutic potential of positive AMPA modulators and their relationship to AMPA receptor subunits. A review of preclinical data. *Psychopharmacology (Berl)* **179**:154–163.

Bleakman D, Lodge D. 1998. Neuropharmacology of AMPA and kainate receptors. *Neuropharmacology* **37**:1187–1204.

Bloch M, Schmidt P, Danaceau M, Adams LF, Rubinow D. 1999. Dehydroepiandrosterone treatment of midlife dysthymia. *Biol Psychiatry* **45**:1533–1541.

Blumberg HP, Wang F, Chepenik LG et al. 2008. Influence of vascular endothelial growth factor variation on human hippocampus morphology. *Biol Psychiatry* **64**:901–903.

Bobon D, Breulet M, Gerard-Vandenhove MA et al. 1988. Is phosphodiesterase inhibition a new mechanism of antidepressant action? A double blind double-dummy study between rolipram and desipramine in hospitalized major and/or endogenous depressives. *Eur Arch Psychiatry Neurol Sci* **238**:2–6.

Boes AD, McCormick LM, Coryell WH, Nopoulos P. 2008. Rostral anterior cingulate cortex volume correlates with depressed mood in normal healthy children. *Biol Psychiatry* **63**:391–397.

Bonfanti L, Strettoi E, Chierzi S et al. 1996. Protection of retinal ganglion cells from natural and axotomy-induced cell death in neonatal transgenic mice overexpressing bcl-2. *J Neurosci* **16**:4186–4194.

Borges K, Dingledine R. 1998. AMPA receptors: molecular and functional diversity. *Prog Brain Res* **116**:153–170.

Botteron KN, Raichle ME, Drevets WC, Heath AC, Todd RD. 2002. Volumetric reduction in left subgenual prefrontal cortex in early onset depression. *Biol Psychiatry* **51**:342–344.

Bourne HR, Nicoll R. 1993. Molecular machines integrate coincident synaptic signals. *Cell* **72** (Suppl.):65–75.

Bowen DM, Najlerahim A, Procter AW, Francis PT, Murphy E. 1989. Circumscribed changes of the cerebral cortex in neuropsychiatric disorders of later life. *Proc Natl Acad Sci USA* **86**:9504–9508.

Bowley MP, Drevets WC, Ongur D, Price JL. 2002. Low glial numbers in the amygdala in major depressive disorder. *Biol Psychiatry* **52**:404–412.

Branski P, Palucha A, Szewczyk B et al. 2008. Antidepressant-like activity of 8-Br-cAMP, a PKA activator, in the forced swim test. *J Neural Transm* **115**:829–830.

Brown ES, Bobadilla L, Rush AJ. 2001. Ketoconazole in bipolar patients with depressive symptoms: a case series and literature review. *Bipolar Disord* **3**:23–29.

Brown GR, McBride L, Bauer MS, Williford WO. 2005. Impact of childhood abuse on the course of bipolar disorder: a replication study in U.S. veterans. *J Affect Disord* **89**:57–67.

Bush G, Luu P, Posner MI. 2000. Cognitive and emotional influences in anterior cingulate cortex. *Trends Cogn Sci* **4**:215–222.

Calzavara R, Mailly P, Haber SN. 2007. Relationship between the corticostriatal terminals from areas 9 and 46 and those from area 8A dorsal and rostral premotor cortex and area 24c: an anatomical substrate for cognition to action. *Eur J Neurosci* **26**:2005–2024.

Cao BJ, Peng NA. 1993. Magnesium valproate attenuates hyperactivity induced by dexamphetamine-chlordiazepoxide mixture in rodents. *Eur J Pharmacol* **237**:177–181.

Carmichael ST, Clugnet M-F, Price JL. 1994. Central olfactory connections in the macaque monkey. *J Comp Neurol* **346**:403–434.

Carmichael ST, Price JL. 1995. Limbic connections of the orbital and medial prefrontal cortex in macaque monkeys. *J Comp Neurol* **363**:615–641.

Carmichael ST, Price JL. 1996. Connectional networks within the orbital and medial prefrontal cortex of macaque monkeys. *J Comp Neurol* **371**:179–207.

Carroll RC, Beattie EC, von Zastrow M, Malenka RC. 2001. Role of AMPA receptor endocytosis in synaptic plasticity. *Nat Rev Neurosci* **2**:315–324.

Carvalho LA, Pariante CM. 2008. In vitro modulation of the glucocorticoid receptor by antidepressants. *Stress* **11**:411–424.

Caspi A, Sugden K, Moffitt TE *et al.* 2003. Influence of life stress on depression: moderation by a polymorphism in the 5-HTT gene. *Science* **301**:386–389.

Chaki S, Hirota S, Funakoshi T *et al.* 2003. Anxiolytic-like and antidepressant-like activities of MCL0129 (1-[(S)-2-(4-fluorophenyl)-2-(4-isopropylpiperadin-1-yl)ethyl]-4-[4-(2-met hoxynaphthalen-1-yl) butyl]piperazine), a novel and potent nonpeptide antagonist of the melanocortin-4 receptor. *J Pharmacol Exp Ther* **304**:818–826.

Chalecka-Franaszek E, Chuang DM. 1999. Lithium activates the serine/threonine kinase Akt-1 and suppresses glutamate-induced inhibition of Akt-1 activity in neurons. *Proc Natl Acad Sci USA* **96**:8745–8750.

Chang K, Barnea-Goraly N, Karchemskiy A *et al.* 2005. Cortical magnetic resonance imaging findings in familial pediatric bipolar disorder. *Biol Psychiatry* **58**:197–203.

Charney DS, Manji HK. 2004. Life stress, genes, and depression: multiple pathways lead to increased risk and new opportunities for intervention. *Sci STKE* 2004 (225):re5.

Chen DF, Schneider GE, Martinou JC, Tonewaga S. 1997. Bcl-2 promotes regeneration of severed axons in mammalian CNS. *Nature* **385**:434–439.

Chen G, Henter ID, Manji HK. 2009. A role for PKC in mediating stress-induced prefrontal cortical structural plasticity and cognitive function. *Proc Natl Acad Sci USA* **106**:17613–17614.

Chen G, Henter ID, Manji HK. 2010a. Translational research in bipolar disorder: emerging insights from genetically based models. *Mol Psychiatry* Feb 9 [Epub ahead of print].

Chen G, Huang LD, Jiang YM, Manji HK. 1999a. The mood-stabilizing agent valproate inhibits the activity of glycogen synthase kinase-3. *J Neurochem* **72**:1327–1330.

Chen G, Manji HK, Hawver DB, Wright CB, Potter WZ. 1994. Chronic sodium valproate selectively decreases protein kinase C alpha and epsilon in vitro. *J Neurochem* **63**:2361–2364.

Chen G, Twyman R, Manji HK. 2010b. p11 and gene therapy for severe psychiatric disorders: a practical goal? *Sci Transl Med* **2**:54–51.

Chen G, Yuan P, Maeng S *et al.* 2007. Bcl-2 and BAG-1, part of the Bcl-2 family of proteins, modulate affective-like behavioral resilience. *American College of Neuropsychopharmacology (ACNP) 47th Annual Meeting*; Dec. 7–11, 2008; Scottsdale, AZ.

Chen G, Zeng WZ, Yuan PX *et al.* 1999b. The mood-stabilizing agents lithium and valproate robustly increase the levels of the neuroprotective protein bcl-2 in the CNS. *J Neurochem* **72**:879–882.

Chen J, Kelz MB, Hope BT, Nakabeppu Y, Nestler EJ. 1997. Chronic Fos-related antigens: stable variants of deltaFosB induced in brain by chronic treatments. *J Neurosci* **17**:4933–4941.

Chen J, Nye HE, Kelz MB *et al.* 1995. Regulation of delta FosB and FosB-like proteins by electroconvulsive seizure and cocaine treatments. *Mol Pharmacol* **48**:880–889.

Chuang DM. 2004. Neuroprotective and neurotrophic actions of the mood stabilizer lithium: can it be used to treat neurodegenerative diseases? *Crit Rev Neurobiol* **16**:83–90.

Chuang DM. 2005. The antiapoptotic actions of mood stabilizers: molecular mechanisms and therapeutic potentials. *Ann N Y Acad Sci* **1053**:195–204.

Chuang DM, Manji HK. 2007. In search of the holy grail for the treatment of neurodegenerative disorders: has a simple cation been overlooked? *Biol Psychiatry* **62**:4–6.

Chuang DM, Priller J. 2006. Potential use of lithium in neurodegenerative disorders. In *Lithium in Neuropsychiatry: The Comprehensive Guide*. Bauer M, Grof P, Muler-Oerlingausen B, eds. London: Taylor & Francis, pp. 381–397.

Churchill L, Zahm DS, Kalivas PW. 1996. The mediodorsal nucleus of the thalamus in rats–I. Forebrain gabaergic innervation. *Neuroscience* **70**:93–102.

Claes S. 2009. Glucocorticoid receptor polymorphisms in major depression. *Ann N Y Acad Sci* **1179**:216–228.

Clark CP, Brown GG, Frank L et al. 2006. Improved anatomic delineation of the antidepressant response to partial sleep deprivation in medial frontal cortex using perfusion-weighted functional MRI. *Psychiatry Res* **146**:213–222.

Collingridge GL. 1994. Long-term potentiation. A question of reliability. *Nature* **371**:652–653.

Collingridge GL, Bliss TV. 1995. Memories of NMDA receptors and LTP. *Trends Neurosci* **18**:54–56.

Conn PJ, Pin JP. 1997. Pharmacology and functions of metabotropic glutamate receptors. *Annu Rev Pharmacol Toxicol* **37**:205–237.

Conway CR, Sheline YI, Chibnall JT et al. 2006. Cerebral blood flow changes during vagus nerve stimulation for depression. *Psychiatry Res* **146**:179–184.

Cooper DM. 2003. Regulation and organization of adenylyl cyclases and cAMP. *Biochem J* **375**:517–529.

Coryell W, Nopoulos P, Drevets W, Wilson T, Andreasen NC. 2005. Subgenual prefrontal cortex volumes in major depressive disorder and schizophrenia: diagnostic specificity and prognostic implications. *Am J Psychiatry* **162**:1706–1712.

Cotter D, Mackay D, Chana G et al. 2002. Reduced neuronal size and glial cell density in area 9 of the dorsolateral prefrontal cortex in subjects with major depressive disorder. *Cereb Cortex* **12**:386–394.

Cotter D, Mackay D, Landau S, Kerwin R, Everall I. 2001. Reduced glial cell density and neuronal size in the anterior cingulate cortex in major depressive disorder. *Arch Gen Psychiatry* **58**:545–553.

Coyle JT, Duman RS. 2003. Finding the intracellular signaling pathways affected by mood disorder treatments. *Neuron* **38**:157–160.

Creson TK, Yuan P, Manji HK, Chen G. 2009. Evidence for involvement of ERK, PI3K, and RSK in induction of Bcl-2 by valproate. *J Mol Neurosci* **37**:123–134.

Critchley HD, Elliott R, Mathias CJ, Dolan RJ. 2000. Neural activity relating to generation and representation of galvanic skin conductance responses: a functional magnetic resonance imaging study. *J Neurosci* **20**:3033–3040.

Critchley HD, Mathias CJ, Josephs O et al. 2003. Human cingulate cortex and autonomic control: converging neuroimaging and clinical evidence. *Brain* **126**:2139–2152.

Czeh B, Simon M, Schmelting B, Hiemke C, Fuchs E. 2005. Astroglial plasticity in the hippocampus is affected by chronic psychosocial stress and concomitant fluoxetine treatment. *Neuropsycho-pharmacology* **31**:1616–1626.

D'Amelio F, Eng LF, Gibbs MA. 1990. Glutamine synthetase immunoreactivity is present in oligodendroglia of various regions of the central nervous system. *Glia* **3**:335–341.

Dall'Olio R, Rimondini R, Gandolfi O. 1994. The NMDA positive modulator D-cycloserine inhibits dopamine-mediated behaviors in the rat. *Neuropharmacology* **33**:55–59.

Damasio AR. 1994. Descartes' error and the future of human life. *Sci Am* **271**:144.

Damasio AR, Tranel D, Damasio H. 1990. Individuals with sociopathic behavior caused by frontal damage fail to respond autonomically to social stimuli. *Behav Brain Res* **41**:81–94.

Dantzer R, O'Connor JC, Freund GG, Johnson RW, Kelley KW. 2008. From inflammation to sickness and depression: when the immune system subjugates the brain. *Nat Rev Neurosci* **9**:46–56.

De Sarno P, Li X, Jope RS. 2002. Regulation of Akt and glycogen synthase kinase-3beta phosphorylation by sodium valproate and lithium. *Neuropharmacology* **43**:1158–1164.

DeBattista C, Belanoff J, Glass S et al. 2006. Mifepristone versus placebo in the treatment of psychosis in patients with psychotic major depression. *Biol Psychiatry* **60**:1343–1349.

DeBattista C, Posener JA, Kalehzan BM, Schatzberg AF. 2000. Acute antidepressant effects of intravenous hydrocortisone and CRH in depressed patients: a double-blind, placebo-controlled study. *Am J Psychiatry* **157**:1334–1337.

Diazgranados N, Ibrahim LA, Brutsche N et al. 2010a. Rapid resolution of suicidal ideation after a single infusion of an N-methyl-D-aspartate antagonist in patients with treatment-resistant major depressive disorder. *J Clin Psychiatry* **71**:1605–1611.

Diazgranados N, Ibrahim L, Brutsche NE et al. 2010b. A randomized add-on trial of an N-methyl-D-aspartate (NMDA) antagonist in treatment-resistant bipolar depression. *Arch Gen Psychiatry* **67**:793–802.

Diorio D, Viau V, Meaney MJ. 1993. The role of the medial prefrontal cortex (cingulate gyrus) in the regulation of hypothalamic-pituitary-adrenal responses to stress. *J Neurosci* **13**:3839–3847.

Donevan SD, Rogawski MA. 1993. GYKI 52466, a 2,3-benzodiazepine, is a highly selective, noncompetitive antagonist of AMPA/kainate receptor responses. *Neuron* **10**:51–59.

Dowlatshahi D, MacQueen GM, Wang JF, Young LT. 1998. Increased temporal cortex CREB concentrations and antidepressant treatment in major depression. *Lancet* **352**:1754–1755.

Drevets WC. 2000. Neuroimaging studies of mood disorders. *Biol Psychiatry* **48**:813–829.

Drevets WC. 2001. Neuroimaging and neuropathological studies of depression: implications for the cognitive-emotional features of mood disorders. *Curr Opin Neurobiol* **11**:240–249.

Drevets WC. 2007. Orbitofrontal cortex function and structure in depression. *Ann N Y Acad Sci* **1121**:499–527.

Drevets WC, Bogers W, Raichle ME. 2002. Functional anatomical correlates of antidepressant drug treatment assessed using PET measures of regional glucose metabolism. *Eur Neuropsychopharmacol* **12**:527–544.

Drevets WC, Gadde K, Krishnan KRR. 2004a. Neuroimaging studies of depression. In *The Neurobiological Foundation of Mental Illness*, 2nd ed. Charney DS, Nestler EJ, Bunney BJ, eds. New York: Oxford University Press, pp. 461–490.

Drevets WC, Gautier C, Lowry T et al. 2001. Abnormal hemodynamic responses to facially expressed emotion in major depression. *Soc Neurosci Abstr* 31.

Drevets WC, Kupfer DJ, Bogers W, Thase M. 2006. Glucose metabolism in dorsal versus ventral striatum differentiates major depressive subtypes. *Soc Neurosci Abstr* **792.8**.

Drevets WC, Price JL. 2005. Neuroimaging and neuropathological studies of mood disorders. In *Biology of Depression: From Novel Insights to Therapeutic Strategies*. Licinio J, Wong M-L, eds. Weinheim: Wiley-VCH Verlag, pp. 427–466.

Drevets WC, Price JL, Simpson JR, Jr et al. 1997. Subgenual prefrontal cortex abnormalities in mood disorders. *Nature* **386**:824–827.

Drevets WC, Raichle ME. 1998. Reciprocal suppression of regional cerebral blood flow during emotional versus higher cognitive processes: implications for interactions between emotion and cognition. *Cognition and Emotion* **12**:353–385.

Drevets WC, Ryan N, Bogers W et al. 2004b. Subgenual prefrontal cortex volume decreased in healthy humans at high familial risk for mood disorders. Annual Meeting of the Society for Neuroscience, San Diego, CA.

Drevets WC, Savitz J, Trimble M. 2008. The subgenual anterior cingulate cortex in mood disorders. *CNS Spectr* **13**:663–681.

Du J, Gray NA, Falke CA et al. 2004. Modulation of synaptic plasticity by antimanic agents: the role of AMPA glutamate receptor subunit 1 synaptic expression. *J Neurosci* **24**:6578–6589.

Du J, Suzuki K, Wei Y et al. 2007. The anticonvulsants lamotrigine, riluzole, and valproate differentially regulate AMPA receptor membrane localization: relationship to clinical effects in mood disorders. *Neuropsychopharmacology* **32**:793–802.

Ducottet C, Griebel G, Belzung C. 2003. Effects of the selective nonpeptide corticotropin-releasing factor receptor 1 antagonist antalarmin in the chronic mild stress model of depression in mice. *Prog Neuropsychopharmacol Biol Psychiatry* **27**:625–631.

Duman RS. 2002. Synaptic plasticity and mood disorders. *Mol Psychiatry* **7** (Suppl. 1):S29–S34.

Duman RS. 2009. Neuronal damage and protection in the pathophysiology and treatment of psychiatric illness: stress and depression. *Dialogues Clin Neurosci* **11**:239–255.

Dunn RT, Kimbrell TA, Ketter TA et al. 2002. Principal components of the Beck Depression Inventory and regional cerebral metabolism in unipolar and bipolar depression. *Biol Psychiatry* **51**:387–399.

Eastwood SL, Harrison PJ. 2000. Hippocampal synaptic pathology in schizophrenia, bipolar disorder and major depression: a study of complexin mRNAs. *Mol Psychiatry* **5**:425–432.

Eastwood SL, Harrison PJ. 2001. Synaptic pathology in the anterior cingulate cortex in schizophrenia and mood disorders. A review and a Western blot study of synaptophysin, GAP-43 and the complexins. *Brain Res Bull* **55**:569–578.

Einat H, Yuan P, Gould TD et al. 2003. The role of the extracellular signal-regulated kinase signaling pathway in mood modulation. *J Neurosci* **23**:7311–7316.

Eisch AJ, Bolanos CA, de Wit J et al. 2003. Brain-derived neurotrophic factor in the ventral midbrain-nucleus accumbens pathway: a role in depression. *Biol Psychiatry* **54**:994–1005.

Elliott R, Rubinsztein JS, Sahakian BJ, Dolan RJ. 2000. Selective attention to emotional stimuli in a verbal go/no-go task: an fMRI study. *Neuroreport* **11**:1739–1744.

Encinas JM, Vaahtokari A, Enikolopov G. 2006. Fluoxetine targets early progenitor cells in the adult brain. *Proc Natl Acad Sci USA* **103**:8233–8238.

Farley S, Apazoglou K, Witkin JM, Giros B, Tzavara ET. 2010. Antidepressant-like effects of an AMPA receptor potentiator under a chronic mild stress paradigm. *Int J Neuropsychopharmacol* **13**:1207–1218.

Farrokhi C, Blanchard DC, Griebel G et al. 2004. Effects of the CRF1 antagonist SSR125543A on aggressive behaviors in hamsters. *Pharmacol Biochem Behav* **77**:465–469.

Feder A, Nestler EJ, Charney DS. 2009. Psychobiology and molecular genetics of resilience. *Nat Rev Neurosci* **10**:446–457.

Ferry AT, Lu XC, Price JL. 2000a. Effects of excitotoxic lesions in the ventral striatopallidal–thalamocortical pathway on odor reversal learning: inability to extinguish an incorrect response. *Exp Brain Res* **131**:320–335.

Ferry AT, Ongur D, An X, Price JL. 2000b. Prefrontal cortical projections to the striatum in macaque monkeys: evidence for an organization related to prefrontal networks. *J Comp Neurol* **25**:447–470.

File SE, Aranko K. 1988. Sodium valproate decreases exploratory behaviour in mice: development of tolerance and cross-tolerance with chlordiazepoxide. *Eur J Pharmacol* **151**:293–299.

Fleischhacker WW, Hinterhuber H, Bauer H et al. 1992. A multicenter double-blind study of three different doses of the new cAMP-phosphodiesterase inhibitor rolipram in patients with major depressive disorder. *Neuropsychobiology* **26**:59–64.

Flores BH, Kenna H, Keller J, Solvason HB, Schatzberg AF. 2006. Clinical and biological effects of mifepristone treatment for psychotic depression. *Neuropsychopharmacology* **31**:628–636.

Frank L, Ventimiglia R, Anderson K, Lindsay RM, Rudge JS. 1996. BDNF down-regulates neurotrophin responsiveness, TrkB protein and TrkB mRNA levels in cultured rat hippocampal neurons. *Eur J Neurosci* **8**:1220–1230.

Frank L, Wiegand SJ, Siuciak JA, Lindsay RM, Rudge JS. 1997. Effects of BDNF infusion on the regulation of TrkB protein and message in adult rat brain. *Exp Neurol* **145**:62–70.

Freedman LJ, Insel TR, Smith Y. 2000. Subcortical projections of area 25 (subgenual cortex) of the macaque monkey. *J Comp Neurol* **421**:172–188.

Friedman E, Hoau Yan W, Levinson D, Connell TA, Singh H. 1993. Altered platelet protein kinase C activity in bipolar affective disorder, manic episode. *Biol Psychiatry* **33**:520–525.

Frysztak RJ, Neafsey EJ. 1994. The effect of medial frontal cortex lesions on cardiovascular conditioned emotional responses in the rat. *Brain Res* **643**:181–193.

Fu CH, Williams SC, Cleare AJ et al. 2004. Attenuation of the neural response to sad faces in major depression by antidepressant treatment: a prospective, event-related functional magnetic resonance imaging study. *Arch Gen Psychiatry* **61**:877–889.

Fukumoto T, Morinobu S, Okamoto Y, Kagaya A, Yamawaki S. 2001. Chronic lithium treatment increases the expression of brain-derived neurotrophic factor in the rat brain. *Psychopharmacology (Berl)* **158**:100–106.

Furukawa K, Mattson MP. 1998. The transcription factor NF-kappaB mediates increases in calcium currents and decreases in NMDA- and AMPA/kainate-induced currents induced by tumor necrosis factor-alpha in hippocampal neurons. *J Neurochem* **70**:1876–1886.

Garcia LS, Comim CM, Valvassori SS et al. 2008. Acute administration of ketamine induces antidepressant-like effects in the forced swimming test and increases BDNF levels in the rat hippocampus. *Prog Neuropsychopharmacol Biol Psychiatry* **32**:140–144.

Garno JL, Goldberg JF, Ramirez PM, Ritzler BA. 2005. Impact of childhood abuse on the clinical course of bipolar disorder. *Br J Psychiatry* **186**:121–125.

Gatt JM, Nemeroff CB, Dobson-Stone C et al. 2009. Interactions between BDNF Val66Met polymorphism and early life stress predict brain and arousal pathways to syndromal depression and anxiety. *Mol Psychiatry* **14**:681–695.

George MS, Ketter TA, Parekh PI et al. 1995. Brain activity during transient sadness and happiness in healthy women. *Am J Psychiatry* **152**:341–351.

Gerber JC 3rd, Choki J, Brunswick DJ, Reivich M, Frazer A. 1983. The effect of antidepressant drugs on regional cerebral glucose utilization in the rat. *Brain Res* **269**:319–325.

Gillath O, Bunge SA, Shaver PR, Wendelken C, Mikulincer M. 2005. Attachment-style differences in the ability to suppress negative thoughts: exploring the neural correlates. *Neuroimage* **28**:835–847.

Gillespie CF, Phifer J, Bradley B, Ressler KJ. 2009. Risk and resilience: genetic and environmental influences on development of the stress response. *Depress Anxiety* **26**:984–992.

Golan H, Levav T, Mendelsohn A, Huleihel M. 2004. Involvement of tumor necrosis factor alpha in hippocampal development and function. *Cereb Cortex* **14**:97–105.

Gold PW, Chrousos GP. 2002. Organization of the stress system and its dysregulation in melancholic and atypical depression: high vs low CRH/NE states. *Mol Psychiatry* **7**:254–275.

Goldberg JF, Burdick KE, Endick CJ. 2004. A preliminary randomized, double-blind, placebo-controlled trial of pramipexole added to mood stabilizers for treatment-resistant bipolar depression. *Am J Psychiatry* **161**:564–566.

Goodwin FK, Jamison KR. 2007. *Manic-depressive Illness: Bipolar Disorders and Recurrent Depression*. Oxford: Oxford University Press.

Gould TD, Chen G, Manji HK. 2004a. In vivo evidence in the brain for lithium inhibition of glycogen synthase kinase-3. *Neuropsychopharmacology* **29**:32–38.

Gould TD, Dow ER, O'Donnell KC, Chen G, Manji HK. 2007. Targeting signal transduction pathways in the treatment of mood disorders: recent insights into the relevance of the

Wnt pathway. *CNS Neurol Disord Drug Targets* **6**:193–204.

Gould TD, Einat H, Bhat R, Manji HK. 2004*b*. AR-A014418, a selective GSK-3 inhibitor, produces antidepressant-like effects in the forced swim test. *Int J Neuropsychopharmacol* **7**:387–390.

Gould TD, Manji HK. 2004. The molecular medicine revolution and psychiatry: bridging the gap between basic neuroscience research and clinical psychiatry. *J Clin Psychiatry* **65**:598–604.

Gould TD, Manji HK. 2005. Glycogen synthase kinase-3: a putative molecular target for lithium mimetic drugs. *Neuropsychopharmacology* **30**:1223–1237.

Gould TD, O'Donnell KC, Dow ER et al. 2008. Involvement of AMPA receptors in the antidepressant-like effects of lithium in the mouse tail suspension test and forced swim test. *Neuropharmacology* **54**:577–587.

Gould TD, Picchini AM, Einat H, Manji HK. 2006. Targeting glycogen synthase kinase-3 in the CNS: implications for the development of new treatments for mood disorders. *Curr Drug Targets* **7**:1399–1409.

Govindarajan A, Rao BS, Nair D et al. 2006. Transgenic brain-derived neurotrophic factor expression causes both anxiogenic and antidepressant effects. *Proc Natl Acad Sci USA* **103**:13208–13213.

Griebel G, Simiand J, Steinberg R et al. 2002. 4-(2-Chloro-4-methoxy-5-methylphenyl)-N-[(1S)-2-cyclopropyl-1-(3-fluoro-4-methylphenyl)ethyl]5-methyl-N-(2-propynyl)-1, 3-thiazol-2-amine hydrochloride (SSR125543A), a potent and selective corticotrophin-releasing factor(1) receptor antagonist. II. Characterization in rodent models of stress-related disorders. *J Pharmacol Exp Ther* **301**:333–345.

Grimm S, Boesiger P, Beck J et al. 2009. Altered negative BOLD responses in the default-mode network during emotion processing in depressed subjects. *Neuropsychopharmacology* **34**:832–843.

Guo Z, Zhou D, Schultz PG. 2000. Designing small-molecule switches for protein–protein interactions. *Science* **288**:2042–2045.

Gurvich N, Klein PS. 2002. Lithium and valproic acid: parallels and contrasts in diverse signaling contexts. *Pharmacol Ther* **96**:45–66.

Habib KE, Weld KP, Rice KC et al. 2000. Oral administration of a corticotropin-releasing hormone receptor antagonist significantly attenuates behavioral, neuroendocrine, and autonomic responses to stress in primates. *Proc Natl Acad Sci USA* **97**:6079–6084.

Hahn CG, Friedman E. 1999. Abnormalities in protein kinase C signaling and the pathophysiology of bipolar disorder. *Bipolar Disord* **1**:81–86.

Hajszan T, Szigeti-Buck K, Sallam NL et al. 2010. Effects of estradiol on learned helplessness and associated remodeling of hippocampal spine synapses in female rats. *Biol Psychiatry* **67**:168–174.

Hall AC, Brennan A, Goold RG et al. 2002. Valproate regulates GSK-3-mediated axonal remodeling and synapsin I clustering in developing neurons. *Mol Cell Neurosci* **20**:257–270.

Hamidi M, Drevets WC, Price JL. 2004. Glial reduction in amygdala in major depressive disorder is due to oligodendrocytes. *Biol Psychiatry* **55**:563–569.

Hasler G, Drevets WC, Gould TD, Gottesman, II, Manji HK. 2006. Toward constructing an endophenotype strategy for bipolar disorders. *Biol Psychiatry* **60**:93–105.

Hasler G, Fromm S, Carlson PJ et al. 2008. Neural response to catecholamine depletion in unmedicated subjects with major depressive disorder in remission and healthy subjects. *Arch Gen Psychiatry* **65**:521–531.

Hasler G, van der Veen JW, Tumonis T et al. 2007. Reduced prefrontal glutamate/glutamine and gamma-aminobutyric acid levels in major depression determined using proton magnetic resonance spectroscopy. *Arch Gen Psychiatry* **64**:193–200.

Hastings RS, Parsey RV, Oquendo MA, Arango V, Mann JJ. 2004. Volumetric analysis of the prefrontal cortex, amygdala, and hippocampus in major depression. *Neuropsychopharmacology* **29**:952–959.

Haznedar MM, Roversi F, Pallanti S et al. 2005. Fronto-thalamo-striatal gray and white matter volumes and anisotropy of their connections in bipolar spectrum illnesses. *Biol Psychiatry* **57**:733–742.

Hebenstreit GF, Fellerer K, Fichte K et al. 1989. Rolipram in major depressive disorder: results of a double-blind comparative study with imipramine. *Pharmacopsychiatry* **22**:156–160.

Hedgepeth C, Conrad L, Zhang Z et al. 1997. Activation of the Wnt signaling pathway: a molecular mechanism for lithium action. *Dev Biol* **185**:82–91.

Heim C, Newport DJ, Bonsall R, Miller AH, Nemeroff CB. 2001. Altered pituitary-adrenal axis responses to provocative challenge tests in adult survivors of childhood abuse. *Am J Psychiatry* **158**:575–581.

Henry TR, Bakay RA, Votaw JR et al. 1998. Brain blood flow alterations induced by therapeutic vagus nerve stimulation in partial epilepsy: I. Acute effects at high and low levels of stimulation. *Epilepsia* **39**:983–990.

Heresco-Levy U, Javitt DC, Gelfin Y et al. 2006. Controlled trial of D-cycloserine adjuvant therapy for treatment-resistant major depressive disorder. *J Affect Disord* **93**:239–243.

Hines LM, Hoffman PL, Bhave S et al. 2006. A sex-specific role of type VII adenylyl cyclase in depression. *J Neurosci* **26**:12609–12619.

Hirayasu Y, Shenton ME, Salisbury DF et al. 1999. Subgenual cingulate cortex volume in first-episode psychosis. *Am J Psychiatry* **156**:1091–1093.

Hiroi N, Marek GJ, Brown JR et al. 1998. Essential role of the fosB gene in molecular, cellular, and behavioral actions of chronic electroconvulsive seizures. *J Neurosci* **18**:6952–6962.

Holick KA, Lee DC, Hen R, Dulawa SC. 2008. Behavioral effects of chronic fluoxetine in BALB/cJ mice do not require adult hippocampal neurogenesis or the serotonin 1A receptor. *Neuropsychopharmacology* **33**:406–417.

Holmes A, Heilig M, Rupniak NM, Steckler T, Griebel G. 2003. Neuropeptide systems as novel therapeutic targets for depression and anxiety disorders. *Trends Pharmacol Sci* **24**:580–588.

Holthoff VA, Beuthien-Baumann B, Zundorf G et al. 2004. Changes in brain metabolism associated with remission in unipolar major depression. *Acta Psychiatr Scand* **110**:184–194.

Hong M, Chen DC, Klein PS, Lee VM-Y. 1997. Lithium reduces tau phosphorylation by inhibition of glycogen synthase kinase-3. *J Biol Chem* **272**:25326–25332.

Hope B, Kosofsky B, Hyman SE, Nestler EJ. 1992. Regulation of immediate early gene expression and AP-1 binding in the rat nucleus accumbens by chronic cocaine. *Proc Natl Acad Sci USA* **89**:5764–5768.

Hope BT, Nye HE, Kelz MB et al. 1994. Induction of a long-lasting AP-1 complex composed of altered Fos-like proteins in brain by chronic cocaine and other chronic treatments. *Neuron* **13**:1235–1244.

Horovitz Z. 1966. The amygdala and depression. In *Antidepressant Drugs*. Garattini S, Dukes, M, eds. Amsterdam: Excerpta Medica, pp. 121–129.

Hunsberger JG, Austin DR, Chen G, Manji HK. 2009a. Cellular mechanisms underlying affective resiliency: the role of glucocorticoid receptor- and mitochondrially-mediated plasticity. *Brain Res* **1293**:76–84.

Hunsberger J, Austin DR, Henter ID, Chen G. 2009b. The neurotrophic and neuroprotective effects of psychotropic agents. *Dialogues Clin Neurosci* **11**:333–348.

Hunsberger JG, Newton SS, Bennett AH et al. 2007. Antidepressant actions of the exercise-regulated gene VGF. *Nat Med* **13**:1476–1482.

Inagaki M, Yoshikawa E, Kobayakawa M et al. 2007. Regional cerebral glucose metabolism in patients with secondary depressive episodes after fatal pancreatic cancer diagnosis. *J Affect Disord* **99**:231–236.

Insel TR, Scolnick EM. 2006. Cure therapeutics and strategic prevention: raising the bar for mental health research. *Mol Psychiatry* **11**:11–17.

Ising M, Horstmann S, Kloiber S et al. 2007. Combined dexamethasone/corticotropin releasing hormone test predicts treatment response in major depression – a potential biomarker? *Biol Psychiatry* **62**:47–54.

Izquierdo A, Wellman CL, Holmes A. 2006. Brief uncontrollable stress causes dendritic retraction in infralimbic cortex and resistance to fear extinction in mice. *J Neurosci* **26**:5733–5738.

Jahn H, Schick M, Kiefer F et al. 2004. Metyrapone as additive treatment in major depression: a double-blind and placebo-controlled trial. *Arch Gen Psychiatry* **61**:1235–1244.

Johnson SA, Wang JF, Sun X et al. 2009. Lithium treatment prevents stress-induced dendritic remodeling in the rodent amygdala. *Neuroscience* **163**:34–39.

Johnston-Wilson NL, Sims CD, Hofmann JP et al. 2000. Disease-specific alterations in frontal cortex brain proteins in schizophrenia, bipolar disorder, and major depressive disorder. The Stanley Neuropathology Consortium. *Mol Psychiatry* **5**:142–149.

Jope RS. 2003. Lithium and GSK-3: one inhibitor, two inhibitory actions, multiple outcomes. *Trends Pharmacol Sci* **24**:441–443.

Jope RS, Roh MS. 2006. Glycogen synthase kinase-3 (GSK3) in psychiatric diseases and therapeutic interventions. *Curr Drug Targets* **7**:1421–1434.

Jutkiewicz EM, Wood SK, Houshyar H et al. 2005. The effects of CRF antagonists, antalarmin, CP154,526, LWH234, and R121919, in the forced swim test and on swim-induced increases in adrenocorticotropin in rats. *Psychopharmacology (Berl)* **180**:215–223.

Kaada BR. 1960. Cingulate, posterior orbital, anterior insular and temporal pole cortex. In *Handbook of Physiology Section I Neurophysiology*, Vol II. Magoun HW, ed. Washington, DC: American Physiological Society, pp. 1345–1372.

Kaidanovich-Beilin O, Milman A, Weizman A, Pick CG, Eldar-Finkelman H. 2004. Rapid antidepressive-like activity of specific glycogen synthase kinase-3 inhibitor and its effect on beta-catenin in mouse hippocampus. *Biol Psychiatry* **55**:781–784.

Karasawa J, Shimazaki T, Kawashima N, Chaki S. 2005. AMPA receptor stimulation mediates the antidepressant-like effect of a group II metabotropic glutamate receptor antagonist. *Brain Res* **1042**:92–98.

Kazama A, Bachevalier J. 2009. Selective aspiration or neurotoxic lesions of orbital frontal areas 11 and 13 spared monkeys' performance on the object discrimination reversal task. *J Neurosci* **29**:2794–2804.

Kegeles LS, Malone KM, Slifstein M et al. 2003. Response of cortical metabolic deficits to serotonergic challenge in familial mood disorders. *Am J Psychiatry* **160**:76–82.

Ketter TA, Kimbrell TA, George MS et al. 2001. Effects of mood and subtype on cerebral glucose metabolism in treatment-resistant bipolar disorder. *Biol Psychiatry* **49**:97–109.

Khairova R, Machado-Vieira R, Du J, Manji HK. 2009. A potential role for pro-inflammatory cytokines in regulating synaptic plasticity in major depressive disorder. *Int J Neuropsychopharmacol* **12**:561–578.

Kim HW, Rapoport SI, Rao JS. 2010. Altered expression of apoptotic factors and synaptic markers in postmortem brain from bipolar disorder patients. *Neurobiol Dis* **37**:596–603.

Kim J, Hajjar K. 2002. Annexin II: a plasminogen-plasminogen activator co-receptor. *Front Biosci* **7**:d341–d348.

Kiselyczyk CL, Qi H, Chen G, Manji H, Svenningsson P. 2009. Phosphorylation of key sites on the AMPA GluR1 subunit is not necessary for the antidepressant-like effect of NR2b subunit antagonists and imipramine in the mouse forced swim test. *SOBP 64th Annual Scientific Convention.* Vancouver, CA.

Kitamura Y, Kosaka T, Kakimura JI et al. 1998. Protective effects of the antiparkinsonian drugs talipexole and pramipexole against 1-methyl-4-phenylpyridinium-induced apoptotic death in human neuroblastoma SH-SY5Y cells. *Mol Pharmacol* **54**:1046–1054.

Klein PS, Melton DA. 1996. A molecular mechanism for the effect of lithium on development. *Proc Natl Acad Sci USA* **93**:8455–8459.

Knapp RJ, Goldenberg R, Shuck C et al. 2002. Antidepressant activity of memory-enhancing drugs in the reduction of submissive behavior model. *Eur J Pharmacol* **440**:27–35.

Knutson B, Bhanji JP, Cooney RE, Atlas LY, Gotlib IH. 2007. Neural responses to monetary incentives in major depression. *Biol Psychiatry* **63**:686–692.

Kondo H, Saleem KS, Price JL. 2005. Differential connections of the perirhinal and parahippocampal cortex with the orbital and medial prefrontal networks in macaque monkeys. *J Comp Neurol* **493**:479–509.

Koo MS, Levitt JJ, Salisbury DF et al. 2008. A cross-sectional and longitudinal magnetic resonance imaging study of cingulate gyrus gray matter volume abnormalities in first-episode schizophrenia and first-episode affective psychosis. *Arch Gen Psychiatry* **65**:746–760.

Kostic V, Jackson-Lewis V, de Bilbao F, Dubois-Dauphin M, Przedborski S. 1997. Bcl-2: prolonging life in a transgenic mouse model of familial amyotrophic lateral sclerosis. *Science* **277**:559–562.

Krishnan KR, Doraiswamy PM, Lurie SN et al. 1991. Pituitary size in depression. [see comments]. *J Clin Endocrinol Metab* **72**:256–259.

Krishnan KR, McDonald WM, Escalona PR et al. 1992. Magnetic resonance imaging of the caudate nuclei in depression: preliminary observations. *Arch Gen Psychiatry* **49**:553–557.

Krishnan V, Graham A, Mazei-Robison MS et al. 2008. Calcium-sensitive adenylyl cyclases in depression and anxiety: behavioral and biochemical consequences of isoform targeting. *Biol Psychiatry* **64**:336–343.

Krishnan V, Nestler EJ. 2008. The molecular neurobiology of depression. *Nature* **455**:894–902.

Kruger S, Seminowicz D, Goldapple K, Kennedy SH, Mayberg HS. 2003. State and trait influences on mood regulation in bipolar disorder: blood flow differences with an acute mood challenge. *Biol Psychiatry* **54**:1274–1283.

Kulkarni J, Garland KA, Scaffidi A et al. 2006. A pilot study of hormone modulation as a new treatment for mania in women with bipolar affective disorder. *Psychoneuroendocrinology* **31**:543–547.

Kumano H, Ida I, Oshima A et al. 2006. Brain metabolic changes associated with predisposition to onset of major depressive disorder and adjustment disorder in cancer patients – a preliminary PET study. *J Psychiatr Res* **41**:591–599.

Kunzel HE, Zobel AW, Nickel T et al. 2003. Treatment of depression with the CRH-1-receptor antagonist R121919: endocrine changes and side effects. *J Psychiatr Res* **37**:525–533.

Kuroda M, Price JL. 1991a. Ultrastructure and synaptic organization of axon terminals from brainstem structures to the mediodorsal thalamic nucleus of the rat. *J Comp Neurol* **313**:539–552.

Kuroda M, Price JL. 1991b. Synaptic organization of projections from basal forebrain structures to the mediodorsal thalamic nucleus of the rat. *J Comp Neurol* **313**:513–533.

Lattanzi L, Dell'Osso L, Cassano P et al. 2002. Pramipexole in treatment-resistant depression: a 16-week naturalistic study. *Bipolar Disord* **4**:307–314.

Lawrence MS, Ho DY, Sun GH, Steinberg GK, Sapolsky RM. 1996. Overexpression of Bcl-2 with herpes simplex virus vectors protects CNS neurons against neurological insults in vitro and in vivo. *J Neurosci* **16**:486–496.

Leverich GS, McElroy SL, Suppes T et al. 2002. Early physical and sexual abuse associated with an adverse course of bipolar illness. *Biol Psychiatry* **51**:288–297.

Li N, Banasr M, Lee B, Duman RS. 2009. Rapid antidepressant actions of ketamine in a CUS/Anhedonia model: role of NR2B and vascular endothelial growth factor. *2009 Neuroscience Meeting*. Chicago, IL.

Li X, Bijur GN, Jope RS. 2002. Glycogen synthase kinase-3beta, mood stabilizers, and neuroprotection. *Bipolar Disorders* **4**:137–144.

Li X, Rosborough KM, Friedman AB, Zhu W, Roth KA. 2007. Regulation of mouse brain glycogen synthase kinase-3 by atypical antipsychotics. *Int J Neuropsychopharmacol* **10**:7–19.

Li X, Tizzano JP, Griffey K et al. 2001. Antidepressant-like actions of an AMPA receptor potentiator (LY392098). *Neuropharmacology* **40**:1028–1033.

Liotti M, Mayberg HS, McGinnis S, Brannan SL, Jerabek P. 2002. Unmasking disease-specific cerebral blood flow abnormalities: mood challenge in patients with remitted unipolar depression. *Am J Psychiatry* **159**:1830–1840.

Liu D, Diorio J, Day JC, Francis DD, Meaney MJ. 2000. Maternal care, hippocampal synaptogenesis and cognitive development in rats. *Nat Neurosci* **3**:799–806.

Liu D, Diorio J, Tannenbaum B et al. 1997. Maternal care, hippocampal glucocorticoid receptors, and hypothalamic-pituitary-adrenal responses to stress. *Science* **277**:1659–1662.

Lochhead PA, Kinstrie R, Sibbet G et al. 2006. A chaperone-dependent GSK3beta transitional intermediate mediates activation-loop autophosphorylation. *Mol Cell* **24**:627–633.

Lopez JF, Palkovits M, Arato M et al. 1992. Localization and quantification of pro-opiomelanocortin mRNA and glucocorticoid receptor mRNA in pituitaries of suicide victims. *Neuroendocrinology* **56**: 491–501.

Lovestone S, Davis DR, Webster MT et al. 1999. Lithium reduces tau phosphorylation: effects in living cells and in neurons at therapeutic concentrations. *Biological Psychiatry* **45**:995–1003.

Lu W, Man H, Ju W et al. 2001. Activation of synaptic NMDA receptors induces membrane insertion of new AMPA receptors and LTP in cultured hippocampal neurons. *Neuron* **29**:243–254.

Lupien SJ, McEwen BS, Gunnar MR, Heim C. 2009. Effects of stress throughout the lifespan on the brain, behaviour and cognition. *Nat Rev Neurosci* **10**:434–445.

Lyoo IK, Kim MJ, Stoll AL et al. 2004. Frontal lobe gray matter density decreases in bipolar I disorder. *Biol Psychiatry* **55**:648–651.

MacFall JR, Payne ME, Provenzale JE, Krishnan KR. 2001. Medial orbital frontal lesions in late-onset depression. *Biol Psychiatry* **49**:803–806.

Machado-Vieira R, Salvadore G, Luckenbaugh DA, Manji HK, Zarate CA, Jr. 2008. Rapid onset of antidepressant action: a new paradigm in the research and treatment of major depressive disorder. *J Clin Psychiatry* **69**:946–958.

Machado-Vieira R, Yuan P, Brutsche N et al. 2009. Brain derived neurotrophic factor and initial antidepressant response to an N-methyl-D-aspartate antagonist. *J Clin Psychiatry* **70**:1662–1666.

Maeda H, Ozawa H, Saito T, Irie T, Takahata N. 1997. Potential antidepressant properties of forskolin and a novel water-soluble forskolin (NKH477) in the forced swimming test. *Life Sci* **61**:2435–2442.

Maeng S, Hunsberger JG, Pearson B et al. 2008a. BAG1 plays a critical role in regulating recovery from both manic-like and depression-like behavioral impairments. *Proc Natl Acad Sci USA* **105**:8766–8771.

Maeng S, Zarate CA Jr. 2007. The role of glutamate in mood disorders: results from the Ketamine in Major Depression study and the presumed cellular mechanism underlying its antidepressant effects. *Curr Psychiatry Rep* **9**:467–474.

Maeng S, Zarate CA Jr, Du J et al. 2008b. Cellular mechanisms underlying the antidepressant effects of ketamine: role of alpha-amino-3-hydroxy-5-methylisoxazole-4-propionic acid receptors. *Biol Psychiatry* **63**:349–352.

Mah L, Zarate CA Jr, Singh J et al. 2007. Regional cerebral glucose metabolic abnormalities in bipolar II depression. *Biol Psychiatry* **61**:765–775.

Malberg JE, Eisch AJ, Nestler EJ, Duman RS. 2000. Chronic antidepressant treatment increases neurogenesis in adult rat hippocampus. *J Neurosci* **20**:9104–9110.

Malison RT, Anand A, Pelton GH et al. 1999. Limited efficacy of ketoconazole in treatment-refractory major depression. *J Clin Psychopharmacol* **19**:466–470.

Malkesman O, Tragon T, Austin DR et al. 2011. Targeting the BH3-interacting domian death agonist to develop mechanistically unique antidepressants. *Mol Psychiatry* doi: 10. 1038/mp. 2011. 77. epub ahead of print.

Manji H, Duman R. 2001. Impairments of neuroplasticity and cellular resilience in severe mood disorder: implications for the development of novel therapeutics. *Psychopharmacol Bull* **35**:5–49.

Manji HK, Drevets WC, Charney DS. 2001a. The cellular neurobiology of depression. *Nat Med* **7**:541–547.

Manji HK, Etcheberrigaray R, Chen G, Olds JL. 1993. Lithium decreases membrane-associated protein kinase C in hippocampus: selectivity for the alpha isozyme. *J Neurochem* **61**:2303–2310.

Manji HK, Lenox RH. 1999. Ziskind-Somerfeld Research Award. Protein kinase C signaling in the brain: molecular transduction of mood stabilization in the treatment of manic-depressive illness. *Biol Psychiatry* **46**:1328–1351.

Manji HK, Lenox RH. 2000. Signaling: cellular insights into the pathophysiology of bipolar disorder. *Biol Psychiatry* **48**:518–530.

Manji HK, Moore GJ, Chen G. 2000. Lithium up-regulates the cytoprotective protein Bcl-2 in the CNS in vivo: a role for neurotrophic and neuroprotective effects in manic depressive illness. *J Clin Psychiatry* **61** (Suppl. 9):82–96.

Manji HK, Moore GJ, Chen G. 2001*b*. Bipolar disorder: leads from the molecular and cellular mechanisms of action of mood stabilizers. *Br J Psychiatry* **41**:107–119.

Manji HK, Quiroz JA, Sporn J et al. 2003. Enhancing neuronal plasticity and cellular resilience to develop novel, improved therapeutics for difficult-to-treat depression. *Biol Psychiatry* **53**:707–742.

Mansbach RS, Brooks EN, Chen YL. 1997. Antidepressant-like effects of CP-154,526, a selective CRF1 receptor antagonist. *Eur J Pharmacol* **323**:21–26.

Martinowich K, Manji H, Lu B. 2007. New insights into BDNF function in depression and anxiety. *Nat Neurosci* **10**:1089–1093.

Mathew SJ, Murrough JW, aan het Rot M et al. 2010. Riluzole for relapse prevention following intravenous ketamine in treatment-resistant depression: a pilot randomized, placebo-controlled continuation trial. *Int J Neuropsychopharmacol* **13**:71–82.

Mayberg HS, Brannan SK, Mahurin RK et al. 1997. Cingulate function in depression: a potential predictor of treatment response. *Neuroreport* **8**:1057–1061.

Mayberg HS, Brannan SK, Tekell JL et al. 2000. Regional metabolic effects of fluoxetine in major depression: serial changes and relationship to clinical response. *Biol Psychiatry* **48**:830–843.

Mayberg HS, Liotti M, Brannan SK et al. 1999. Reciprocal limbic-cortical function and negative mood: converging PET findings in depression and normal sadness. *Am J Psychiatry* **156**:675–682.

Mayberg HS, Lozano AM, Voon V et al. 2005. Deep brain stimulation for treatment-resistant depression. *Neuron* **45**:651–660.

McAllister KH. 1994. D-cycloserine enhances social behavior in individually-housed mice in the resident-intruder test. *Psychopharmacology (Berl)* **116**:317–325.

McBride SA, Slotnick B. 1997. The olfactory thalamocortical system and odor reversal learning examined using an asymmetrical lesion paradigm in rats. *Behav Neurosci* **111**:1273–1284.

McClung CA, Nestler EJ. 2003. Regulation of gene expression and cocaine reward by CREB and DeltaFosB. *Nat Neurosci* **6**:1208–1215.

McDonald C, Bullmore ET, Sham PC et al. 2004. Association of genetic risks for schizophrenia and bipolar disorder with specific and generic brain structural endophenotypes. *Arch Gen Psychiatry* **61**:974–984.

McEwen BS, Magarinos AM. 2001. Stress and hippocampal plasticity: implications for the pathophysiology of affective disorders. *Hum Psychopharmacol* **16**:S7–S19.

McGowan PO, Sasaki A, D'Alessio AC et al. 2009. Epigenetic regulation of the glucocorticoid receptor in human brain associates with childhood abuse. *Nat Neurosci* **12**:342–348.

Meloni D, Gambarana C, De Montis MG et al. 1993. Dizocilpine antagonizes the effect of chronic imipramine on learned helplessness in rats. *Pharmacol Biochem Behav* **46**:423–426.

Merry DE, Korsmeyer SJ. 1997. Bcl-2 gene family in the nervous system. *Annu Rev Neurosci* **20**:245–267.

Mickley GA, Schaldach MA, Snyder KJ et al. 1998. Ketamine blocks a conditioned taste aversion (CTA) in neonatal rats. *Physiol Behav* **64**:381–390.

Miller AH, Maletic V, Raison CL. 2009. Inflammation and its discontents: the role of cytokines in the pathophysiology of major depression. *Biol Psychiatry* **65**:732–741.

Miller B, Saleem KS, Price JL. 2008. *Cingulate cortex connections with prefrontal cortex circuits in monkeys. Program 465.11. Neuroscience Meeting Planner*. Society for Neuroscience, Washington, DC.

Mitra R, Jadhav S, McEwen BS, Vyas A, Chattarji S. 2005. Stress duration modulates the spatiotemporal patterns of spine formation in the basolateral amygdala. *Proc Natl Acad Sci USA* **102**:9371–9376.

Miu P, Jarvie KR, Radhakrishnan V et al. 2001. Novel AMPA receptor potentiators LY392098 and LY404187: effects on recombinant human AMPA receptors in vitro. *Neuropharmacology* **40**:976–983.

Moghaddam B, Adams B, Verma A, Daly D. 1997. Activation of glutamatergic neurotransmission by ketamine: a novel step in the pathway from NMDA receptor blockade to dopaminergic and cognitive disruptions associated with the prefrontal cortex. *J Neurosci* **17**:2921–2927.

Monteggia LM, Barrot M, Powell CM et al. 2004. Essential role of brain-derived neurotrophic factor in adult hippocampal function. *Proc Natl Acad Sci USA* **101**:10827–10832.

Moore G, Cortese B, Glitz D et al. 2009. Chronic lithium increases prefrontal and subgenual prefrontal gray matter in patients with bipolar disorder: a longitudinal high resolution volumetric MRI study. *J Clin Psychiatry* **70**:699–705.

Moore GJ, Bebchuk JM, Hasanat K et al. 2000*a*. Lithium increases N-acetyl-aspartate in the human brain: in vivo evidence in support of bcl-

2's neurotrophic effects? *Biol Psychiatry* **48**:1–8.

Moore GJ, Bebchuk JM, Wilds IB, Chen G, Manji HK. 2000b. Lithium-induced increase in human brain grey matter. *Lancet* **356**:1241–1242.

Morgan MA, LeDoux JE. 1995. Differential contribution of dorsal and ventral medial prefrontal cortex to the acquisition and extinction of conditioned fear in rats. *Behav Neurosci* **109**:681–688.

Moryl E, Danysz W, Quack G. 1993. Potential antidepressive properties of amantadine, memantine and bifemelane. *Pharmacol Toxicol* **72**:394–397.

Munoz-Montano JR, Moreno FJ, Avila J, Diaz-Nido J. 1997. Lithium inhibits Alzheimer's disease-like tau protein phosphorylation in neurons. *FEBS Lett* **411**:183–188.

Murgatroyd C, Patchev AV, Wu Y et al. 2009. Dynamic DNA methylation programs persistent adverse effects of early-life stress. *Nat Neurosci* **12**:1559–1566.

Murphy BE, Filipini D, Ghadirian AM. 1993. Possible use of glucocorticoid receptor antagonists in the treatment of major depression: preliminary results using RU 486. *J Psychiatry Neurosci* **18**:209–213.

Murphy DL. 1977. Animal models for mania. In *Animal Models in Psychiatry and Neurology*. Hanin I, Usdin E, eds. Oxford: Pergammon Press, pp. 211–223.

Murphy FC, Sahakian BJ, Rubinsztein JS et al. 1999. Emotional bias and inhibitory control processes in mania and depression. *Psychol Med* **29**:1307–1321.

Murray CJ, Lopez AD. 1996. Evidence-based health policy – lessons from the Global Burden of Disease Study. *Science* **274**:740–743.

Murray LA, Whitehouse WG, Alloy LB. 1999. Mood congruence and depressive deficits in memory: a forced-recall analysis. *Memory* **7**:175–196.

Nahas Z, Teneback C, Chae JH et al. 2007. Serial vagus nerve stimulation functional MRI in treatment-resistant depression. *Neuropsychopharmacology* **32**:1649–1660.

Nestler EJ, Barrot M, DiLeone RJ et al. 2002. Neurobiology of depression. *Neuron* **34**:13–25.

Nestler EJ, Kelz MB, Chen J. 1999. DeltaFosB: a molecular mediator of long-term neural and behavioral plasticity. *Brain Res* **835**:10–17.

Neumann H, Schweigreiter R, Yamashita T et al. 2002. Tumor necrosis factor inhibits neurite outgrowth and branching of hippocampal neurons by a rho-dependent mechanism. *J Neurosci* **22**:854–862.

Neumeister A, Drevets WC, Belfer I et al. 2006a. Effects of an alpha 2C-adrenoreceptor gene polymorphism on neural responses to facial expressions in depression. *Neuropsychopharmacology* **31**:1750–1756.

Neumeister A, Hu XZ, Luckenbaugh DA et al. 2006b. Differential effects of 5-HTTLPR genotypes on the behavioral and neural responses to tryptophan depletion in patients with major depression and controls. *Arch Gen Psychiatry* **63**:978–986.

Neumeister A, Nugent AC, Waldeck T et al. 2004. Neural and behavioral responses to tryptophan depletion in unmedicated patients with remitted major depressive disorder and controls. *Arch Gen Psychiatry* **61**:765–773.

Neumeister A, Wood S, Bonne O et al. 2005. Reduced hippocampal volume in unmedicated, remitted patients with major depression versus control subjects. *Biol Psychiatry* **57**:935–937.

Newton SS, Collier EF, Hunsberger J et al. 2003. Gene profile of electroconvulsive seizures: induction of neurotrophic and angiogenic factors. *J Neurosci* **23**:10841–10851.

Newton SS, Thome J, Wallace TL et al. 2002. Inhibition of cAMP response element-binding protein or dynorphin in the nucleus accumbens produces an antidepressant-like effect. *J Neurosci* **22**:10883–10890.

Nibuya M, Morinobu S, Duman RS. 1995. Regulation of BDNF and trkB mRNA in rat brain by chronic electroconvulsive seizure and antidepressant drug treatments. *J Neurosci* **15**:7539–7547.

Nibuya M, Nestler EJ, Duman RS. 1996. Chronic antidepressant administration increases the expression of cAMP response element binding protein (CREB) in rat hippocampus. *J Neurosci* **16**:2365–2372.

Nickola TJ, Ignatowski TA, Reynolds JL, Spengler RN. 2001. Antidepressant drug-induced alterations in neuron-localized tumor necrosis factor-alpha mRNA and alpha(2)-adrenergic receptor sensitivity. *J Pharmacol Exp Ther* **297**:680–687.

Nielsen EO, Varming T, Mathiesen C et al. 1999. SPD 502: a water-soluble and in vivo long-lasting AMPA antagonist with neuroprotective activity. *J Pharmacol Exp Ther* **289**:1492–1501.

Noble W, Planel E, Zehr C et al. Inhibition of glycogen synthase kinase-3 by lithium correlates with reduced tauopathy and degeneration in vivo. *Proc Natl Acad Sci USA* **102**:6990–6995.

Nugent AC, Milham MP, Bain EE et al. 2006. Cortical abnormalities in bipolar disorder investigated with MRI and voxel-based morphometry. *Neuroimage* **30**:485–497.

Nye HE, Nestler EJ. 1996. Induction of chronic Fos-related antigens in rat brain by chronic morphine administration. *Mol Pharmacol* **49**:636–645.

O'Brien WT, Harper AD, Jove F et al. 2004. Glycogen synthase kinase-3beta haploinsufficiency mimics the behavioral and molecular effects of lithium. *J Neurosci* **24**:6791–6798.

O'Donnell JM, Frith S. 1999. Behavioral effects of family-selective inhibitors of cyclic nucleotide phosphodiesterases. *Pharmacol Biochem Behav* **63**:185–192.

Ochs G, Penn RD, York M *et al.* 2000. A phase I/II trial of recombinant methionyl human brain derived neurotrophic factor administered by intrathecal infusion to patients with amyotrophic lateral sclerosis. *Amyotroph Lateral Scler Other Motor Neuron Disord* **1**:201–206.

Olausson P, Jentsch JD, Tronson N *et al.* 2006. DeltaFosB in the nucleus accumbens regulates food-reinforced instrumental behavior and motivation. *J Neurosci* **26**:9196–9204.

Ongur D, An X, Price JL. 1998*a*. Prefrontal cortical projections to the hypothalamus in macaque monkeys. *J Comp Neurol* **401**:480–505.

Ongur D, Drevets WC, Price JL. 1998*b*. Glial reduction in the subgenual prefrontal cortex in mood disorders. *Proc Natl Acad Sci USA* **95**:13290–13295.

Ongur D, Ferry AT, Price JL. 2003. Architectonic subdivision of the human orbital and medial prefrontal cortex. *J Comp Neurol* **460**:425–449.

Osuch EA, Ketter TA, Kimbrell TA *et al.* 2000. Regional cerebral metabolism associated with anxiety symptoms in affective disorder patients. *Biol Psychiatry* **48**:1020–1023.

Padovan CM, Guimaraes FS. 2004. Antidepressant-like effects of NMDA-receptor antagonist injected into the dorsal hippocampus of rats. *Pharmacol Biochem Behav* **77**:15–19.

Papp M, Moryl E. 1993. New evidence for the antidepressant activity of MK-801, a non-competitive antagonist of NMDA receptors. *Pol J Pharmacol* **45**:549–553.

Park M, Penick EC, Edwards JG, Kauer JA, Ehlers MD. 2004. Recycling endosomes supply AMPA receptors for LTP. *Science* **305**:1972–1975.

Paul IA, Skolnick P. 2003. Glutamate and depression: clinical and preclinical studies. *Ann N Y Acad Sci* **1003**:250–272.

Pezawas L, Meyer-Lindenberg A, Drabant EM *et al.* 2005. 5-HTTLPR polymorphism impacts human cingulate–amygdala interactions: a genetic susceptibility mechanism for depression. *Nat Neurosci* **8**:828–834.

Phelps EA, Delgado MR, Nearing KI, LeDoux JE. 2004. Extinction learning in humans: role of the amygdala and vmPFC. *Neuron* **43**:897–905.

Phelps LE, Brutsche N, Moral JR *et al.* 2009. Family history of alcohol dependence and initial antidepressant response to an N-methyl-D-aspartate antagonist. *Biol Psychiatry* **65**:181–184.

Pierre S, Eschenhagen T, Geisslinger G, Scholich K. 2009. Capturing adenylyl cyclases as potential drug targets. *Nat Rev Drug Discov* **8**:321–335.

Pitkanen A, Mathiesen C, Ronn LC, Moller A, Nissinen J. 2007. Effect of novel AMPA antagonist, NS1209, on status epilepticus. An experimental study in rat. *Epilepsy Res* **74**:45–54.

Pizzagalli DA, Oakes TR, Fox AS, *et al.* 2004. Functional but not structural subgenual prefrontal cortex abnormalities in melancholia. *Mol Psychiatry* **9**:325, 393–405.

Pizzagalli D, Pascual-Marqui RD, Nitschke JB *et al.* 2001. Anterior cingulate activity as a predictor of degree of treatment response in major depression: evidence from brain electrical tomography analysis. *Am J Psychiatry* **158**:405–415.

Plotsky PM, Owens MJ, Nemeroff CB. *et al* 1998. Psychoneuro-endocrinology of depression. Hypothalamic-pituitary-adrenal axis. *Psychiatr Clin North Am* **21**:293–307.

Polanczyk G, Caspi A, Williams B *et al.* 2009. Protective effect of CRHR1 gene variants on the development of adult depression following childhood maltreatment: replication and extension. *Arch Gen Psychiatry* **66**:978–985.

Post RM, Gerner RH, Carman JS *et al.* 1978. Effects of a dopamine agonist piribedil in depressed patients: relationship of pretreatment homovanillic acid to antidepressant response. *Arch Gen Psychiatry* **35**:609–615.

Preskorn SH, Baker B, Kolluri S *et al.* 2008. An innovative design to establish proof of concept of the antidepressant effects of the NR2B subunit selective N-methyl-D-aspartate antagonist, CP-101,606, in patients with treatment-refractory major depressive disorder. *J Clin Psychopharmacol* **28**:631–637.

Price JL, Drevets WC. 2010. Neurocircuitry of mood disorders. *Neuropsychopharmacology* **35**:192–216.

Price RB, Nock MK, Charney DS, Mathew SJ. 2009. Effects of intravenous ketamine on explicit and implicit measures of suicidality in treatment-resistant depression. *Biol Psychiatry* **66**:522–526.

Przegalinski E, Tatarczynska E, Deren-Wesolek A, Chojnacka-Wojcik E. 1997. Antidepressant-like effects of a partial agonist at strychnine-insensitive glycine receptors and a competitive NMDA receptor antagonist. *Neuropharmacology* **36**:31–37.

Quiroz J, Post R. 2009. Novel treatments in bipolar disorder: future directions. In *Bipolar Disorder: A Clinician's Guide to Treatment Management*. Yatham LN, Kusumakar V, eds. Florence, KY: Routledge, pp. 591–617.

Quiroz JA, Singh J, Gould TD *et al.* 2004. Emerging experimental therapeutics for bipolar disorder: clues from the molecular pathophysiology. *Mol Psychiatry* **9**:756–776.

Radley JJ, Rocher AB, Rodriguez A *et al.* 2008. Repeated stress alters dendritic spine morphology in the rat medial prefrontal cortex. *J Comp Neurol* **507**:1141–1150.

Raghupathi R, Fernandez SC, Murai H *et al*. 1998. BCL-2 overexpression attenuates cortical cell loss after traumatic brain injury in transgenic mice. *J Cereb Blood Flow Metab* **18**:1259–1269.

Raichle ME, MacLeod AM, Snyder AZ *et al*. 2001. A default mode of brain function. *Proc Natl Acad Sci USA* **98**:676–682.

Rajkowska G, Miguel-Hidalgo JJ, Wei J *et al*. 1999. Morphometric evidence for neuronal and glial prefrontal cell pathology in major depression. *Biol Psychiatry* **45**:1085–1098.

Rajkowska G, O'Dwyer G, Teleki Z *et al*. 2007. GABAergic neurons immunoreactive for calcium binding proteins are reduced in the prefrontal cortex in major depression. *Neuropsychopharmacology* **32**:471–482.

Rao S, Rajesh KR, Joseph T. 1991. Effect of antiepileptic drugs valproic acid, carbamazepine and ethosuccimide on exploratory behaviour in mice. *Indian J Exp Biol* **29**:127–130.

Rauch SL, Drevets WC. 2008. Neuroimaging and neuroanatomy of stress-induced and fear circuitry disorders: the agenda for future research. In *Stress-Induced and Fear Circuitry Disorders: Refining the Research Agenda for DSM-V*. Andrews G, Charney DS, Sirovatka PJ, Regier DA, eds. Washington, DC: American Psychiatric Press, pp. 235–278.

Rayasam GV, Tulasi VK, Sodhi R, Davis JA, Ray A. 2009. Glycogen synthase kinase 3: more than a namesake. *Br J Pharmacol* **156**:885–898.

Reif A, Fritzen S, Finger M *et al*. 2006. Neural stem cell proliferation is decreased in schizophrenia, but not in depression. *Mol Psychiatry* **11**:514–522.

Rempel-Clower N, Barbas H. 1998. Topographic organization of connections between the hypothalamus and prefrontal cortex in the rhesus monkey. *J Comp Neurol* **398**:393–419.

Ren M, Senatorov VV, Chen RW, Chuang DM. 2003. Postinsult treatment with lithium reduces brain damage and facilitates neurological recovery in a rat ischemia/reperfusion model. *Proc Natl Acad Sci USA* **100**:6210–6215.

Reynolds JL, Ignatowski TA, Sud R, Spengler RN. 2004. Brain-derived tumor necrosis factor-alpha and its involvement in noradrenergic neuron functioning involved in the mechanism of action of an antidepressant. *J Pharmacol Exp Ther* **310**:1216–1225.

Riedel G, Platt B, Micheau J. 2003. Glutamate receptor function in learning and memory. *Behav Brain Res* **140**:1–47.

Roberts AC, Robbins TW, Everitt BJ *et al*. 1990. The effects of excitotoxic lesions of the basal forebrain on the acquisition, retention and serial reversal of visual discriminations in marmosets. *Neuroscience* **34**:311–329.

Rogawski MA. 2006. Diverse mechanisms of antiepileptic drugs in the development pipeline. *Epilepsy Res* **69**:273–294.

Roh MS, Cui FJ, Ahn YM, Kang UG. 2009. Up-regulation of cocaine- and amphetamine-regulated transcript (CART) in the rat nucleus accumbens after repeated electroconvulsive shock. *Neurosci Res* **65**:210–213.

Roh MS, Eom TY, Zmijewska AA *et al*. 2005. Hypoxia activates glycogen synthase kinase-3 in mouse brain in vivo: protection by mood stabilizers and imipramine. *Biol Psychiatry* **57**:278–286.

Rosoklija G, Toomayan G, Ellis SP *et al*. 2000. Structural abnormalities of subicular dendrites in subjects with schizophrenia and mood disorders: preliminary findings. *Arch Gen Psychiatry* **57**:349–356.

Roth TL, Lubin FD, Funk AJ, Sweatt JD. 2009. Lasting epigenetic influence of early-life adversity on the BDNF gene. *Biol Psychiatry* **65**:760–769.

Russchen FT, Bakst I, Amaral DG, Price JL. 1985. The amygdalostriatal projections in the monkey. An anterograde tracing study. *Brain Res* **329**:241–257.

Sadoul R. 1998. Bcl-2 family members in the development and degenerative pathologies of the nervous system. *Cell Death Differ* **5**:805–815.

Sairanen M, Lucas G, Ernfors P, Castren M, Castren E. 2005. Brain-derived neurotrophic factor and antidepressant drugs have different but coordinated effects on neuronal turnover, proliferation, and survival in the adult dentate gyrus. *J Neurosci* **25**:1089–1094.

Salinska E, Stafiej A. 2003. Metabotropic glutamate receptors (mGluRs) are involved in early phase of memory formation: possible role of modulation of glutamate release. *Neurochem Int* **43**:469–474.

Salvadore G, Cornwell BR, Colon-Rosario V *et al*. 2009. Increased anterior cingulate cortical activity in response to fearful faces: a neurophysiological biomarker that predicts rapid antidepressant response to ketamine. *Biol Psychiatry* **65**:289–295.

Sanacora G, Kendell SF, Levin Y *et al*. 2007. Preliminary evidence of riluzole efficacy in antidepressant-treated patients with residual depressive symptoms. *Biol Psychiatry* **61**:822–825.

Sanacora G, Mason GF, Rothman DL *et al*. 1999. Reduced cortical gamma-aminobutyric acid levels in depressed patients determined by proton magnetic resonance spectroscopy. *Arch Gen Psychiatry* **56**:1043–1047.

Sanacora G, Zarate CA, Krystal JH, Manji HK. 2008. Targeting the glutamatergic system to develop novel, improved therapeutics for mood disorders. *Nat Rev Drug Discov* **7**:426–437.

Santarelli L, Saxe M, Gross C et al. 2003. Requirement of hippocampal neurogenesis for the behavioral effects of antidepressants. *Science* **301**:805–809.

Sassi RB, Nicoletti M, Brambilla P et al. 2002. Increased gray matter volume in lithium-treated bipolar disorder patients. *Neurosci Lett* **329**:243–245.

Saunders J, Williams J. 2003. Antagonists of the corticotropin releasing factor receptor. *Prog Med Chem* **41**:195–247.

Savitz J, Nugent AC, Bogers W et al. 2010. Amygdala volume in depressed patients with bipolar disorder assessed using high resolution 3T MRI: the impact of medication. *Neuroimage* **49**:2966–2976.

Schlaepfer TE, Cohen MX, Frick C et al. 2008. Deep brain stimulation to reward circuitry alleviates anhedonia in refractory major depression. *Neuropsychopharmacology* **33**:368–377.

Schloesser RJ, Huang J, Klein PS, Manji HK. 2008. Cellular plasticity cascades in the pathophysiology and treatment of bipolar disorder. *Neuropsychopharmacology* **33**:110–133.

Schmidt HD, Duman RS. 2008. Peripheral BDNF administration increases adult hippocampal neurogenesis and produces antidepressant-like behavioral responses in rodent models of anxiety and depression. 2008 Neuroscience, Society of Neuroscience Annual Meeting, Washington, DC, Nov 15–19, 2008.

Scott AI, Perini AF, Shering PA, Whalley LJ. 1991. In-patient major depression: is rolipram as effective as amitriptyline? *Eur J Clin Pharmacol* **40**:127–129.

Semba J, Kuroda Y, Takahashi R. 1989. Potential antidepressant properties of subchronic GABA transaminase inhibitors in the forced swimming test in mice. *Neuropsychobiology* **21**:152–156.

Sen S, Duman R, Sanacora G. 2008. Serum brain-derived neurotrophic factor, depression, and antidepressant medications: meta-analyses and implications. *Biol Psychiatry* **64**:527–532.

Seymour PA, Schmidt AW, Schulz DW. 2003. The pharmacology of CP-154,526, a non-peptide antagonist of the CRH1 receptor: a review. *CNS Drug Rev* **9**:57–96.

Shansky RM, Hamo C, Hof PR, McEwen BS, Morrison JH. 2009. Stress-induced dendritic remodeling in the prefrontal cortex is circuit specific. *Cereb Cortex* **19**:2479–2484.

Shekhar A, Truitt W, Rainnie D, Sajdyk T. 2005. Role of stress, corticotrophin releasing factor (CRF) and amygdala plasticity in chronic anxiety. *Stress* **8**:209–219.

Sheline YI, Barch DM, Donnelly JM et al. 2001. Increased amygdala response to masked emotional faces in depressed subjects resolves with antidepressant treatment: an fMRI study. *Biol Psychiatry* **50**:651–658.

Sheline YI, Gado MH, Kraemer HC. 2003. Untreated depression and hippocampal volume loss. *Am J Psychiatry* **160**:1516–1518.

Shirayama Y, Chen AC, Nakagawa S, Russell DS, Duman RS. 2002. Brain-derived neurotrophic factor produces antidepressant effects in behavioral models of depression. *J Neurosci* **22**:3251–3261.

Shulman RG, Rothman DL, Behar KL, Hyder F. 2004. Energetic basis of brain activity: implications for neuroimaging. *Trends Neurosci* **27**:489–495.

Siegle GJ, Carter CS, Thase ME. 2006. Use of FMRI to predict recovery from unipolar depression with cognitive behavior therapy. *Am J Psychiatry* **163**:735–738.

Siegle GJ, Steinhauer SR, Thase ME, Stenger VA, Carter CS. 2002. Can't shake that feeling: event-related fMRI assessment of sustained amygdala activity in response to emotional information in depressed individuals. *Biol Psychiatry* **51**:693–707.

Silvestre JS, Nadal R, Pallares M, Ferre N. 1997. Acute effects of ketamine in the holeboard, the elevated-plus maze, and the social interaction test in Wistar rats. *Depress Anxiety* **5**:29–33.

Simen BB, Duman CH, Simen AA, Duman RS. 2006. TNF alpha signaling in depression and anxiety: behavioral consequences of individual receptor targeting. *Biol Psychiatry* **59**:775–785.

Simpson GM, El Sheshai A, Loza N et al. 2005. An 8-week open-label trial of a 6-day course of mifepristone for the treatment of psychotic depression. *J Clin Psychiatry* **66**:598–602.

Singer BH, Jutkiewicz EM, Fuller CL et al. 2009. Conditional ablation and recovery of forebrain neurogenesis in the mouse. *J Comp Neurol* **514**:567–582.

Siuciak JA, Lewis DR, Wiegand SJ, Lindsay RM. 1997. Antidepressant-like effect of brain-derived neurotrophic factor (BDNF). *Pharmacol Biochem Behav* **56**:131–137.

Siuciak JA, McCarthy SA, Chapin DS, Martin AN. 2008. Behavioral and neurochemical characterization of mice deficient in the phosphodiesterase-4B (PDE4B) enzyme. *Psychopharmacology (Berl)* **197**:115–126.

Skolnick P, Miller R, Young A, Boje K, Trullas R. 1992. Chronic treatment with 1-aminocyclopropanecarboxylic acid desensitizes behavioral responses to compounds acting at the N-methyl-D-aspartate receptor complex. *Psychopharmacology (Berl)* **107**:489–496.

Song L, De Sarno P, Jope RS. 2002. Central role of Glycogen Synthase

Kinase-3beta in endoplasmic reticulum stress-induced caspase-3 activation. *J Biol Chem* **277**:44701–44708.

Sporn J, Ghaemi SN, Sambur MR et al. 2000. Pramipexole augmentation in the treatment of unipolar and bipolar depression: a retrospective chart review. *Ann Clin Psychiatry* **12**:137–140.

Stambolic V, Ruel L, Woodgett J. 1996. Lithium inhibits glycogen synthase kinase-3 activity and mimics wingless signalling in intact cells. *Curr Biol* **6**:1664–1668.

Stellwagen D, Beattie EC, Seo JY, Malenka RC. 2005. Differential regulation of AMPA receptor and GABA receptor trafficking by tumor necrosis factor-alpha. *J Neurosci* **25**:3219–3228.

Stellwagen D, Malenka RC. 2006. Synaptic scaling mediated by glial TNF-alpha. *Nature* **440**:1054–1059.

Stockmeier CA, Mahajan GJ, Konick LC et al. 2004. Cellular changes in the postmortem hippocampus in major depression. *Biol Psychiatry* **56**:640–650.

Sullivan RM, Gratton A. 1999. Lateralized effects of medial prefrontal cortex lesions on neuroendocrine and autonomic stress responses in rats. *J Neurosci* **19**:2834–2840.

Svenningsson P, Bateup H, Qi H et al. 2007. Involvement of AMPA receptor phosphorylation in antidepressant actions with special reference to tianeptine. *Eur J Neurosci* **26**:3509–3517.

Svenningsson P, Chergui K, Rachleff I et al. 2006. Alterations in 5-HT1B receptor function by p11 in depression-like states. *Science* **311**:77–80.

Svenningsson P, Tzavara ET, Witkin JM et al. 2002. Involvement of striatal and extrastriatal DARPP-32 in biochemical and behavioral effects of fluoxetine (Prozac). *Proc Natl Acad Sci USA* **99**:3182–3187.

Swaab DF, Bao AM, Lucassen PJ. 2005. The stress system in the human brain in depression and neurodegeneration. *Ageing Res Rev* **4**:141–194.

Sweatt JD. 2009. Experience-dependent epigenetic modifications in the central nervous system. *Biol Psychiatry* **65**:191–197.

Szabo S, Gould TD, Manji HK. 2004. Neurotransmitters, receptors, signal transduction pathways and second messengers. In *American Psychiatric Publishing Textbook of Psychopharmacology*. Schatzberg AF, Nemeroff CB, eds. Washington, DC: American Psychiatric Press, pp. 3–52.

Takahashi M, Terwilliger R, Lane C et al. 1999. Chronic antidepressant administration increases the expression of cAMP-specific phosphodiesterase 4A and 4B isoforms. *J Neurosci* **19**:610–618.

Takata K, Kitamura Y, Kakimura J, Kohno Y, Taniguchi T. 2000. Increase of bcl-2 protein in neuronal dendritic processes of cerebral cortex and hippocampus by the antiparkinsonian drugs, talipexole and pramipexole. *Brain Res* **872**:236–241.

Tan Y, Hori N, Carpenter DO. 2003. The mechanism of presynaptic long-term depression mediated by group I metabotropic glutamate receptors. *Cell Mol Neurobiol* **23**:187–203.

Tanis KQ, Duman RS. 2007. Intracellular signaling pathways pave roads to recovery for mood disorders. *Ann Med* **39**:531–544.

Taylor Tavares JV, Clark L, Furey ML et al. 2008. Neural basis of abnormal response to negative feedback in unmedicated mood disorders. *Neuroimage* **42**:1118–1126.

Teves D, Videen TO, Cryer PE, Powers WJ. 2004. Activation of human medial prefrontal cortex during autonomic responses to hypoglycemia. *Proc Natl Acad Sci USA* **101**:6217–6221.

Thome J, Sakai N, Shin K et al. 2000. cAMP response element-mediated gene transcription is upregulated by chronic antidepressant treatment. *J Neurosci* **20**:4030–4036.

Todtenkopf MS, Vincent SL, Benes FM. 2005. A cross-study meta-analysis and three-dimensional comparison of cell counting in the anterior cingulate cortex of schizophrenic and bipolar brain. *Schizophr Res* **73**:79–89.

Trullas R, Skolnick P. 1990. Functional antagonists at the NMDA receptor complex exhibit antidepressant actions. *Eur J Pharmacol* **185**:1–10.

Tsankova NM, Berton O, Renthal W et al. 2006. Sustained hippocampal chromatin regulation in a mouse model of depression and antidepressant action. *Nat Neurosci* **9**:519–525.

Tsankova N, Renthal W, Kumar A, Nestler EJ. 2007. Epigenetic regulation in psychiatric disorders. *Nat Rev Neurosci* **8**:355–367.

Tyring S, Gottlieb A, Papp K et al. 2006. Etanercept and clinical outcomes, fatigue, and depression in psoriasis: double-blind placebo-controlled randomised phase III trial. *Lancet* **367**:29–35.

Uranova N, Orlovskaya D, Vikhreva O et al. 2001. Electron microscopy of oligodendroglia in severe mental illness. *Brain Res Bull* **55**:597–610.

Uranova NA, Vostrikov VM, Orlovskaya DD, Rachmanova VI. 2004. Oligodendroglial density in the prefrontal cortex in schizophrenia and mood disorders: a study from the Stanley Neuropathology Consortium. *Schizophr Res* **67**:269–275.

Van Laere K, Nuttin B, Gabriels L et al. 2006. Metabolic imaging of anterior capsular stimulation in refractory obsessive-compulsive disorder: a key role for the subgenual anterior cingulate and ventral striatum. *J Nucl Med* **47**:740–747.

Victor TA, Furey MA, Fromm S, Ohman A, Drevets WC. 2010.

Relationship of emotional processing to masked faces in the amygdala to mood state and treatment in major depressive disorder. *Arch Gen Psychiatry* 67:1128–1138.

Vidal-Gonzalez I, Vidal-Gonzalez B, Rauch SL, Quirk GJ. 2006. Microstimulation reveals opposing influences of prelimbic and infralimbic cortex on the expression of conditioned fear. *Learn Mem* 13:728–733.

Vostrikov VM, Uranova NA, Orlovskaya DD. 2007. Deficit of perineuronal oligodendrocytes in the prefrontal cortex in schizophrenia and mood disorders. *Schizophr Res* 94:273–280.

Vyas A, Bernal S, Chattarji S. 2003. Effects of chronic stress on dendritic arborization in the central and extended amygdala. *Brain Res* 965:290–294.

Vyas A, Jadhav S, Chattarji S. 2006. Prolonged behavioral stress enhances synaptic connectivity in the basolateral amygdala. *Neuroscience* 143:387–393.

Vyas A, Mitra R, Shankaranarayana Rao BS, Chattarji S. 2002. Chronic stress induces contrasting patterns of dendritic remodeling in hippocampal and amygdaloid neurons. *J Neurosci* 22:6810–6818.

Vythilingam M, Heim C, Newport J et al. 2002. Childhood trauma associated with smaller hippocampal volume in women with major depression. *Am J Psychiatry* 159:2072–2080.

Wallace DL, Han MH, Graham DL et al. 2009. CREB regulation of nucleus accumbens excitability mediates social isolation-induced behavioral deficits. *Nat Neurosci* 12:200–209.

Wallace DL, Vialou V, Rios L et al. 2008. The influence of DeltaFosB in the nucleus accumbens on natural reward-related behavior. *J Neurosci* 28:10272–10277.

Wallace TL, Stellitano KE, Neve RL, Duman RS. 2004. Effects of cyclic adenosine monophosphate response element binding protein overexpression in the basolateral amygdala on behavioral models of depression and anxiety. *Biol Psychiatry* 56:151–160.

Warner-Schmidt JL, Duman RS. 2007. VEGF is an essential mediator of the neurogenic and behavioral actions of antidepressants. *Proc Natl Acad Sci USA* 104:4647–4652.

Warner-Schmidt JL, Flajolet M, Maller A et al. 2009. Role of p11 in cellular and behavioral effects of 5-HT4 receptor stimulation. *J Neurosci* 29:1937–1946.

Watanabe Y, Gould E, Daniels DC, Cameron H, McEwen BS. 1992. Tianeptine attenuates stress-induced morphological changes in the hippocampus. *Eur J Pharmacol* 222:157–162.

Watkins J, Collingridge G. 1994. Phenylglycine derivatives as antagonists of metabotropic glutamate receptors. *Trends Pharmacol Sci* 15:333–342.

Weaver IC. 2009. Epigenetic effects of glucocorticoids. *Semin Fetal Neonatal Med* 14:143–150.

Weaver IC, Cervoni N, Champagne FA et al. 2004. Epigenetic programming by maternal behavior. *Nat Neurosci* 7:847–854.

Weaver IC, Champagne FA, Brown SE et al. 2005. Reversal of maternal programming of stress responses in adult offspring through methyl supplementation: altering epigenetic marking later in life. *J Neurosci* 25:11045–11054.

Weaver IC, D'Alessio AC, Brown SE et al. The transcription factor nerve growth factor-inducible protein a mediates epigenetic programming: altering epigenetic marks by immediate-early genes. *J Neurosci* 27:1756–1768.

Weaver IC, Meaney MJ, Szyf M. 2006. Maternal care effects on the hippocampal transcriptome and anxiety-mediated behaviors in the offspring that are reversible in adulthood. *Proc Natl Acad Sci USA* 103:3480–3485.

Webster MJ, Knable MB, Johnston-Wilson N et al. 2001. Immunohistochemical localization of phosphorylated glial fibrillary acidic protein in the prefrontal cortex and hippocampus from patients with schizophrenia, bipolar disorder, and depression. *Brain Behav Immun* 15:388–400.

Wellman CL. 2001. Dendritic reorganization in pyramidal neurons in medial prefrontal cortex after chronic corticosterone administration. *J Neurobiol* 49:245–253.

Weng G, Bhalla US, Iyengar R. 1999. Complexity in biological signaling systems. *Science* 284:92–96.

Werme M, Messer C, Olson L et al. 2002. Delta FosB regulates wheel running. *J Neurosci* 22:8133–8138.

Williams LM, Brammer MJ, Skerrett D et al. 2000. The neural correlates of orienting: an integration of fMRI and skin conductance orienting. *Neuroreport* 11:3011–3015.

Witkin JM, Marek GJ, Johnson BG, Schoepp DD. 2007. Metabotropic glutamate receptors in the control of mood disorders. *CNS Neurol Disord Drug Targets* 6:87–100.

Wolkowitz OM, Reus VI, Chan T et al. 1999. Antiglucocorticoid treatment of depression: double-blind ketoconazole. *Biol Psychiatry* 45:1070–1074.

Wood GE, Young LT, Reagan LP, Chen B, McEwen BS. 2004. Stress-induced structural remodeling in hippocampus: prevention by lithium treatment. *Proc Natl Acad Sci USA* 101:3973–3978.

Wu J, Gillin JC, Buchsbaum MS et al. 1992. Effect of sleep deprivation on brain metabolism of depressed patients. *Am J Psychiatry* 149:538–543.

Xu J, Culman J, Blume A, Brecht S, Gohlke P. 2003. Chronic treatment with a low dose of lithium protects the brain against ischemic injury by reducing apoptotic death. *Stroke* **34**:1287–1292.

Yang L, Lindholm K, Konishi Y, Li R, Shen Y. 2002. Target depletion of distinct tumor necrosis factor receptor subtypes reveals hippocampal neuron death and survival through different signal transduction pathways. *J Neurosci* **22**:3025–3032.

Yang L, Matthews RT, Schulz JB *et al.* 1998. 1-Methyl-4-phenyl-1,2,3,6-tetrahydropyride neurotoxicity is attenuated in mice overexpressing Bcl-2. *J Neurosci* **18**:8145–8152.

Yildiz A, Guleryuz S, Ankerst DP, Ongur D, Renshaw PF. 2008. Protein kinase C inhibition in the treatment of mania: a double-blind, placebo-controlled trial of tamoxifen. *Arch Gen Psychiatry* **65**:255–263.

Yoshimizu T, Chaki S. 2004. Increased cell proliferation in the adult mouse hippocampus following chronic administration of group II metabotropic glutamate receptor antagonist, MGS0039. *Biochem Biophys Res Commun* **315**:493–496.

Yoshimizu T, Shimazaki T, Ito A, Chaki S. 2006. An mGluR2/3 antagonist, MGS0039, exerts antidepressant and anxiolytic effects in behavioral models in rats. *Psychopharmacology (Berl)* **186**:587–593.

Young AH, Gallagher P, Watson S *et al.* 2004. Improvements in neurocognitive function and mood following adjunctive treatment with mifepristone (RU-486) in bipolar disorder. *Neuropsychopharmacology* **29**:1538–1545.

Young LT, Wang JF, Woods CM, Robb JC. 1999. Platelet protein kinase C alpha levels in drug-free and lithium-treated subjects with bipolar disorder. *Neuropsychobiology* **40**:63–66.

Yucel K, Taylor VH, McKinnon MC *et al.* 2008. Bilateral hippocampal volume increase in patients with bipolar disorder and short-term lithium treatment. *Neuropsychopharmacology* **33**:361–367.

Zachariou V, Bolanos CA, Selley DE *et al.* 2006. An essential role for DeltaFosB in the nucleus accumbens in morphine action. *Nat Neurosci* **9**:205–211.

Zarate CA, Quiroz J, Payne J, Manji HK. 2002. Modulators of the glutamatergic system: implications for the development of improved therapeutics in mood disorders. *Psychopharmacol Bull* **36**:35–83.

Zarate CA, Du J, Quiroz J *et al.* 2003. Regulation of cellular plasticity cascades in the pathophysiology and treatment of mood disorders: role of the glutamatergic system. *Ann N Y Acad Sci* **1003**:273–291.

Zarate CA Jr, Manji HK. 2008. Bipolar disorder: candidate drug targets. *Mt Sinai J Med* **75**:226–247.

Zarate CA Jr, Payne JL, Quiroz J *et al.* 2004a. An open-label trial of riluzole in patients with treatment-resistant major depression. *Am J Psychiatry* **161**:171–174.

Zarate CA Jr, Payne JL, Singh J *et al.* 2004b. Pramipexole for bipolar II depression: a placebo-controlled proof of concept study. *Biol Psychiatry* **56**:54–60.

Zarate CA Jr, Quiroz JA, Singh JB *et al.* 2005. An open-label trial of the glutamate-modulating agent riluzole in combination with lithium for the treatment of bipolar depression. *Biol Psychiatry* **57**:430–432.

Zarate CA Jr, Singh JB, Carlson PJ *et al.* 2006. A randomized trial of an N-methyl-D-aspartate antagonist in treatment-resistant major depression. *Arch Gen Psychiatry* **63**:856–864.

Zarate CA Jr, Singh JB, Carlson PJ *et al.* 2007. Efficacy of a protein kinase C inhibitor (Tamoxifen) in the treatment of acute mania: a pilot study. *Bipolar Disord* **9**:561–570.

Zeller E, Stief HJ, Pflug B, Sastre-y-Hernandez M. 1984. Results of a phase II study of the antidepressant effect of rolipram. *Pharmacopsychiatry* **17**:188–190.

Zhang F, Phiel CJ, Spece L, Gurvich N, Klein PS. 2003. Inhibitory phosphorylation of glycogen synthase kinase-3 (GSK-3) in response to lithium. Evidence for autoregulation of GSK-3. *J Biol Chem* **278**:33067–33077.

Zhang HT. 2009. Cyclic AMP-specific phosphodiesterase-4 as a target for the development of antidepressant drugs. *Curr Pharm Des* **15**:1688–1698.

Zhang HT, Huang Y, Jin SL *et al.* 2002. Antidepressant-like profile and reduced sensitivity to rolipram in mice deficient in the PDE4D phosphodiesterase enzyme. *Neuropsychopharmacology* **27**:587–595.

Zhang HT, Huang Y, Masood A *et al.* Anxiogenic-like behavioral phenotype of mice deficient in phosphodiesterase 4B (PDE4B). *Neuropsychopharmacology* **33**:1611–1623.

Zhang TY, Meaney MJ. 2010. Epigenetics and the environmental regulation of the genome and its function. *Annu Rev Psychol* **61**:439–466, C431–433.

Zhou R, Gray NA, Yuan P *et al.* 2005. The anti-apoptotic, glucocorticoid receptor cochaperone protein BAG-1 is a long-term target for the actions of mood stabilizers. *J Neurosci* **25**:4493–4502.

Zobel AW, Nickel T, Kunzel HE *et al.* 2000. Effects of the high-affinity corticotropin-releasing hormone receptor 1 antagonist R121919 in major depression: the first 20 patients treated. *J Psychiatr Res* **34**:171–181.

Chapter 4

Schizophrenia

Darrick T. Balu and Donald C. Goff

History of drug discovery for treating schizophrenia

To this day, the pharmacological management of schizophrenia is based upon a serendipitous discovery over 50 years ago of the antipsychotic effects of chlorpromazine. Chlorpromazine (Thorazine; GlaxoSmithKline, Philadelphia, PA), the first effective pharmacological treatment for schizophrenia, was developed initially as an antihistamine to reduce intraoperative autonomic stress. A French naval surgeon, Henri Laborit, recognized its calming effects and, in 1952, convinced Deniker and Delay to study it in psychiatric patients, in whom it was found to be remarkably effective for psychosis. This serendipitous discovery led to Food and Drug Administration (FDA) approval in 1954 and rapidly transformed the care of many individuals with schizophrenia from lifelong inpatient confinement to outpatient treatment in the community. In an early NIMH-funded multicenter study of more than 400 patients acutely ill with schizophrenia, three phenothiazines (chlorpromazine, thioridazine, and fluphenazine) produced moderate or greater improvement in 75% of patients compared with a 23% rate of improvement with placebo (Lasky et al. 1962).

The discovery by Carlsson and Lindquist (1963) that the new antipsychotic drugs increased dopamine turnover, combined with the observation that dopamine agonists produce psychosis in healthy subjects, established excess dopamine activity as the dominant etiologic model for schizophrenia. Subsequently, the D_2 receptor affinity of all antipsychotic agents was shown to correlate with clinical potency (Seeman et al. 1976). Drug discovery for schizophrenia treatments at that time was directed at identifying agents with comparable properties inferred by indirect criteria such as protection against apomorphine-induced canine vomiting or improvement in the conditioned avoidance response, while at the same time seeking increased potency and attenuated neurological side effects (Janssen and Awouters, 1994). The dopamine hypothesis was sufficiently compelling that exploration of other drug targets was not pursued for several decades. Haloperidol, which was approved by the FDA in 1967, was the tenth and final first-generation dopamine D_2 blocker marketed in the USA for the treatment of schizophrenia.

In another serendipitous advance, clozapine, a dibenzodiazepine derivative of the tricyclic antidepressant imipramine, which had failed to exhibit antidepressant and antipsychotic efficacy in animal models, was found in clinical trials to possess antipsychotic efficacy superior to that of existing agents. In 1988, Kane et al. reported results from a pivotal study of clozapine demonstrating greater efficacy compared with chlorpromazine for psychosis, agitation, negative symptoms, and mood in the absence of neurological side effects or prolactin elevation, proving that more effective antipsychotics could be developed. This finding ushered in an era of intensive research by pharmaceutical companies competing to develop additional atypical or second-generation antipsychotics. Although experimental evidence suggested that a high $5-HT_2/D_2$ ratio was the mechanism for the therapeutic advantages of clozapine (Meltzer 1989), a series of second-generation drugs developed on the basis of favorable $5-HT_2/D_2$ ratios failed to outperform representative first-generation agents in large publicly funded multicenter trials (Jones et al. 2006; Lieberman et al. 2005a; Sikich et al. 2008). Moreover, although these second-generation antipsychotics produced fewer extrapyramidal side effects than their first-generation counterparts, they introduced other serious

---

Translational Neuroscience, ed. James E. Barrett, Joseph T. Coyle and Michael Williams. Published by Cambridge University Press. © Cambridge University Press 2012.

problems including weight gain, hyperlipidosis, and glucose intolerance (Meltzer 2007).

It was not until the past 15 years that investigators began to focus on other components of schizophrenia rather than just the antipsychotic-responsive positive symptoms (i.e., hallucinations, delusion, and thought disorder). Negative symptoms including apathy, poverty of thought, anhedonia, lack of drive, disorganization, and social isolation were observed to co-vary independently from positive symptoms and be much more enduring. Patients suffering from schizophrenia also have significant impairments in memory, problem solving, and executive functions (Heinrichs and Zakzanis 1998; Mesholam-Gately et al. 2009). Of these characteristic symptoms, only psychosis responds to current treatments, whereas the cognitive deficits and negative symptoms are primarily responsible for the chronic disability associated with the illness and correlate inversely with outcome (Arango et al. 2004). In addition to the increased awareness of other behavioral symptoms, progress in both structural and functional imaging, as well as in neuroanatomical data, has made it apparent that there are substantial perturbations in cortical connectivity in schizophrenia.

Introduction

Despite decades of research exploring the neuropathology and biochemistry of schizophrenia, few therapies in current practice have followed from a translational medicine approach. This lack of success reflects the daunting complexity of the illness. Clinical heterogeneity represents one obstacle, because patients with schizophrenia exhibit considerable diversity in their expression of a wide range of symptoms. A translational medicine approach has also been hampered by the fact that the neurobiological processes underlying schizophrenia are not well understood.

However, recent advances in research on schizophrenia have significantly changed the manner in which translational research is being conducted in this field. Although there is a lack of gross morphological change observed in the brains of schizophrenic patients, there is substantial evidence that this disorder is one of impaired synaptic connectivity, which has been observed in numerous humans postmortem as well as in functional and structural brain imaging studies (Andero et al. 2011). Moreover, the recent explosion of human genetic studies has greatly increased our understanding of the biological mechanisms underlying schizophrenia. Genetic studies of schizophrenia have revealed many common genes contributing very small risk and rare copy number variants (CNVs) contributing greater risk, but with variable penetrance.

It is these neuropathological, genetic, and behavioral abnormalities observed in schizophrenia that can be "translated" into animal models and then used to understand the pathophysiology of the disorder, nominate therapeutic targets, and ultimately test their safety and efficacy. Given that schizophrenia is a complex and heterogeneous psychiatric disorder, it is not possible to model it in its entirety. Therefore, animal models are generated that recapitulate only certain aspects of schizophrenia. Early animal models involved various pharmacological manipulations to reproduce particular phenotypes of schizophrenia, whereas more recent models have used the wealth of human genetic data to manipulate these risk genes in various species.

This chapter outlines the major neuropathological and behavioral abnormalities associated with schizophrenia, because it is these alterations that one looks to produce in models of the disease. Next, it discusses the risk genes most implicated in the pathophysiology of schizophrenia and outlines their roles in regulating aspects of neuroplasticity thought to be perturbed in this disease. The following sections describe the pharmacological and genetic animal models that are being used in translational research. The final section highlights novel therapeutic targets currently being investigated for treating schizophrenia.

Neurobiology
Synaptic changes and dysconnectivity

Improper synaptic connectivity now appears to be one of the hallmark pathological characteristics of schizophrenia. The abnormalities in neural connectivity are present in multiple regions of the brain that are important for regulating cognitive function, sensory processing, and affect. One of the most consistent structural abnormalities found in schizophrenia is the volumetric reduction of the medial temporal lobe (hippocampal formation, subiculum, parahippocampal gyrus) and of the neocortex (Ross et al. 2006) that coincide with increased volume of the lateral ventricles. Because these volumetric reductions are associated with increased cell packing density but not with changes in neuronal number, they are likely due to decreased amounts of cortical neuropil (the axon terminals, dendrites and dendritic spines, and glial processes that occupy the interneuronal spaces) (Selemon and Goldman-Rakic 1999). Several lines of evidence support this notion. Postmortem studies have found changes in cortical molecular markers that suggest that both neuronal and/or axonal integrity are compromised (Bertolino *et al.* 1996; Buckley *et al.* 1994) and that the number of synapses (Stanley *et al.* 1995) is reduced in schizophrenia. In addition, the complexity of dendritic branching, total dendritic length, and dendritic spine density of pyramidal neurons is reduced in the prefrontal cortex (PFC) of patients with schizophrenia (Garey *et al.* 1998; Glantz and Lewis 2000; Kalus *et al.* 2000; Rajkowska *et al.* 1998). The number of puncta immunoreactive for spinophilin, a marker of dendritic spines, is reduced in the primary auditory cortex in schizophrenia (Sweet *et al.* 2009). Because dendritic spines are the principal structural targets of excitatory neurotransmission, these findings suggest that the disruptions in dendritic morphology alter the cortical and/or thalamic circuitry in schizophrenia, which in turn might be the neurobiological substrate underlying the cognitive and sensory dysfunctions observed in patients (Lewis and Gonzalez-Burgos 2008).

Neuroimaging studies have also provided evidence for impaired connectivity in schizophrenia. Functional magnetic resonance imaging (fMRI) has shown abnormalities in the activation of the dorsolateral PFC (DLPFC), medial temporal lobe, hippocampus, anterior cingulate, striatum, and thalamus (Niznikiewicz *et al.* 2003), which are associated with impaired working memory (Potkin *et al.* 2009). Diffusion tensor (DT) imaging evaluates the organization and coherence of white matter fiber tracts that serve as anatomical connections between proximal and distant brain regions, thereby creating functional networks. Deficits in white matter tracts appear to be present in the early stages of schizophrenia, even in neuroleptic-naïve patients (Kyriakopoulos and Frangou 2009). Finally, event-related potentials (ERPs) reveal disruption in cortical processing of sensory stimuli regardless of modality (Javitt 2009). Thus, the preponderance of evidence supports the notion that schizophrenia is a progressive disorder that diffusely affects the corticolimbic system.

Neurotransmitter systems

Dopaminergic activity

As described in the Introduction, the model of excessive dopamine activity stems from the observation that sufficient doses of catecholamine releasers (amphetamines) administered over a sufficient period produce psychosis in healthy individuals and trigger relapse in patients with schizophrenia. In 1991, Davis *et al.* modified the initial model of dopamine hyperactivity and argued that a primary deficit in prefrontal cortical dopamine resulted in negative symptoms and produced a reciprocal increase in striatal dopamine. This model has subsequently been supported by the demonstration of increased presynaptic dopamine in the brains of patients with schizophrenia and increased release of striatal dopamine in response to challenge with amphetamine (Howes and Kapur 2009). Family members and individuals at risk for psychosis have an intermediate degree of dopamine activity. This model posits that vulnerability to psychosis involves excessive dopamine release under stress. Dopamine release can be elevated through many mechanisms, including NMDA receptor (NMDAR) blockade (Kegeles *et al.* 2000), γ-amino butyric acid (GABA)ergic interneuron dysfunction, sensitization by stress or by psychostimulants (Lieberman *et al.* 1997), and cannabis abuse (Howes and Kapur 2009). Excessive dopaminergic activity in the hippocampus has been conjectured to cause inappropriate blocking of sensory input and misinterpretation of previously coded memories (Lisman and Otmakhova 2001). This defect might link perceptions or memories to inappropriate affective salience (Kapur 2003) and might hinder reality testing and correction of distorted memories or beliefs. Although early studies did not produce consistent results, evidence now supports an increased density of D_1 receptors in the PFC of medication-naïve patients that corresponds to cognitive deficits and is believed to represent an upregulation in response to diminished dopamine release (Abi-Dargham *et al.* 2002).

GABAergic activity

One of the first neurochemical abnormalities described in postmortem studies in schizophrenia was a reduction in the activity of cortical glutamate decarboxylase of 67 kDa (GAD67), the enzyme that synthesizes GABA (Spokes 1979). More recent studies have revealed a much more selective effect primarily on the parvalbumin (PV+)-expressing, fast-firing GABAergic interneurons in the intermediate layers of the cortex and in subsectors of the hippocampus that provide recurrent inhibition to the pyramidal cells (Benes 1999; Hashimoto *et al.* 2008; Lewis *et al.* 2005). Thus, reduction in the expression of GAD67, PV, and the GABA transporter has been demonstrated in this neuronal population. That the downregulation of these presynaptic markers reflects reduced activity of these GABAergic neurons is inferred by the compensatory upregulation of postsynaptic α_2 containing $GABA_A$ receptors (Volk *et al.* 2002).

Glutamatergic activity

The hypothesis that dysregulation of glutamate transmission contributes to the pathophysiology of schizophrenia is supported by several converging lines of evidence. Dissociative anesthetics such as ketamine and phencyclidine (PCP), which are NMDAR channel blockers, produce the full range of schizophrenia symptoms and cognitive deficits in healthy subjects and exacerbate symptoms in treated patients (Jentsch and Roth 1999). Subsequent studies showed that low-dose ketamine could produce in normal volunteers the physiological abnormalities associated with schizophrenia, including abnormal ERPs (Umbricht *et al.* 2000), eye-tracking abnormalities (Radant *et al.* 1998), and enhanced subcortical dopamine release (Kegeles *et al.* 2000). Cerebrospinal fluid (CSF) levels of the endogenous glycine modulatory site (GMS) antagonist, kynurenic acid, are elevated in patients with schizophrenia (Erhardt *et al.* 2001). On the other hand, the GMS agonist, D-serine, is reduced in the CSF and serum of patients with schizophrenia (Hashimoto *et al.* 2003, 2005). Moreover, there is a preponderance of glutamate-related schizophrenia risk genes (Harrison and Weinberger 2005) and postmortem findings of glutamate receptor abnormalities (Goff and Coyle 2001).

Integrating the postmortem, genetic, and animal modeling results has suggested a plausible pathological circuit in schizophrenia (Coyle *et al.* 2010). Hypofunction of corticolimbic NMDARs could be due to elevated levels of endogenous inhibitors, such as kynurenic acid or *N*–ethyl aspartyl glutamate (NAAG), reduced availability of the endogenous co-agonist D-serine, heritable abnormalities in NR2B expression, or reductions in the fast-firing PV+- GABAergic interneurons in the intermediate layers of the cortex. This reduction in glutamatergic activity results in downregulation of GAD67 and PV expression, and disinhibition of the postsynaptic pyramidal cells (Lisman *et al.* 2008). Disinhibition of glutamatergic output from the ventral hippocampus would drive the firing of dopaminergic neurons in the ventral tegmental area and enhanced subcortical dopamine release, which in PET studies correlates with psychosis (Grace, 2010). Thus, in this model, psychosis is a downstream event. Obviously, the pathophysiology of schizophrenia is much more complex than suggested by this simplified model. Indeed, a number of putative risk genes encode transcriptional factors that affect brain development and synaptic plasticity (Margolis and Ross 2010). Nevertheless, it does yield a host of potential targets for therapeutic intervention.

Intermediate phenotypes

As previously mentioned, schizophrenia is a heterogeneous syndrome that lacks any single defining symptom or sign. One approach to classify such complex psychiatric disorders is by identifying intermediate phenotypes (Walters and Owen 2007). These are heritable, individually measured traits or markers that alone represent only a component of the disease and may be useful in genetic linkage studies. Valid intermediate phenotypes will associate with schizophrenia in population studies, be present but less prominent in first-degree family members of probands with schizophrenia, and will be found in both members of twins discordant for schizophrenia (Ross *et al.* 2006). A variety of behavioral and electrophysiological intermediate phenotypes have been associated with schizophrenia. Many of these intermediate phenotypes are tractable in rodents and are therefore prime candidates for use in translational research, which is the topic of this section.

Electrophysiological measures
Auditory evoked related potentials

Electroencephalography (EEG) has been widely used to study sensory processing deficits in schizophrenia, with EEG responses to auditory stimuli recorded and averaged to yield ERPs. Human ERPs are characterized by a positive voltage deflection occurring approximately 50 ms after the stimulus (P50) and a negative voltage deflection occurring 100 ms after the stimulus (N100), whereas the novelty-elicited P300 positive deflection occurs 300 ms poststimulus. Patients with schizophrenia have deficits in P50, N100, and P300 ERP amplitudes. They also have a reduced ability to detect changes in the auditory environment, called mismatch negativity (MMN) (Amann et al. 2010). Analogous EEG measurements can be recorded from a variety of rodent species. These EEG recordings are sensitive to pharmacological and genetic manipulations posited to be involved in the pathophysiology and treatment of schizophrenia (Amann et al. 2010). Dopamine agonists, like amphetamine, as well as NMDAR antagonists (ketamine, phencyclidine, and MK-801) reduce the P20 and N40 amplitudes in mice (analogous to the P50 and N100 in humans). On the other hand, antipsychotics increase these amplitudes, or if administered prior to dopamine agonists or NMDAR antagonists, can block their effects. Ketamine and MK-801 have also been shown to reduce MMN amplitude in both mice and rats (Amann et al. 2010).

Oscillatory activity

Frequency oscillations (slowest to fastest frequencies: delta, theta, alpha, beta, and gamma) represent the coordinated firing of clusters of neurons and are thought to help synchronize activity within and between brain regions. The theta and gamma bands are abnormal in patients with schizophrenia, and these deficits have been linked to the disease via heritability studies (Hall et al. 2009; Hong et al. 2008). Animal models of oscillatory deficits are relatively new to the field. It has been shown that ketamine and amphetamine reduce evoked theta, whereas NMDAR antagonists increase basal gamma activity similar to that seen in schizophrenia. Moreover, these oscillations are responsive to antipsychotic drugs (Amann et al. 2010).

Prepulse inhibition

Prepulse inhibition (PPI) of the acoustic startle reflex refers to the neurological phenomenon in which a weaker prestimulus (prepulse) inhibits the reaction to a subsequent strong startling stimulus. It is well documented that patients with schizophrenia show deficits in PPI that correlate clinically to symptoms such as thought disorder and distractibility (Turetsky et al. 2007). This paradigm is extremely amenable to use in rodents, because it is one of the few tests that is largely conserved across all vertebrate species (Geyer et al. 2002). There is an extensive literature that demonstrates the sensitivity of this assay to drugs that modulate dopaminergic and glutamatergic signaling, antipsychotics, and genetic models that are linked to the pathophysiology of schizophrenia (Geyer et al. 2001, 2002).

Cognitive abnormalities

The cognitive symptoms in schizophrenia are related to impairments in working memory, attention, learning, executive function, and other prefrontal-dependent cognitive tasks. Based on imaging and lesion studies, working memory and behavioral flexibility have been associated with the DLPFC in humans (Goldman-Rakic 1994), with the mPFC being the homologous structure in rodents. In mice, the mPFC is required for spatial working memory tasks, attentional set shifting and reversal learning, and conditioned associative learning, tasks that are similar to those administered to human subjects (Kellendonk et al. 2009). Therefore, working memory tasks that engage the DLPFC in humans can be modified for translational research in rodents.

Latent inhibition

Latent inhibition (LI) refers to an animal's unconscious capacity to ignore stimuli that experience has shown are irrelevant to its needs. LI deficits in patients with schizophrenia have been used as evidence of a selective attention deficit in the disorder because it reflects an organism's ability to ignore irrelevant stimuli (Lubow and Gewitz 1995). Experimental evidence suggests that the mesolimbic-dopaminergic systems play a major role in regulating LI (Amann et al. 2010). One of the major strengths of the LI task is that it can be applied across mammalian species. Administration of amphetamine disrupts LI in rodents and humans, an effect that is reversed by antipsychotics (Amann et al. 2010).

Social abnormalities

Patients with schizophrenia also have deficits in social interaction and exhibit social withdrawal, a subset of the negative symptoms of the disease. A number of tasks have been developed to assess proper sociability in mice that test for social approach and social avoidance and for social dominance behaviors (Amann et al. 2010).

Genetics

Even though schizophrenia has a strong genetic component (heritability of approximately 0.8) as evidenced by family and twin studies, the genetics are complex, with no single gene producing a strong effect. Rather, schizophrenia appears to be the result of multiple genes of moderate effect interacting with each other and the environment to produce a phenotype (Purcell et al. 2009). Linkage and association studies have now implicated several loci in the genome that appear to contain genes conferring risk of schizophrenia (Ross et al. 2006). In addition, a large number of single nucleotide polymorphisms (SNPs) in functionally relevant risk genes were found to be associated with individual schizophrenia intermediate phenotypes, with a subset of these SNPs being associated with multiple phenotypes (Greenwood et al. 2011). Recent research suggests that highly penetrant de novo CNVs (deletions and/or duplications) also contribute to the genetic risk for schizophrenia (Purcell et al. 2009).

Although initial genetic studies provided evidence suggestive of associations between schizophrenia and putative risk genes, the strength of these associations has recently been called into question because hypothesis-neutral, genome-wide association studies (GWAS) have not confirmed these risk gene associations. However, an important limitation of GWAS is that they examine hundreds of thousands to millions of SNPs requiring a substantial correction for multiple comparisons that can compromise statistical power (Cannon 2010). Thus, there is debate as to whether negative GWAS findings invalidate the results of candidate gene association studies or they are insufficiently powered (Cannon 2010).

DISC1

The DISC locus was identified via a balanced (1;11) (q42.1; q14.3) chromosomal translocation in a large Scottish pedigree that segregates in a highly significant manner with a broad range of psychiatric illnesses, including schizophrenia, bipolar disorder, and major depression (St Clair et al. 1990). The chromosomal translocation occurs between exons 8 and 9 of the DISC1 gene on chromosome 1, which has not yet been found in any other families (Ross et al. 2006). Evidence for this chromosomal association with psychiatric illness has been supported with studies from various populations and from multiple independent association studies supporting DISC1 as a risk factor for psychiatric illness (Chubb et al. 2008). Numerous studies have also reported evidence of linkage or association between the DISC1 locus and impaired cognitive function in both normal individuals and patients with schizophrenia (Chubb et al. 2008), deficits that are consistent with dysfunction of the DLPFC and hippocampus. DISC1 haplotypes, including the putative functional SNP (Ser704Cys), are also associated with reduced gray matter volume in the hippocampus and cortex (Callicott et al. 2005; Hashimoto et al. 2006; Thomson et al. 2005). In addition to cognition, DISC1 variants also affect the level of social anhedonia (Tomppo et al. 2009). The molecular mechanism of the DISC1 translocation is still uncertain and remains controversial. Possible outcomes include haploinsufficiency or a dominant/negative product, or both, of the C-terminally truncated mutant protein encoded from exons 1–8 (Sawa and Snyder 2005). An additional implication of the balanced translocation is the production of unique fusion transcripts (Zhou et al. 2008, 2010).

DISC1 is a truly multifunctional scaffolding protein with a diverse cellular distribution. In vitro and in silico data suggest a network of potential protein interaction partners including 127 proteins and 158 interactions that are involved in processes related to cell cycle/division, cytoskeletal stability and organization, intracellular transport, and synaptic function (Camargo et al. 2007). A preponderance of evidence supports a critical role of DISC1 protein interactions for proper functioning of the centrosome and links perturbation of this system to abnormal cortical development (Andero et al. 2011). DISC1 also regulates cortical and hippocampal neurogenesis, although the roles it plays in these processes are complex and depend on numerous factors including brain region and stage of development. Impaired DISC1 signaling during development contributes to the alterations of dopaminergic and GABAergic signaling in the PFC (Niwa et al. 2010). Finally, DISC1 is a regulator of NMDAR-dependent activity changes in dendritic spine morphology (Hayashi-Takagi et al. 2010).

Neuregulin

Neuregulin 1 (NRG1) was first identified as a candidate schizophrenia risk gene by extensive fine mapping of the 8p locus (*NRG1* lies in the 8p12–8p21 region) and haplotype-association analysis of affected Icelandic families. Many studies since then from diverse populations have supported the genetic association between *NRG1* and schizophrenia and identified 80 SNPs (Alaerts *et al.* 2009; Mei and Xiong 2008; Walker *et al.* 2010). Nevertheless, some studies have shown poor associations (Iwata *et al.* 2004; Rosa *et al.* 2007; Thiselton *et al.* 2004). Several meta-analyses examining the strength of association between *NRG1* and schizophrenia have provided mixed results (Li *et al.* 2006; Gong *et al.* 2009). Functional polymorphisms associated with schizophrenia have been identified that influence NRG1 expression in the brain postmortem (Nicodemus *et al.* 2009; Tan *et al.* 2007). Brain-imaging studies have found genotype–phenotype effects with allelic variants of *NRG1* and *ErbB4*. These effects include decreased activation of the temporal and frontal lobe regions, increased development of psychotic symptoms, and decreased premorbid IQ (Hall *et al.* 2006), as well as deficits in white matter integrity in unaffected subjects carrying *NRG1* risk SNPs (McIntosh *et al.* 2008; Winterer *et al.* 2008). In healthy subjects carrying an *ErbB4* schizophrenia risk haplotype, left temporal lobe white matter abnormalities were found that correlated with impaired working memory (Konrad *et al.* 2009).

NRG1 belongs to a family of growth factors that signals through ErbB tyrosine kinase receptors (ErbB1–4), with the ErbB4 isoform best characterized for its CNS function. NRG1 is most known for its importance during brain development, where it regulates cell proliferation, myelination, neuronal migration, axon guidance, and synapse formation (Balu and Coyle 2011). NRG1 signaling during development is also important for determining the dopaminergic tone of the PFC in adulthood (Kato *et al.* 2011). In adult brain, NRG1-ErB4 signaling regulates glutamatergic, GABAergic, and dopaminergic neurotransmission, all of which are implicated in the etiology of schizophrenia (Balu and Coyle 2011).

Dysbindin

Evidence for dystrobrevin-binding protein 1 gene (DTNBP1; dysbindin) as a putative schizophrenia risk gene came from systematic linkage disequilibrium mapping across a linkage region on 6p in the 270 multiply affected pedigrees from the Irish Study of High Density Schizophrenia Families (Straub *et al.* 2002). Subsequent reanalysis of these data found a single high-risk haplotype containing eight SNPs covering 30 kb (van den Oord *et al.* 2003). As of 2008, there have been 45 follow-up association studies, 18 of them with positive results (Allen *et al.* 2008). Although there are inconsistencies in the reported alleles/haplotypes between studies (Desbonnet *et al.* 2009), the associations do cluster in eight commonly typed SNPs that yield six common haplotypes (Riley *et al.* 2009). These inconsistent findings have triggered skepticism of their validity (Strohmaier *et al.* 2010). Several studies have described an association between DTNBP1 SNPs and haplotypes with a higher level of negative and cognitive symptoms in schizophrenia (DeRosse *et al.* 2006; Fanous *et al.* 2005; Wessman *et al.* 2009; Wirgenes *et al.* 2009). These findings are in agreement with other evidence of DTNBP1 haplotypes influencing prefrontal brain function (Donohoe *et al.* 2007; Fallgatter *et al.* 2010; Luciano *et al.* 2009; Markov *et al.* 2010), as well as an association of a DTNBP1 haplotype with significant reductions of cortical gray matter volumes (Donohoe *et al.* 2010).

Dysbindin-1 is widely distributed in the brain (Guo *et al.* 2009) and is concentrated in synapses of brain areas commonly affected in schizophrenia, including the hippocampus, striatum, and cortex (Benson *et al.* 2001; Talbot *et al.* 2006). In mice, dysbindin-1 protein levels are developmentally regulated, with higher levels observed during embryonic and early postnatal periods than in young adulthood (Ghiani *et al.* 2010). Dysbindin is important for cytoskeletal function (Benson *et al.* 2001) and intracellular membrane trafficking and organelle biogenesis. In the presynaptic neuron, dysbindin increases glutamate release, whereas postsynaptically it inhibits the surface expression of NR2A but not NR2B containing NMDARs (Tang *et al.* 2009). Dysbindin negatively regulates the surface expression of dopamine type-2 (D_2) but not D_1 receptors, which in turn modulates GABAergic transmission (Ji *et al.* 2009).

Akt1

The first evidence for an association between variants of V-akt murine thymoma viral oncogen homolog 1 (*AKT1*) and schizophrenia came in 2004

(Emamian et al. 2004). Since then, the association between *AKT1* and schizophrenia has been replicated in multiple independent studies from diverse populations (Ikeda et al. 2004; Schwab et al. 2005; Tan et al. 2008; Thiselton et al. 2008; Xu et al. 2007), although not all studies have replicated this association (Ide et al. 2006; Liu et al. 2006; Ohtsuki et al. 2004; Turunen et al. 2007). Individuals carrying an *AKT1* haplotype associated with schizophrenia had significantly reduced Akt1 protein levels in the PFC compared with noncarriers (Karege et al. 2010). Healthy subjects who were minor allele (G/A) carriers of the synonymous coding SNP rs1130233 in *AKT1* (associated with increased risk for schizophrenia in a family-based associated study) had impaired cognitive performance, reduced protein levels of Akt1 in peripheral lymphoblasts, inefficient task-related activation of the DLPFC, and reduced gray matter volume in the bilateral caudate and right PFC (Tan et al. 2008).

Akt1 is a serine/threonine kinase of which there are two other isoforms (Akt2, Akt3), each with its own distinct physiological function (Cho et al. 2001a, 2001b). Akt receives inputs from many extracellular stimuli, including neurotrophic factors and neuronal activity. This kinase regulates numerous downstream cellular processes including protein synthesis, apoptosis, and activity-dependent plasticity (Brazil and Hemmings 2001). Akt is also directly downstream of dopamine receptor activation and is important for proper dopaminergic neurotransmission and dopamine-dependent behaviors (Emamian et al. 2004; Lai et al. 2006).

BDNF

The most extensively studied SNP in the gene encoding brain-derived neurotrophic factor (BDNF) is rs6265, which produces a G/A amino acid substitution (valine to methionine) at codon 66 (Val66Met). Val66Met is a functional polymorphism that affects the activity-dependent secretion of BDNF in neuronal cell cultures (Chen et al. 2006). Allele status affects human hippocampal function and episodic memory (Dempster et al. 2005; Egan et al. 2003). Association studies between Val66Met and schizophrenia have generated conflicting results (Gratacòs et al. 2007; Hong et al. 2003; Jonsson et al. 2006; Kanazawa et al. 2007; Neves-Pereira et al. 2005; Xie et al. 2007; Xu et al. 2007), suggesting the existence of an association, albeit of low increased risk and likely including multiple causal variants. Association between the *BDNF* alleles and brain morphology in schizophrenia has indicated that, compared with Val-homozygotes, Met-allele carriers tend to have reduced gray matter volumes in the hippocampus (Takahashi et al. 2008) and cortex (Ho et al. 2006). In patients with schizophrenia, Met-carriers had greater reductions in frontal gray matter volume and excessive increases in lateral ventricle and sulcal CSF volume over time compared with Val-homozygotes (Ho et al. 2007).

BDNF is a neurotrophic factor that, by signaling through its high-affinity receptor, tropomysin receptor kinase B (TrkB), regulates a vast array of processes during development and in the adult brain (Binder and Scharfman 2004). BDNF and TrkB are critical for the proper development of GABAergic interneurons in the cortex (Gorba and Wahle 1999). In the adult brain, they are important regulators of GABAergic (Sakata et al. 2009) and glutamatergic (Minichiello 2009) neurotransmission in regions of the brain that are perturbed in schizophrenia.

NMDA receptor

Recent genetic studies support a role for NMDARs in the etiology of schizophrenia. Most of the evidence is derived from association studies, although this strategy has come under criticism by advocates of the "unbiased" GWAS strategy. Meta-analysis has strongly implicated the gene encoding the NR2B subunit, D-amino acid oxidase (DAAO), which regulates the availability of D-serine, as well as G72, a gene encoding a protein that binds to and inhibits DAAO (Allen et al. 2008; Lisman et al. 2008). Furthermore, analysis of SNPs shown to be associated with intermediate phenotypes revealed extensive evidence for pleiotropy across multiple genes involved either directly or indirectly in glutamate signaling, suggesting a strong role for this pathway in mediating susceptibility to schizophrenia (Greenwood et al. 2011).

The heterotetrameric NMDAR is a critical postsynaptic mediator of activity-dependent synaptic plasticity. It is composed of two NR1 subunits and two NR2 subunits, all of which contribute to form the pore of the ion channel that is characterized by high Ca^{2+} permeability. NMDAR activation requires postsynaptic depolarization and the binding of two agonists, glutamate, and either glycine or

D-serine, at the (Gms Tsien 2000). The influx of Ca^{2+} triggers a cascade of intracellular events that regulates many types of neuroplasticity (Greer and Greenberg 2008; Wayman *et al.* 2008), including long-term potentiation (LTP), dendritic patterning, spine elaboration, and synaptogenesis, which are perturbed in schizophrenia and animal models of the disease.

Schizophrenia is a disorder of complex genetics that is the product of multiple risk genes with moderate effects, combined with environmental interactions. There is substantial evidence that schizophrenia is associated with perturbations in synaptogenesis and neuroplasticity, processes regulated by the aforementioned risk genes. Not only is a single risk gene involved in numerous signaling cascades, but also multiple risk genes may converge to affect the same signaling pathways and biological processes. These genes regulate glutamatergic, GABAergic, and dopaminergic transmission, all of which are dysregulated in schizophrenia. Therefore, disturbances in one of these genes could have significant effects on brain function, resulting in an intermediate phenotype, as has been demonstrated with allelic variants, whereas the presence of two or more risk alleles could have multiplicative effects. To determine how dysregulation of common biological functions underlies the etiology of schizophrenia, work needs to be done to delineate exactly which pathways are convergent, when during brain development their cross talk is critical, and where they intersect intracellularly. This task is made difficult by the complex transcriptional and translational regulation and by the time- and brain region-dependent expression of many of these proteins.

Animal models of schizophrenia
Pharmacological models
Neurodevelopmental manipulations

Considerable evidence points to a developmental component to schizophrenia, including in utero and perinatal risk factors, deficits in cognition and behavior prior to onset of the illness, linkage with genes involved with brain development, and histopathological findings consistent with abnormal neuronal migration, dendritic arborization, and circuit formation (Fatemi and Folsom 2009; Jaaro-Peled *et al.* 2009). A review of susceptibility genes identified broad categories of genes involved in neuroplasticity, neurodevelopment, and maintenance of brain microcircuits. Environmental insults in the second and third trimesters associated with increased risk include viral (influenza and rubella) and parasitic (toxoplasmosis) infections, starvation, elevated maternal concentrations of homocysteine and proinflammatory cytokine (interleukin [IL]-8), preeclampsia, and exposure to toxins. Increasingly, interactions between genetic risk and environmental factors are being identified, including an interaction between catechol-O-methyltransferase (COMT) genotype and cannabis use and between familial liability and in utero exposure to infection or maternal depression (Gilmore *et al.* 2004). Reduced expression of reelin mRNA in the PFC and hippocampus in schizophrenia is consistent with early deficits in neurodevelopment and neuroplasticity, particularly of GABAergic interneurons (Eastwood and Harrison 2006).

Neurodevelopmental models posit that errors in brain development, including progenitor cell proliferation, neuronal migration, synapse formation, myelination, and pruning, are the fundamental causes of the illness (Fatemi and Folsom 2009). If aberrant brain development cannot be prevented, this model would tend to predict that pharmacological approaches in adulthood are unlikely to correct the underlying defects but rather produce compensatory changes to minimize the consequences of abnormal brain circuits.

Many animal developmental models for schizophrenia reproduce gestational risk factors including maternal exposure to stress, infection, malnutrition, antimitotic agents, irradiation, and placental insufficiency (Carpenter and Koenig 2008). In one of the most compelling developmental animal models for schizophrenia, administration of the proinflammatory cytokine-releasing agent, polyinosinic: polycytidylic acid (polyI:C) on gestational days 2–6 in mice produces offspring that appear normal at birth but exhibit abnormalities consistent with schizophrenia at 10–12 weeks, including increased locomotor activity in response to amphetamine, decreased PPI, and deficits in working memory (Meyer *et al.* 2005). Deficits in depolarization-induced hippocampal glutamate release (Ibi *et al.* 2009) and dysregulation of neurotrophic factors (Gilmore *et al.* 2003) have also been observed in offspring. Other studies suggest that the timing and the balance between proinflammatory and anti-inflammatory cytokines are critical in determining behavioral outcomes (Meyer *et al.* 2009). Inflammatory cytokines are released in response to several forms of maternal stress that increase risk for schizophrenia in offspring, including infection and preeclampsia. This model may have greater validity for drug discovery than approaches using lesioning or pharmacological challenges in mature animals, at least for a subgroup of patients who may have developed their illness following this developmental path.

It will be important to identify not only the specific elements of early brain development that are disrupted by perinatal risk factors but also the elements of brain development in young adulthood that trigger the expression of symptoms of schizophrenia. It remains unclear whether a neurodevelopmental error is present in all individuals with schizophrenia and, if so, when the first behavioral evidence of such a lesion becomes manifest. Torrey *et al.* (1994) examined developmental histories of monozygotic twin pairs discordant for schizophrenia and found that roughly one-third of individuals demonstrated a behavioral or cognitive divergence from their twin prior to their early teens, suggesting that a distinct developmental clinical course may not characterize the majority of cases of schizophrenia. A study of performance on standardized tests routinely administered to schoolchildren indicated that the decline in mean cognitive performance, most marked in language comprehension, was first apparent between ages 13 and 16 years (Fuller *et al.* 2002). Cognitive deficits are almost uniformly found in individuals with the schizophrenic prodrome prior to onset of sustained psychosis. Early in the prodrome, impairment may be most evident in processing speed and executive function, with progression by the time psychosis emerges to impairment in all domains characteristic of schizophrenia (Frommann *et al.* 2010). The period during which cognitive decline and psychosis appear correlates with maturation of GABAergic interneurons and mesocortical dopamine tracts, pruning of glutamatergic synapses, and myelination, all of which enhance cognitive efficiency. It is unclear whether these developmental processes are abnormal in schizophrenia or merely serve to reveal an underlying earlier defect in brain formation.

Therapeutic approaches implied by developmental models include prevention of environmental risk factors during pregnancy, including viral infection (via immunization and isolation), malnutrition (specifically folate supplementation), toxins, preeclampsia, and birth complications. Individuals at heightened risk may in the future be identified by genetic profile, particularly maternal genes related to cytokine regulation and folate metabolism. It is also possible that interventions might be based on specific environmental risks; for example, the antioxidant N-acetylcysteine (NAC) has been shown to prevent maternal inflammatory cytokine release in response to a lipopolysaccharide challenge in mice (Beloosesky *et al.* 2009) and is currently in clinical trials to prevent brain injury resulting from chorioamnionitis. Another approach implied by the developmental model is to intervene to prevent pathological expression of underlying neurodevelopmental deficits, possibly by modifying synaptic pruning in adolescents at risk for the cognitive deficits of schizophrenia or to prevent psychosis in early adulthood by targeting dopamine systems. Much more information is needed regarding biological mechanisms, clinical markers, and genetic risk factors before such approaches can be seriously contemplated as public health measures.

Although the developmental model primarily implies a strategy of prevention, recent attention has also focused on approaches to facilitate neuroplasticity and synaptogenesis in individuals in whom deficits in brain function are already manifest. Abnormalities in neuroplasticity have been demonstrated using repetitive transcranial magnetic stimulation (rTMS) in medicated and unmedicated patients with schizophrenia (Daskalakis *et al.* 2008). It is posited that abnormalities in neuroplasticity during crucial periods of brain development may contribute to dysfunctional circuits in adults with schizophrenia. Following puberty, activation of D_1 receptors promotes NMDAR-dependent LTP in the PFC, whereas activation of D_2 receptors on inhibitory interneurons attenuates LTP (Goto *et al.* 2010), suggesting that D_2 antagonists or D_1 agonists might promote PFC neuroplasticity. Early results with cognitive remediation aimed at enhancing neuroplasticity via auditory discrimination training have been promising (Fisher *et al.* 2009); response correlated with elevation of serum BDNF (Vinogradov *et al.* 2009). It is hoped that neuroplasticity may be enhanced using such strategies, possibly in combination with medications that facilitate neuroplasticity via LTP (Nitsche *et al.* 2004) or that stimulate BDNF release (Angelucci *et al.* 2005). Another approach involves the development of drugs targeting compounds involved in brain formation and response to injury, such as activity-dependent neuroprotection protein (Gozes 2007).

Genetic models

The power of mouse genetics combined with the recent knowledge gleaned from human association and GWA studies has greatly improved our understanding of the underlying neurobiology of schizophrenia. The ability to manipulate mouse genetics provides the tools needed to establish causal relationships between genotype and intermediate phenotype, identify novel therapeutic targets, and determine whether drugs aimed at these targets are capable of reversing or preventing behavioral and neurochemical abnormalities.

DISC1

Although a DISC1 knockout mouse has yet to be generated, seven DISC1 mutant mouse models have been created, ranging from ENU-induced missense DISC1 mutants, to truncated human DISC1 transgenics and bacterial artificial chromosome (BAC) expressing mice (Jaaro-Peled 2009). All of them display a range of behavioral (disrupted PPI; impaired cognitive performance and sociability) and neuroanatomical (enlarged lateral ventricles, reduced spine density and number of parvalbumin interneurons) abnormalities relevant to schizophrenia (for extensive review see Desbonnet et al. 2009; Jaaro-Peled 2009; Jaaro-Peled et al. 2010). However, one important feature to take into account is that the mouse DISC1 is only ~60% identical to the human DISC1 at both the nucleotide and amino acid levels (Ma et al. 2002).

NRG1/ErbB4

NRG1-ErbB4 signaling has been perturbed in mouse models by knocking down NRG1 and ErbB receptors and targeting mutations of specific ErbB receptor domains. Many of these models recapitulate the behavioral (disrupted PPI and hyperactivity) and structural brain abnormalities (lateral ventricle enlargement and reduced dendritic spine density) that are observed in schizophrenia (for extensive review see Desbonnet et al. 2009; Jaaro-Peled et al. 2010).

Dysbindin

Sandy mice arose from spontaneous mutation and carry a mutant *DNTBP1* allele encoding a protein with an in-frame 22-residue deletion (Li et al. 2003). These null mice display behavioral abnormalities consistent with certain schizophrenia intermediate phenotypes, including deficits in social interaction (Feng et al. 2008), enhanced stimulant sensitization (Bhardwaj et al. 2009), and various cognitive deficits (Bhardwaj et al. 2009; Cox et al. 2009; Jentsch et al. 2009; Takao et al. 2008). Dysbindin null mice also have deficits in auditory-evoked response adaptation, PPI, evoked γ-activity, and fast-phasic inhibition (Carlson et al. 2011).

Akt1

Mice lacking Akt1 display behavioral and neuronal abnormalities pertinent to schizophrenia, such as impaired PPI, cognitive deficits, enhanced locomotor activity produced by amphetamine, altered hippocampal synaptic plasticity, and reduced dendritic spine density (Balu et al. 2012; Desbonnet et al. 2009).

NMDAR function

Many mutant mice have been generated that display NMDAR hypofunction, including but not limited to NR1 hypomorphs (90% reduction in NR1), glycine transporter-1 (GlyT1), and SynGAP (NMDAR interactor) heterozygote mutants, mice carrying point mutations in the GMS, and SR and glial glutamate and aspartate transporter (GLAST) knockouts (Desbonnet et al. 2009). In general, mutants with disruptions in NMDAR signaling demonstrate phenotypes consistent with intermediate schizophrenia phenotypes such as cognitive and social deficits, disruptions in PPI, deficits in neuroplasticity, and dendritic abnormalities (Basu et al. 2009; Desbonnet et al. 2009; DeVito et al. 2011; Balu et al. 2012). Given that the NMDA receptor sits between the presynaptic and postsynaptic risk genes described above, it may be the critical mediator of synaptic dysconnection in schizophrenia.

CNV-based models

There is a strong genetic link between the 22q11.2 chromosomal microdeletion (also known as velocardiofacial syndrome or DiGeorge syndrome) and schizophrenia. Most of the microdeletions are either 3 megabases (Mb) (~60 known genes) or 1.5 Mb in size (~35 known genes), and most of the genes affected are expressed in the brain (Karayiorgou et al. 2010). The phenotype of this syndrome is highly variable, but almost all patients suffer from craniofacial abnormalities and display a wide range of cognitive deficits. Approximately 30% of adult patients are diagnosed with psychiatric disorders, with the relative risk for developing schizophrenia ~20 to 25 times higher than that of the general population. Due to the high risk conferred by this genetic lesion, mouse models of this deletion have been created to better understand which genes are critical for the development of schizophrenia. Mice with deletions of varying lengths in the syntenic region of chromosome 16 largely have deficits in PPI, and some show deficits in working memory and learned fear (Karayiorgou *et al.* 2010). Moreover, mice have been generated with heterozygous deletion of individual genes located within the chromosomal deletion, and these genes (*Dgcr8*, *Gnb1l*, *Prodh*, and *Zdhhc8*) have been shown to be important for PPI, neuronal architecture, microRNA processing, hippocampal-PFC synchrony, and cortical short-term plasticity (Karayiorgou *et al.* 2010).

Novel therapeutic targets

Drug targets for schizophrenia are increasingly being identified on the basis of genetic linkage and gene expression studies. Although no individual gene has more than a small effect, it is possible to identify synergistic factors or pathways using this approach. For example, the first study to analyze CNVs in schizophrenia identified several biologically meaningful categories, including genes involved in neurodevelopment (including NRG1) and glutamate signaling (including nitric oxide signaling and LTP) (Walsh *et al.* 2008). Glutamate, GABA, and dopamine are the neurotransmitters most strongly implicated by susceptibility genes (Harrison and Weinberger 2005). Others have examined the growing list of implicated genes and identified groups linked to infectious agents (Carter 2009) and oligodendrocyte function (Karoutzou *et al.* 2008). Postmortem gene expression studies have also identified genes that fall into several categories, including GABA and glutamate transmission, mitochondrial metabolic function, oligodendrocytes, synaptic integrity, and neurotrophic factors (BDNF) (Altar *et al.* 2009; Hakak *et al.* 2001). Many of these genes have been explored with knockout models that have successfully captured varying aspects of the illness (Carpenter and Koenig 2008). Drug discovery has targeted candidate genes identified on the basis of gene linkage combined with relevance to existing models of schizophrenia.

Non-D_2 receptors

The antipsychotic effects of the D_2-receptor blockade are believed to result from diminished activity of the ventral tegmental neurons projecting to mesolimbic areas, whereas diminished nigrostriatal dopaminergic activity results in neurological side effects. Preservation of the former remains a goal for novel antipsychotics – one that can be partially realized by addition of 5-HT_{2A} antagonism, by a high dissociation constant for binding to the D_2 receptor, or by partial agonist activity at the D_2 receptor. It is also possible that atypical agents preferentially bind to D_2 and D_3 receptors in the thalamus and temporal cortex compared with the striatum (Bressan *et al.* 2003; Pilowsky *et al.* 1997). Targeting D_3 receptors may modulate limbic dopamine activity with less effect on ventral tegmental or nigrostriatal neuronal firing (Gurevich *et al.* 1997). Amisulpride has been reported to preferentially block D_3 receptors, to which has been attributed its favorable clinical profile of efficacy for positive and negative symptoms with minimal extrapyramidal symptoms (Kerwin 2000). Despite considerable interest in D_4 antagonists following the discovery of the high affinity of clozapine for this receptor, trials of selective D_4 antagonists have been disappointing (Kramer *et al.* 1997; Truffinet *et al.* 1999). Dopamine activity can also be modulated by muscarinic acetylcholine receptors. Xanomeline, a muscarinic M1 and M2 agonist, decreased ventral tegmental dopamine neuron firing and blocked dopamine agonist disruption of conditioned avoidance response and sensory gating (Stanhope *et al.* 2001). A placebo-controlled add-on pilot study of xanomeline in 20 patients with schizophrenia provided evidence suggestive of efficacy for psychosis, negative symptoms, and memory (Shekhar *et al.* 2008).

Glutamatergic receptors

As described above, NMDAR hypofunction could result in excessive dopamine release that may account for psychotic symptoms, whereas disruption of inhibitory interneurons is expected to produce excessive glutamate release, aberrant spread of excitatory transmission, and loss of neuronal network synchronization necessary for working memory and other cognitive functions (e.g., gamma oscillations). This model suggests several therapeutic targets that would either enhance NMDA channel opening or reduce glutamate release.

Because excessive NMDAR channel opening and calcium influx can be neurotoxic, agonists at the NMDAR are not a viable therapeutic option. Instead, modulatory factors that influence NMDAR channel opening have provided pharmacological targets, including the GMS, redox status, neurosteroids, and the voltage-dependent magnesium block. GMS agonists, like glycine, D-serine, and D-alanine, despite poor penetrance of the blood–brain barrier, have demonstrated efficacy in several small trials, most consistently for negative symptoms. A meta-analysis found significant efficacy for glycine treatment of negative symptoms (Tuominen *et al.* 2005). D-cycloserine (DCS), a partial agonist at the GMS that readily crosses the blood–brain barrier, demonstrated efficacy for negative symptoms when added to first-generation antipsychotics in one placebo-controlled trial (Goff *et al.* 1999*b*), but results have been less than consistent (Tuominen *et al.* 2005). A large multicenter placebo-controlled add-on trial (CONSIST: The Cognitive and Negative Symptoms in Schizophrenia Trial) failed to confirm efficacy for either glycine or DCS, but interpretation of these results is clouded by the fact that it was a failed trial with significant site differences, including variability in patient compliance between inpatient and outpatient clinics (Buchanan *et al.* 2007). However, a recent meta-analysis of strategies to enhance NMDAR-mediated neurotransmission in schizophrenia reported the striking finding that NMDAR-enhancing molecules (glycine, DCS, D-serine, sarcosine, and D-alanine) as a whole exerted statistically significant effects on total psychopathology, depressive symptoms, negative symptoms, cognitive symptoms, positive symptoms, and general psychopathology in descending order of effect size (Tsai and Lin 2010).

Clozapine and possibly other second-generation antipsychotics, unlike first-generation agents, decrease behavioral effects of NMDAR antagonists. In patients with schizophrenia, clozapine attenuates the psychomimetic effects of ketamine (Malhotra *et al.* 1997); glycine serum concentrations were found to predict the response of negative symptoms to clozapine (Sumiyoshi *et al.* 2005). Similarly, elevation by olanzapine of glutamate concentrations in the cingulate gyrus measured by magnetic resonance spectroscopy (MRS) correlated with improvement of negative symptoms (Goff *et al.* 2002). GMS full agonists have not demonstrated efficacy when added to clozapine (Evins *et al.* 2000; Tsai *et al.* 1999), and DCS significantly worsened negative symptoms when added to clozapine (Goff *et al.* 1999*a*), possibly because the partial agonism of DCS at the GMS diminished activation by clozapine. In the CONSIST trial, a significant interaction was found with class of antipsychotic (first vs. second generation); response to glycine and DCS was greater when they were added to first-generation antipsychotics, but the number of subjects treated with first-generation agents was small (Buchanan *et al.* 2007).

A more promising approach for activation of the GMS involves inhibition of the glycine transporter (GlyT1) (Javitt 2009). Sarcosine, a naturally occurring precursor of glycine that competes for the glycine transporter, has displayed efficacy for positive and negative symptoms in a series of small trials (Lane *et al.* 2005, 2008). The meta-analysis by Tsai and Lin (2010) found it effective on total psychopathology, negative symptoms, and general psychopathology. Although several GlyT1 inhibitors are currently in development, undesirable side effects of sarcosine-derived GlyT1 inhibitors have also been noted (ataxia, hypoactivity, and decreased respiration), prompting the development of novel classes of non-sarcosine-based inhibitors of GlyT1 (Lindsley *et al.* 2006). Another approach to enhancing agonist occupation of the GMS is the combination of supplemental D-serine with a DAAO inhibitor (Hashimoto *et al.* 2009), which has displayed promising results in animal models.

NMDAR channel opening is also modified by redox status and can be enhanced by reducing oxidative stress. The antioxidant NAC improved negative symptoms in patients with schizophrenia in a placebo-controlled add-on trial (Berk *et al.* 2008) and improved MMN (Lavoie *et al.* 2008). However, NAC may also affect the concentration of synaptic glutamate by increasing the concentration of cysteine, a competitor of glutamate for the cystine-glutamate antiporter (Baker *et al.* 2008). The neurosteroid pregnenolone has also been reported to improve negative symptoms and cognition, possibly via the steroid modulator site of the NMDAR complex. Removal of the dose-dependent magnesium blockade of the NMDAR represents another strategy for enhancing the channel opening. Activation of the α-amino-3-hydroxyl-5-methyl-4-isoxazole-propionate (AMPA)-gated calcium channel initiates rapid depolarization and hence facilitates NMDAR opening. The low-potency, short half-life AMPA-positive modulator CX516 improved cognitive functioning when added to clozapine in a placebo-controlled pilot trial (Goff *et al.* 2001), but this therapeutic effect was not replicated in a multicenter trial (Goff *et al.* 2008*b*).

In addition to disrupting synchronization of neural circuits, hypofunction of NMDARs on inhibitory interneurons would also be expected to result in excessive glutamatergic transmission due to diminished inhibitory input. Several approaches have been taken to compensate for such a defect in glutamate modulation. Lamotrigine has been shown to attenuate excessive glutamate release in animal models and blocked psychosis, negative symptoms, and cognitive deficits produced by ketamine in healthy subjects (Anand *et al.* 2000; Large *et al.* 2005). Early studies reported improvement of psychosis with the addition of lamotrigine to clozapine in patients with chronic symptoms (Dursun and McIntosh 1999; Tiihonen *et al.* 2003), although two large multicenter trials failed to demonstrate therapeutic effects on positive or negative symptoms, whereas cognition improved with lamotrigine in one multicenter trial (Goff *et al.* 2007). A meta-analysis performed by Tiihonen *et al.* (2009) examined the effects of lamotrigine within clozapine-treated subjects, including the two large negative trials, and found significant efficacy for psychosis. Another strategy to reduce glutamate release targets presynaptic metabotropic glutamate receptors (mGluRs). The metabotropic type II agonist LY354754 attenuated working memory deficits produced by ketamine in healthy subjects (Krystal *et al.* 2005). The mGluR2/3 agonist prodrug LY2140023 significantly improved positive and negative symptoms when administered as monotherapy in one study advantaged by minimal placebo response (Patil *et al.* 2007) but failed in a replication study that was compromised by a large placebo response.

Researchers have recently approached the NMDAR hypofunction model from a different vantage point, focusing on impairment of LTP and neuroplasticity. A large number of animal studies have demonstrated enhancement of learning and memory consolidation with DCS – an effect that is rapidly lost with repeated dosing (Parnas *et al.* 2005). Memory consolidation is selectively impaired by NMDAR antagonists and has been shown to be selectively impaired in patients with schizophrenia (Holt *et al.* 2009; Manoach *et al.* 2004). In mice, a single low dose of DCS significantly enhanced recovery of motor function and memory following closed head injury (Yaka *et al.* 2007) and enhanced hippocampal LTP in the CA1 region. In healthy human subjects, DCS 100 mg/day significantly enhanced cortical motor neuroplasticity measured by TMS without adverse effects (Nitsche *et al.* 2004) – a paradigm similar to the measurement of neuroplasticity that was found by Daskalakis *et al.* (2008) to be impaired in schizophrenia. An 8-week pilot trial of once-weekly dosing with DCS in patients with schizophrenia found improvement of negative symptoms measured 7 days after the last DCS dose (Goff *et al.* 2008a). In addition, a single dose of DCS enhanced memory consolidation tested after a delay of 7 days (Goff *et al.* 2008a). Intermittent administration of GMS agonists to avoid tachyphylaxis represents a promising approach, particularly in combination with cognitive behavioral therapies or cognitive remediation.

α7 nACh receptors

The involvement of nicotinic acetylcholine receptors (nAChRs) in the pathophysiology of schizophrenia was initially suggested by behavioral and biochemical data, including the fact that nicotine has been shown to improve cognitive function differentially in patients with schizophrenia compared with healthy controls (Jubelt *et al.* 2008). In particular, α7 nAChRs have been linked genetically and via postmortem studies to schizophrenia. Preliminary studies with the α7 nAChR partial agonist 3-(2,4 dimethoxy) benzylidene-anabaseine (DMXBA) demonstrated improved performance on the Repeatable Battery for the Assessment of Neuropsychological Status (RBANS) (Olincy *et al.* 2006) and improvements on the Scale for the Assessment of Negative Symptoms (SANS) total score (Freedman *et al.* 2008).

GABA$_A$ receptors

A final treatment approach based on the circuit model involving the putative impairment of inhibitory interneurons targets GABAergic output from the inhibitory interneuron synapsing at GABA$_A$ receptors on pyramidal cells (Lisman *et al.* 2008). Postmortem studies have reported reduced cortical GABA concentrations and reduced activity of the enzyme that synthesizes GABA, glutamate decarboxylase, in schizophrenia (Lewis *et al.* 2004). A compensatory upregulation of postsynaptic GABA$_A$ receptors has also been demonstrated in the cortex of patients with schizophrenia. A pilot add-on trial of MK-0777, a selective agonist at GABA$_A$ receptors containing α2 subunits, found improvement of memory and enhanced gamma band power (Lewis *et al.* 2008), although a larger trial recently failed to replicate these results.

Antiapoptotic targets

Postmortem studies in schizophrenia have consistently revealed a loss of neuropil without gliosis and without loss of pyramidal neurons. Proton MRS has revealed significant reduction of NAA in the PFC of patients with chronic schizophrenia compared with patients having a first episode of schizophrenia and healthy controls (Ohrmann et al. 2007). One potential mechanism for these findings is apoptosis ("programmed cell death") selectively affecting glia and interneurons, as apoptosis is noteworthy in not causing reactive gliosis. However, the presence of apoptosis has not been confirmed; markers of apoptosis were absent in the temporal lobe of patients with chronic schizophrenia examined postmortem (Jarskog et al. 2004).

Whereas gray matter loss has been described in patients with the schizophrenic prodrome prior to antipsychotic exposure (Pantelis et al. 2003), comparison of medication-naïve patients with medicated first-episode patients suggests progression of gray matter loss associated with illness progression and antipsychotic exposure (Leung et al. 2009). Antipsychotics (typical and atypical) have been associated with reductions in cortical gray matter and in number of glia in monkeys (Dorph-Petersen et al. 2005; Konopaske et al. 2007) and with increased caspase-3 concentrations (Jarskog et al. 2007), increased lipid peroxidation (Parikh et al. 2003), and reduced nerve growth factor (Pillai et al. 2006) in rats. Cahn et al. (2002) found that gray matter loss at 1 year in first-episode patients correlated with cumulative antipsychotic exposure, negative symptoms, and measures of functioning. Salisbury et al. (2007) reported that ERP amplitude during the MMN task decreased significantly over a mean 1.7-year period in first-episode schizophrenia patients and correlated with volume loss in the left Heschl gyrus. Whereas olanzapine and haloperidol were similar in their toxic effects on glia in monkeys (Dorph-Petersen et al. 2005), a large clinical trial reported by Lieberman and colleagues (2005b) found marked gray matter volume reduction with haloperidol and not with olanzapine after 1 year of exposure in first-episode schizophrenia patients, although in patients treated with olanzapine, loss of brain volume correlated with worsening of negative symptoms. These complex findings suggest that several potential mechanisms for gray matter loss may occur in patients with schizophrenia or in a poor-outcome subgroup characterized by progressive worsening of negative symptoms and may represent the interplay between the natural course of the illness and treatment effects.

Identification of factors that trigger apoptosis is critical if interventions to halt progression are to be developed. Apoptosis can result from the activation of three broad pathways: the mitochondrial (intrinsic) pathway, the tumor necrosis factor receptor (extrinsic) pathway, and the inflammatory pathway (Jarskog et al. 2005); release of caspase 3 is a final common pathway. Apoptotic activation can be restricted to synapses or dendrites; for example, application of glutamate can cause a localized activation of caspase 3 in synaptic terminals (Mattson et al. 1998). Neurotrophic factors such as BDNF play a critical role in protecting against apoptosis (McAllister 2001). The BDNF genotype associated with reduced BDNF activity significantly predicted gray matter loss in first-episode schizophrenia patients (Ho et al. 2007). Several environmental factors that promote apoptosis have been linked to schizophrenia, including perinatal hypoxia and infection. Markers of increased vulnerability to apoptosis have also been reported in patients with chronic disease, including abnormalities of cytokine and interferon levels, elevated oxidative stress (Tsai et al. 1998), mitochondrial dysfunction (Goff et al. 1995), glutamate dysregulation (Goff and Coyle 2001), and deficits of neurotrophic factors (Parikh et al. 2003).

In the CNS, microglia are the major immune cells that mediate an inflammatory response to infection and other stressors via release of proinflammatory cytokines, nitric oxide, and reactive oxygen species (Rock et al. 2004). In some instances, microglial activation occurs in response to neuronal dysfunction (e.g., ischemia), and microglia are recruited to limit further CNS damage (Hanisch and Kettenmann 2007). The selective serotonin reuptake inhibitor fluoxetine recently was shown in a rat cerebral ischemia model to protect against postischemic brain injury by suppressing microglial activation (Lim et al. 2009). Two nuclear imaging studies have demonstrated neuroinflammation in patients with schizophrenia compared with controls using a peripheral benzodiazepine receptor ligand, PK11195, which measures microglial activation (Doorduin et al. 2009; van Berckel et al. 2008). S100β, which is expressed by astrocytes in response to microglial activation, is consistently elevated in both serum and

CSF of patients with schizophrenia regardless of medication status (Schroeter *et al.* 2009). In contrast to this glial marker, a marker of neuronal damage (neuron-specific enolase) is not increased in patients with schizophrenia (Steiner *et al.* 2006). In a review of 62 studies, Potvin *et al.* (2008) concluded that an inflammatory syndrome characterized by elevated levels of inflammatory cytokines is present in patients with schizophrenia. Elevated IL-6 levels consistently have been found in CSF and serum from medicated and unmedicated patients with schizophrenia, although atypical antipsychotics may reduce the ratio of inflammatory to anti-inflammatory cytokines (Sugino *et al.* 2009). The inflammatory cytokines activate several pathways relevant to schizophrenia. IL-6 activates NADPH oxidase (Behrens *et al.* 2008), resulting in an increase in oxidative stress. The proinflammatory cytokines interferon-γ and tumor necrosis factor-α activate a key enzyme of tryptophan metabolism, indolamine 2,3-dioxygenase (O'Connor *et al.* 2009), increasing the production of the psychotomimetic, kynurenic acid (Muller 2010). Two studies have found elevated levels of kynurenic acid in the CSF of patients with schizophrenia compared with controls (Erhardt *et al.* 2001; Nilsson *et al.* 2005). Trials with the anti-inflammatory cyclooxygenase-2 inhibitor celecoxib have produced mixed results in patients with schizophrenia, with modest improvement in psychotic symptoms found in two placebo-controlled trials (Akhondzadeh *et al.* 2007; Muller *et al.* 2002).

Oxidative stress resulting from an imbalance between the generation of reactive oxygen and nitrogen species and a deficiency of endogenous antioxidants can decrease NMDAR activity; cause peroxidation of lipids, proteins, and DNA; disrupt mitochondrial energy metabolism; and can ultimately result in cell injury and death. The brain is particularly vulnerable to oxidative injury due to its high utilization of oxygen, high content of oxidizable polyunsaturated fatty acids, and the presence of redox-active metals (Cu and Fe). The primary defense against oxidative stress involves superoxide dismutase, catalase, and glutathione (GSH). GSH protects against oxidative injury as a cofactor with antioxidant enzymes and as a direct scavenger of free radicals; reduced activity of GSH has been linked to schizophrenia via polymorphisms in several key genes for GSH synthesis (Do *et al.* 2009). GSH levels were lower in CSF and PFC in patients with schizophrenia compared with controls (Do *et al.* 2000). In addition, low concentrations of GSH in the brain measured by MRS predicted negative symptoms in patients with schizophrenia (Matsuzawa *et al.* 2008). A recent placebo-controlled add-on trial of the GSH precursor NAC in patients with chronic schizophrenia demonstrated significant improvement of negative symptoms (Berk *et al.* 2008). Thioredoxin, a marker of oxidative stress, was elevated in the serum of first-episode patients and in patients experiencing acute psychotic episodes compared with patients with chronic disease and healthy controls (Zhang *et al.* 2009). The mean number of neurons in the hippocampus of elderly patients with schizophrenia exhibiting 8-hydroxy, 2'deoxyguanasine (8-OHdG), a marker of DNA oxidative damage, was elevated 10-fold compared with controls (Nishioka and Arnold 2004). In addition, abnormalities of mitochondrial function, a major source of free radicals, have been identified in a subgroup of patients with schizophrenia, including elevation of CSF lactate concentrations (Regenold *et al.* 2009). Excessive glutamate release resulting from impairment of inhibitory interneurons can also result in apoptosis mediated by oxidative stress (Coyle and Puttfarcken 1993).

Conclusions and future directions

As highlighted throughout this chapter, schizophrenia is a disorder of complex genetics that is the product of multiple risk genes with moderate effects, combined with environmental interactions. As basic science research further interprets the human genetic findings, it is becoming apparent that many of these risk genes converge on common signaling pathways that are important regulators of neurodevelopment and adult neuroplasticity (Mitchell 2011). Elucidating the functions of putative schizophrenia risk gene products under normal conditions and how their functions are altered in schizophrenia, as well as understanding how they interact with each other and environmental risk factors, will provide new insight into the pathophysiology of schizophrenia. Moreover, this information will likely lead to an emergence of novel targets for therapeutic intervention directed at reversing deficiencies in neuroplasticity with hopefully improved clinical outcomes.

The large array of etiological models and complex genetics implies that no single approach is likely to treat all aspects of the illness or to be appropriate for all patients with schizophrenia. Schizophrenia likely results from combinations of environmental disruptions of early brain development, genetic vulnerability, and neurotoxicity. An element of a patient's genetic, clinical, or neuroimaging profile that contributes to symptoms or cognitive impairment might be identified and could serve as a pharmacological target for a personalized medicine approach. Although pharmacological approaches tend to be blunt, combinations of psychosocial interventions (cognitive–behavior therapy, cognitive remediation, or vocational rehabilitation) plus pharmacological agents that promote neuroplasticity may ultimately be more successful.

In addition to improving the models used in basic science research, work is needed to optimize clinical trial design to provide the greatest opportunity to detect novel drugs with improved clinical outcomes for the negative and cognitive symptoms and more tolerable side-effect profiles. Promising novel treatments frequently are successful in early proof-of-concept trials but subsequently fail in larger replication studies. Clinical trials of new agents for schizophrenia are plagued by high rates of placebo response and subject attrition, poor adherence, and surreptitious substance use. Increasingly, active comparators with well-established efficacy have failed against placebo in industry-sponsored trials. If discoveries in the neuroscience of schizophrenia are to be successfully translated to clinical therapeutics, new approaches to clinical trials are needed to improve assay sensitivity, which could be accomplished by enriching subject samples on the basis of genotype or employing more sensitive biomarkers.

References

Abi-Dargham A, Mawlawi O, Lombardo I *et al.* 2002. Prefrontal dopamine D1 receptors and working memory in schizophrenia. *J Neurosci* **22**:3708–3719.

Akhondzadeh S, Tabatabaee M, Amini H *et al.* 2007. Celecoxib as adjunctive therapy in schizophrenia: a double-blind, randomized and placebo-controlled trial. *Schizophr Res* **90**:179–185.

Alaerts M, Ceulemans S, Forero D *et al.* 2009. Support for NRG1 as a susceptibility factor for schizophrenia in a northern Swedish isolated population. *Arch Gen Psychiatry* **66**:828–837.

Allen NC, Bagade S, McQueen MB *et al.* 2008. Systematic meta-analyses and field synopsis of genetic association studies in schizophrenia: the SzGene database. *Nat Genet* **40**:827–834.

Altar CA, Vawter MP, Ginsberg SD. 2009. Target identification for CNS diseases by transcriptional profiling. *Neuropsychopharmacology* **34**:18–54.

Amann LC, Gandal MJ, Halene TB *et al.* 2010. Mouse behavioral endophenotypes for schizophrenia. *Brain Res Bull* **83**:147–161.

Anand A, Charney DS, Oren DA *et al.* 2000. Attenuation of the neuropsychiatric effects of ketamine with lamotrigine. *Arch Gen Psychiatry* **57**:270–276.

Andero R, Heldt SA, Ye K *et al.* 2011. Effect of 7,8-dihydroxyflavone, a small-molecule TrkB agonist, on emotional learning. *Am J Psychiatry* **168**:163–172.

Angelucci F, Brene S, Mathe AA. 2005. BDNF in schizophrenia, depression and corresponding animal models. *Mol Psychiatry* **10**:345–352.

Arango C, Buchanan RW, Kirkpatrick B, Carpenter WT. 2004. The deficit syndrome in schizophrenia: implications for the treatment of negative symptoms. *Eur Psychiatry* **19**:21–26.

Baker DA, Madayag A, Kristiansen LV *et al.* 2008. Contribution of cystine-glutamate antiporters to the psychotomimetic effects of phencyclidine. *Neuropsychopharmacology* **33**:1760–1772.

Balu DT, Carlson GC, Talbot K *et al.* 2012. Akt1 deficiency in schizophrenia and impairment of hippocampal plasticity and function. *Hippocampus* **22**:230–240.

Balu DT, Coyle JT. 2011. Neuroplasticity signaling pathways linked to the pathophysiology of schizophrenia. *Neurosci Biobehav Rev* **35**:848–870.

Balu DT, Basu AC, Corradi JP, Cacace AM, Coyle JT. 2012. The NMDA receptor co-agonists, D-serine and glycine, regulate neuronal dendritic architecture in the somatosensory cortex. *Neurobiol Dis* **45**:671–682.

Basu AC, Tsai GE, Ma CL *et al.* 2009. Targeted disruption of serine racemase affects glutamatergic neurotransmission and behavior. *Mol Psychiatry* **14**:719–727.

Behrens MM, Ali SS, Dugan LL. 2008. Interleukin-6 mediates the increase in NADPH-oxidase in the ketamine model of schizophrenia. *J Neurosci* **28**:13957–13966.

Beloosesky R, Weiner Z, Khativ N *et al.* 2009. Prophylactic maternal n-acetylcysteine before lipopolysaccharide suppresses fetal inflammatory cytokine responses. *Am J Obstet Gynecol* **200**: e661–e665.

Benes FM. 1999. Evidence for altered trisynaptic circuitry in schizophrenic hippocampus. *Biol Psychiatry* **46**:589–599.

Benson MA, Newey SE, Martin-Rendon E, Hawkes R, Blake DJ. 2001. Dysbindin, a novel coiled-coil-containing protein that interacts with the dystrobrevins in muscle and brain. *J Biol Chem* **276**:24232–24241.

Berk M, Copolov D, Dean O *et al.* 2008. N-acetyl cysteine as a glutathione precursor for schizophrenia – a double-blind, randomized, placebo-controlled trial. *Biol Psychiatry* **64**:361–368.

Bertolino A, Nawroz S, Mattay VS *et al.* 1996. Regionally specific pattern of neurochemical pathology in schizophrenia as assessed by multislice proton magnetic resonance spectroscopic imaging. *Am J Psychiatry* **153**:1554–1563.

Bhardwaj SK, Baharnoori M, Sharif-Askari B *et al.* 2009. Behavioral characterization of dysbindin-1 deficient sandy mice. *Behav Brain Res* **197**:435–441.

Binder DK, Scharfman HE. 2004. Brain-derived neurotrophic factor. *Growth Factors* **22**:123–131.

Brazil DP, Hemmings BA. 2001. Ten years of protein kinase B signalling: a hard Akt to follow. *Trends Biochem Sci* **26**:657–664.

Bressan RA, Erlandsson K, Jones HM *et al.* 2003. Optimizing limbic selective D2/D3 receptor occupancy by risperidone: a [123I]-epidepride SPET study. *J Clin Psychopharmacol* **23**:5–14.

Buchanan RW, Javitt DC, Marder SR *et al.* 2007. The Cognitive and Negative Symptoms in Schizophrenia Trial (CONSIST): the efficacy of glutamatergic agents for negative symptoms and cognitive impairments. *Am J Psychiatry* **164**:1593–1602.

Buckley PF, Moore C, 1994. 1H-magnetic resonance spectroscopy of the left temporal and frontal lobes in schizophrenia: clinical, neurodevelopmental, and cognitive correlates. *Biol Psychiatry* **36**:792–800.

Cahn W, Hulshoff Pol HE, Lems EB *et al.* 2002. Brain volume changes in first-episode schizophrenia: a 1-year follow-up study. *Arch Gen Psychiatry* **59**:1002–1010.

Callicott JH, Straub RE, Pezawas L *et al.* 2005. Variation in DISC1 affects hippocampal structure and function and increases risk for schizophrenia. *Proc Natl Acad Sci USA* **102**:8627–8632.

Camargo LM, Collura V, Rain JC *et al.* 2007. Disrupted-in-Schizophrenia 1 Interactome: evidence for the close connectivity of risk genes and a potential synaptic basis for schizophrenia. *Mol Psychiatry* **12**:74–86.

Cannon TD. 2010. Candidate gene studies in the GWAS era: the MET proto-oncogene, neurocognition, and schizophrenia. *Am J Psychiatry* **167**:369–372.

Carlson GC, Talbot K, Halene TB *et al.* 2011. Dybindin-1 mutant mice implicate reduced fast-phasic inhibition as a final common disease mechanism in schizophrenia. *Proc Natl Acad Sci USA* **108**:E962–E970.

Carlsson A, Lindquist M. 1963. Effect of chlorpromazine or haloperidol on the formation of 3-methoxytyramine and normetanephrine in mouse brain. *Acta Pharmacol Toxicol* **20**: 140–144.

Carpenter WT, Koenig JI. 2008. The evolution of drug development in schizophrenia: past issues and future opportunities. *Neuropsychopharmacology* **33**:2061–2079.

Carter CJ. 2009. Schizophrenia susceptibility genes directly implicated in the life cycles of pathogens: cytomegalovirus, influenza, herpes simplex, rubella, and *Toxoplasma gondii*. *Schizophr Bull* **35**:1163–1182.

Chen ZY, Jing D, Bath KG *et al.* 2006. Genetic variant BDNF (Val66Met) polymorphism alters anxiety-related behavior. *Science* **314**:140–143.

Cho H, Mu J, Kim JK *et al.* 2001. Insulin resistance and a diabetes mellitus-like syndrome in mice lacking the protein kinase Akt2 (PKB beta). *Science* **292**: 1728–1731.

Cho H, Thorvaldsen JL, Chu Q, Feng F, Birnbaum MJ. 2001. Akt1/PKBalpha is required for normal growth but dispensable for maintenance of glucose homeostasis in mice. *J Biol Chem* **276**:38349–38352.

Chubb JE, Bradshaw NJ, Soares DC, Porteous DJ, Millar JK. 2008. The DISC locus in psychiatric illness. *Mol Psychiatry* **13**:36–64.

Cox MM, Tucker AM, Tang J *et al.* 2009. Neurobehavioral abnormalities in the dysbindin-1 mutant, sandy, on a C57BL/6J genetic background. *Genes Brain Behav* **8**:390–397.

Coyle JT, Balu D, Benneyworth M, Basu A, Roseman A. 2010. Beyond the dopamine receptor: novel therapeutic targets for treating schizophrenia. *Dialogues Clin Neurosci* **12**:359–382.

Coyle JT, Puttfarcken P. 1993. Oxidative stress, glutamate, and neurodegenerative disorders. *Science* **262**:689–695.

Daskalakis ZJ, Christensen BK, Fitzgerald PB, Chen R. 2008. Dysfunctional neural plasticity in patients with schizophrenia. *Arch Gen Psychiatry* **65**:378–385.

Davis K, Kahn R, Ko G, Davidson M. 1991. Dopamine in schizophrenia: a review and reconceptualization. *Am J Psychiatry* **148**:1474–1486.

Dempster E, Toulopoulou T, McDonald C *et al.* 2005. Association between BDNF val66 met genotype and episodic memory. *Am J Med Genet B Neuropsychiatr Genet* **134B**:73–75.

DeRosse P, Funke B, Burdick KE *et al.* 2006. Dysbindin genotype and negative symptoms in schizophrenia. *Am J Psychiatry* **163**:532–534.

Desbonnet L, Waddington JL, Tuathaigh CM. 2009. Mice mutant for genes associated with schizophrenia: common phenotype or distinct endophenotypes? *Behav Brain Res* **204**:258–273.

DeVito LM, Balu DT, Kanter BR et al. 2011. Serine racemase deletion disrupts memory for order and alters cortical dendritic morphology. *Genes Brain Behav* **10**:210–222.

Do KQ, Cabungcal JH, Frank A, Steullet P, Cuenod M. 2009. Redox dysregulation, neurodevelopment, and schizophrenia. *Curr Opin Neurobiol* **19**:220–230.

Do KQ, Trabesinger AH, Kirsten-Kruger M et al. 2000. Schizophrenia: glutathione deficit in cerebrospinal fluid and prefrontal cortex in vivo. *Eur J Neurosci* **12**:3721–3728.

Donohoe G, Frodl T, Morris D et al. 2010. Reduced occipital and prefrontal brain volumes in dysbindin-associated schizophrenia. *Neuropsychopharmacology* **35**:368–373.

Donohoe G, Morris DW, Clarke S et al. 2007. Variance in neurocognitive performance is associated with dysbindin-1 in schizophrenia: a preliminary study. *Neuropsychologia* **45**:454–458.

Doorduin J, de Vries EF, Willemsen AT et al. 2009. Neuroinflammation in schizophrenia-related psychosis: a PET study. *J Nucl Med* **50**:1801–1807.

Dorph-Petersen KA, Pierri JN, Perel JM et al. 2005. The influence of chronic exposure to antipsychotic medications on brain size before and after tissue fixation: a comparison of haloperidol and olanzapine in macaque monkeys. *Neuropsychopharmacology* **30**:1649–1661.

Dursun SM, McIntosh D. 1999. Clozapine plus lamotrigine in treatment-resistant schizophrenia [letter]. *Arch Gen Psychiatry* **56**:950.

Eastwood SL, Harrison PJ. 2006. Cellular basis of reduced cortical reelin expression in schizophrenia. *Am J Psychiatry* **163**:540–542.

Egan MF, Kojima M, Callicott JH et al. 2003. The BDNF val66met polymorphism affects activity-dependent secretion of BDNF and human memory and hippocampal function. *Cell* **112**:257–269.

Emamian ES, Hall D, Birnbaum MJ, Karayiorgou M, Gogos JA. 2004. Convergent evidence for impaired AKT1-GSK3beta signaling in schizophrenia. *Nat Genet* **36**:131–137.

Erhardt S, Blennow K, Nordin C et al. 2001. Kynurenic acid levels are elevated in the cerebrospinal fluid of patients with schizophrenia. *Neurosci Lett* **313**:96–98.

Evins A, Fitzgerald S, Wine L, Roselli R, Goff D. 2000. A placebo controlled trial of glycine added to clozapine in schizophrenia. *Am J Psychiatry* **157**:826–828.

Fallgatter AJ, Ehlis AC, Herrmann MJ et al. 2010. DTNBP1 (dysbindin) gene variants modulate prefrontal brain function in schizophrenic patients – support for the glutamate hypothesis of schizophrenias. *Genes Brain Behav* **9**:489–497.

Fanous AH, van den Oord EJ, Riley BP et al. 2005. Relationship between a high-risk haplotype in the DTNBP1 (dysbindin) gene and clinical features of schizophrenia. *Am J Psychiatry* **162**:1824–1832.

Fatemi SH, Folsom TD. 2009. The neurodevelopmental hypothesis of schizophrenia, revisited. *Schizophr Bull* **35**:528–548.

Feng YQ, Zhou ZY, He X et al. 2008. Dysbindin deficiency in sandy mice causes reduction of snapin and displays behaviors related to schizophrenia. *Schizophr Res* **106**:218–228.

Fisher M, Holland C, Merzenich MM, Vinogradov S. 2009. Using neuroplasticity-based auditory training to improve verbal memory in schizophrenia. *Am J Psychiatry* **166**:805–811.

Freedman R, Olincy A, Buchanan RW et al. 2008. Initial phase 2 trial of a nicotinic agonist in schizophrenia. *Am J Psychiatry* **165**:1040–1047.

Frommann I, Pukrop R, Brinkmeyer J et al. 2010. Neuropsychological profiles in different at-risk states of psychosis: executive control impairment in the early – and additional memory dysfunction in the late – prodromal state. *Schizophr Bull* Jan 6 [epub ahead of print].

Fuller R, Nopoulos P, Arndt S et al. 2002. Longitudinal assessment of premorbid cognitive functioning in patients with schizophrenia through examination of standardized scholastic test performance. *Am J Psychiatry* **159**:1183–1189.

Garey LJ, Ong WY, Patel TS et al. 1998. Reduced dendritic spine density on cerebral cortical pyramidal neurons in schizophrenia. *J Neurol Neurosurg Psychiatry* **65**:446–453.

Geyer MA, Krebs-Thomson K, Braff DL, Swerdlow NR. 2001. Pharmacological studies of prepulse inhibition models of sensorimotor gating deficits in schizophrenia: a decade in review. *Psychopharmacology (Berl)* **156**:117–154.

Geyer MA, McIlwain KL, Paylor R. 2002. Mouse genetic models for prepulse inhibition: an early review. *Mol Psychiatry* **7**:1039–1053.

Ghiani CA, Starcevic M, Rodriguez-Fernandez IA et al. 2010. The dysbindin-containing complex (BLOC-1) in brain: developmental regulation, interaction with SNARE proteins and role in neurite outgrowth. *Mol Psychiatry* **15**:115, 204–215.

Gilmore JH, Fredrik Jarskog L, Vadlamudi S, Lauder JM. 2004. Prenatal infection and risk for schizophrenia: IL-1beta, IL-6, and TNFalpha inhibit cortical neuron dendrite development. *Neuropsychopharmacology* **29**:1221–1229.

Gilmore JH, Jarskog LF, Vadlamudi S. 2003. Maternal infection regulates

BDNF and NGF expression in fetal and neonatal brain and maternal-fetal unit of the rat. *J Neuroimmunol* **138**:49–55.

Glantz LA, Lewis DA. 2000. Decreased dendritic spine density on prefrontal cortical pyramidal neurons in schizophrenia. *Arch Gen Psychiatry* **57**:65–73.

Goff DC, Cather C, Gottlieb JD *et al.* 2008a. Once-weekly d-cycloserine effects on negative symptoms and cognition in schizophrenia: an exploratory study. *Schizophr Res* **106**:320–327.

Goff DC, Coyle JT. 2001. The emerging role of glutamate in the pathophysiology and treatment of schizophrenia. *Am J Psychiatry* **158**:1367–1377.

Goff D, Henderson D, Evins A, Amico E. 1999a. A placebo-controlled crossover trial of D-cycloserine added to clozapine in patients with schizophrenia. *Biol Psychiatry* **45**:512–514.

Goff DC, Hennen J, Tsai G *et al.* 2002. Modulation of brain and serum glutamatergic concentrations following a switch from conventional neuroleptics to olanzapine. *Biol Psychiatry* **51**:493–497.

Goff DC, Keefe R, Citrome L *et al.* 2007. Lamotrigine as add-on therapy in schizophrenia: results of 2 placebo-controlled trials. *J Clin Psychopharmacol* **27**: 582–589.

Goff DC, Lamberti JS, Leon AC *et al.* 2008b. A placebo-controlled add-on trial of the ampakine, CX516, for cognitive deficits in schizophrenia. *Neuropsychopharmacology* **33**:465–472.

Goff D, Leahy L, Berman I *et al.* 2001. A placebo-controlled pilot study of the ampakine, CX516, added to clozapine in schizophrenia. *J Clin Psychopharmacology* **21**:484–487.

Goff DC, Tsai G, Beal MF, Coyle JT. 1995. Tardive dyskinesia and substrates of energy metabolism in CSF. *Am J Psychiatry* **152**:1730–1736.

Goff DC, Tsai G, Levitt J *et al.* 1999b. A placebo-controlled trial of D-cycloserine added to conventional neuroleptics in patients with schizophrenia. *Arch Gen Psychiatry* **56**:21–27.

Goldman-Rakic PS. 1994. Working memory dysfunction in schizophrenia. *J Neuropsychiatry Clin Neurosci* **6**:348–357.

Gong YG, Wu CN, Xing QH *et al.* 2009. A two-method meta-analysis of Neuregulin 1(NRG1) association and heterogeneity in schizophrenia. *Schizophr Res* **111**:109–114.

Gorba T, Wahle P. 1999. Expression of TrkB and TrkC but not BDNF mRNA in neurochemically identified interneurons in rat visual cortex in vivo and in organotypic cultures. *Eur J Neurosci* **11**:1179–1190.

Goto Y, Yang CR, Otani S. 2010. Functional and dysfunctional synaptic plasticity in prefrontal cortex: roles in psychiatric disorders. *Biol Psychiatry* **67**:199–207.

Gozes I. 2007. Activity-dependent neuroprotective protein: from gene to drug candidate. *Pharmacol Ther* **114**:146–154.

Grace AA. 2010. Dopamine system dysregulation by the ventral subiculum as the common pathophysiological basis for schizophrenia psychosis, psychostimulant abuse, and stress. *Neurotox Res* **18**:367–376.

Gratacòs M, González JR, Mercader JM *et al.* 2007. Brain-derived neurotrophic factor Val66Met and psychiatric disorders: meta-analysis of case-control studies confirm association to substance-related disorders, eating disorders, and schizophrenia. *Biol Psychiatry* **61**:911–922.

Greenwood TA, Lazzeroni LC, Murray SS *et al.* 2011. Analysis of 94 candidate genes and 12 endophenotypes for schizophrenia from the Consortium on the Genetics of Schizophrenia. *Am J Psychiatry*. Apr 15. [Epub ahead of print]

Greer PL, Greenberg ME. 2008. From synapse to nucleus: calcium-dependent gene transcription in the control of synapse development and function. *Neuron* **59**:846–860.

Guo AY, Sun J, Riley BP, Thiselton DL, Kendler KS, Zhao Z. 2009. The dystrobrevin-binding protein 1 gene: features and networks. *Mol Psychiatry* **14**:18–29.

Gurevich EV, Bordelon Y, Shapiro RM *et al.* 1997. Mesolimbic dopamine D3 receptors and use of antipsychotics in patients with schizophrenia. *Arch Gen Psychiatry* **54**:225–232.

Hakak Y, Walker JR, Li C *et al.* 2001. Genome-wide expression analysis reveals dysregulation of myelination-related genes in chronic schizophrenia. *Proc Natl Acad Sci USA* **98**:4746–4751.

Hall J, Whalley HC, Job DE *et al.* 2006. A neuregulin 1 variant associated with abnormal cortical function and psychotic symptoms. *Nat Neurosci* **9**:1477–1478.

Hall MH, Taylor G, Sham P *et al.* 2009. The early auditory gamma-band response is heritable and a putative endophenotype of schizophrenia. *Schizophr Bull* Nov 27. [Epub ahead of print]

Hanisch UK, Kettenmann H. 2007. Microglia: active sensor and versatile effector cells in the normal and pathologic brain. *Nat Neurosci* **10**:1387–1394.

Harrison PJ, Weinberger DR. 2005. Schizophrenia genes, gene expression, and neuropathology: on the matter of their convergence [erratum: *Mol Psychiatry* 2005;**10**:420. doi:10.1038/sj.mp.4001630]. *Mol Psychiatry* **10**:48–60.

Hashimoto K, Engberg G, Shimizu E *et al.* 2005. Reduced D-serine to total serine ratio in the cerebrospinal fluid of drug naive schizophrenic patients. *Prog Neuropsychopharmacol Biol Psychiatry* **29**:767–769.

Hashimoto K, Fujita Y, Horio M et al. 2009. Co-administration of a D-amino acid oxidase inhibitor potentiates the efficacy of D-serine in attenuating prepulse inhibition deficits after administration of dizocilpine. *Biol Psychiatry* **65**:1103–1106.

Hashimoto K, Fukushima T, Shimizu E et al. 2003. Decreased serum levels of D-serine in patients with schizophrenia: evidence in support of the N-methyl-D-aspartate receptor hypofunction hypothesis of schizophrenia. *Arch Gen Psychiatry* **60**:572–576.

Hashimoto R, Numakawa T, Ohnishi T et al. 2006. Impact of the DISC1 Ser704Cys polymorphism on risk for major depression, brain morphology and ERK signaling. *Hum Mol Genet* **15**:3024–3033.

Hashimoto T, Bazmi HH, Mirnics K et al. 2008. Conserved regional patterns of GABA-related transcript expression in the neocortex of subjects with schizophrenia. *Am J Psychiatry* **165**:479–489.

Hayashi-Takagi A, Takaki M, Graziane N et al. 2010. Disrupted-in-Schizophrenia 1 (DISC1) regulates spines of the glutamate synapse via Rac1. *Nat Neurosci* **13**:327–332.

Heinrichs RW, Zakzanis KK. 1998. Neurocognitive deficit in schizophrenia: a quantitative review of the evidence. *Neuropsychology* **12**:426–445.

Ho BC, Andreasen NC, Dawson JD, Wassink TH. 2007. Association between brain-derived neurotrophic factor Val66Met gene polymorphism and progressive brain volume changes in schizophrenia. *Am J Psychiatry* **164**:1890–1899.

Ho BC, Milev P, O'Leary DS et al. 2006. Cognitive and magnetic resonance imaging brain morphometric correlates of brain-derived neurotrophic factor Val66Met gene polymorphism in patients with schizophrenia and healthy volunteers. *Arch Gen Psychiatry* **63**:731–740.

Holt DJ, Lebron-Milad K, Milad MR et al. 2009. Extinction memory is impaired in schizophrenia. *Biol Psychiatry* **65**:455–463.

Hong CJ, Yu YW, Lin CH, Tsai SJ. 2003. An association study of a brain-derived neurotrophic factor Val66Met polymorphism and clozapine response of schizophrenic patients. *Neurosci Lett* **349**:206–208.

Hong LE, Summerfelt A, Mitchell BD et al. 2008. Sensory gating endophenotype based on its neural oscillatory pattern and heritability estimate. *Arch Gen Psychiatry* **65**:1008–1016.

Howes OD, Kapur S. 2009. The dopamine hypothesis of schizophrenia: version III – the final common pathway. *Schizophr Bull* **35**:549–562.

Ibi D, Nagai T, Kitahara Y et al. 2009. Neonatal polyI: C treatment in mice results in schizophrenia-like behavioral and neurochemical abnormalities in adulthood. *Neurosci Res* **64**:297–305.

Ide M, Ohnishi T, Murayama M et al. 2006. Failure to support a genetic contribution of AKT1 polymorphisms and altered AKT signaling in schizophrenia. *J Neurochem* **99**:277–287.

Ikeda M, Iwata N, Suzuki T et al. 2004. Association of AKT1 with schizophrenia confirmed in a Japanese population. *Biol Psychiatry* **56**:698–700.

Iwata N, Suzuki T, Ikeda M et al. 2004. No association with the neuregulin 1 haplotype to Japanese schizophrenia. *Mol Psychiatry* **9**:126–127.

Jaaro-Peled H. 2009. Gene models of schizophrenia: DISC1 mouse models. *Prog Brain Res* **179**:75–86.

Jaaro-Peled H, Ayhan Y, Pletnikov MV, Sawa A. 2010. Review of pathological hallmarks of schizophrenia: comparison of genetic models with patients and nongenetic models. *Schizophr Bull* **36**:301–313.

Jaaro-Peled H, Hayashi-Takagi A, Seshadri S et al. 2009. Neurodevelopmental mechanisms of schizophrenia: understanding disturbed postnatal brain maturation through neuregulin-1-ErbB4 and DISC1. *Trends Neurosci* **32**:485–495.

Janssen PA, Awouters FH. 1994. Is it possible to predict the clinical effects of neuroleptics from animal data? Part V: From haloperidol and pipamperone to risperidone. *Arzneimittelforschung* **44**:269–277.

Jarskog LF, Gilmore JH, Glantz LA et al. 2007. Caspase-3 activation in rat frontal cortex following treatment with typical and atypical antipsychotics. *Neuropsychopharmacology* **32**:95–102.

Jarskog LF, Glantz LA, Gilmore JH, Lieberman JA. 2005. Apoptotic mechanisms in the pathophysiology of schizophrenia. *Prog Neuropsychopharmacol Biol Psychiatry* **29**:846–858.

Jarskog LF, Selinger ES, Lieberman JA, Gilmore JH. 2004. Apoptotic proteins in the temporal cortex in schizophrenia: high Bax/Bcl-2 ratio without caspase-3 activation. *Am J Psychiatry* **161**:109–115.

Javitt DC. 2009. Glycine transport inhibitors for the treatment of schizophrenia: symptom and disease modification. *Curr Opin Drug Discov Devel* **12**:468–478.

Jentsch J, Roth R. 1999. The neuropsychopharmacology of phencyclidine: from NMDA receptor hypofunction to the dopamine hypothesis of schizophrenia. *Neuropsychopharmacology* **20**:201–225.

Jentsch JD, Trantham-Davidson H, Jairl C et al. 2009. Dysbindin modulates prefrontal cortical glutamatergic circuits and working memory function in mice. *Neuropsychopharmacology* **34**:2601–2608.

Ji Y, Yang F, Papaleo F et al. 2009. Role of dysbindin in dopamine receptor trafficking and cortical GABA function. *Proc Natl Acad Sci USA* **106**:19593–19598.

Jones PB, Barnes TR, Davies L et al. 2006. Randomized controlled trial of the effect on quality of life of second- vs first-generation antipsychotic drugs in schizophrenia: Cost Utility of the Latest Antipsychotic Drugs in Schizophrenia Study (CUtLASS 1). *Arch Gen Psychiatry* **63**:1079–1087.

Jonsson EG, Edman-Ahlbom B, Sillen A et al. 2006. Brain-derived neurotrophic factor gene (BDNF) variants and schizophrenia: an association study. *Prog Neuropsychopharmacol Biol Psychiatry* **30**:924–933.

Jubelt LE, Barr RS, Goff DC et al. 2008. Effects of transdermal nicotine on episodic memory in non-smokers with and without schizophrenia. *Psychopharmacology (Berl)* **199**:89–98.

Kalus P, Müller TJ, Zuschratter W, Senitz D. 2000. The dendritic architecture of prefrontal pyramidal neurons in schizophrenic patients. *Neuroreport* **11**:3621–3625.

Kanazawa T, Glatt SJ, Kia-Keating B, Yoneda H, Tsuang MT. 2007. Meta-analysis reveals no association of the Val66Met polymorphism of brain-derived neurotrophic factor with either schizophrenia or bipolar disorder. *Psychiatr Genet* **17**:165–170.

Kane J, Honigfeld G, Singer J, Meltzer H. 1988. Clozapine for the treatment-resistant schizophrenic: a double-blind comparison with chlorpromazine. *Arch Gen Psychiatry* **45**:789–796.

Kapur S. 2003. Psychosis as a state of aberrant salience: a framework linking biology, phenomenology, and pharmacology in schizophrenia. *Am J Psychiatry* **160**:13–23.

Karayiorgou M, Simon TJ, Gogos JA. 2010. 22q11.2 microdeletions: linking DNA structural variation to brain dysfunction and schizophrenia. *Nat Rev Neurosci* **11**:402–416.

Karege F, Perroud N, Schurhoff F et al. 2010. Association of AKT1 gene variants and protein expression in both schizophrenia and bipolar disorder. *Genes Brain Behav* **9**:503–511.

Karoutzou G, Emrich HM, Dietrich DE. 2008. The myelin-pathogenesis puzzle in schizophrenia: a literature review. *Mol Psychiatry* **13**:245–260.

Kato T, Abe Y, Sotoyama H et al. 2011. Transient exposure of neonatal mice to neuregulin-1 results in hyperdopaminergic states in adulthood: implication in neurodevelopmental hypothesis for schizophrenia. *Mol Psychiatry* **16**:307–320.

Kegeles LS, Abi-Dargham A, Zea-Ponce Y et al. 2000. Modulation of amphetamine-induced striatal dopamine release by ketamine in humans: implications for schizophrenia. *Biol Psychiatry* **48**:627–640.

Kellendonk C, Simpson EH, Kandel ER. 2009. Modeling cognitive endophenotypes of schizophrenia in mice. *Trends Neurosci* **32**:347–358.

Kerwin R. 2000. From pharmacological profiles to clinical outcomes. *Int Clin Psychopharmacol* **15** (Suppl. 4):S1–S4.

Konopaske GT, Dorph-Petersen KA, Pierri JN et al. 2007. Effect of chronic exposure to antipsychotic medication on cell numbers in the parietal cortex of macaque monkeys. *Neuropsychopharmacology* **32**:1216–1223.

Konrad A, Vucurevic G, Musso F et al. 2009. ErbB4 genotype predicts left frontotemporal structural connectivity in human brain. *Neuropsychopharmacology* **34**:641–650.

Kramer MS, Last B, Getson A, Reines SA. 1997. The effects of a selective D4 dopamine receptor antagonist (L-745,870) in acutely psychotic inpatients with schizophrenia. D4 Dopamine Antagonist Group. *Arch Gen Psychiatry* **54**:567–572.

Krystal JH, Abi-Saab W, Perry E et al. 2005. Preliminary evidence of attenuation of the disruptive effects of the NMDA glutamate receptor antagonist, ketamine, on working memory by pretreatment with the group II metabotropic glutamate receptor agonist, LY354740, in healthy human subjects. *Psychopharmacology (Berl)* **179**:303–309.

Kyriakopoulos M, Frangou S. 2009. Recent diffusion tensor imaging findings in early stages of schizophrenia. *Curr Opin Psychiatry* **22**:168–176.

Lai WS, Xu B, Westphal KG et al. 2006. Akt1 deficiency affects neuronal morphology and predisposes to abnormalities in prefrontal cortex functioning. *Proc Natl Acad Sci USA* **103**:16906–16911.

Lane HY, Chang YC, Liu YC, Chiu CC, Tsai GE. 2005. Sarcosine or D-serine add-on treatment for acute exacerbation of schizophrenia: a randomized, double-blind, placebo-controlled study. *Arch Gen Psychiatry* **62**:1196–1204.

Lane HY, Liu YC, Huang CL et al. 2008. Sarcosine (N-methylglycine) treatment for acute schizophrenia: a randomized, double-blind study. *Biol Psychiatry* **63**:9–12.

Large CH, Webster EL, Goff DC. 2005. The potential role of lamotrigine in schizophrenia. *Psychopharmacology (Berl)* **181**:415–436.

Lasky J, Klett C, Caffey E et al. 1962. A comparison evaluation of chlorpromazine, chlorprothixene, fluphenazine, reserpine, thioridazine, and triflupromazine. *Dis Nerv Syst* **23**:1–8.

Lavoie S, Murray MM, Deppen P et al. 2008. Glutathione precursor, N-acetyl-cysteine, improves mismatch negativity in schizophrenia patients. *Neuropsychopharmacology* **33**:2187–2199.

Leung M, Cheung C, Yu K et al. 2009. Gray matter in first-episode schizophrenia before and after antipsychotic drug treatment. Anatomical likelihood estimation meta-analyses with sample size weighting. *Schizophr Bull* Sep 16 [epub ahead of print].

Lewis DA, Cho RY, Carter CS et al. 2008. Subunit-selective modulation of GABA type A receptor neurotransmission and cognition in schizophrenia. *Am J Psychiatry* **165**:1585–1593.

Lewis DA, Gonzalez-Burgos G. 2008. Neuroplasticity of neocortical circuits in schizophrenia. *Neuropsychopharmacology* **33**:141–165.

Lewis DA, Hashimoto T, Volk DW. 2005. Cortical inhibitory neurons and schizophrenia. *Nat Rev Neurosci* **6**:312–324.

Lewis DA, Volk DW, Hashimoto T. 2004. Selective alterations in prefrontal cortical GABA neurotransmission in schizophrenia: a novel target for the treatment of working memory dysfunction. *Psychopharmacology (Berl)* **174**:143–150.

Li D, Collier DA, He L. 2006. Meta-analysis shows strong positive association of the neuregulin 1 (NRG1) gene with schizophrenia. *Hum Mol Genet* **15**:1995–2002.

Li W, Zhang Q, Oiso N et al. 2003. Hermansky-Pudlak syndrome type 7 (HPS-7) results from mutant dysbindin, a member of the biogenesis of lysosome-related organelles complex 1 (BLOC-1). *Nat Genet* **35**:84–89.

Lieberman J, Sheitman B, Kinon B. 1997. Neurochemical sensitization in the pathophysiology of schizophrenia: deficits and dysfunction in neuronal regulation and plasticity. *Neuropsychopharmacology* **17**:205–229.

Lieberman JA, Stroup TS, McEvoy JP et al. 2005a. Effectiveness of antipsychotic drugs in patients with chronic schizophrenia. *N Engl J Med* **353**:1209–1223.

Lieberman JA, Tollefson GD, Charles C et al. 2005b. Antipsychotic drug effects on brain morphology in first-episode psychosis. *Arch Gen Psychiatry* **62**:361–370.

Lim CM, Kim SW, Park JY et al. 2009. Fluoxetine affords robust neuroprotection in the postischemic brain via its anti-inflammatory effect. *J Neurosci Res* **87**:1037–1045.

Lindsley CW, Wolkenberg SE, Kinney GG. 2006. Progress in the preparation and testing of glycine transporter type-1 (GlyT1) inhibitors. *Curr Top Med Chem* **6**:1883–1896.

Lisman JE, Coyle JT, Green RW et al. 2008. Circuit-based framework for understanding neurotransmitter and risk gene interactions in schizophrenia. *Trends Neurosci* **31**:234–242.

Lisman JE, Otmakhova NA. 2001. Storage, recall, and novelty detection of sequences by the hippocampus: elaborating on the SOCRATIC model to account for normal and aberrant effects of dopamine. *Hippocampus* **11**:551–568.

Liu YL, Fann CS, Liu CM et al. 2006. Absence of significant associations between four AKT1 SNP markers and schizophrenia in the Taiwanese population. *Psychiatr Genet* **16**:39–41.

Lubow RE, Gewirtz JC. 1995. Latent inhibition in humans: data, theory, and implications for schizophrenia. *Psychol Bull* **117**: 87–103.

Luciano M, Miyajima F, Lind PA et al. 2009. Variation in the dysbindin gene and normal cognitive function in three independent population samples. *Genes Brain Behav* **8**:218–227.

Ma L, Liu Y, Ky B et al. 2002. Cloning and characterization of Disc1, the mouse ortholog of DISC1 (Disrupted-in-Schizophrenia 1). *Genomics* **80**:662–672.

Malhotra A, Adler C, Kennison S et al. 1997. Clozapine blunts N-methyl-D-aspartate antagonist-induced psychosis: a study with ketamine. *Biol Psychiatry* **42**:664–668.

Manoach DS, Cain MS, Vangel MG et al. 2004. A failure of sleep-dependent procedural learning in chronic, medicated schizophrenia. *Biol Psychiatry* **56**:951–956.

Margolis RL, Ross CA. 2010. Neuronal signaling pathways: genetic insights into the pathophysiology of major mental illness. *Neuropsychopharmacology* **35**:350–351.

Markov V, Krug A, Krach S et al. 2010. Impact of schizophrenia-risk gene dysbindin 1 on brain activation in bilateral middle frontal gyrus during a working memory task in healthy individuals. *Hum Brain Mapp* **31**:266–275.

Matsuzawa D, Obata T, Shirayama Y et al. 2008. Negative correlation between brain glutathione level and negative symptoms in schizophrenia: a 3T 1H-MRS study . *PLoS One* **3**:**e1944**.

Mattson MP, Keller JN, Begley JG. 1998. Evidence for synaptic apoptosis. *Exp Neurol* **153**:35–48.

McAllister AK. 2001. Neurotrophins and neuronal differentiation in the central nervous system. *Cell Mol Life Sci* **58**:1054–1060.

McIntosh AM, Moorhead TW, Job D et al. 2008. The effects of a neuregulin 1 variant on white matter density and integrity. *Mol Psychiatry* **13**:1054–1059.

Mei L, Xiong WC. 2008. Neuregulin 1 in neural development, synaptic plasticity and schizophrenia. *Nat Rev Neurosci* **9**:437–452.

Meltzer HY. 1989. Clinical studies on the mechanism of action of clozapine: the dopamine-serotonin hypothesis of schizophrenia. *Psychopharmacology* (Berl) **99** (Suppl.):S18–S27.

Meltzer HY. 2007. Illuminating the molecular basis for some antipsychotic drug-induced metabolic burden. *Proc Natl Acad Sci USA* **104**:3019–3020.

Mesholam-Gately RI, Giuliano AJ, Goff KP, Faraone SV, Seidman LJ. 2009. Neurocognition in first-episode schizophrenia: a meta-analytic review. *Neuropsychology* **23**:315–336.

Meyer U, Feldon J, Schedlowski M, Yee BK. 2005. Towards an immuno-precipitated neurodevelopmental animal model of schizophrenia. *Neurosci Biobehav Rev* **29**:913–947.

Meyer U, Feldon J, Yee BK. 2009. A review of the fetal brain cytokine imbalance hypothesis of schizophrenia. *Schizophr Bull* **35**:959–972.

Minichiello L. 2009. TrkB signalling pathways in LTP and learning. *Nat Rev Neurosci* **10**:850–860.

Mitchell KJ. 2011. The genetics of neurodevelopmental disease. *Curr Opin Neurobiol* **21**:197–203.

Muller N. 2010. COX-2 inhibitors as antidepressants and antipsychotics: clinical evidence. *Curr Opin Investig Drugs* **11**:31–42.

Muller N, Riedel M, Scheppach C et al. 2002. Beneficial antipsychotic effects of celecoxib add-on therapy compared to risperidone alone in schizophrenia. *Am J Psychiatry* **159**:1029–1034.

Neves-Pereira M, Cheung JK, Pasdar A et al. 2005. BDNF gene is a risk factor for schizophrenia in a Scottish population. *Mol Psychiatry* **10**:208–212.

Nicodemus KK, Law AJ, Luna A et al. 2009. A 5'¢ promoter region SNP in NRG1 is associated with schizophrenia risk and type III isoform expression. *Mol Psychiatry* **14**:741–743.

Nilsson LK, Linderholm KR, Engberg G et al. 2005. Elevated levels of kynurenic acid in the cerebrospinal fluid of male patients with schizophrenia. *Schizophr Res* **80**:315–322.

Nishioka N, Arnold SE. 2004. Evidence for oxidative DNA damage in the hippocampus of elderly patients with chronic schizophrenia. *Am J Geriatr Psychiatry* **12**:167–175.

Nitsche MA, Jaussi W, Liebetanz D et al. 2004. Consolidation of human motor cortical neuroplasticity by D-cycloserine. *Neuropsychopharmacology* **29**:1573–1578.

Niwa M, Kamiya A, Murai R et al. 2010. Knockdown of DISC1 by in utero gene transfer disturbs postnatal dopaminergic maturation in the frontal cortex and leads to adult behavioral deficits. *Neuron* **65**:480–489.

Niznikiewicz MA, Kubicki M, Shenton ME. 2003. Recent structural and functional imaging findings in schizophrenia. *Curr Opin Psychiatry* **16**:123–147.

O'Connor JC, Andre C, Wang Y et al. 2009. Interferon-gamma and tumor necrosis factor-alpha mediate the upregulation of indoleamine 2,3-dioxygenase and the induction of depressive-like behavior in mice in response to bacillus Calmette-Guerin. *J Neurosci* **29**:4200–4209.

Ohrmann P, Siegmund A, Suslow T et al. 2007. Cognitive impairment and in vivo metabolites in first-episode neuroleptic-naive and chronic medicated schizophrenic patients: a proton magnetic resonance spectroscopy study. *J Psychiatr Res* **41**:625–634.

Ohtsuki T, Inada T, Arinami T. 2004. Failure to confirm association between AKT1 haplotype and schizophrenia in a Japanese case-control population. *Mol Psychiatry* **9**:981–983.

Olincy A, Harris JG, Johnson LL et al. 2006. Proof-of-concept trial of an alpha7 nicotinic agonist in schizophrenia. *Arch Gen Psychiatry* **63**:630–638.

Pantelis C, Velakoulis D, McGorry PD et al. 2003. Neuroanatomical abnormalities before and after onset of psychosis: a cross-sectional and longitudinal MRI comparison. *Lancet* **361**:281–288.

Parikh V, Evans DR, Khan MM, Mahadik SP. 2003. Nerve growth factor in never-medicated first-episode psychotic and medicated chronic schizophrenic patients: possible implications for treatment outcome. *Schizophr Res* **60**:117–123.

Parikh V, Khan MM, Mahadik SP. 2003. Differential effects of antipsychotics on expression of antioxidant enzymes and membrane lipid peroxidation in rat brain. *J Psychiatr Res* **37**:43–51.

Parnas AS, Weber M, Richardson R. 2005. Effects of multiple exposures to D-cycloserine on extinction of conditioned fear in rats. *Neurobiol Learn Mem* **83**:224–231.

Patil ST, Zhang L, Martenyi F et al. 2007. Activation of mGlu2/3 receptors as a new approach to treat schizophrenia: a randomized Phase 2 clinical trial. *Nat Med* **13**:1102–1107.

Pillai A, Terry AV Jr, Mahadik SP. 2006. Differential effects of long-term treatment with typical and atypical antipsychotics on NGF and BDNF levels in rat striatum and hippocampus. *Schizophr Res* **82**:95–106.

Pilowsky LS, Mulligan RS, Acton PD et al. 1997. Limbic selectivity of clozapine. *Lancet* **350**:490–491.

Potkin SG, Turner JA, Brown GG et al. 2009. Working memory and DLPFC inefficiency in schizophrenia: the FBIRN study. *Schizophr Bull* **35**:19–31.

Potvin S, Stip E, Sepehry AA et al. 2008. Inflammatory cytokine alterations in schizophrenia: a systematic quantitative review. *Biol Psychiatry* **63**:801–808.

Purcell SM, Wray NR, Stone JL et al. (International Schizophrenia Consortium) 2009. Common polygenic variation contributes to risk of schizophrenia and bipolar disorder. *Nature* **460**:748–752.

Radant AD, Bowdle TA, Cowley DS et al. 1998. Does ketamine-mediated N-methyl-D-aspartate receptor antagonism cause schizophrenia-like oculomotor abnormalities? *Neuropsychopharmacology* **19**:434–444.

Rajkowska G, Selemon LD, Goldman-Rakic PS. 1998. Neuronal and glial somal size in the prefrontal cortex: a postmortem morphometric study of schizophrenia and Huntington disease. *Arch Gen Psychiatry* **55**:215–224.

Regenold WT, Phatak P, Marano CM et al. 2009. Elevated cerebrospinal fluid lactate concentrations in patients with bipolar disorder and schizophrenia: implications for the mitochondrial dysfunction hypothesis. *Biol Psychiatry* **65**:489–494.

Riley B, Kuo PH, Maher BS et al. 2009. The dystrobrevin binding protein 1 (DTNBP1) gene is associated with schizophrenia in the Irish Case Control Study of Schizophrenia (ICCSS) sample. *Schizophr Res* **115**:245–253.

Rock RB, Gekker G, Hu S et al. 2004. Role of microglia in central nervous system infections. *Clin Microbiol Rev* **17**:942–964.

Rosa A, Gardner M, Cuesta MJ et al. 2007. Family-based association study of neuregulin-1 gene and psychosis in a Spanish sample. *Am J Med Genet B Neuropsychiatr Genet* **144B**:954–957.

Ross CA, Margolis RL, Reading SA, Pletnikov M, Coyle JT. 2006. Neurobiology of schizophrenia. *Neuron* **52**:139–153.

Sakata K, Woo NH, Martinowich K et al. 2009. Critical role of promoter IV-driven BDNF transcription in GABAergic transmission and synaptic plasticity in the prefrontal cortex. *Proc Natl Acad Sci USA* **106**:5942–5947.

Salisbury DF, Kuroki N, Kasai K, Shenton ME, McCarley RW. 2007. Progressive and interrelated functional and structural evidence of post-onset brain reduction in schizophrenia. *Arch Gen Psychiatry* **64**:521–529.

Sawa A, Snyder SH. 2005. Genetics. Two genes link two distinct psychoses. *Science* **310**:1128–1129.

Schroeter ML, Abdul-Khaliq H, Krebs M, Diefenbacher A, Blasig IE. 2009. Neuron-specific enolase is unaltered whereas S100B is elevated in serum of patients with schizophrenia – original research and meta-analysis. *Psychiatry Res* **167**:66–72.

Schwab SG, Hoefgen B, Hanses C et al. 2005. Further evidence for association of variants in the AKT1 gene with schizophrenia in a sample of European sib-pair families. *Biol Psychiatry* **58**:446–450.

Seeman P, Lee T, Chau-Wong M. 1976. Antipsychotic drug doses and neuroleptic/dopamine receptors. *Nature* **261**:717–719.

Selemon LD, Goldman-Rakic PS. 1999. The reduced neuropil hypothesis: a circuit based model of schizophrenia. *Biol Psychiatry* **45**:17–25.

Shekhar A, Potter WZ, Lightfoot J et al. 2008. Selective muscarinic receptor agonist xanomeline as a novel treatment approach for schizophrenia. *Am J Psychiatry* **165**:1033–1039.

Sikich L, Frazier JA, McClellan J et al. 2008. Double-blind comparison of first- and second-generation antipsychotics in early-onset schizophrenia and schizo-affective disorder: findings from the Treatment of Early-Onset Schizophrenia Spectrum Disorders (TEOSS) Study. *Am J Psychiatry* **165**:1420–1431.

Spokes EG. 1979. An analysis of factors influencing measurements of dopamine, noradrenaline, glutamate decarboxylase and choline acetylase in human post-mortem brain tissue. *Brain* **102**:333–346.

St Clair D, Blackwood D, Muir W et al. 1990. Association within a family of a balanced autosomal translocation with major mental illness. *Lancet* **336**:13–16.

Stanhope KJ, Mirza NR, Bickerdike MJ et al. 2001. The muscarinic receptor agonist xanomeline has an antipsychotic-like profile in the rat. *J Pharmacol Exp Ther* **299**: 782–792.

Stanley JA, Williamson PC, Drost DJ et al. 1995. An in vivo study of the prefrontal cortex of schizophrenic patients at different stages of illness via phosphorus magnetic resonance spectroscopy. *Arch Gen Psychiatry* **52**:399–406.

Steiner J, Bielau H, Bernstein HG, Bogerts B, Wunderlich MT. 2006. Increased cerebrospinal fluid and serum levels of S100B in first-onset schizophrenia are not related to a degenerative release of glial fibrillary acidic protein, myelin basic protein and neurone-specific enolase from glia or neurones. *J Neurol Neurosurg Psychiatry* **77**:1284–1287.

Straub RE, Jiang Y, MacLean CJ et al. 2002. Genetic variation in the 6p22.3 gene DTNBP1, the human ortholog of the mouse dysbindin gene, is associated with schizophrenia. *Am J Hum Genet* **71**:337–348.

Strohmaier J, Frank J, Wendland JR et al. 2010. A reappraisal of the association between Dysbindin (DTNBP1) and schizophrenia in a large combined case-control and family-based sample of German ancestry. *Schizophr Res* **118**: 98–105.

Sugino H, Futamura T, Mitsumoto Y, Maeda K, Marunaka Y. 2009. Atypical antipsychotics suppress production of proinflammatory cytokines and up-regulate interleukin-10 in lipopolysaccharide-treated mice. *Prog Neuropsychopharmacol Biol Psychiatry* **33**:303–307.

Sumiyoshi T, Jin D, Jayathilake K, Lee M, Meltzer HY. 2005. Prediction of the ability of clozapine to treat negative symptoms from plasma glycine and serine levels in schizophrenia. *Int J Neuropsychopharmacol* **8**:451–455.

Sweet RA, Henteleff RA, Zhang W, Sampson AR, Lewis DA. 2009. Reduced dendritic spine density in auditory cortex of subjects with schizophrenia. *Neuropsychopharmacology* **34**:374–389.

Takahashi T, Suzuki M, Tsunoda M et al. 2008. Association between the brain-derived neurotrophic factor Val66Met polymorphism and brain morphology in a Japanese sample of schizophrenia and healthy comparisons. *Neurosci Lett* **435**:34–39.

Takao K, Toyama K, Nakanishi K et al. 2008. Impaired long-term memory retention and working memory in sdy mutant mice with a deletion in Dtnbp1, a susceptibility gene for schizophrenia. *Mol Brain* **1**:11.

Talbot K, Cho DS, Ong WY et al. 2006. Dysbindin-1 is a synaptic and microtubular protein that binds brain snapin. *Hum Mol Genet* **15**:3041–3054.

Tan HY, Nicodemus KK, Chen Q et al. 2008. Genetic variation in AKT1 is linked to dopamine-associated prefrontal cortical structure and function in humans. *J Clin Invest* **118**:2200–2208.

Tan W, Wang Y, Gold B et al. 2007. Molecular cloning of a brain-specific, developmentally regulated neuregulin 1 (NRG1) isoform and identification of a functional promoter variant associated with schizophrenia. *J Biol Chem* **282**:24343–24351.

Tang TT, Yang F, Chen BS et al. 2009. Dysbindin regulates hippocampal LTP by controlling NMDA receptor surface expression. *Proc Natl Acad Sci USA* **106**:21395–21400.

Thiselton DL, Vladimirov VI, Kuo PH et al. 2008. AKT1 is associated with schizophrenia across multiple symptom dimensions in the Irish study of high density schizophrenia families. *Biol Psychiatry* **63**:449–457.

Thiselton DL, Webb BT, Neale BM et al. 2004. No evidence for linkage or association of neuregulin-1 (NRG1) with disease in the Irish study of high-density schizophrenia families (ISHDSF). *Mol Psychiatry* **9**:777–783; image 729.

Thomson PA, Harris SE, Starr JM et al. 2005. Association between genotype at an exonic SNP in DISC1 and normal cognitive aging. *Neurosci Lett* **389**:41–45.

Tiihonen J, Hallikainen T, Ryynanen OP et al. 2003. Lamotrigine in treatment-resistant schizophrenia: a randomized placebo-controlled crossover trial. *Biol Psychiatry* **54**:1241–1248.

Tiihonen J, Wahlbeck K, Kiviniemi V. 2009. The efficacy of lamotrigine in clozapine-resistant schizophrenia: a systematic review and meta-analysis. *Schizophr Res* **109**:10–14.

Tomppo L, Hennah W, Lahermo P et al. 2009. Association between genes of Disrupted-in-schizophrenia 1 (DISC1) interactors and schizophrenia supports the role of the DISC1 pathway in the etiology of major mental illnesses. *Biol Psychiatry* **65**:1055–1062.

Torrey EF, Taylor EH, Bracha HS et al. 1994. Prenatal origin of schizophrenia in a subgroup of discordant monozygotic twins. *Schizophr Bull* **20**:423–432.

Truffinet P, Tamminga CA, Fabre LF et al. 1999. Placebo-controlled study of the D4/5-HT2A antagonist fananserin in the treatment of schizophrenia. *Am J Psychiatry* **156**:419–425.

Tsai G, Goff D, Chang R et al. 1998. Markers of glutamatergic neurotransmission and oxidative stress associated with tardive dyskinesia. *Am J Psychiatry* **9**:1207–1213.

Tsai GE, Lin PY. 2010. Strategies to enhance N-methyl-D-aspartate receptor-mediated neurotransmission in schizophrenia, a critical review and meta-analysis. *Curr Pharm Des* **16**:522–537.

Tsai G, Yang P, Chung L-C et al. 1999. D-serine added to clozapine for the treatment of schizophrenia. *Am J Psychiatry* **156**:1822–1825.

Tsien JZ. 2000. Linking Hebb's coincidence-detection to memory formation. *Curr Opin Neurobiol* **10**:266–273.

Tuominen HJ, Tiihonen J, Wahlbeck K. 2005. Glutamatergic drugs for schizophrenia: a systematic review and meta-analysis. *Schizophr Res* **72**:225–234.

Turetsky BI, Calkins ME, Light GA et al. 2007. Neurophysiological endophenotypes of schizophrenia: the viability of selected candidate measures. *Schizophr Bull* **33**:69–94.

Turunen JA, Peltonen JO, Pietilainen OP et al. 2007. The role of DTNBP1, NRG1, and AKT1 in the genetics of schizophrenia in Finland. *Schizophr Res* **91**:27–36.

Umbricht D, Schmid L, Koller R et al. 2000. Ketamine-induced deficits in auditory and visual context-dependent processing in healthy volunteers: implications for models of cognitive deficits in schizophrenia. *Arch Gen Psychiatry* **57**:1139–1147.

van Berckel BN, Bossong MG, Boellaard R et al. 2008. Microglia activation in recent-onset schizophrenia: a quantitative (R)-[11C]PK11195 positron emission tomography study. *Biol Psychiatry* **64**:820–822.

van den Oord EJ, Sullivan PF, Jiang Y et al. 2003. Identification of a high-risk haplotype for the dystrobrevin binding protein 1 (DTNBP1) gene in the Irish study of high-density schizophrenia families. *Mol Psychiatry* **8**:499–510.

Vinogradov S, Fisher M, Holland C et al. 2009. Is serum brain-derived neurotrophic factor a biomarker for cognitive enhancement in schizophrenia? *Biol Psychiatry* **66**:549–553.

Volk DW, Pierri JN, Fritschy JM et al. 2002. Reciprocal alterations in pre- and post-synaptic inhibitory markers at chandelier cell inputs to pyramidal neurons in schizophrenia. *Cereb Cortex* **12**:1063–1070.

Walker RM, Christoforou A, Thomson PA et al. 2010. Association analysis of Neuregulin 1 candidate regions in schizophrenia and bipolar disorder. *Neurosci Lett* **478**:9–13.

Walsh T, McClellan JM, McCarthy SE et al. 2008. Rare structural variants disrupt multiple genes in neurodevelopmental pathways in schizophrenia. *Science* **320**:539–543.

Walters JT, Owen MJ. 2007. Endophenotypes in psychiatric genetics. *Mol Psychiatry* **12**:886–890.

Wayman GA, Lee YS, Tokumitsu H, Silva AJ, Soderling TR. 2008. Calmodulin-kinases: modulators of neuronal development and plasticity. *Neuron* **59**:914–931.

Wessman J, Paunio T, Tuulio-Henriksson A et al. 2009. Mixture model clustering of phenotype features reveals evidence for association of DTNBP1 to a specific subtype of schizophrenia. *Biol Psychiatry* **66**:990–996.

Winterer G, Konrad A, Vucurevic G et al. 2008. Association of 5'¢ end neuregulin-1 (NRG1) gene variation with subcortical medial frontal microstructure in humans. *Neuroimage* **40**:712–718.

Wirgenes KV, Djurovic S, Agartz I et al. 2009. Dysbindin and d-amino-acid-oxidase gene polymorphisms associated with positive and negative symptoms in schizophrenia. *Neuropsychobiology* **60**:31–36.

Xie Z, Srivastava DP, Photowala H et al. 2007. Kalirin-7 controls activity-dependent structural and functional plasticity of dendritic spines. *Neuron* **56**:640–656.

Xu MQ, St Clair D, Ott J, Feng GY, He L. 2007. Brain-derived neurotrophic factor gene C-270T and Val66Met functional polymorphisms and risk of schizophrenia: a moderate-scale population-based study and meta-analysis. *Schizophr Res* **91**:6–13.

Xu MQ, Xing QH, Zheng YL et al. 2007. Association of AKT1 gene polymorphisms with risk of schizophrenia and with response to antipsychotics in the Chinese population. *J Clin Psychiatry* **68**:1358–1367.

Yaka R, Biegon A, Grigoriadis N et al. 2007. D-cycloserine improves functional recovery and reinstates long-term potentiation (LTP) in a mouse model of closed head injury. *FASEB J* **21**:2033–2041.

Zhang XY, Chen da C, Xiu MH et al. 2009. The novel oxidative stress marker thioredoxin is increased in first-episode schizophrenic patients. *Schizophr Res* **113**:151–157.

Zhou X, Chen Q, Schaukowitch K, Kelsoe JR, Geyer MA. 2010. Insoluble DISC1-Boymaw fusion proteins generated by DISC1 translocation. *Mol Psychiatry* **15**:669–672.

Zhou X, Geyer MA, Kelsoe JR. 2008. Does disrupted-in-schizophrenia (DISC1) generate fusion transcripts? *Mol Psychiatry* **13**:361–363.

Chapter 5

Addictive disorders

Charles P. O'Brien

Translational research on addictive disorders has several built-in advantages over research on other mental disorders. First, we know that the origin of the disorder is a specific drug, and, in most cases, we know the specific receptors involved. Second, we can identify circuits in the brain that are activated by the drug. Knowing where the drug has its initial action is helpful, although it does not necessarily point to the circuits involved in the clinically important symptoms of loss of control and the persistent tendency to relapse to drug taking despite a conscious desire to stop. Third, and perhaps most important, we have animal models of drug taking that have face validity; that is, the animals' behavior is similar to human drug-taking behavior. These models also have predictive validity in that medications that suppress drug taking in animals tend to have similar effects when tested in human subjects. Thus, using animal models of relapse or reinstatement of drug taking can allow us to identify neural circuits involved in the pressure to relapse (O'Brien and Gardner 2005).

The fundamental basis of addiction is learning which is mediated by neuroplasticity. This fact was first discovered by Abraham Wikler using animal models that he developed based on his clinical observations of addicts in the Lexington Kentucky Prison Hospital. Wikler showed that withdrawal symptoms in rats could be experimentally conditioned to environmental cues (Wikler and Pescor 1967). Conditioned withdrawal was later demonstrated in monkeys and was followed by studies focusing on drugs as reinforcers of operant or self-directed behaviors (Goldberg and Schuster 1970). These findings were soon translated to human addiction when symptoms of opiate withdrawal were conditioned in the human laboratory. This phenomenon was demonstrated by pairing opiate withdrawal with a novel stimulus, the odor of peppermint, which then acquired the ability to produce signs and symptoms of opioid withdrawal. Conditioned withdrawal responses in heroin addicts included tachycardia, reduced skin temperature, nausea, retching, and, in certain paradigms, changes in pupillary diameter (O'Brien et al. 1977). Subjective states such as craving and euphoria were also produced in patients by presenting drug-associated cues such as pictures or videos of addicts taking drugs (O'Brien et al. 1976). Conditioned brain responses such as dopamine release in response to drug-related cues were first demonstrated in animal models (Weiss et al. 1992). Subsequently, as brain-imaging techniques developed, human studies also found conditioned brain responses in patients addicted to cocaine, nicotine, opioid, alcohol, and marijuana (Childress et al. 1999). The conditioned responses in most of these studies involved changes in regional cerebral blood flow as measured by positron emission tomography (PET) (O^{15}-labeled water) or functional magnetic resonance imaging (fMRI). The human brain regions activated by drug-associated cues were the same limbic structures known to be activated in animals by drugs of abuse. These studies in human subjects showed that cues associated with the drugs by a learned response activated the same brain circuits that previously had been demonstrated to be activated by a pharmacological mechanism. This conditioned activation was demonstrated in addicts who had been free of drugs for at least 30 days and yet still showed brain reward system activation when presented with stimuli associated with their drugs of choice.

This clear research finding has major clinical implications. Medical insurance usually covers the detoxification process, the cleansing of drugs from the body. Conditioning research based on animal

Translational Neuroscience, ed. James E. Barrett, Joseph T. Coyle and Michael Williams. Published by Cambridge University Press. © Cambridge University Press 2012.

models demonstrates that the learned responses persist long after the drug has disappeared and that treatment to prevent relapse must therefore continue for months or years.

Studies conducted using animal microdialysis showing a conditioned dopamine (DA) release were replicated in drug-free human cocaine addicts who were presented with cocaine cues while in a PET scanner. In this experiment, the indirect evidence of DA release was obtained by measuring the binding of C^{11} raclopride to dopamine D_2 receptors in the striatum. This binding was competitively inhibited by presumed endogenous DA release in response to cocaine cues (Volkow *et al.* 2006). To date, the translation of circuitry and neurotransmitter findings from animal models to humans has been excellent.

The animal model of drug self-administration (intravenous or oral) is very useful for determining which drugs humans might take to excess. Drugs that are readily self-administered by animals are likely to be abused by humans. The most commonly used animals are rats and monkeys. Inbred mouse strains have been used in the search for genes that might influence specific drug-taking behavior. Because of their small size, chronic venous cannulation for continued self-administration in mice is difficult but has led to important genetic findings (Rocha *et al.* 1998).

Publications describing animal models, however, often fail to measure the *vulnerability factor*, so prominent among human drug users. Most humans who try abused drugs such as ethanol, nicotine, heroin, or cocaine do *not* go on to become addicted. Some humans are very vulnerable to the development of addiction whereas others are resistant. However, most studies using animal models have the implied assumption that *all* subjects will take the drug equally. Tricks may be used to get the animal to initiate drug taking, such as water deprivation or adding a sweetener to the water containing the drug. In studies using intravenous self-administration, putting a small bit of food on the lever controlling the intravenous infusion may be needed to encourage the rat to begin bar pressing. Once initiated, self-administration of highly rewarding drugs continues, but not all animals show progression to levels similar to human addiction (Deroche-Gamonet *et al.* 2004; Vanderschuren and Everitt 2004). In some studies, individual variation in the rapidity of developing self-administration has been the focus, and some variation among animals has usually been found. This variation in vulnerability to development of addiction behavior has not received attention proportionate to its importance in human subjects.

Another problem with translation of animal models to the clinic is the focus on the immediate effects of the drug rather than on the changes in the brain that develop with repeated administration and produce the tendency to relapse long after the drug has disappeared from the body. This tendency does not mean that brain changes that underlie direct and immediate effects such as adaptation or tolerance are unimportant. Nevertheless, insufficient recognition is given to the fact that such adaptive changes are completely normal and do *not* imply the presence of addiction. This situation may be an example of "searching for lost keys under the street light" because it is much easier to study the changes in the brain underlying tolerance than it is to study the brain substrates of individuals involved in chronic, relapsing, compulsive drug taking.

Over the past 15 years, animal models have improved, perhaps in response to criticism from clinicians. An increasing number of published reports go beyond drug taking and focus on the neurological changes that may underlie the *return* to drug taking after a period of abstinence. One of the most intriguing series of studies is that of Shaham and colleagues who observed that longer periods of time between the initiation of abstinence from cocaine and the testing for relapse lead to stronger reinstatement of drug-seeking behavior. This group coined the term *incubation* for the process that increases relapse potential over time and correlated it with changes in brain-derived neurotrophic factor (Schoenbaum *et al.* 2007).

Validity of animal models

Information learned from animal models of drug-taking behavior has taught us that virtually all drugs that are taken to excess by humans have as one of their direct effects the activation of what is known as the *reward system* of the brain. Anatomically, this system is composed of circuits in a part of the brain that appeared early in mammalian evolution called the *limbic system*. Structures that play key roles in reward include the ventral tegmental area, the nucleus accumbens (NAC), the amygdala, the insula, the frontal lobe, the arcuate nucleus, the bed nucleus (stria terminalis), and others. When animals are prepared with stimulating electrodes in positions that will activate these circuits, they will work (press a lever or turn a wheel) to activate them electrically and ignore natural rewards such as food and sex (Olds 1976). By their behavior, the animals are telling us that activation of these circuits is very rewarding. An important neurotransmitter (among others) in this region is dopamine (DA), which can be measured in the extracellular fluid of freely behaving animals using microdialysis. Extracellular DA is reliably increased in the NAC and amygdala by the important drugs abused by humans. These include cocaine, methamphetamine, nicotine, opioids, ethanol, and marijuana.

Ample evidence therefore exists that drugs that activate the reward system are self-administered by animals and are likely to be abused by humans. This relationship is so reliable that animal models are now used as one measure of assessing a new medication's abuse liability prior to marketing. Even before a new medication is approved for marketing, it is important to know the likelihood of abuse and the need for restrictions on prescribing. Prior to the era of careful premarketing testing for abuse liability, some medications were approved with loose regulations until clinical experience demonstrated their potential to be abused. Data on abuse liability are now obtained from animal models much earlier in the drug development process. Such data now influence decisions on the need for restrictive scheduling by the US Drug Enforcement Administration before a new medication becomes generally available for prescribing by physicians. This fact is a practical example of the benefits of translational research in the addiction area.

Strategies for medication-assisted treatment of addictive disorders

Treatment of addiction usually begins with *detoxification*. Detoxification refers to the cleansing of the body of drugs by means of their being metabolized in the liver or excreted by the kidneys. The patient can be given medication to treat withdrawal symptoms produced as the drug concentration falls and its receptors become vacant. The signs and symptoms of withdrawal are usually opposite to the changes produced by the acute effects of the drug, appearing as a kind of "rebound." For example, opioids directly inhibit gut contractions, an effect that usually produces symptoms of constipation; in withdrawal from opioids, the gut rebounds and becomes hyperactive, producing the symptoms of diarrhea. In animal models, withdrawal symptoms are similar to those in human patients. Treatment of withdrawal can be accomplished by administering a drug in the same class as the drug of dependence and then tapering the dosage over days. Most clinicians transfer the patient from the drug of abuse to a long-acting drug in the same class to gradually wean the patient with less discomfort. Thus, in treating dependence on a short-acting barbiturate, the clinician may use a long-acting barbiturate to prevent or reduce withdrawal symptoms.

Animal models can be used to test the effectiveness of different medications for withdrawal that are in the same pharmacological category as the drug of abuse. An important current use of animal models is the search for better medications for the treatment of ethanol withdrawal. Such studies in animal models have led to some novel treatments for ethanol withdrawal, a condition that is clinically important and life-threatening. Moreover, we have clinical evidence of sensitization to ethanol withdrawal such that repeated episodes of withdrawal may produce progressively more severe symptoms. This phenomenon cannot be studied experimentally in humans, but it has been the subject of productive research using models of ethanol withdrawal in rodents (Becker and Lopez 2004).

Cross-tolerance as a therapeutic strategy

Tolerance is the reduction in drug effect that occurs with repeat dosing such that the body adapts and has a decreased response to each administration over time. Tolerance develops rapidly to many drugs of abuse so that persons with addiction may require a daily dose that is so high that it would be fatal to a non-tolerant person. Cross-tolerance refers to the fact that tolerance to one drug confers tolerance to all drugs in the same class.

The first treatment to use cross-tolerance as a maintenance strategy was discovered in heroin addiction by Vincent Dole and colleagues in the early 1960s. Dole tested several opioid drugs in a search for a medication that reduced the symptoms of heroin addiction. He found that methadone, a synthetic opioid, reduced heroin craving and withdrawal symptoms and allowed the addict to function normally in society (Dole and Nyswander 1965). This treatment was based on a fundamental pharmacological concept and developed in the human laboratory before being translated to clinical programs. Former heroin addicts can function normally for years while taking a level daily dose of oral methadone. Drug craving and withdrawal are blocked, and, if the patient injects heroin, the effects are minimized because of cross-tolerance between methadone and heroin. A patient maintained on the appropriate dose of methadone experiences little immediate effect from the medication and would require a costly amount of heroin to experience any euphoria (Dole *et al.* 1966). The successful development of methadone maintenance served as a model for other opioid maintenance treatments such as buprenorphine. Buprenorphine is a partial agonist instead of a full agonist like methadone, but it has many similar benefits (Comer *et al.* 2001).

Maintenance treatment for opioid addiction was followed by maintenance for nicotine addiction using nicotine chewing gum, patch, or nasal spray. The mechanism appears to be analogous to that of methadone. The medically supplied nicotine reduces withdrawal symptoms and craving for cigarettes (Jorenby *et al.* 1999). Thus far the maintenance approach has not been successful for alcohol or stimulant addiction.

Receptor antagonists to block drug effects

Researchers have been working for decades to learn the mechanism of action of important medications such as opioids. This research was partly motivated by the search for medications that would relieve pain without having the potential to produce addiction. In the case of opioid receptors, some molecules had strong affinity for the receptor but did not produce the chain of events that led to typical opioid effects. The concept of receptor antagonists was born using combinations of in vitro and in vivo animal models. Some of the first generation antagonists such as nalorphine were used as antidotes to reverse the effects of an opioid overdose but were not pure antagonists. That is, they had some opioid-like effects. Subsequent research led to the synthesis of pure antagonists such as naloxone and naltrexone (Martin *et al.* 1973). A family of opioid receptors was identified by translation from in vitro and in vivo models, and the human versions of these receptors were ultimately cloned (Pert and Snyder 1973; Simon *et al.* 1973; Terenius 1973). Natural ligands for these receptors were identified, again using both in vivo and in vitro models (Hughes *et al.* 1975). The 1970s was a remarkable decade in the history of biology because the endogenous opioid system was discovered and the term "endogenous morphine" or endorphin was coined. Later, an endogenous cannabinoid system was discovered (Devane *et al.* 1992). It was hoped that these discoveries could be translated into improved treatment of pain and addiction. Although improved understanding has clearly occurred, better treatments have not naturally followed.

Naltrexone is an example of a relatively pure antagonist at μ, ∂, and κ opioid receptors. It was initially thought to be an ideal treatment for opioid addiction. A person stabilized on a dose of naltrexone could not feel the euphoric effect of a heroin injection because the receptors were blocked. Animals trained to administer opioids would stop self-administering and not reinstate self-injection if maintained on naltrexone. It was hoped that addicts could also be maintained on this medication, which had minimal side effects and no possibility of producing dependence or abuse. Numerous studies were conducted in the 1970s and 1980s in an effort to translate this excellent pharmacological efficacy into clinical efficacy (O'Brien *et al.* 1975). Unfortunately, human patients could not be required to take the medication as was done in animal models. Motivation to remain abstinent from opioids was necessary. Few human heroin addicts were willing even to try naltrexone and fewer still would remain on it for more than a few weeks. The first difficulty was that detoxification from opioids was necessary before beginning naltrexone treatment. Naltrexone has such high affinity for opioid receptors that it would immediately displace typical opioids from the receptor site and precipitate acute withdrawal symptoms. After detoxification was accomplished, the opioid-free patient could receive his first dose of naltrexone. The patient would experience none of the opioid agonist effects similar to methadone. Patients accustomed to the comforting antianxiety effects of opioids would be uncomfortable taking naltrexone in comparison to an agonist like methadone. If a patient taking naltrexone for maintenance attempted to get high by injecting heroin or another opioid, the effects would be blocked, producing a feeling of frustration and unpleasant conditioned withdrawal symptoms precipitated by the cues of injection. Only addicts with strong motivation to remain drug free are likely to respond to naltrexone. This group of patients includes physicians and other medical professionals who have become addicted to opioids and risk losing their medical license if they relapse. After detoxification and appropriate evaluation, such patients can return to work while taking naltrexone. In the absence of naltrexone, the physicians are at high risk of relapse due to the great availability of opioids in a hospital setting. While taking naltrexone, recovering physicians can safely handle opioids because they would experience virtually no effect if they relapsed and took a dose (O'Brien et al. 1986). The knowledge that one is taking naltrexone may also have the effect of reducing craving.

Results of a few studies of parolees with a history of opioid addiction suggest that they represent another group that could benefit from a favorable response to opioid antagonist treatment. These parolees and probationers share with opioid-addicted physicians the risk of severe consequences if they relapse. Thus, they would have a reason to adhere to naltrexone prescription (Cornish et al. 1997). For the majority of opioid addicts, however, the clear pharmacological efficacy of naltrexone demonstrated in animal models did not translate into the clinical situation for which it had been developed. The human variable of motivation for abstinence could not be modeled in animals.

The partial agonist strategy

Another approach to the treatment of opioid addiction that was developed in preclinical laboratories involves the use of partial opioid agonists. The only medication of this type that has achieved Food and Drug Administration approval for the treatment of opioid addiction is buprenorphine (Johnson et al. 1992). This medication was originally used for its analgesic properties. It activates μ receptors as a partial agonist, which means that although it has high affinity for μ receptors, it does not fully activate them. Its opioid effects are limited to the equivalent of 40 mg to 50 mg of methadone. Higher doses produce no greater effect. It also acts as an antagonist at κ-opioid receptors and as an agonist at nociceptin receptors. These characteristics, elucidated in animal models, enable buprenorphine to be used in a fashion similar to that of methadone, that is, as a maintenance medication, except in cases with a high tolerance to opioids. Buprenorphine has a long half-life, and, because of its high binding affinity for the μ receptor, buprenorphine blocks access to the receptor by opiates such as heroin (morphine). In this context buprenorphine has an effect similar to that of naltrexone, but unlike naltrexone, it has partial agonist properties that provide a moderate opioid effect that patients report as comforting.

Buprenorphine has also benefited from what might be called enlightened legislation. As a partial agonist, it was not placed in schedule II with full μ agonists such as methadone. It was placed in schedule III where it can be prescribed by physicians who have obtained certification by taking a brief course on the medication's unique properties. The federal law was changed in 2000, making it possible for the first time since 1914 to treat addiction in a private physician's office. Through this process, treatment of opioid addiction became available to many more people, and adherence to a methadone program was no longer the only maintenance option.

Another translation from basic pharmacology was the idea to combine buprenorphine with naloxone (4:1 ratio) to discourage people from injecting it (Comer et al. 2005). Naloxone is not well absorbed when the buprenorphine/naloxone combination is taken as prescribed, that is, by allowing it to dissolve under the tongue. Thus the sublingual route does not antagonize the μ opioid effects of buprenorphine, and the patient benefits from the moderate opioid effect. However, if the patient decides to "cheat" by injecting the combination, naloxone via the intravenous route will block or diminish the μ effects of buprenorphine and even produce withdrawal symptoms if the patient is dependent on another opioid. This strategy is thought to limit the abuse of buprenorphine because most of it is prescribed in the combination form with naloxone.

Medication strategies for nicotine addiction

The first medication strategy for smokers was based on the agonist maintenance concept that was successfully used with methadone for opioid addiction. Nicotine was provided in the form of chewing gum and later made available as a skin patch and a nasal spray. Nicotine taken by a route other than smoking allows the dependent smoker to maintain a nicotine level without exposure to the harmful tars and other substances contained in tobacco smoke. By transferring their dependence to non-smoked nicotine, smokers could block nicotine withdrawal symptoms as they gradually reduced nicotine intake through the gum or patch. Randomized, controlled trials showed that more smokers were able to achieve abstinence with the aid of nicotine replacement, but relapse rates within 6 to 12 months remained high (Fiore et al. 1994).

The next advance in the treatment of tobacco dependence was the serendipitous discovery that the antidepressant bupropion reduced craving for cigarettes and improved abstinence rates. This medication blocks the reuptake of norepinephrine and DA into presynaptic nerve cells, thus prolonging the actions of these neurotransmitters at the synapse. It is not known how this process influences the desire for cigarettes, but the medication has shown efficacy in multiple double-blind trials for smoking cessation (Hays et al. 2001). Bupropion can be given along with nicotine replacement. Nicotine treatment immediately reduces withdrawal symptoms when smoking is terminated or reduced. Bupropion becomes active in the second week and reduces the rate of relapse.

The next major advance was perhaps the best example of a pharmaceutical laboratory using knowledge of the actions of nicotine and its interaction with specific receptors and creating a partial agonist at these receptors. The result, varenicline, is a molecule that has partial agonist properties at nicotinic receptors. Specifically, varenicline is a partial agonist at α4β2 nicotinic acetylcholine receptors and a full agonist at the α7 sub-type. Development of this product was translation at the most basic level, and it has proven to be the most successful aid to the treatment of nicotine addiction thus far available. The clinical effects are analogous to the effects of buprenorphine in opioid addicts. The medication reduces nicotine withdrawal symptoms and reduces craving for cigarettes. The abstinence rates at 12 months are significantly higher for smokers randomized to varenicline than for those randomized to other medications (Gonzales et al. 2006).

A new strategy aimed at blocking an endogenous system activated by a drug of abuse

In the late 1970s, the race was on to understand the normal function of the endogenous opioid system. One way to study it was to use an antagonist to block the receptors and see which functions were impaired in animal models. Harold Altshuler, in a poster presented at the 1979 meeting of the College on Problems of Drug Dependence, reported on 10 of 22 rhesus monkeys that avidly self-administered intravenous ethanol (Altshuler et al. 1980). He tested them with naloxone and naltrexone to determine whether the endogenous opioid system was involved. Both antagonists produced a clear dose-related suppression of the self-administration of ethanol in these animals. Subsequent research on alcohol drinking in rodent models also found that naltrexone could block ethanol self-administration (Volpicelli et al. 1986). Based solely on these results from animal models, the addiction research team at the Philadelphia Veterans Administration Medical Center obtained an Investigational New Drug application in 1983 to test naltrexone in humans addicted to alcohol. In initial open studies, some alcoholics reported a loss of anticipated pleasure when they drank alcohol and they seemed more amenable to rehabilitation. A double-blind clinical trial was then conducted in 70 male veterans with chronic alcoholism under treatment in an intensive day-hospital program. In addition to 12-step (Alcoholics Anonymous) groups, each patient received either placebo or 50 mg per day of naltrexone for 3 months. The dose of 50 mg was chosen because this dose effectively blocked the average dose of heroin in studies of heroin addiction (Volpicelli et al. 1990). Those addicted to alcohol who were randomized to naltrexone showed significantly less relapse to heavy drinking than did the controls. They reported less craving for alcohol and, if they did drink, they reported less euphoria or "high" (Volpicelli et al. 1992). The results were met with much skepticism from clinicians because endogenous opioids were not thought to be involved in alcohol drinking, despite the data from animal studies.

Eventually, investigators at Yale led by Stephanie O'Malley conducted a similar trial among patients who were alcoholics and found the same outcome: significantly less relapse in patients randomly assigned to naltrexone (O'Malley et al. 1992). Based on these two studies translated from animal models, the Food and Drug Administration approved the addition of alcoholism to the indications for naltrexone. Translational research on the endogenous opioid system in alcohol drinking has continued and has led to important new findings with implications for clinical practice.

In rodent models of alcohol drinking, the phenomenon of clinical relapse can be studied by terminating alcohol availability, thus forcing the animals to become abstinent. When alcohol is again made available, the rats will reinstate alcohol drinking if they are given mild foot shock stress or if they are exposed to environmental cues that had previously been associated with alcohol availability. It was found that treatment with naltrexone during the abstinence period blocked the effect of alcohol-associated cues in producing reinstatement of alcohol drinking, but it had little effect on stress-induced drinking.

In rats studied using microdialysis, the DA level was increased in the NAC when the rat drank alcohol, but this DA increase was blocked by pretreatment with naltrexone. These results are explained by the effects of alcohol on the release of endogenous opioids, which in turn cause the augmentation of DA release. But a learning mechanism is also involved. Rats that previously received alcohol in the chamber showed increased levels of DA in the NAC as soon as they were placed in the chamber and before alcohol became available (Gonzales and Weiss 1998). Thus, for the rats with alcohol drinking experience, the DA increase (reward) was both a conditioned response and a pharmacological response. This finding parallels the human data in which alcohol cues (bar scenes, pictures of alcoholic beverages) produce activation in the reward system of the brain as measured by fMRI (Myrick et al. 2004). In both the rats and the humans addicted to alcohol, the activation of the reward system is blocked by pretreatment with naltrexone (Myrick et al. 2008).

Beginning with the earliest clinical trials of naltrexone in the 1980s, it was apparent that patients with alcoholism gave variable treatment responses. Some patients showed a large effect, ranging from frequent heavy drinking before naltrexone to total abstinence or only occasional drinking while receiving the medication. Other patients showed no benefit and continued to drink while taking naltrexone. This finding suggests genetic variability, which was supported by family history studies. Patients with the greatest density of relatives with alcoholism had the poorest response to placebo in clinical trials but had a good response to naltrexone (Monterosso et al. 2001).

Reactivity to ethanol also seems to be influenced by family history of alcoholism. Based on the original animal studies, it was hypothesized in 1983 that ethanol activated the endogenous opioid system and this was a mechanism underlying at least a portion of alcohol reward. Subsequent research suggested that this effect is variable and influenced by heredity.

Volunteers with a positive family history showed a significantly greater high or euphoria from a standard dose of alcohol compared with subjects with a negative family history. This euphoria was blocked by pretreatment with naltrexone (King et al. 1997). This laboratory observation was paralleled by results from clinical trials of patients with alcoholism randomized to naltrexone. Patients randomized to naltrexone reported less euphoria or high from alcohol when they drank (Volpicelli et al. 1995). This finding was also paralleled in rodent studies in which naltrexone blocked DA increase when alcohol was administered and also reduced the behavior of alcohol self-administration (Gonzales and Weiss 1998).

The reward or high experienced by drinkers with a positive family history for alcoholism is postulated to be based on endorphin activation, but direct measurement of endogenous opioids in the brain is not possible. A study by Gianoulakis of family history-positive and family history-negative drinkers showed major differences in plasma β-endorphin response to ethanol (Bart et al. 2005; Gianoulakis et al. 1996), but plasma β-endorphin is known to be of pituitary origin. Clinicians could rely only on family history as a marker of which alcoholic patients were likely to have a good response to naltrexone.

A candidate gene search focused on the genes known to code for various aspects of the endogenous opioid system. A variant of the gene for the μ opioid receptor (A118G) was identified and found to have important functional effects. It had a frequency of about 20% in persons of European ancestry (Bart et al. 2005) and was associated with greater stimulation or high from a given ethanol blood level compared with subjects with the standard allele (Ray and Hutchison 2004). This increased high from ethanol was blocked by pretreatment with naltrexone (Ray and Hutchison 2007). A functional allele for the μ opioid receptor in male rhesus monkeys also is associated with greater alcohol preference, effect, and consumption (Barr et al. 2007).

Male social drinkers with the A118G allele showed an increased DA release in response to alcohol compared with subjects with the standard allele as measured by C^{11}-labeled raclopride in a PET study. DA release was observed in the ventral striatum. Humanized mouse lines with a "knock-in" μ opioid receptor for the A118G allele showed a fourfold greater DA response to ethanol compared with mice with the standard human allele (Ramchandani et al. 2011).

Thus, we note remarkable consistency in translation across "knock-in" mouse strains, monkey models, normal human subjects, and patients with alcoholism. The most significant finding in this series of translational research studies is that in genetic analyses of two sets of data from clinical trials, the patients with the A118G allele had significantly better clinical outcome if they were randomized to naltrexone instead of to placebo (Anton *et al.* 2008; Oslin *et al.* 2003).

The preceding series of studies suggests a biological subtype of alcoholism characterized by an increased response to ethanol in the endogenous opioid system. This subtype could be identified by genotype. Clinical trials are now in progress involving genotyping of patients with alcoholism prior to randomization in a balanced design. If the prospective trials show a significant advantage for patients with the A118G allele when they are randomized to naltrexone, genotype can be used in the future as a predictor of clinical response to a specific medication for a subtype of alcoholism.

Activation of inhibitory systems

Studies of the reward system in animals have identified inhibitory circuits that tend to have an anti-impulsive effect and to put brakes on reward-motivated behavior. γ-Aminobutyric acid (GABA) is the primary inhibitory neurotransmitter in the brain; therefore, GABA circuits have been studied in animal models. Based on the known inhibitory pathways, activation of GABA function should inhibit reward from drugs such as cocaine with the result that self-administration by animals should decline. The first GABA-enhancing drug to be studied in the context of cocaine self-administration was baclofen, a $GABA_B$ agonist (Roberts *et al.* 1996; Shoptaw *et al.* 2003). Roberts and colleagues published several studies beginning in 1996 reporting that baclofen reduced cocaine self-administration. The observation was replicated by other groups and eventually tested in human cocaine addicts with mixed results.

Shoptaw and colleagues (2003) in a small study found cocaine use somewhat reduced in cocaine addicts randomized to baclofen or placebo, but differences were not statistically significant. Haney *et al.* (2006) in a human laboratory study showed that baclofen reduced the intake of a low dose of smoked cocaine but did not significantly diminish the subjective effects of the drug. In a brain-imaging study, Childress and colleagues showed that baclofen blocked the limbic system activation produced by cocaine-related cues (Childress *et al.* 2002). A multisite trial of cocaine in actively using cocaine addicts (Kahn *et al.* 2009) showed no significant benefit from baclofen in reducing cocaine-positive urine samples. Baclofen was not tested in patients already abstinent to determine if relapse could be prevented. The translation of findings on the effects of baclofen from laboratory to clinical trials is complicated by issues of dosage. The human studies mentioned above were conducted with a maximum dose of 60 mg per day. Higher doses were avoided due to complaints of sedation. However, individual cases of cocaine addiction (Kampman K, personal communication, December 2009) and alcoholism (Ameisen 2005) have reported success with much higher doses (up to 280 mg/day). The dose was increased slowly to allow tolerance to sedation to develop. Franklin and colleagues (2009) reported reduction of cigarette smoking in a controlled trial at 80 mg baclofen per day. Thus the question of translation of baclofen effects from animal models to the clinic remains unsettled.

Another means of increasing GABA-based inhibition is vigabatrin, a medication that irreversibly blocks the enzyme that metabolizes GABA, causing high concentrations of the transmitter to accumulate. Vigabatrin is approved for the treatment of seizure disorders. In a series of studies of drug-taking behavior, Dewey and colleagues showed that vigabatrin reduces or blocks the self-administration of cocaine, amphetamine, alcohol, opioids, or nicotine. It has been studied in two controlled clinical trials for the treatment of cocaine addiction in human subjects. In the first trial, conducted in Mexico, vigabatrin significantly reduced self-reported cocaine use and cocaine-positive urine samples compared with placebo-treated patients. End-of-trial abstinence from cocaine was also significantly higher for the group randomized to vigabatrin (Brodie *et al.* 2009). The results of the multisite trial conducted in the USA have not yet been reported. The early results suggest that the effects of vigabatrin on reducing cocaine reward and self-administration in animal models may be successfully translated to human cocaine addicts. Conclusions must be only tentative until the results from large-sample clinical trials are published.

Future goals: understanding plasticity

Because learned addictive behavior is thought to result from neuroplasticity underlying the conditioned responses described in this chapter, it seems logical to consider that influencing mechanisms of neuroplasticity could also be a means of countering these learned addictive behaviors. An interesting animal model of this approach is illustrated by a series of experiments from the laboratory of Peter Kalivas. Using rats trained to self-administer cocaine, Kalivas and colleagues reported a reduction in glutamate levels in the brains of animals exposed to long-term cocaine and a disruption of glutamate homeostasis. Following withdrawal from chronic cocaine, they observed a marked imbalance in glutamate homeostasis with both cystine–glutamate exchange and glutamate uptake being reduced in the nucleus accumbens (Baker *et al.* 2003). The imbalance in glutamate homeostasis is associated with a reduction in basal extracellular glutamate levels and a potentiated release of synaptic glutamate during drug seeking (McFarland *et al.* 2003). In addition, researchers also observed a basal increase in the AMPA to NMDA current ratio and a loss of both long-term potentiation and long-term depression (Moussawi *et al.* 2009).

These observations on glutamate homeostasis suggest therapeutic implications. Cystine can be administered to animals withdrawn from chronic cocaine use using N-acetylcysteine as a carrier, or glutamate uptake can be increased by the antibiotic ceftriaxone. By restoring glutamate homeostasis in this manner, reinstatement of cocaine seeking is prevented. The treated animals also showed a restored ability to induce long-term potentiation and long-term depression as well as normalization of the AMPA:NMDA ratio. The treatment also prevents changes in neuronal spine head diameter induced during cocaine seeking (Moussawi *et al.* 2009).

Taken together, the data above suggest the possibility that normalization of glutamate homeostasis in addicts might restore the ability to induce synaptic plasticity in the accumbens, which in turn could facilitate establishing behaviors that might compete with drug seeking. Early clinical trials to test this approach have begun. Exogenous N-acetylcysteine is used for the treatment of hepatic failure in acetaminophen overdose. Thus, it is available to be administered to cocaine addicts tested by presentation of the cocaine-related cues described earlier. Cue-induced craving is one aspect of cocaine addiction that lends itself to rapid testing of the preclinical findings in human subjects. In a double-blind study, cocaine addicts treated with N-acetylcysteine reported reduced desire for cocaine compared with the control group when presented with cues associated with cocaine (LaRowe *et al.* 2007). In another human study, N-acetylcysteine was found to reduce cigarette smoking (Knackstedt and Kalivas 2009). Further clinical trials are in progress.

Conclusions

As stated in the introduction, numerous animal models of drug-taking behavior have been used to increase understanding of addiction. Moreover, this increased understanding has led directly to new treatment approaches, novel and unexpected medications, and improved treatment results. Therefore, society has strong reasons to support basic research on addiction. Applied research in the absence of a strong preclinical background is likely to be wasteful and unsuccessful.

References

Altshuler HL, Phillips PA, Feinhandler DA. 1980. Alteration of ethanol self-administration by naltrexone. *Life Sci* **26**:679–688.

Ameisen O. 2005. Complete and prolonged suppression of symptoms and consequences of alcohol-dependence using high-dose baclofen: a self-case report of a physician. *Alcohol Alcohol* **40**:147–150.

Anton RF, Oroszi G, O'Malley S *et al.* 2008. An evaluation of mu-opioid receptor (OPRM1) as a predictor of naltrexone response in the treatment of alcohol dependence: results from the Combined Pharmacotherapies and Behavioral Interventions for Alcohol Dependence (COMBINE) study. *Arch Gen Psychiatry* **65**:135–144.

Baker DA, McFarland K, Lake RW *et al.* 2003. Neuroadaptations in cystine–glutamate exchange underlie cocaine relapse. *Nat Neurosci* **6**:743–749.

Barr CS, Schwandt M, Lindell SG *et al.* 2007. Association of a functional polymorphism in the mu-opioid receptor gene with alcohol response and consumption in male rhesus macaques. *Arch Gen Psychiatry* **64**:369–376.

Bart G, Kreek MJ, Ott J *et al.* 2005. Increased attributable risk related to a functional mu-opioid receptor gene polymorphism in association with alcohol dependence in central Sweden. *Neuropsychopharmacology* **30**:417–422.

Becker HC, Lopez MF. 2004. Increased ethanol drinking after repeated chronic ethanol exposure and withdrawal experience in C57BL/6 mice. *Alcohol Clin Exp Res* **28**:1829–1838.

Brodie JD, Case BG, Figueroa E et al. 2009. Randomized, double-blind, placebo-controlled trial of vigabatrin for the treatment of cocaine dependence in Mexican parolees. *Am J Psychiatry* **166**:1269–1277.

Childress AR, Franklin, T, Listerud J, Acton P, O'Brien CP. 2002. Neuroimaging of cocaine craving states: cessation, stimulant administration, and drug cue paradigms. In: *Neuropsychopharmacology: Fifth Generation of Progress.* Davis KL, Charney D, Coyle JT, Nemeroff C, eds. Philadelphia: Lippincott Williams & Wilkins.

Childress AR, Mozley PD, McElgin W et al. 1999. Limbic activation during cue-induced cocaine craving. *Am J Psychiatry* **156**:11–18.

Comer S, Walker E, Collins E. 2005. Buprenorphine/naloxone reduces the reinforcing and subjective effects of heroin in heroin-dependent volunteers. *Psychopharmacology (Berl)* **181**:664–675.

Comer SD, Collins ED, Fischman MW. 2001. Buprenorphine sublingual tablets: effects on IV heroin self-administration by humans. *Psychopharmacology (Berl)* **154**:28–37.

Cornish JW, Metzger D, Woody GE et al. 1997. Naltrexone pharmacotherapy for opioid dependent federal probationers. *J Subst Abuse Treat* **14**:529–534.

Deroche-Gamonet V, Belin D, Piazza PV. 2004. Evidence for addiction-like behavior in the rat. *Science* **305**:1014–1017.

Devane WA, Hanus L, Breuer A et al. 1992. Isolation and structure of a brain constituent that binds to the cannabinoid receptor. *Science* **258**:1946–1949.

Dole VP, Nyswander M. 1965. A medical treatment for diacetylmorphine (heroin) addiction: a clinical trial with methadone hydrochloride. *J Am Med Assoc* **193**:80–84.

Dole VP, Nyswander ME, Kreek MJ. 1966. Narcotic blockade – a medical technique for stopping heroin use by addicts. *Arch Intern Med* **118**:304–309.

Fiore MC, Smith SS, Jorenby DE, Baker TB. 1994. The effectiveness of the nicotine patch for smoking cessation. *J Am Med Assoc* **271**:1940–1946.

Franklin T, Harper D, Kampman K et al. 2009. The GABA B agonist baclofen reduces cigarette consumption in a preliminary double-blind placebo-controlled smoking reduction study. *Drug Alcohol Depend* **103**:30–36.

Gianoulakis C, Krishnan B, Thavundayil J. 1996. Enhanced sensitivity of pituitary beta-endorphin to ethanol in subjects at high risk of alcoholism [published erratum appears in *Arch Gen Psychiatry* 1996 Jun;53:555]. *Arch Gen Psychiatry* **53**:250–257.

Goldberg SR, Schuster CR. 1970. Conditioned morphine-induced abstinence changes: persistence in post morphine-dependent monkeys. *J Exper Analys Behav* **14**:33–46.

Gonzales D, Rennard SI, Nides M et al. 2006. Varenicline, an alpha4beta2 nicotinic acetylcholine receptor partial agonist, vs sustained-release bupropion and placebo for smoking cessation: a randomized controlled trial. *J Am Med Assoc* **296**:47–55.

Gonzales RA, Weiss F. 1998. Suppression of ethanol-reinforced behavior by naltrexone is associated with attenuation of the ethanol-induced increase in dialysate dopamine levels in the nucleus accumbens. *J Neurosci* **18**:10663–10671.

Haney M, Hart CL, Foltin RW. 2006. Effects of baclofen on cocaine self-administration: opioid- and nonopioid-dependent volunteers. *Neuropsychopharmacology* **31**:1814–1821.

Hays JT, Hurt RD, Rigotti NA et al. 2001. Sustained-release bupropion for pharmacologic relapse prevention after smoking cessation. a randomized, controlled trial. *Ann Intern Med* **135**:423–433.

Hughes J, Smith TW, Kosterlitz HW et al. 1975. Identification of two related pentapeptides from the brain with potent opiate agonist activity. *Nature* **258**:577–580.

Johnson RE, Jaffe JH, Fudala PJ. 1992. A controlled trial of buprenorphine treatment for opioid dependence. *J Am Med Assoc* **267**:2750–2755.

Jorenby DE, Leschow SJ, Nides MA et al. 1999. A controlled trial of sustained-release bupropion, a nicotine patch, or both for smoking cessation. *N Engl J Med* **340**:685–691.

Kahn R, Biswas K, Childress AR et al. 2009. Multi-center trial of baclofen for abstinence initiation in severe cocaine-dependent individuals. *Drug Alcohol Depend* **103**:59–64.

King A, Volpicelli J, Frazer A, O'Brien C. 1997. Effect of naltrexone on subjective alcohol response in subjects at high and low risk for future alcohol dependence. *Psychopharmacology (Berl)* **129**:15–22.

Knackstedt LA, Kalivas PW. 2009. Glutamate and reinstatement. *Curr Opin Pharmacol* **9**:59–64.

LaRowe SD, Myrick H, Hedden S et al. 2007. Is cocaine desire reduced by N-acetylcysteine? *Am J Psychiatry* **164**:1115–1117.

Martin W, Jasinski D, Mansky P. 1973. Naltrexone, an antagonist for the treatment of heroin dependence. *Arch Gen Psych* **28**:784–791.

McFarland K, Lapish CC, Kalivas PW. 2003. Prefrontal glutamate release into the core of the nucleus accumbens mediates cocaine-induced reinstatement of drug-seeking behavior. *J Neurosci* **23**:3531–3537.

Monterosso JR, Flannery BA, Pettinati HM *et al.* 2001. Predicting treatment response to naltrexone: the influence of craving and family history. *Am J Addict* **10**:258–268.

Moussawi K, Pacchioni A, Moran M *et al.* 2009. N-acetylcysteine reverses cocaine-induced metaplasticity. *Nat Neurosci* **12**:182–189.

Myrick H, Anton RF, Li X *et al.* 2004. Differential brain activity in alcoholics and social drinkers to alcohol cues: relationship to craving. *Neuropsychopharmacology* **29**:393–402.

Myrick H, Anton RF, Li X *et al.* 2008. Effect of naltrexone and ondansetron on alcohol cue-induced activation of the ventral striatum in alcohol-dependent people. *Arch Gen Psychiatry* **65**:466–475.

O'Brien C, Gardner E. 2005. Critical assessment of how to study addiction and its treatment: human and non-human animal models. *Pharmacol Ther* **108**:18–58.

O'Brien CP, Greenstein RA, Mintz J, Woody GE. 1975. Clinical experience with naltrexone. *Am J Drug Alcohol Abuse* **2**:365–377.

O'Brien CP, Greenstein R, Testa T, Woody G. 1976. Experimental analysis of narcotic use in humans. *Psychopharmacol Bull* **12**:9–10.

O'Brien CP, Testa T, O'Brien TJ, Brady JP, Wells B. 1977. Conditioned narcotic withdrawal in humans. *Science* **195**:1000–1002.

O'Brien CP, Woody GE, McLellan AT. 1986. A new tool in the treatment of impaired physicians. *Phila Med* **82**:442–446.

Olds J. 1976. Brain stimulation and the motivation of behavior. *Prog Brain Res* **45**:401–426.

O'Malley SS, Jaffe AJ, Chang G *et al.* 1992. Naltrexone and coping skills therapy for alcohol dependence: a controlled study. *Arch Gen Psychiatry* **49**:881–887.

Oslin DW, Berrettini W, Kranzler HR *et al.* 2003. A functional polymorphism of the mu-opioid receptor gene is associated with naltrexone response in alcohol-dependent patients. *Neuropsychopharmacology* **28**:1546–1552.

Pert CB, Snyder SH. 1973. Properties of opiate-receptor binding in rat brain. *Proc Natl Acad Sci USA* **70**:2243–2247.

Ramchandani VA, Umhau J, Pavon FJ *et al.* 2011. A genetic determinant of the striatal response to alcohol in men. *Mol Psychiatry* **16**:809–817.

Ray LA, Hutchison KE. 2004. A polymorphism of the mu-opioid receptor gene (OPRM1) and sensitivity to the effects of alcohol in humans. *Alcohol Clin Exp Res* **28**:1789–1795.

Ray LA, Hutchison KE. 2007. Effects of naltrexone on alcohol sensitivity and genetic moderators of medication response: a double-blind placebo-controlled study. *Arch Gen Psychiatry* **64**:1069–1077.

Roberts DC, Andrews MM, Vickers GJ. 1996. Baclofen attenuates the reinforcing effects of cocaine in rats. *Neuropsychopharmacology* **15**:417–423.

Rocha BA, Fumagalli F, Gainetdinov RR *et al.* 1998. Cocaine self-administration in dopamine-transporter knockout mice. *Nat Neurosci* **1**:132–137.

Schoenbaum G, Stalnaker TA, Shaham Y. 2007. A role for BDNF in cocaine reward and relapse. *Nat Neurosci* **10**:935–936.

Shoptaw S, Yang X, Rotheram-Fuller EJ *et al.* 2003. Randomized placebo-controlled trial of baclofen for cocaine dependence: preliminary effects for individuals with chronic patterns of cocaine use. *J Clin Psychiatry* **64**:1440–1448.

Simon EJ, Hiller JM, Edelman I. 1973. Stereospecific binding of the potent narcotic analgesic (^{3}H)etorphine to rat-brain homogenate. *Proc Natl Acad Sci USA* **70**:1947–1949.

Terenius L. 1973. Stereospecific interaction between narcotic analgesics and a synaptic plasma membrane fraction of rat cerebral cortex. *Acta Pharmacol Toxicol* **32**:317–320.

Vanderschuren LJ, Everitt BJ. 2004. Drug seeking becomes compulsive after prolonged cocaine self-administration. *Science* **305**:1017–1019.

Volkow ND, Wang GJ, Telang F *et al.* 2006. Cocaine cues and dopamine in dorsal striatum: mechanism of craving in cocaine addiction. *J Neurosci* **26**:6583–6588.

Volpicelli JR, Alterman AI, Hayashida M, O'Brien CP. 1992. Naltrexone in the treatment of alcohol dependence. *Arch Gen Psychiatry* **49**:876–880.

Volpicelli JR, Davis MA, Olgin JE. 1986. Naltrexone blocks the post-shock increase of ethanol consumption. *Life Sci* **38**:841–847.

Volpicelli JR, O'Brien CP, Alterman AI, Hayashida M. 1990. Naltrexone and the treatment of alcohol dependence: initial observations. In *Opioids, Bulimia, Alcohol Abuse and Alcoholism*. Reid LB, ed. New York: Springer-Verlag, pp. 195–214.

Volpicelli JR, Watson NT, King AC, Sherman CE, O'Brien CP. 1995. Effect of naltrexone on alcohol "high" in alcoholics. *Am J Psychiatry* **152**:613–615.

Weiss F, Paulus MP, Lorang MT, Koob GF. 1992. Increases in extracellular dopamine in the nucleus accumbens by cocaine are inversely related to basal levels: effects of acute and repeated administration. *J Neurosci* **12**:4372–4380.

Wikler A, Pescor F. 1967. Classical conditioning of a morphine abstinence phenomenon, reinforcement of opioid-drinking behavior and relapse in morphine-addicted rats. *Psychopharmacologia* **10**:255–284.

Chapter 6

Section summary and perspectives: Translational medicine in psychiatry

Joseph T. Coyle

Historically, translational research in psychiatry has focused on animal models, which were based on the biochemical and behavioral effects of the psychotropic medications that were originally discovered by serendipity to have therapeutic effects in patients. For example, a robust predictor of antipsychotic efficacy was the ability of the novel agent to prevent apomorphine-induced vomiting in dogs, like the first antipsychotic chlorpromazine, as a behavioral measure of D_2 receptor antagonism (Rotrosn et al. 1972). Subsequently, with the characterization of the dopamine D_2 receptor by ligand-binding methods, a highly significant correlation between the antipsychotic potency of these drugs and their affinity for the dopamine D_2 receptor was demonstrated, thereby providing a simple ligand binding measure for predicting antipsychotic activity (Creese et al. 1976). Similarly, a variety of behavioral tests that relied on the biogenic amine potentiating effects of imipramine, the first clinically effective tricyclic antidepressant, were used to identify other potential antidepressants (Lapin and Oxenkrug 1969).

A logical consequence of this strategy was that the identification of potential new drugs would lead to drugs with the same primary mechanism of action as the founding drug. This situation has in fact taken place, with current antipsychotic (Jones et al. 2006; Lieberman et al. 2005) and antidepressant medications (Trivedi et al. 2006) having negligible differences in efficacy compared with older generations of these drugs that are now off patent. The increasing prevalence of patients who are poorly responsive or unresponsive to existing antipsychotics (Leucht et al. 2007) and antidepressants (Thase 2009), respectively, may result from the limited targets of therapeutic action for both of these two classes of medication.

As the preceding chapters indicate, over the last decade, considerable progress has been made in the development of translational research related to serious psychiatric disorders that moves beyond the circular logic dominating prior treatment discovery efforts. These advances have been based to a considerable extent on the elucidation of disorder-related neuropathology, the characterization of intermediate phenotypes identified by brain imaging and electrophysiological biomarkers, and the identification of putative risk genes. Most evidence indicates that psychiatric disorders are disorders of complex genetics like hypertension and diabetes in which multiple common risk alleles interact with the environment to produce the disorder (Tiwari et al. 2010; Toro et al. 2010). Through the use of the recombinant DNA strategies, this information has permitted the development of mutant mouse models that recapitulate the endophenotype of the disorders of interest (Nestler and Hyman 2010). An endophenotype represents a heritable component of the disorder that can be observed in first-degree relatives and not the full manifestation of the disorder, consistent with the complex genetics of psychiatric disorders. Validation of the endophenotype derives from the results of behavioral analysis and the demonstration of shared biomarkers such as impaired prepulse inhibition, dysregulation of the hypothalamic-pituitary-adrenal axis, or structural brain changes.

Schizophrenia

Although pharmacological challenge studies designed to mimic symptoms in controls or to reduce symptoms in affected individuals address the acute symptomatic manifestations of a psychiatric disorder, they nevertheless have the potential for illuminating more fundamental aspects of the pathophysiology as is the case for ketamine and schizophrenia (DeVito et al. 2011). The fact that ketamine, a use-dependent,

---

Translational Neuroscience, ed. James E. Barrett, Joseph T. Coyle and Michael Williams. Published by Cambridge University Press. © Cambridge University Press 2012.

noncompetitive NMDA receptor antagonist, could reproduce the positive, negative, and subtle cognitive symptoms of schizophrenia as well as its attendant neurophysiological abnormalities shone light on glutamate, a neurotransmitter system different from dopamine that dominated hypotheses about the etiology of schizophrenia (Goff and Coyle 2001). The plausibility of a role for N-methyl-D-aspartic acid (NMDA) receptors in the pathophysiology of schizophrenia gained traction as several genetic loci of risk for schizophrenia, which encode genes that directly or indirectly affect NMDA receptor function, were identified in linkage and association studies (for review, Balu and Coyle 2011). These include the NMDA receptor subunit, NR2B, G72, D-amino acid oxidase and serine racemase, which affect the availability of the co-agonist, D-serine, and neuregulin. The apparent hypofunction of NMDA receptors prompted a series of placebo-controlled clinical trials in patients with schizophrenia on stable doses of antipsychotics with drugs that act as agonists at the glycine modulatory site (GMS) on the NMDA receptor, thereby enhancing its function. These showed significant improvement in multiple symptom domains including negative symptoms and cognitive functions (Tsai and Lin 2010).

The NMDA receptors most sensitive to low-dose ketamine appear to reside on fast-firing, parvalbumin (PV)-positive GABAergic interneurons in the intermediate levels of the cortex that provide feedback inhibition to the pyramidal neurons (Gonzalez-Burgos et al. 2010). A "pathological circuit" emerged from these studies that could account for the GABAergic pathology in schizophrenia such as loss of PV and GAD67 and disinhibition of subcortical dopamine release, causing psychosis (Lisman et al. 2008). The pathological circuit thus offers a number of potential targets of intervention aside from the NMDA receptors on the PV+GABAergic neurons. These include GlyT1 inhibitors and D-amino acid inhibitors to increase endogenous agonist levels at the GMS on the NMDA receptor, mGluR5 agonists to potentiate NMDA receptor function, $GABA_A$ receptor agonists or positive allosteric modulators to compensate for reduced PV+-GABAergic neuronal activity, and mGluR2/3 agonists to reduce disinhibited glutamatergic subcortical projections (Coyle et al. 2010).

As emphasized in Chapter 4 by Balu and Goff, many of the putative risk genes for schizophrenia appear to play a role in brain development so that the pathology observed in the mature brain often represents the end stage of a disrupted developmental process. In particular, several studies indicate that schizophrenia exhibits atrophic pyramidal cell somata, reduced dendritic complexity, and reduced spine density in the cortex and limbic system (Glantz and Lewis 2000; Penzes et al. 2011). Monitoring the normal role of such genes in brain development or the impact of allelic variants associated with risk for disease in humans is simply not feasible whereas such studies are readily carried out in mice. Furthermore, the preclinical studies allow the discovery of gene–gene interactions so that "pathways of pathology" can be uncovered. D-serine-NMDA receptor function, crucial in the acute symptomatic manifestations of schizophrenia, also plays a critical role in the developmental elaboration of dendrites and spine formation (McKinney 2010). Thus, serine racemase null mutant mice exhibit reduced dendritic complexity and spine density in prefrontal pyramidal neurons (DeVito et al. 2011). DISC1 (Lee et al. 2011) and neuregulin (Krivosheya et al. 2008), strong risk genes for schizophrenia, also converge on pathways responsible for dendritic elaboration and spine formation. The hypotrophic neurons with reduced dendritic complexity and reduced spines account for the decreased cortical volume and ventricular enlargement characteristic of schizophrenia. Notably, these structural changes correlate best with the negative symptoms and cognitive impairments of schizophrenia (Ho et al. 2003).

Another strategy that transcends the dopamine D_2 receptor circular logic is to create animal models of schizophrenia based on histological homologies. For example, using cortical atrophy/ventricular enlargement as a biomarker for schizophrenia, investigators have replicated the cortical deficits of schizophrenia by the exposure of rat fetuses to the mitotoxin, methylazoxymethanol acetate, resulting in rats with reduced cortical volume and cognitive/behavioral deficits reminiscent of schizophrenia (Johnston et al. 1979; Lodge and Grace 2009). By timing the treatment with methylazoxymethanol acetate to late in gestation in rats, it is possible to cause mild, selective loss of GABAergic interneurons analogous to the pathology of schizophrenia. Because late gestational influenza infection is an established risk factor for schizophrenia (Brown and Patterson 2011), Patterson (2009) has shown that late gestational exposure of mice to influenza results in a histopathological and behavioral phenocopy of schizophrenia. Notably, the neurodevelopmental damage to the cortex caused by maternal viral infection does not result from the virus infecting the fetal brain but rather by the mounting of an inflammatory cellular response in the infected mother. This finding is intriguing because genes located in the major histocompatability complex are risk genes for schizophrenia as well as multiple sclerosis (Stefansson *et al.* 2009). Nevertheless, the behavioral correlates in rodent models for schizophrenia are relatively nonspecific and could apply equally to other severe forms of developmental disorders. Thus, impairments in prepulse inhibition (Powell *et al.* 2009), hyperactivity, impairments in spatial memory, and social deficits are also observed in intellectual disability and in autism spectrum disorder, not just schizophrenia.

The fact that risk genes for schizophrenia are salient for brain development or that fetal brain insults mimic the cortical and behavioral pathology of schizophrenia has led to a certain degree of pessimism that these deficits could be ameliorated in the mature brain. However, recent research using mutant mouse models has provided encouraging results to counter this pessimism (Ehninger *et al.* 2008). For example, Rett syndrome is a disorder that affects primarily young women and shares clinical features with autism but is associated with progressive cortical atrophy, scoliosis, breathing abnormalities, and early death (Chahrour and Zoghbi 2007). The disorder results from loss of function mutations, often spontaneous, of methyl CpG binding protein 2 (MeCP2), which is located on the X chromosome. MeCP2 binds to methylated DNA and represses gene expression. Inactivation of the murine MeCP2 results in a mouse with a phenotype that closely matches that of human Rett syndrome, including cortical atrophy, scoliosis, breathing abnormalities, and death by about 15 weeks postpartum in males. Cobb *et al.* (2010) created a mouse in which MeCP2 was "knocked out" but had another MeCP2 gene construct "knocked in" so that it could be conditionally expressed when the mouse was treated with tamoxifen. Despite the severe phenotype of the MeCP2 knockout, it was dramatically reversed within days of imminent death when the expression of MeCP2 was restored. This example and others suggest that with the proper intervention the cellular pathology of psychiatric disorders with prominent developmental features might be reversed well after birth.

Anxiety disorders

Animal models of disorders like schizophrenia that are manifest primarily by cognitive symptoms such as disorganized thinking and hallucinations are based on rather tenuous behavioral inferences such as hyperactivity and stereotypic behavior and are equivalent to psychosis because it is reduced by antipsychotic drugs (Magnusson *et al.* 1988). More compelling behavioral models have been developed for the anxiety disorders. As reviewed in Chapter 2, the neural circuitry and the synaptic mechanisms of conditioned fear have been worked out in great detail in the rodent (for other reviews, LeDoux 2003; Myers and Davis 2007). Conditioned fear is produced in experimental animals, for example, by repeatedly coupling an electric shock with a warning tone. Subsequent presentation of the tone alone causes freezing in the rodent. Severity of the anxiety is inferred by the duration of freezing. Repeated presentation of the tone without an electric shock results in gradual "extinction" of freezing. Extinction in this paradigm is not a passive process like "forgetting" but requires the activation of NMDA receptors in the amygdala. Administration of drugs that block NMDA receptors prevents extinction whereas administration of drugs that enhance NMDA receptor function at the GMS such as D-cycloserine accelerates extinction by facilitating memory consolidation (Davis *et al.* 2006).

The extension of this behavioral model to human anxiety disorders has face validity. Conditioned fear has been demonstrated in human subjects (Schiller *et al.* 2008), and extinction of specific phobias such as acrophobia by exposure therapy is an effective form of behavioral therapy (Choy *et al.* 2007). That circuitry similar to that delineated in the rodent is relevant to human anxiety disorders is supported by the results of functional imaging studies demonstrating robust activation of the amygdala when phobic subjects are exposed to the feared object (Caseras *et al.* 2010). Ressler *et al.* (2004) demonstrated the therapeutic implications of the model by showing that co-administration of D-cycloserine with behavioral therapy to subjects with acrophobia resulted in a significant increase in their tolerance to heights that persisted long after the intervention compared with those who received placebo and behavioral therapy. The potential value of using drugs that enhance NMDA receptor function including D-cycloserine, D-serine, and glycine transport inhibitors in other disorders, in which enhanced neuroplasticity would likely contribute to therapeutic effects such as the treatment of addictions, is currently being explored (Myers *et al.* 2011).

Mood disorders

For 40 years, studies to understand the mechanism of therapeutic action of the antidepressants stopped at the surface of the neuronal membrane, focusing on the biogenic amine transporters and their post-synaptic biogenic amine receptors (Charney 1998). However, as reviewed in Chapter 3 by Quiroz *et al.*, the last decade has witnessed an explosion of new information about the downstream events activated by the biogenic amine G-protein-coupled receptors as a consequence of reduced uptake/inactivation of their neurotransmitter. An important target of this cascade is the cAMP response element binding protein (CREB) that induces the expression of functionally related genes, the effects of which are neurotrophic, including brain-derived neurotrophic factor (BDNF). Although it has long been known that schizophrenia is associated with loss of cortical volume and increased size of the lateral ventricles, the pathology of the mood disorders was thought to be primarily functional. However, with careful scrutiny with neuroimaging studies, it became apparent that reductions in the amygdala, orbital-frontal cortex, and hippocampal volumes occurred in major depressive disorder (Lorenzetti *et al.* 2009). In the case of bipolar disorder, volumetric studies have disclosed additional reductions in prefrontal cortex, medial temporal cortex, and the limbic structures (Kempton *et al.* 2011). Microscopic examination of the cingulate cortex has revealed significant reductions in glia but no change in neuronal number in mood disorders in contrast to schizophrenia, where the glia appear to be unaffected and the neurons are atrophic (Rajkowska and Miguel-Hidalgo 2007).

Behavioral models most predictive of antidepressant activity have long been based on recurrent stress paradigms, which cause behaviors analogous to depression such as "despair" in the Porsolt swim test and anhedonia (Porsolt *et al.* 1977; Rygula *et al.* 2005). Chronic recurrent stress also replicates the macro- and microscopic brain structural changes found in depression, including the reduced hippocampal volume, atrophy of the apical dendrites of the pyramidal neurons in the prefrontal cortex, and reduced number of glial fibrillary acidic protein-positive astrocytes (Banasr *et al.* 2010; Goldwater *et al.* 2009). The dentate gyrus of the hippocampus is one of the few brain regions where neurogenesis persists throughout life. Chronic stress also inhibits hippocampal neurogenesis (for review, Samuels and Hen 2011). An abundance of evidence demonstrates that all of the effective antidepressant treatments including electroconvulsive therapy reverse the behavioral, neurochemical, and cellular pathology resulting from the recurrent stress. However, recovery requires the restoration of neurogenesis in the dentate gyrus of the hippocampus. The key mediator of this treatment response is BDNF (Schmidt and Duman 2007). Its levels and that of its receptor, tyrosine kinase B, are reduced in postmortem studies in the hippocampus of suicide victims and in the hippocampus of the stress models of depression (Pandey *et al.* 2008). Antidepressant treatment induces increased expression of BDNF through the cAMP-PKA-CREB pathway. Notably, BDNF expression is downregulated by the proinflammatory IL–1β-NFkB pathway (Barrientos *et al.* 2003). Thus, it has become apparent that the underlying neural pathology observed in affective disorders with region-selective atrophy and loss of glia is entirely consistent with the final common pathways of action of the mood stabilizers and antidepressants in terms of the expression of trophic factors that stimulate neurogenesis and restore neuronal vitality.

In Chapter 3, the recent clinical evidence that blockade of NMDA receptors with ketamine produces a rapid, robust, and persistent reduction in the symptoms of major depressive disorder (MDD) is also reviewed. This therapeutic effect of ketamine, especially in cases of major depression unresponsive to traditional antidepressant treatment (approximately 50% of MDD patients are unresponsive), suggests the existence of a pathophysiology for depression unrelated to the classical biogenic amine hypothesis (Diazgranados *et al.* 2010; Zarate *et al.* 2006). Li *et al.* (2010) have developed the evidence that the acute NMDA receptor blockade activates the mammalian target of rapamycin pathway via rebound AMPA receptor activation, thereby promoting synaptogenesis in the prefrontal cortex, the region affected by dendritic atrophy in stress models of major depression.

What are the neurochemical processes that might bridge the gap between NMDA receptors and depression? Meta-analyses of studies on community and clinical samples of MDD have revealed that plasma levels of inflammatory markers including IL-6, IL-1, TNF-α, and C-reactive protein are significantly elevated in MDD (Dowlati *et al.* 2010; Howren *et al.*

2009). The proinflammatory cytokines induce indole amine 2,3-dioxygenase, which catabolizes tryptophan into the kynurenine pathway (Dantzer *et al.* 2011). Elevated levels of indole amine 2,3-dioxygenase reduce the level of plasma tryptophan, which ultimately attenuates the synthesis of serotonin in the brain because tryptophan hydroxylase is not saturated by tryptophan. Perhaps of greater significance are the downstream metabolites of tryptophan, kynurenine and quinolinic acid. Kynurenine has anxiogenic effects whereas quinolinic acid, an NMDA receptor agonist, is prodepressive and at high concentrations has excitotoxic effects.

Research on the neurobiology of bipolar disorder has been both blessed and cursed by the existence of two drugs that were found serendipitously to be effective in preventing recurrence of the mood disturbances. These two drugs – lithium and valproic acid – could not be more different, the one being a cation and the other an organic acid. Such chemical diversity gives power for identifying final common pathways of therapeutic effects (Coyle and Duman 2003). Identification of such a pathway could also shed light on the underlying pathophysiology of bipolar disorder. The curse is that both drugs exert their therapeutic effects at very high concentrations, not characteristic of the more typical ligand–receptor interaction of drugs. As Quiroz *et al.* illustrate in Chapter 3, understanding their sites of action has been greatly facilitated by the explosion of knowledge about intracellular signaling pathways that ultimately regulate gene expression. Considerable evidence now supports the notion that Li+ likely exerts its effects through inhibition of GSK-3β whereas valproic acid inhibits histone deacetylase. Through convergent intracellular signaling pathways, the mood stabilizers have effects on diverse cellular processes including energy metabolism, neuroplasticity, neurogenesis, and neuronal resilience. Importantly, these pathways interact with potential risk genes for bipolar disorder such as *CLOCK* (Roybal *et al.* 2007) and provide alternative targets for intervention such as inhibition of PKC with tamoxifen (Zarate and Manji 2009).

Substance abuse

The area of substance abuse research as reviewed in Chapter 5 has probably made the most substantial advances over the last decade of any major area of clinical neuroscience. Historically, substance abuse has been shrouded in stigma and considered to be the result of moral weakness. But, substance abuse research has had one important advantage for understanding its pathophysiology over other psychiatric disorders – the substances themselves. This fact permitted investigators not only to probe the behavioral mechanisms of substance abuse but more fundamentally to identify the neural circuitry responsible for drug taking, drug seeking, dependence, and withdrawal. It became evident that drug abuse, regardless of the type of drug (opiates, nicotine, stimulants, and ethanol), engaged a common circuit for reward.

It is not surprising, given the long-lasting effects of drug addiction on behavior, that it would be associated not only with functional but also structural changes in the brain associated with sensitization. Studies in experimental animals in models of chronic administration reveal robust structural changes but differences in direction depending on the type of drug (Russo *et al.* 2010). Chronic administration of cocaine is associated with increases in spine density and dendritic complexity in medium spiny neurons in the nucleus accumbens, in pyramidal neurons in the prefrontal cortex, and in dopamine neurons in the ventral tegmental area. In contrast, chronic administration of opiates is associated with decreases in spine density and dendritic complexity of medium spiny neurons in the nucleus accumbens and of prefrontal pyramidal neurons and shrinkage of dopamine neurons in the ventral tegmental area. However, it remains unresolved whether these structural changes mediate sensitization or are simply epiphenomena.

Understanding how drugs of abuse work in the brain does not necessarily tell us how to help addicts to resist resuming substance abuse after a period of abstinence, the core problem in treating addicts. Relapse in substance abuse can occur weeks, months, or years after the addict has been abstinent. In examining the natural history of relapse, it became apparent that stress and/or exposure to the social/physical context of their substance abuse could produce an overwhelming desire to obtain the drug despite the well-known adverse risk (Koob and Volkow 2010). This flooding desire for the drug is known as "craving." Functional brain imaging studies have demonstrated that craving results in activation of the ventral striatum just as if the subject had actually taken the drug. Through clever behavioral paradigms such as place preference and self-administration, investigators have been able to tease out the neurocircuitry of craving in experimental animals (Aguilar *et al.* 2009; Bossert *et al.* 2011).

The endorphins appear to be important in the reinforcing effects of abused substances aside from opiates including stimulants, nicotine, and alcohol. Indeed, administration of the opiate receptor antagonist, naltrexone, in clinical trials significantly reduced relapse in abstinent cigarette smokers and alcohol abusers. Although the success rate was low, the protective effect was significant. As stated in Chapter 5, the μ-opiate receptor, which naltrexone blocks, has a common allelic variant at amino acid 40 (Asn40Asp). Individuals with at least one copy of the Asp40 allele are much more responsive to naltrexone treatment than are those homozygous for Asn40, who are unresponsive to naltrexone treatment (Anton *et al.* 2008). This differential response may reflect the fact that those harboring the Asp40 allele release more endogenous opioids in response to ethanol consumption than do those homozygous for Asn40. This enhanced endogenous opioid response to alcohol may put such individuals at greater risk for alcoholism and plausibly distinguishes two types of alcoholism. This pharmacogenetic finding provides the first taste of "individualized medicine" in psychiatry whereby diagnostic and treatment decisions will be informed by the patient's genotype.

Neuroplasticity

Until the turn of the century, psychiatric disorders were largely considered "functional," with little evidence of structural changes in the nervous system with the possible exception of schizophrenia. Biogenic amine neurotransmitters were the major focus of translational research, given their role in mediating the therapeutic effects of antipsychotic and antidepressant medications. In contrast, translational research in psychiatry over the last decade has repeatedly encountered a mechanism, neural plasticity, which appears to be a core pathological feature of serious mental disorders and a pathway for therapeutic intervention. The aphorism, "insanity is doing the same thing over and over and expecting a different outcome," aptly characterizes the synaptic pathology of serious mental disorders including schizophrenia (Balu and Coyle 2011; Lewis 2009), mood disorders (Duman 2002), anxiety disorders (Davis *et al.* 2006), and substance abuse (Russo *et al.* 2010), where maladaptive responses such as delusions, phobias, and addictions persist despite overwhelming evidence of their futility.

In the case of schizophrenia, reduced dendritic complexity, spine density, and NMDA receptor hypofunction point to maladaptive developmental and neural plastic processes. In depression, atrophic dendrites, arrested neurogenesis, and reduced levels of BDNF are counteracted by antidepressant and mood-stabilizing drug effects through the activation of neurotrophic gene expression by CREB. Anxiety states can be learned, and they are associated with heightened reactivity of the amygdala to the feared objects or situations. Conversely, extinction of the pathological response results from changes in synaptic efficacy mediated by the NMDA receptor. Finally, addiction is a consequence of repeated exposure to the abused substance causing functional and structural changes in the synaptic connections in components of the reward circuit. The challenge for future research will be how to target treatments to modify the synaptic pathology unique to each group of disorders.

Future directions

The future of translational research in psychiatry faces several challenges and opportunities. There is no question that genetics and molecular strategies will dominate the stage for the foreseeable future. The following sections represent recent advances that will likely play a major role in translational research in psychiatry.

Elimination of current diagnostic schemata

As Hyman recently pointed out (Hyman 2010), refinements of the currently used diagnostic schemata, the *Diagnostic and Statistical Manual of Mental Disorders* (DSM–V) and the *International Classification of Diseases* (ICD–10), have focused largely on developing operationalized diagnostic criteria with high inter-rater reliability. Unfortunately, the focus on reliability occurred when the understanding of mental disorders was rudimentary. However, advances in psychiatric genetics, brain imaging, and neuroscience are eroding our confidence in the validity of these diagnostic distinctions. For example, as previously noted, the same CNV may be associated with an increased risk for autism and schizophrenia (Sebat *et al.* 2009), and other risk genes are shared between schizophrenia and bipolar disorder (O'Dushlaine *et al.* 2011). In this regard, the National Institutes of Health has a new initiative, the Research Domain Criteria Project, which will develop new ways of classifying disorders "based on dimensions of observable behavior and neurobiologic measures" (Cuthbert and Insel 2010). The project is inherently translational because the constructs, which may bear little relationship to existing diagnoses, will range across levels of analysis including genes, molecules, cells, circuits, and behavior. Thus, the diagnostic landscape in psychiatric research will likely change radically over the next decade.

Genome-wide association studies

Association studies using plausible candidate genes have foundered on the shoals of irreproducible results because of underpowered studies that are vulnerable to both false positive and false negative statistical results. To avoid the inherent biases of choosing to study "the usual suspects" as the risk genes in association studies, the field has moved to genome-wide association studies (GWAS), in which hundreds of thousands of single nucleotide polymorphisms on a DNA array permit the agnostic survey of the entire genome for potential gene associations (Allen *et al.* 2008). The hundreds of thousands of comparisons inherent in this strategy require very large numbers of affected subjects and suitable controls (10^4 to greater than 10^5) to achieve the requisite degree of statistical significance. An unfortunate consequence of this more rigorous approach was that many of the results identifying putative risk genes in prior underpowered association studies were not replicated in GWAS.

The statistical challenge for identifying unequivocal risk genes can only be resolved by cooperation among research groups to achieve the requisite number of subjects in individual studies or by meta-analysis of comparably executed studies. Examples of this approach are the recent reports of the analysis of combined GWAS in Alzheimer's disease in which over 40 000 subjects were involved (Hollingworth *et al.* 2011; Naj *et al.* 2011). The studies by Naj *et al.* (2011) on late-onset Alzheimer's disease confirmed the five previously identified risk genes and identified five additional risk genes. The new risk genes do not link closely to the amyloid hypothesis but rather are involved in immune system function, cholesterol metabolism, and synaptic dysfunction (Morgan 2011). These surprising new pathological pathways demonstrate the power of the agnostic approach taken with GWAS that avoids the exclusive focus on a single pathological process such as amyloidosis. However, identification of a risk gene is only the first step because sequencing is required to determine the particular allelic variant conferring risk, and expression studies must be performed to determine how the variant affects the expression or function of the gene product.

Copy number variants

An unanticipated by-product of the GWAS in autism and schizophrenia was the discovery of an elevated prevalence of copy number variants (CNVs) in their genomes compared with those of controls (Sebat *et al.* 2007; Levinson *et al.* 2011). CNVs refer to microdeletions, inversions, and reduplications in the genome. The CNVs are rare, often highly penetrant, and occasionally involve de novo mutations. Notably, some "hotspots" for CNVs have been found to be shared between autism spectrum disorder and schizophrenia (Sebat *et al.* 2009). Thus, diagnostic distinctions revered for decades are now breaking down, with the evidence of the same risk genes occurring in more than one disorder. Furthermore, the low prevalence of CNVs in bipolar disorder may distinguish it from schizophrenia (Grozeva *et al.* 2010). Transgenic studies will be required to determine how individual genes in a CNV contribute to the phenotype.

MicroRNAs

MicroRNAs (miRNAs) are single-stranded RNAs of approximately 22 nucleotides in length whose genes are located in noncoding regions of the genome. MicroRNAs are generated in a multistep process (Coyle 2009). The primary transcript (pre-miRNA) is processed within the nucleus to yield a ~70 nucleotide hairpin, from which the mature miRNA is generated in the cytoplasm by cleavage by the nuclease Dicer. After incorporation into the RNA-induced silencing complex, the miRNA binds to the complementary sequences in the 3'-untranslated region of the target mRNA. The complex activates endonuclease, which degrades the mRNA or directly blocks translation, both of which prevent the expression of the protein. Individual miRNAs can affect the expression of dozens of functionally related proteins. Several hundred miRNAs have been identified, half of which are expressed predominantly or exclusively in the brain. Given the recency of their discovery in mammalian brain, our understanding of their role in psychiatric disorders is rudimentary, although their roles in schizophrenia and bipolar disorder have been suggested (Kim *et al.* 2010).

Epigenetics

Epigenetics refers to changes in gene expression caused by mechanisms other than changes in the underlying DNA sequence. It includes any structural adaptation in chromosomal regions that mediate altered rates of gene transcription. Chromatin remodeling is a process whereby the activity of a particular gene is controlled by the structure of chromatin in proximity to the gene. Chromatin remodeling involves multiple covalent modifications of histones such as acetylation, phosphorylation, and methylation. Epigenetic regulation is crucial for nervous system development. It is responsible for imprinting, a transgenerational process that affects the phenotypic characteristics of the disorder based on whether the responsible gene is transmitted from the father or the mother, as is the case in any Angelman syndrome (Nicholls and Knepper 2001). Epigenetic regulation occurs in the mature nervous system and appears to account for stable changes in gene expression under normal circumstances as well as pathological states such as substance abuse. However, behavioral epigenetics is in its infancy, with fewer than 100 publications on the topic by 2011. Despite this limited database, findings accumulated thus far in substance abuse, adverse childhood experiences, and fetal drug exposure indicate that research in this area will have a tremendous impact on translational psychiatry.

Human induced pluripotent stem cells (hiPSCs)

Human induced pluripotent stem cells (hiPCSs) are a type of pluripotent stem cell generated from an adult somatic cell such as a fibroblast by inducing the expression of certain stem cell genes and proteins. hiPSCs were first produced in 2007. The advantage of hiPSCs is that they can be obtained from patients with a neuropsychiatric disorder, propagated, and differentiated into nervous tissue in vitro so that the pathophysiology of the disorder can be characterized (Vaccarino *et al.* 2011). With this method, the broad array of techniques for studying nervous tissue from experimental animals but ethically impossible for studying the living human brain can now be applied to living human brain tissue. Brennand *et al.* (2011) directly reprogrammed fibroblasts from schizophrenic patients into hiPSCs and subsequently differentiated these disorder-specific hiPSCs into neurons. hiPSC-derived neurons showed diminished neuronal connectivity in conjunction with decreased neurite number, PSD95-protein levels, and glutamate receptor expression compared with controls, which was consistent with alterations reported for schizophrenia.

Conclusions

It has been nearly 40 years since a mechanistically novel drug has been introduced for the treatment of a serious mental disorder. Like Moses wandering in the desert, neuropsychopharmacologists have been anticipating all this time the discovery of novel therapeutics based on increasingly sophisticated models of psychiatric disorders informed by brain imaging, postmortem studies, assorted biomarkers, and genetics. It is sobering to note that the autosomal dominant mutant gene responsible for Huntington's disease was identified nearly 20 years ago and was soon introduced in mice where it reproduced the pathology (Huntington's Disease Collaborative Research Group 1993; Mangiarini *et al.* 1996). Yet, plausible treatments for Huntington's disease remain on the distant horizon. Translational research in psychiatry faces much more complex challenges. Perhaps, like the serendipity of the founding years of clinical psychopharmacology, good luck and the informed mind may serve as the catalyst for future substantive advances in translational research in psychiatry.

References

Aguilar MA, Rodríguez-Arias M, Miñarro J. 2009. Neurobiological mechanisms of the reinstatement of drug-conditioned place preference. *Brain Res Rev* **59**:253–277.

Allen NC, Bagade S, McQueen MB *et al.* 2008. Systematic meta-analyses and field synopsis of genetic association studies in schizophrenia: the SzGene database. *Nat Genet* **40**:827–834.

Anton RF, Oroszi G, O'Malley S *et al.* 2008. An evaluation of mu-opioid receptor (OPRM1) as a predictor of naltrexone response in the treatment of alcohol dependence: results from the Combined Pharmacotherapies and Behavioral Interventions for Alcohol Dependence (COMBINE) study. *Arch Gen Psychiatry* **65**:135–144.

Balu DT, Coyle JT. 2011. Neuroplasticity signaling pathways linked to the pathophysiology of schizophrenia. *Neurosci Biobehav Rev* **35**:848–870.

Banasr M, Chowdhury GM, Terwilliger R et al. 2010. Glial pathology in an animal model of depression: reversal of stress-induced cellular, metabolic and behavioral deficits by the glutamate-modulating drug riluzole. *Mol Psychiatry* **15**:501–511.

Barrientos RM, Sprunger DB, Campeau S et al. 2003. Brain-derived neurotrophic factor mRNA downregulation produced by social isolation is blocked by intrahippocampal interleukin-1 receptor antagonist. *Neuroscience* **121**:847–853.

Bossert JM, Stern AL, Theberge FR et al. 2011. Ventral medial prefrontal cortex neuronal ensembles mediate context-induced relapse to heroin. *Nat Neurosci* **14**:420–422.

Brennand KJ, Simone A, Jou J et al. 2011. Modelling schizophrenia using human induced pluripotent stem cells. *Nature* **473**:221–225.

Brown AS, Patterson PH. 2011. Maternal infection and schizophrenia: implications for prevention. *Schizophr Bull* **37**:284–290.

Caseras X, Mataix-Cols D, Trasovares MV et al. 2010. Dynamics of brain responses to phobic-related stimulation in specific phobia subtypes. *Eur J Neurosci* **32**:1414–1422.

Chahrour M, Zoghbi HY. 2007. The story of Rett syndrome: from clinic to neurobiology. *Neuron* **56**:422–437.

Charney DS. 1998. Monoamine dysfunction and the pathophysiology and treatment of depression. *J Clin Psychiatry* **59** (Suppl. 14):11–14.

Choy Y, Fyer AJ, Lipsitz JD. 2007. Treatment of specific phobia in adults. *Clin Psychol Rev* **27**:266–286.

Cobb S, Guy J, Bird A. 2010. Reversibility of functional deficits in experimental models of Rett syndrome. *Biochem Soc Trans* **38**:498–506.

Coyle JT. 2009. MicroRNAs suggest a new mechanism for altered brain gene expression in schizophrenia. *Proc Natl Acad Sci USA* **106**:2975–2976.

Coyle JT, Balu D, Benneyworth M, Basu A, Roseman A. 2010. Beyond the dopamine receptor: novel therapeutic targets for treating schizophrenia. *Dialogues Clin Neurosci* **12**:359–382.

Coyle JT, Duman RS. 2003. Finding the intracellular signaling pathways affected by mood disorder treatments. *Neuron* **38**:157–160.

Creese I, Burt DR, Snyder SH. 1976. Dopamine receptor binding predicts clinical and pharmacological potencies of antischizophrenic drugs. *Science* **192**:481–483.

Cuthbert B, Insel T. 2010. The data of diagnosis: new approaches to psychiatric classification. *Psychiatry* **73**:311–314.

Dantzer R, O'Connor JC, Lawson MA, Kelley KW. 2011. Inflammation-associated depression: from serotonin to kynurenine. *Psychoneuroendocrinology* **36**:426–436.

Davis M, Ressler K, Rothbaum BO, Richardson R. 2006. Effects of D-cycloserine on extinction: translation from preclinical to clinical work. *Biol Psychiatry* **60**:369–375.

DeVito LM, Balu DT, Kanter BR et al. 2011. Serine racemase deletion disrupts memory for order and alters cortical dendritic morphology. *Genes Brain Behav* **10**:210–222.

Diazgranados N, Ibrahim L, Brutsche NE et al. 2010. A randomized add-on trial of an N-methyl-D-aspartate antagonist in treatment-resistant bipolar depression. *Arch Gen Psychiatry* **67**:793–802.

Dowlati Y, Herrmann N, Swardfager W et al. 2010. A meta-analysis of cytokines in major depression. *Biol Psychiatry* **67**:446–457.

Duman RS. 2002. Synaptic plasticity and mood disorders. *Mol Psychiatry* **7**(Suppl. 1):S29–S34.

Ehninger D, Li W, Fox K, Stryker MP, Silva AJ. 2008. Reversing neurodevelopmental disorders in adults. *Neuron* **60**:950–960.

Glantz LA, Lewis DA. 2000. Decreased dendritic spine density on prefrontal cortical pyramidal neurons in schizophrenia. *Arch Gen Psychiatry* **57**:65–73.

Goff DC, Coyle JT. 2001. The emerging role of glutamate in the pathophysiology and treatment of schizophrenia. *Am J Psychiatry* **158**:1367–1377.

Goldwater DS, Pavlides C, Hunter RG et al. 2009. Structural and functional alterations to rat medial prefrontal cortex following chronic restraint stress and recovery. *Neuroscience* **164**:798–808.

Gonzalez-Burgos G, Hashimoto T, Lewis DA. 2010. Alterations of cortical GABA neurons and network oscillations in schizophrenia. *Curr Psychiatry Rep* **12**:335–344.

Grozeva D, Kirov G, Ivanov D et al. 2010. Rare copy number variants: a point of rarity in genetic risk for bipolar disorder and schizophrenia. *Arch Gen Psychiatry* **67**:318–327.

Ho BC, Andreasen NC, Nopoulos P et al. 2003. Progressive structural brain abnormalities and their relationship to clinical outcome: a longitudinal magnetic resonance imaging study early in schizophrenia. *Arch Gen Psychiatry* **60**:585–594.

Hollingworth P, Harold D, Sims R *et al.* 2011. Common variants at ABCA7, MS4A6A/MS4A4E, EPHA1, CD33 and CD2AP are associated with Alzheimer's disease. *Nat Genet* **43**:429–435.

Howren MB, Lamkin DM, Suls J. 2009. Associations of depression with C-reactive protein, IL-1, and IL-6: a meta-analysis. *Psychosom Med* **71**:171–186.

Huntington's Disease Collaborative Research Group. 1993. A novel gene containing a trinucleotide repeat that is expanded and unstable on Huntington's disease chromosomes. *Cell* **72**:971–983.

Hyman SE. 2010. The diagnosis of mental disorders: the problem of reification. *Annu Rev Clin Psychol* **6**:155–179.

Johnston MV, Grzanna R, Coyle JT. 1979. Methylazoxymethanol treatment of fetal rats results in abnormally dense noradrenergic innervation of neocortex. *Science* **203**:369–371.

Jones PB, Barnes TR, Davies L *et al.* 2006. Randomized controlled trial of the effect on quality of life of second- vs first-generation antipsychotic drugs in schizophrenia: Cost Utility of the Latest Antipsychotic Drugs in Schizophrenia Study (CUtLASS 1). *Arch Gen Psychiatry* **63**:1079–1087.

Kempton MJ, Salvador Z, Munafò MR *et al.* 2011. Structural neuroimaging studies in major depressive disorder: meta-analysis and comparison with bipolar disorder. *Arch Gen Psychiatry* **68**:675–690.

Kim AH, Reimers M, Maher B *et al.* 2010. MicroRNA expression profiling in the prefrontal cortex of individuals affected with schizophrenia and bipolar disorders. *Schizophr Res* **124**:183–191.

Koob GF, Volkow ND. 2010. Neurocircuitry of addiction. *Neuropsychopharmacology* **35**:217–238.

Krivosheya D, Tapia L, Levinson JN *et al.* 2008. ErbB4-neuregulin signaling modulates synapse development and dendritic arborization through distinct mechanisms. *J Biol Chem* **283**:32944–32956.

Lapin IP, Oxenkrug GF. 1969. Intensification of the central serotoninergic processes as a possible determinant of the thymoleptic effect. *Lancet* **1**:132–136.

LeDoux J. 2003. The emotional brain, fear and the amygdale. *Cell Mol Neurobiol* **23**:727–738.

Lee FH, Fadel MP, Preston-Maher K *et al.* 2011. Disc1 point mutations in mice affect development of the cerebral cortex. *J Neurosci* **31**:3197–3206.

Leucht S, Busch R, Kissling W, Kane JM. 2007. Early prediction of antipsychotic nonresponse among patients with schizophrenia. *J Clin Psychiatry* **68**:352–360.

Levinson DF, Duan J, Oh S *et al.* 2011. Copy number variants in schizophrenia: confirmation of five previous findings and new evidence for 3q29 microdeletions and VIPR2 duplications. *Am J Psychiatry* **168**:302–316.

Lewis DA. 2009. Neuroplasticity of excitatory and inhibitory cortical circuits in schizophrenia. *Dialogues Clin Neurosci* **11**:269–280.

Li N, Lee B, Liu RJ *et al.* 2010. mTOR-dependent synapse formation underlies the rapid antidepressant effects of NMDA antagonists. *Science* **329**:959–964.

Lieberman JA, Stroup TS, McEvoy JP. 2005. Effectiveness of antipsychotic drugs in patients with chronic schizophrenia. *N Engl J Med* **353**:1209–1223.

Lisman JE, Coyle JT, Green RW *et al.* 2008. Circuit-based framework for understanding neurotransmitter and risk gene interactions in schizophrenia. *Trends Neurosci* **31**:234–242.

Lodge DJ, Grace AA. 2009. Gestational methylazoxymethanol acetate administration: a developmental disruption model of schizophrenia. *Behav Brain Res* **204**:306–312.

Lorenzetti V, Allen NB, Fornito A *et al.* 2009. Structural brain abnormalities in major depressive disorder: a selective review of recent MRI studies. *J Affect Disord* **117**:1–17.

Magnusson O, Fowler CJ, Mohringe B, Wijkström A, Ogren SO. 1988. Comparison of the effects of haloperidol, remoxipride and raclopride on "pre"- and postsynaptic dopamine receptors in the rat brain. *Naunyn Schmiedebergs Arch Pharmacol* **337**:379–384.

Mangiarini L, Sathasivam K, Seller M *et al.* 1996. Exon 1 of the HD gene with an expanded CAG repeat is sufficient to cause a progressive neurological phenotype in transgenic mice. *Cell* **87**:493–506.

McKinney RA. 2010. Excitatory amino acid involvement in dendritic spine formation, maintenance and remodelling. *J Physiol* **588** (Pt 1):107–116.

Morgan K. 2011. Commentary: Three new pathways leading to Alzheimer's disease. *Neuropath Appl Neurobiol* **37**:353–357.

Myers KM, Carlezon WA Jr, Davis M. 2011. Glutamate receptors in extinction and extinction-based therapies for psychiatric illness. *Neuropsychopharmacology* **36**:274–293.

Myers KM, Davis M. 2007. Mechanisms of fear extinction. *Mol Psychiatry* **12**:120–150.

Naj AC, Jun G, Beecham GW *et al.* 2011. Common variants at MS4A4/MS4A6E, CD2AP, CD33 and EPHA1 are associated with late-onset Alzheimer's disease. *Nat Genet* **43**:436–441.

Nestler EJ, Hyman SE. 2010. Animal models of neuropsychiatric disorders. *Nat Neurosci* **13**: 1161–1169.

Nicholls RD, Knepper JL. 2001. Genome organization, function, and imprinting in Prader-Willi and Angelman syndromes. *Annu Rev Genomics Hum Genet* **2**:153–175.

O'Dushlaine C, Kenny E, Heron E *et al.* 2011. Molecular pathways involved in neuronal cell adhesion and membrane scaffolding contribute to schizophrenia and bipolar disorder susceptibility. *Mol Psychiatry* **16**:286–292.

Pandey GN, Ren X, Rizavi HS *et al.* 2008. Brain-derived neurotrophic factor and tyrosine kinase B receptor signalling in post-mortem brain of teenage suicide victims. *Int J Neuropsychopharmacol* **11**:1047–1061.

Patterson PH. 2009. Immune involvement in schizophrenia and autism: etiology, pathology and animal models. *Behav Brain Res* **204**:313–321.

Penzes P, Cahill ME, Jones KA, VanLeeuwen JE, Woolfrey KM. 2011. Dendritic spine pathology in neuropsychiatric disorders. *Nat Neurosci* **14**:285–293.

Porsolt RD, Bertin A, Jalfre M. 1977. Behavioral despair in mice: a primary screening test for antidepressants. *Arch Int Pharmacodyn Ther* **229**:327–336.

Powell SB, Zhou X, Geyer MA. 2009. Prepulse inhibition and genetic mouse models of schizophrenia. *Behav Brain Res* **204**:282–294.

Rajkowska G, Miguel-Hidalgo JJ. 2007. Gliogenesis and glial pathology in depression. *CNS Neurol Disord Drug Targets* **6**:219–233.

Ressler KJ, Rothbaum BO, Tannenbaum L *et al.* 2004. Cognitive enhancers as adjuncts to psychotherapy: use of D-cycloserine in phobic individuals to facilitate extinction of fear. *Arch Gen Psychiatry* **61**:1136–1144.

Rotrosen J, Wallach MB, Angrist B, Gershon S. 1972. Antagonism of apomorphine-induced stereotypy and emesis in dogs by thioridazine, haloperidol, and pimozide. *Psychopharmacologia* **26**:185–194.

Roybal K, Theobold D, Graham A *et al.* 2007. Mania-like behavior induced by disruption of CLOCK. *Proc Natl Acad Sci USA* **104**:6406–6411.

Russo SJ, Dietz DM, Dumitriu D *et al.* 2010. The addicted synapse: mechanisms of synaptic and structural plasticity in nucleus accumbens. *Trends Neurosci* **33**:267–276.

Rygula R, Abumaria N, Flügge G *et al.* 2005. Anhedonia and motivational deficits in rats: impact of chronic social stress. *Behav Brain Res* **162**:127–134.

Samuels BA, Hen R. 2011. Neurogenesis and affective disorders. *Eur J Neurosci* **33**:1152–1159.

Schiller D, Cain CK, Curley NG *et al.* 2008. Evidence for recovery of fear following immediate extinction in rats and humans. *Learn Mem* **15**:394–402.

Schmidt HD, Duman RS. 2007. The role of neurotrophic factors in adult hippocampal neurogenesis, antidepressant treatments and animal models of depressive-like behavior. *Behav Pharmacol* **18**:391–418.

Sebat J, Lakshmi B, Malhotra D *et al.* 2007. Strong association of de novo copy number mutations with autism. *Science* **316**:445–449.

Sebat J, Levy DL, McCarthy SE. 2009. Rare structural variants in schizophrenia: one disorder, multiple mutations; one mutation, multiple disorders. *Trends Genet* **25**:528–535.

Stefansson H, Ophoff RA, Steinberg S *et al.* 2009. Common variants conferring risk of schizophrenia. *Nature* **460**:744–747.

Thase ME. 2009. Pharmacotherapeutic treatment strategies for antidepressant nonresponse. *J Clin Psychiatry* **70**:e42.

Tiwari AK, Zai CC, Müller DJ, Kennedy JL. 2010. Genetics in schizophrenia: where are we and what next? *Dialogues Clin Neurosci* **12**:289–303.

Toro R, Konyukh M, Delorme R *et al.* 2010. Key role for gene dosage and synaptic homeostasis in autism spectrum disorders. *Trends Genet* **26**:363–372.

Tsai GE, Lin PY. 2010. Strategies to enhance N-methyl-D-aspartate receptor-mediated neurotransmission in schizophrenia, a critical review and meta-analysis. *Curr Pharm Des* **16**:522–537.

Trivedi MH, Fava M, Wisniewski SR *et al.* 2006. Medication augmentation after the failure of SSRIs for depression. *N Engl J Med* **354**:1243–1252.

Vaccarino FM, Stevens HE, Kocabas A *et al.* 2011. Induced pluripotent stem cells: a new tool to confront the challenge of neuropsychiatric disorders. *Neuropharmacology* **60**:1355–1363.

Zarate CA, Manji HK. 2009. Protein kinase C inhibitors: rationale for use and potential in the treatment of bipolar disorder. *CNS Drugs* **23**:569–582.

Zarate CA Jr, Singh JB, Carlson PJ *et al.* 2006. A randomized trial of an N-methyl-D-aspartate antagonist in treatment-resistant major depression. *Arch Gen Psychiatry* **63**:856–864.

Chapter 7

Historical perspectives on the discovery and development of drugs to treat neurological disorders

Michael Williams and Joseph T. Coyle

Introduction

Neurodegeneration is a key hallmark of most neurological diseases. These include Alzheimer's disease (AD, see Chapter 8; Ittner and Gotz 2011; Querfurth and LaFerla 2010), Parkinson's disease (PD, see Chapter 11; Meissner et al. 2011; Mounsey and Teismann 2011; Toulouse and Sullivan 2008), multiple sclerosis (MS, see Chapter 10; Peterson and Fujinami 2007), amyotrophic lateral sclerosis (ALS, see Chapter 12; Geser et al. 2009; Kiernan et al. 2011; Wijesekera and Leigh 2009), Huntington's disease (HD; Zuccato et al. 2010), and frontotemporal lobar degeneration (Rabinovici and Miller 2010). Neurodegeneration is also a major factor affecting the prognosis of stroke (Kleinschnitz et al. 2010), chronic pain (Reichling and Levine 2011), and epilepsy (Yang et al. 2008).

Neurodegeneration has a multifactorial etiology with accumulating evidence across the various disease states for both genetic and environmental contributions (Coppede and Migliore 2009; Feany 2010). Although the diseases differ in regard to their postulated initiating events, which are multiple, complex, and largely unresolved, they may converge on common final pathway(s) that are triggered by the misfolding of key cellular proteins manifest as the amyloidopathies, tauopathies, a-synucleopathies, and TDP-43 proteinopathies (Geser et al. 2010). It remains unclear, however, whether protein misfolding is the initiating event for disease occurrence or is the result of other causes that include environmental factors such as toxins (Coppede and Migliore 2009); inflammation (Glass et al. 2010); oxidative stress (Lin and Beal 2006); mitochondrial dysfunction including apoptosis, autophagy/mitophagy (Choi et al. 2011; Correia et al. 2011; Johri et al. 2011; Keane et al. 2011; Mounsey and Teismann 2011; Readnower et al. 2011; Schapira 2007; Schon et al. 2010; Tranah 2011; Yang et al. 2008), and reduced ATP production (Volonte et al. 2003); ubiquitination (Chechanover and Brundin 2003; Huang and Figueiredo-Pereira 2009; Rogers et al. 2010); trauma; and impaired brain glucose/energy metabolism (Beal 2005; Choi et al. 2011; Correia et al. 2011; Johri et al. 2011; Keane et al. 2011; Liu et al. 2009). Thus, putative molecular targets based on both genome-wide association studies (GWAS) and postmortem assessment of brain pathology have not effectively distinguished between cause and effect, except in the case of HD (Zuccato et al. 2010), making the search for effective disease treatments problematic.

The incidence and prevalence of neurodegenerative diseases are projected to rise dramatically as the result of increased longevity and growth in the global population. The prevalence of AD in 2010 was estimated to be approximately 36 million individuals with a cost of more than $600 billion. By 2050, the prevalence of AD will grow to 115 million (Thies and Bleiler 2011; World Alzheimer Report 2009); that has the potential to bankrupt healthcare systems worldwide if no effective treatments are developed.

Neurodegenerative disease research has become, to varying degrees, "AD-centric," with an expectation that the elucidation of the basic mechanisms involved in the cause of AD will facilitate understanding of the pathological processes in other neurodegenerative diseases.

Historical perspective

Many neurogenerative diseases were formally identified in the nineteenth and early twentieth centuries and immortalized those who published the original descriptions of the diseases. However, these diseases had been known for hundreds to thousands of years.

Translational Neuroscience, ed. James E. Barrett, Joseph T. Coyle and Michael Williams. Published by Cambridge University Press. © Cambridge University Press 2012.

For instance, what Parkinson described as the "shaking palsy," which was designated PD in 1817, may have been recognized in Ayurvedic medicine as "Kampavata" some 5000 years BC. Similarly, whereas AD was definitively described in 1907, dementia was well known before the eighteenth century and was eloquently described by Jonathan Swift in the form of the Struldbrugs in *Gulliver's Travels*. Thus, it is interesting to note that, as the research community searches for causal factors for neurodegenerative diseases, historical semantics notwithstanding, these disorders existed long before the advent of the pollutants, chemical and psychological, associated with modern society.

Although the definitive causes of AD (Citron 2010; Holtzman *et al.* 2011; Ittner and Gotz 2011; Palop and Mucke 2010; Querfurth and LaFerla 2010), PD (Obeso *et al.* 2010; Olanow and Pruisner 2009; Toulouse and Sullivan 2008), MS (Artemiadis *et al.* 2011; Ascherio and Munger 2010; Serafini *et al.* 2010), and ALS (McGeer and Steele 2011) remain unknown, for each disease there is abundant evidence for both familial and sporadic forms that involve genetic and environmental factors. In contrast, HD has a single genetic component (Zuccato *et al.* 2010) that can be associated with specific modifier genes (Khoshnan and Patterson 2011).

Environmental factors

Among the environmental factors reputed to contribute to the risk of AD are the use of aluminum cooking utensils, vehicle exhaust, overuse of antibiotics, head trauma, surgical anesthesia, stress, infective agents, diet, intracranial atherosclerosis, recreational drug use, diabetes/metabolic syndrome, and an absence of intellectual stimuli. However, the majority of these factors have yet to provide "evidence of even moderate scientific quality ... to support the association of any modifiable factor ... with reduced risk of AD" (Kolata 2010). Environmental factors thought to contribute to PD risk include pesticide and fungicide exposure (Lai *et al.* 2002), prion infection (Olanow and Pruisner 2009), diabetes (Schernhammer *et al.* 2011), brain trauma, mitochondrial dysfunction, oxidative stress (Bueler 2009; Mitsumoto 2007; Mounsey and Teismann 2011), neuroinflammation (Hirsch and Hunot 2009), and defects in ubiquitin-proteasome function (McNaught *et al.* 2001). For MS, environmental associations include decreased sunlight; hormone imbalance; trauma or stress; smoking; solvent exposure; and infections, specifically by measles, rubella, and Epstein–Barr viruses (Ascherio and Munger 2007, 2010; Kurtzke *et al.* 1982; Marrie 2004). For ALS, associations include head trauma, military service (Haley 2003), and environmental toxins (McGeer and Steele 2011; Mitchell 2000). Whereas HD is unequivocally an autosomal dominant disorder (Zuccato *et al.* 2010), environmental factors including diet and pollution can modify the age of onset (U.S.–Venezuela Collaborative Research Project and Wexler 2004) as can inflammation (Khoshnan and Patterson 2011), mitochondrial dysfunction, and oxidative stress (Weydt *et al.* 2009).

Current treatments

Currently available treatments for neurodegenerative diseases are almost exclusively palliative. In AD, they are focused on the cholinergic deficit (Bartus 2000; Coyle *et al.* 1983) and alterations in glutamate function related to neurotoxicity (Hynd *et al.* 2004). AD drugs include the cholinesterase inhibitors donepezil, rivastigmine, and galantamine and the N-methyl-D-aspartic acid (NMDA) antagonist, memantine, all of which have modest to questionable efficacy (Kaduszkiewicz *et al.* 2005; Raina *et al.* 2008), highlighting the need for new therapies, especially those with disease-modifying properties. For PD, palliative treatments include dopamine (DA) replacement therapies (Olanow *et al.* 2009), including the DA precursor, L-dopa, administered in combination with a peripheral decarboxylase inhibitor and, less frequently, catechol-O-methyltransferase (COMT) inhibitors (e.g., entacapone and tolcapone) to prevent rapid metabolism of the DA formed from L-dopa. Although it is effective in improving symptomatic aspects of the disease, L-dopa suffers from a loss of efficacy due to disease progression together with severe motor fluctuations (on-off effects) and dyskinesias. The shortcomings of L-dopa have been addressed by sustained release formulations, in combination with monoamine oxidase-B (MAO-B) inhibitors and COMT inhibitors and by directly acting DA agonists, in both acute and slow-release forms, that include bromocriptine, apomorphine, pergolide, ropinirole, and pramipexole (Mounsey and Teismann 2011; Toulouse and Sullivan 2008). However, as with AD, these approaches are palliative rather than disease modifying (Obeso *et al.* 2010).

MS can be treated with corticosteroids and disease-modifying treatments that include the interferons, β1a and β1b; glatiramer acetate, a polypeptide mixture that functions as a decoy to protect myelin from immune system attack; the immune suppressant, mitoxantrone; the α4 integrin antibody, natalizumab (Peterson and Fujinami 2007); and the orally active sphingosine-1-phosphate receptor agonist, fingolimod (Brinkmann et al. 2010). Cannabinoids can prevent MS progress by downregulating the adhesion molecules, intercellular adhesion molecule-1 (ICAM-1) and vascular cell adhesion molecule-1 (VCAM-1) (Mestre et al., 2009), in addition to treating the pain, tremor and spasticity, spasms, and sleep and bladder disturbances associated with MS (Pertwee 2002; Zajicek and Apostu 2011).

Riluzole is the only drug approved for the treatment of ALS. It is thought to produce its effects by inhibiting glutamate release and enhancing its uptake, blocking NMDA receptors, and stabilizing voltage-sensitive sodium channels. Nevertheless, its effects on disease progression and mortality are modest. Other approaches to treating ALS include nonsteroidal anti-inflammatory agents (NSAIDs); copaxone, an immunomodulator used in MS; the antibiotics ceftriaxone and minocycline that may function as caspase inhibitors; talampanel (GYKI 53405), a noncompetitive AMPA antagonist; and Coenzyme Q_{10} (Maragakis and Rothstein 2011; Wijesekera and Leigh 2009).

Tetrabenazine, a vesicular monoamine transporter 2 (VMAT2), an inhibitor that blocks DA release, is the only drug currently approved for the treatment of the chorea associated with HD, although neuroleptics and benzodiazepines are also used (Zuccato et al. 2010).

Hurdles to new therapeutics

Finding drugs that can attenuate or reverse neurodegenerative disease progression has been challenging in the absence of a complete understanding of the underlying causes. In this regard, a key issue has been the ability to translate numerous preclinical findings to the clinic, making validated translational research *the* critical challenge in drug discovery in the area of neurodegeneration. Limitations in the predictivity and validity of animal models (Jucker 2010; Nestler and Hyman 2010), especially those involving transgenic models thought to recapitulate the pathological processes and biomarkers (Flood et al. 2011; Lovestone 2010; Olsson et al. 2011; Ptolemy and Rifai 2010) of human disease, represent major confounding issues, especially in regard to the confirmation of the latter in additional patient cohorts (Ioannidis and Panagiotou 2011).

Current approaches establish the diagnoses of AD and PD only after the diseases are well advanced. The early pathology of AD is now thought to begin approximately 10–20 years before clinical symptoms are apparent (Braskie et al. 2011; Morris and Price 2001), stimulating the development of new diagnostic guidelines (DeKosky et al. 2011; Dubois et al. 2010; Jack et al. 2011; McKhann et al. 2011; Sperling et al. 2011) that update existing guidelines (McKhann et al. 1984). The premotor or preclinical symptoms of PD, which include olfactory dysfunction, depression, sleep abnormalities, pain, constipation, and cardiac sympathetic denervation (O'Sullivan et al. 2008), precede the onset of motor symptoms by 4–7 years, by which time 70% of the nigrostriatal DA neurons involved in the disease have been lost (Wu et al. 2011). Thus, the pathological processes leading to PD may predate preclinical PD by decades (Sherer 2011; Wu et al. 2011).

Biomarkers

Biomarkers represent any measure that can be used to indicate the presence of a disease state. Genetic biomarkers can be diagnostic as in the case of HD or identify risk for disease such as APOε in AD. Other biomarkers reflect the disease process including symptom scales, cerebrospinal fluid (CSF) and blood analytes, or images of brain changes.

Biomarkers are critical both for making an accurate diagnosis of each of the neurodegenerative diseases and for assessing their status and response to treatment (Doody et al. 2011). They are crucial for clinical trials from their initial design, to patient recruitment, to establishing objective end points (Lang 2010). Additionally, biomarkers are considered useful in linking the effects of putative new disease treatments active in animal models to the clinical setting and in understanding the contributions of genetics and environmental factors to disease occurrence and progression (Lesage and Brice 2009; Migliore and Coppede 2009; Olsson et al. 2011; Van Broeckhoven 2010). The National Institutes of Health AD Neuroimaging Initiative (ADNI) is focused on identifying biomarkers for AD (Miller 2009) and PD (Sherer 2011), including CSF analytes and pathological changes that can be visualized by positron emission tomography (PET), magnetic resonance imaging (MRI), and computer-assisted tomography (CAT) scans.

Biomarkers for neurodegenerative diseases include behavioral assessments such as the AD Assessment Scale-Cognitive for AD (ADAS-Cog) (Doody *et al.* 2010; Mitchell 2009), the Unified Parkinson's Disease Rating Scale (UPDRS) for PD (Olanow *et al.* 2009), and the Unified Huntington's Disease Rating Scale (UHDRS) for HD (Zuccato *et al.* 2010); analyte analysis from CSF and plasma (Flood *et al.* 2011; Olsson *et al.* 2011); and, more recently, brain imaging (CAT, MRI, functional MRI, PET, and diffusion tensor imaging) to assess volume and tissue changes as well as the use of molecular probes like [^{11}C]-PIB, which reportedly binds specifically to fibrillar Aβ plaques as a measure of amyloid load (Rabinovici *et al.* 2007). Despite considerable efforts, none of these biomarkers is as predictive as needed. Thus, although decreased levels of Aβ$_{42}$ in the CSF (less than 500 pg/ml; Castellano *et al.* 2011) are thought to reflect an increased brain Aβ$_{42}$ load (Jack *et al.* 2010; Shaw *et al.* 2009), its predictive value is viewed as having "limited diagnostic usefulness" (Zetterberg *et al.* 2010). CSF tau and hyperphosphorylated tau (p-tau), inflammatory markers of oxidative stress, e.g., cytokines (Olson and Humpel 2010; Swardfager *et al.* 2010), and markers of cell death are undergoing validation as AD biomarkers (Albert *et al.* 2011). However, like CSF Aβ$_{42}$, the diagnostic value of CSF t-tau and p-tau$_{181}$ has been questioned (Fagan *et al.* 2009; Mattsson *et al.* 2009). A composite measure of CSF Aβ$_{42}$, t-tau, and p-tau$_{181}$ levels used to develop an "AD signature" (De Meyer *et al.* 2010) has also provided mixed outcomes (De Meyer *et al.* 2010; Diniz *et al.* 2008; Mattsson *et al.* 2009; Mihaescu *et al.* 2010), with AD positive signatures occurring in cognitively normal subjects and, in addition, a potential for overlap between patients with AD or PD (Shi *et al.* 2011*b*). These findings are consistent with observations that older individuals having a "significant amyloid burden" can be assessed as cognitively normal (Aizenstein *et al.* 2008; Fagan *et al.* 2009; Zetterberg *et al.* 2010), raising questions as to the predictive accuracy of the diagnosis (Sperling *et al.* 2011).

Genetics of neurodegenerative diseases

Neurodegenerative disease-associated genes continue to be identified at an ever-increasing rate using GWAS in cohorts of affected individuals. On the basis of the null hypothesis, many of the genes identified by GWAS should provide information to reaffirm current approaches or to generate alternative hypotheses as to the cause of disease. To a major degree, however, rather than objectively informing research efforts, these findings have often been integrated into existing hypotheses with alternative hypotheses not receiving appropriate attention. Also, the possibility that such associations may not be disease specific is not always taken into account. For instance, although the PARK6/*PINK1* gene coding for the mitochondrial protein, PTEN (phosphatase and tensin homolog)-induced putative kinase 1, has been associated with PD (Gao and Hong 2011; Mounsey and Teismann 2011), it is also implicated in heart failure (Billia *et al.* 2011). Added to such considerations are the failures to replicate initial findings that are an additional hurdle to the transition of gene products and their associated pathways to use as tractable new drug targets.

Genetic factors

GWAS have identified many candidate and risk genes and loci. For AD, more than 120 AD-associated gene loci have been reported that are thought to be either causal or risk factors for AD (Bertram *et al.* 2007; Feulner *et al.* 2010). Seventeen of these have been replicated (Table 7.1), of which four have been "unequivocally associated with AD" (Feulner *et al.* 2010). These include *APP* (amyloid precursor protein), *PSEN1* (presenilin 1), and *PSEN2* (presenilin 2), early-onset genes associated with early-onset/familial AD (EOAD/FAD) and involved with Aβ clearance. The fourth, *APOE* (apolipoprotein-E), is involved in both Aβ clearance (Castellano *et al.* 2011) and cholesterol metabolism and is a major risk gene for late onset AD (LOAD). The remaining 13 genes are associated with LOAD. Despite the presence of hyperphosphorylated tau in AD brain and its focus as a key part of current approaches to AD drug discovery (Brunden *et al.* 2009), there has been no reported association of the tau gene, *MAPT* (microtubule-associated protein tau), with AD.

Chapter 7: Historical perspectives on the discovery and development of drugs to treat neurological disorders

Table 7.1. Gene associations with Alzheimer's disease identified to date.*

Early-onset AD (EOID) genes

APP	Amyloid precursor protein
PSEN1	Presenilin 1
PSEN2	Presenilin 2

Late-onset AD (LOAD) genes

Apo-E	Apolipoprotein-E
ADAM10	Disintegrin and metalloproteinase domain-containing protein-10
ATXN1	Ataxin-1
CD 33	Myeloid transmembrane receptor
GWA14Q34	???
DGAP1	Homolog of rasGTPase activating proteins
PICALM	Phosphatidylinositol-binding clathrin assembly protein
CLU	Clusterin/apolipoprotein-J
CR1	Complement component (3b/4b) receptor 1
BIN1	Bridging integrator 1
CD2AP	CD2-associated protein
MS44A/ MS4A6E	Membrane-spanning 4A gene family
EPHA1	Ephrin receptor A1
ABCA7	ATP-binding cassette subfamily A member 7

* Information summarized from Bertram et al. (2007); Feulner et al. (2010); Hollingworth et al. (2011); Naj et al. (2011).

Table 7.2. Gene associations with Parkinson's disease.*

Early-onset Parkinson's disease (20–40 years)

PARK1/ SNCA	α-Synuclein
PARK2/ PRKN	Parkin
PARK4	α-Synuclein
PARK6	PINK1 (gene coding for a mitochondrial protein)
PARK7	DJ-1 (putative oncogene, redox-sensitive molecular chaperone)

Late-onset Parkinson's disease (50+ years)

PARK3	??
PARK5	UCH-L1 (ubiquitin C-terminal hydrolase-L1)

Other genes associated with Parkinson's disease

PARK8	LRRK2 (leucine-rich repeat kinase 2)
PARK9	????
PARK10	?????
PARK11	??????
ACMSD/ TMEM163	Aminocarboxymuconate semialdehyde decarboxylase/transmembrane protein 163
ATP13A2	Lysosomal type 5 P-type ATPase
BST1	Bone marrow stromal cell antigen 1
CCDC62/ HIP1R	Coiled-coil domain containing 62/ Huntingtin interacting protein 1 related
FBX07	E3 ligase related to ubiquitination
GIGYF2	Grb10-interacting GYF protein-2
HLA-DRB5	Major GAK cyclin G-associated kinase
MAPT	Microtubule-associated protein tau; saitohin
MCCC1	Peptidase M20 domain containing 1
MED13	Mediator complex subunit 13/ thyroid hormone receptor associated protein 1
Omi/HTRA	Ultrahigh temperature requirement A serine peptidase
PANK2	Pantothenate kinase
PLA2G6	Calcium-independent group VI phospholipase A_2

Several loci and genes (Table 7.2) implicated in cellular bioenergetics, oxidative stress, and mitochondrial function have been associated with the risk for PD (Elbaz et al. 2011; Gao and Hong 2011; Gasser 2010; Lesage and Brice 2009; Lill et al. 2011; Mounsey and Teismann 2011). Although MS was not considered to be hereditary, genetic variations in the major histocompatibility complex alleles, DR15 and DQ6 (Compston and Coles 2008; McElroy and Oksenberg 2008), have been associated with the risk for the disease (Table 7.3). Approximately 12 putative

Table 7.2. (cont.)

PGC-1a	Peroxisome proliferator-activated receptor-γ coactivator-1a
PM20D1	Peptidase M20 domain containing 1
PRKRA	Activator of protein kinase PKA
SYT11/ RAB25	Synaptotagmin XI/ras-related protein Rab-25
STK39	Serine threonine kinase 39
TAF1	TATA binding protein-associated factor-1

* Information summarized from Elbaz *et al.* (2011); Gao and Hong (2011); Lesage and Brice (2009); Lill *et al.* (2011); Mounsey and Teismann (2011); Satake *et al.* (2009); Schneider *et al.* (2009); Simón-Sánchez *et al.* (2009); Zheng *et al.* (2010).

genes and loci for ALS have been identified (Table 7.3; Wijesekera and Leigh 2009). Of these, 110 involve mutations in *SOD1* (superoxide dismutase 1), which is involved in free radical accumulation. The association of TDP-43 with ALS (Geser *et al.* 2009) has been viewed as an important advance in the understanding of ALS (Maragakis and Rothstein 2011), despite its association with frontotemporal lobar degeneration with ubiquitin-immunoreactive inclusions (FLTD-U) – the latter is a discrete neurodegenerative disease that can occur in the absence or presence of ALS. HD is an autosomal dominant inherited disorder involving a trinucleotide repeat mutation in a single gene, *HTT*, that encodes for the brain-specific protein, Huntingtin (Htt). The trinucleotide sequence, CAG, codes for glutamine and normally varies in expression from 6 to 35 repeats, resulting in the production of Htt in individuals who are normal with respect to HD. A CAG repeat of 36 or greater leads to mutant Htt, mHtt, which is associated with neuronal damage and loss. Genes altering the progression of HD have been described, including *GluR6*, *GRIN2B*, *UCHL1*, *ASK*1 (Zuccato *et al.* 2010), and PGC-1α (Table 7.3) (Weydt *et al.* 2009).

In addition to the genes and loci already identified for neurodegenerative diseases, it is anticipated that there are yet-to-be discovered recessive mutations, mutations in miRNAs, promoter, and regulatory regions, copy number variants, and gene dosage effects that will contribute to disease etiology and progression (Van Broeckhoven 2010).

Alzheimer's disease – the amyloid and tau hypotheses

Based on AD neuropathology and genetic associations, the majority of research efforts in the search for novel AD therapeutics over the past 15 years have focused almost exclusively on the amyloid and tau hypotheses (Brunden *et al.* 2009; Ittner and Gotz 2011; Palop and Mucke 2010; Querfurth and LaFerla 2010). Whether these core hallmarks of AD are causative, disease by-products, or the result of an endogenous protective response (Castellani *et al.* 2006, 2008; Lee *et al.* 2007; Maltsev *et al.* 2011) is currently unknown.

Efforts to reduce brain amyloid accumulation have focused on inhibiting the enzymes responsible for amyloid production, the β-secretases (Hunt and Turner 2009) and γ-secretases (Oehlrich *et al.* 2011) as well as mechanisms for enhancing amyloid clearance (Citron 2010; Kurz and Perneczky 2011) that include anti-Aβ antibodies (Lemere and Masliah 2010), metal chelating agents (Maynard *et al.* 2005), and immunoglobulins (Weksler *et al.* 2005). Brain amyloid clearance has been associated with ApoE isoforms, with the E4 isoform being associated with a reduction in brain amyloid clearance (Castellano *et al.* 2011).

Additional drug discovery efforts have focused on inhibiting the various kinases thought to be responsible for tau hyperphosphorylation (Brunden *et al.* 2009), inhibiting tau aggregation (Deng *et al.* 2009; Liu *et al.* 2004; Wischik *et al.* 2010), and improving mitochondrial transition pore function (Blum *et al.* 2011; Donmez *et al.* 2010; Readnower *et al.* 2011). The mitochondrial transition pore (MTP) was identified as the mechanism by which latrepirdine (dimebon) produced its therapeutic benefit in an impressive phase II trial in AD patients (Doody *et al.* 2008). Because it failed a subsequent phase III trial (Sabbagh and Berk 2010), the efficacy of dimebon and the role of the MTP in AD are now being questioned. Transcranial laser therapy can improve mitochondrial function, brain ATP levels, and normalized Aβ neuropathology in an AD transgenic mouse model (De Taboada *et al.* 2011).

Despite clinical trials of several drug candidates, little progress has been made in clinically validating the role of amyloid accumulation or tau hyperphosphorylation in being key to AD causality or in discovering viable new therapeutics for the treatment of AD (Williams 2009). Among the phase III failures are the putative γ-secretase inhibitors tarenflurbil (Green

Table 7.3. Gene associations with multiple sclerosis, amyotrophic lateral sclerosis, and Huntington's disease.[*]

Multiple sclerosis	
DR15 and DQ6	Major histocompatibility complex

Amyotrophic lateral sclerosis	
SOD1	Superoxide dismutase 1
ALS2/alsin	Alsin protein
SETX	Helicase senataxin
FUS	RNA-binding protein FUS (fused in sarcoma)
VAPB	Vesicle-associated membrane protein-associated protein B/C/synaptobrevin 1 binding protein
ANG	Angiogenin, ribonuclease, RNase A family 5
DCTN1	Dopachrome tautomerase
CHMP2B	Chromatin modifying protein 2B
ATXN2	Ataxin 2
TARDBP/ TDP-43	Hyperphosphorylated, ubiquitinated, and cleaved TAR DNA binding protein
FIG4	Polyphosphoinositide phosphatase/SAC domain-containing protein 3
OPTN	Optineurin

Huntington's disease	
HTT	Huntingtin
ASK1	Rabidopsis Skp1 (S-phase kinase associated protein)-like – human homolog p19skp1 encodes a kinetochore protein involved in cell cycle progression
GluR6	Kainate receptor subunit glutamate receptor 6
GRIN2B	Glutamate receptor, ionotropic, N-methyl D-aspartate 2B
PGC-1α	Peroxisome proliferator-activated receptor-g coactivator-1a
UCHL1	Ubiquitin carboxyl-terminal esterase L1/ ubiquitin thiolesterase

[*] Compston and Coles (2008); Geser et al. (2009); McElroy and Oksenberg (2008); Weydt et al. (2009); Wijesekera and Leigh (2009); Zuccato et al. (2010).

et al. 2009) and semagacestat (Cummings 2010; Schor 2011), neither of which had significant efficacy in AD, the former due to low potency and lack of brain penetration (Imbimbo and Giardina 2011) and the latter due to "worsening of clinical measures of cognition and the ability to perform activities of daily living" (Extance 2010) and an increased incidence of skin cancer (Schor 2011). The latter was ascribed (Imbimbo and Giardina 2011) to semagacestat facilitating the accumulation of the neurotoxic precursor of Aβ, CTFβ (the carboxy-terminal fragment of APP), and concomitant inhibition of Notch processing. The Notch pathway is highly conserved and is involved in neural development and carcinogenesis.

AN1792, the first of the Aβ antibodies, was discontinued in phase II trials due to cases of aseptic meningoencephalitis (Morgan 2011). However, a 6-year follow-up study noted that while AN1792 effectively cleared plaques from AD brain, it did not prevent progressive neurodegeneration (Holmes et al. 2008). A second-generation Aβ antibody, bapineuzumab, was associated with reports of vasogenic edema (Panza et al. 2010; Wilcock 2010) and was found in controversial "exploratory analyses" in AD patients lacking the APOE-ε4 allele to have positive outcomes compared with placebo (Wilcock 2010). Together with second-generation vaccines like solanezumab, bapineuzumab continues to advance in clinical trials with expected phase III data in 2012, the outcomes of which will be crucial in validating the amyloid hypothesis and in defining a path for the development of effective AD therapeutics. More recently, a bispecific monoclonal antibody to β-secretase (Atwal et al. 2011) and the transferrin receptor on the blood–brain barrier (Yu et al. 2011) that uses receptor-mediated transcytosis to cross the blood–brain barrier reduced brain amyloid load in transgenic mice and may represent a novel approach to overcoming long-standing issues as to whether biologics can achieve therapeutic levels in the brain. The transferrin receptor approach has also been used to deliver a TNFα chimeric antibody, cTfRMAb-TNFR, to the brain where it should have neuroprotective effects (Zhou et al. 2011).

Alzheimer's disease and anti-inflammatory drugs

On the basis of the association of activated microglia with amyloid plaques in patients with AD and the finding that patients with rheumatoid arthritis had a decreased incidence of AD that was ascribed to the use of NSAIDs like indomethacin, it was suggested that inflammation plays a causative role in AD (McGeer and McGeer 2006; McGeer et al. 2006). A small, randomized controlled trial reported that indomethacin could indeed protect AD patients from cognitive decline (Rogers et al. 1993). However, subsequent studies with both approved NSAIDs (Aisen et al. 2003; de Jong et al. 2008; Reines et al. 2004; Soininen et al. 2007) and experimental agents with similar mechanisms have consistently provided equivocal results, suggesting that the inflammatory component of AD may involve more complex mechanisms than those readily addressed via COX inhibition (Sastre and Gentleman 2010). In open-label trials of the soluble TNFα p75 receptor fusion protein, etanercept, given via a perispinal extrathecal injection, was reported to be effective in the treatment of AD (Tobinick and Gross 2008a, 2008b). As already noted, the TNFα chimeric antibody, cTfRMAb-TNFR, has neuroprotective effects (Zhou et al. 2011). Chronic infusion of the dominant negative TNF inhibitor, DN-TNF XENP345, decreased lipopolysaccharide (LPS)-induced Aβ accumulation in transgenic mice (McAlpine et al. 2009). The TNFα inhibitor, infliximab, given intracerebroventricularly to APP/PS1 transgenic mice decreased TNF-α levels with accompanying reductions in Aβ and tau phosphorylation (Shi et al. 2011a) while inhibition of 5-lipoxygenase, which is upregulated in AD brain, attenuated Aβ formation (Chu and Pratico 2011).

Alzheimer's disease and metabolic syndrome

Type II diabetes is also a risk factor for AD (Maher and Schubert 2009; Moreira et al. 2007) through the development of insulin resistance and the dysregulation of glucose metabolism (Correia et al. 2011) that are manifest as a reduction in cerebral glucose metabolic rate (Baker et al. 2011). Insulin can regulate Aβ degradation via changes in the insulin degrading enzyme (IDE; Qui and Folstein 2006; Zhao et al. 2004) that have been associated with AD severity (Miners et al. 2009). This observation led to the concept of a brain-specific form of diabetes, "Type 3 diabetes," (de la Monte et al. 2006; Hoyer 2004; Steen et al. 2005), which involves both a decrease in the effects of insulin on Aβ processing and insulin-related cerebrovascular dysfunction (Iadecola 2004; Takeda et al. 2010).

New approaches to treat Parkinson's disease

These include direct DA receptor agonists, calcium channel blockers (Ilijic et al. 2011), and neuroprotective agents (Schapira 2010). The latter include the selective MAO-B inhibitors selegiline, rasagailine, safinamide, and zonisamide (Obeso et al. 2010; Rascol et al. 2011); the antioxidants Coenzyme Q_{10} (Shults et al. 2002) and oxyresveratrol (Chao et al. 2008); selenium; vitamins C and E (Toulouse and Sullivan 2008); a propargylamine analog of selegiline that lacks MAO inhibitor activity, TCH346 (Waldmeier et al. 2000); the mixed lineage kinase inhibitor, CEP1347 (Saporito et al. 2002); the selective LRRK2 inhibitor, LRRK2-IN-1 (Deng et al. 2011); the NMDA modulator, riluzole (Obinu et al. 2002); omega-3 fatty acids (Bousquet et al. 2011); NSAIDs; nicotinic agonists; and adenosine A_{2A} receptor antagonists (Richardson et al. 1997).

Consumption of NSAIDs (Gao et al. 2011; Hirsch and Hunot 2009; Powers et al. 2008), nicotine in the form of cigarette smoking (Thacker et al. 2007), and caffeine in the form of coffee and chocolate (Jankovic 2008) is inversely related to the incidence of PD (Ross et al. 2000), with a combination of all three being estimated to produce an 87% reduction in PD risk (Powers et al. 2008). The effect of caffeine consumption on PD was supported by a prospective study of 8000 Japanese-American men, aged 45–68 years, from the Honolulu Heart Program that showed that higher caffeine consumption in the form of coffee was associated with a reduced incidence of PD (Ross et al. 2000). Ongoing drug discovery efforts have demonstrated that selective adenosine A_{2A} receptor antagonists could, because of their co-localization with DA D_2 receptors in striatopallidal neurons, function as both indirect DA agonists and neuroprotectants (Chen and Chern 2011; Richardson et al. 1997; Schwarzschild et al. 2006; Xu et al. 2005).

Deep brain stimulation (Benabid et al. 2009), repetitive transcranial magnetic stimulation (Koch 2010), and cell replacement therapy, the latter including fetal neurons and various types of stem cell and gene therapies (Bjorklund and Bjorklund 2011; Jarraya et al. 2009; LeWitt et al. 2011) are also under evaluation for the treatment of PD. Current approaches to gene therapy involve the use of adeno-associated viral vector serotype 2 (AAV2) to deliver (1) aromatic amino acid decarboxylase

(AADC) to facilitate conversion of L-dopa to DA; (2) glutamic acid decarboxylase (GAD) to enhance production of GABA and increase inhibitory tone; (3) a tricistronic vector encoding for tyrosine hydroxylase, the enzyme responsible for dopa formation, AADC, and GTP cyclohydrolase hydroxylase (Jarraya et al. 2009), that is involved in the synthesis of tetrahydrobiopterin, an essential cofactor for dopa decarboxylase activity; (4) the neurotrophic factor, neurturin (CERE-120) (Marks et al. 2008); and (5) glial-derived neurotrophic factor (GDNF), all of which are in the process of being assessed for PD treatment (Obeso et al. 2010; Richardson et al. 2011).

Clinical score card for neurodegenerative diseases

Despite the intense efforts to find drugs effective in the treatment of AD, many of the compounds targeted toward the Aβ hypothesis have failed in either phase II or III clinical trials irrespective of whether these were small molecules or biologics. This result has been interpreted to reflect (1) insufficient understanding of the mechanism(s) of action of the new chemical entities and biologics being tested and (2) shortcomings in the drug-like properties of the compounds advanced to the clinic (Cummings 2010; Sabbagh and Berk 2010) – a "right target, wrong compound" failure metric (Selkoe 2011). The latter raises serious questions, however, regarding the objectivity of the criteria used to select compounds for advancement to the clinic as well as the inclusion in clinical trials of patients with AD who were too advanced in their disease progression to benefit from any type of disease-modifying therapeutic intervention.

Popper (2002) proposed that deductive reasoning in the experimental situation would lead to "predictions ... [being] ... tested and the [hypothesis] ... rejected if these ... are not shown to be correct" (Trist 2011). In the context of this logic, the clinical results with semagacestat that have "challenged the primacy of Aβ in AD pathophysiology" (Cummings 2010) together with the negative results with tarenflurbil and AN1792 have collectively failed to validate the hypothesis that amyloid is causative in AD (Castellani et al. 2006, 2008; Lee et al. 2007; Williams 2009) and are now leading to a reassessment of the amyloid hypothesis. Researchers are now questioning whether amyloid deposits and tau hyperphosphorylation are intrinsic protective responses to the disease rather than their cause (Castellani et al. 2006, 2008). In this vein, Hardy (2009), an originator of the amyloid hypothesis of AD, has questioned whether a critical reappraisal of its role in disease causality is now necessary and has advocated efforts to better understand the normal physiological role(s) of amyloid, its formation, and its removal. In this context, Aβ has been reported to have antimicrobial properties (Soscia et al. 2010).

For PD, newer DA replacement therapies have also had mixed results, with compounds that showed a convincing absence of dyskinesias in nonhuman primate models failing to replicate these advantages in patients with PD. For instance, although the D1 agonist, adrogolide, was clinically efficacious (Rascol et al. 1999), it elicited dyskinesias similar to those seen with L-dopa (Rascol et al. 2001). Similarly, putative neuroprotective agents like TCH346 (Olanow et al. 2006) and CEP1347 (Parkinson Study Group PRECEPT Investigators, 2007) that had robust activity in preclinical models of PD (Waldmeier et al. 2006) failed to demonstrate efficacy in PD as did riluzole, a TTX-sensitive calcium channel blocker (Bensimon et al. 2009). Adenosine A_{2A} receptor antagonists have had a long, still unresolved path toward approval. Istradefylline (KW-6002), the first-in-class compound, has been in clinical trials since 1996 and was effective as adjunctive therapy to L-dopa, demonstrating a clinically meaningful reduction in "off" time, without an increase in "on" time with associated dyskinesias (Stacy et al. 2008). However, subsequent results (Fernandez et al. 2010) revealed that istradefylline failed to improve motor symptoms relative to placebo in patients with early PD. These issues with istradefylline were widely ascribed to its limited potency and selectivity for the A_{2A} receptor. Second-generation compounds with greater potency and receptor selectivity including vipadenant, preladenant (SCH-420,814), SYN-115, ST-15335, SEP 89068, PS 246518, and DT-1133 are being advanced in the clinic. Vipadenant was recently discontinued due to toxicity issues whereas preladenant was reported to reduce off time and motor fluctuations in patients with PD on L-dopa therapy (Hauser et al. 2011).

In a phase II trial (Marks et al. 2010), CERE-120 (AAV2-neurturin) failed to show superiority to the sham surgery used for its administration when assessed at 12 months using the UPDRS motor score. In contrast, AAV2-*GAD* improved the UPDRS score (Le Witt et al. 2011).

Chapter 7: Historical perspectives on the discovery and development of drugs to treat neurological disorders

Table 7.4. Convergence points in neurodegenerative disease states.

	Alzheimer's disease	Parkinson's disease	Multiple sclerosis	Amyotrophic lateral sclerosis	Huntington's disease
Genes					
MHC		✓	✓	✓	
PGC-1a		✓			✓
Proteins					
Amyloid	✓	✓	✓		
Tau	✓	✓			
TDP-43	✓	✓		✓	
Clusterin	✓				✓
Myelin	✓		✓		
Targets/pathways					
Proteasome/ubiquitination	✓	✓	✓	✓	
Adenosine A$_{2A}$ receptor	✓	✓			
Dopamine receptors	✓	✓			
mTOR	✓	✓			
MTP/mitochondria	✓	✓	✓	✓	✓
Disease associations					
Diabetes	✓	✓			
Inflammation	✓	✓	✓	✓	✓
Prion infection	✓	✓			

MHC, major histocompatibility complex; mTOR, mammalian target of rapamycin.

Common themes in neurodegenerative disease drug discovery

Irrespective of the particular disease with which neurodegeneration is associated, a number of similarities or convergence points appear to be emerging (Table 7.4) that may provide a broader context for understanding these diseases and identifying and advancing treatments. In considering the proposed genetic and environmental risks and causes of the neurodegenerative diseases discussed above, it is clear that, although each disease has distinctive hallmarks, there are also common features. The following points are key in assessing progress in neurodegenerative disease drug discovery:

1. The causes of the majority of neurodegenerative diseases, with the possible exception of mHtt in HD, remain unknown.
2. The only drugs currently available to treat neurodegenerative diseases are palliative. There are no disease-modifying treatments for any neurodegenerative disease except MS.
3. Drug discovery efforts for neurodegenerative diseases suffer from major translational limitations due to the following issues:
    a. Animal models that are generally neither validated nor sufficiently predictive of the human disease to effectively transition compounds from animal models to the

clinic (Morrissette *et al.* 2009; Nestler and Hyman 2010).

b. An inability to reliably diagnose the various neurodegenerative diseases at a sufficiently early stage to allow for the testing of novel therapeutics that may have a positive impact by attenuating disease progression. Thus, efficacy, or a lack thereof, of disease-modifying drugs cannot be objectively and convincingly determined. This factor may account for the failures of semagacestat, tarenflurbil, and AN1792 in AD trials.

c. A lack of validated, predictive biomarkers to use in conjunction with points (a) and (b) to accurately diagnose the disease, to assess its progression, and to monitor the effects of therapeutics.

4. Many of the newer gene associations and possible drug targets for neurodegeneration are also associated with other disease states including cancer, immune disorders, and heart failure (Billia *et al.* 2011). Thus, their utility as tractable targets for drug discovery in the field of neurodegeneration has yet to be proven. They may also produce unacceptable side effects because of these other associations.

5. Recent targets for drug discovery for neurodegenerative diseases involve protein–protein interactions, for which small-molecule-based drug discovery is still in its infancy.

6. Given the nature of the diseases and the lack of other apparent options for restoration of lost cells, CNS gene and stem cell therapies may currently be the best option at advanced stages of the diseases.

7. Several major pharmaceutical companies have withdrawn from CNS drug discovery due to concerns regarding the cost and failure rate of clinical trials (ECNP Summit Report 2011).

8. Patient advocacy groups, private not-for-profit foundations (e.g., Michael J. Fox Foundation), and private philanthropy organizations (High Q Foundation for Huntington's Disease), as in other disease areas, e.g. multiple myeloma (MMRF; Prokesch 2011), are altering the clinical research paradigm because such organizations are less "risk aversive" (Harford 2011) in funding approaches that lie outside current approaches and in enabling clinical trials.

9. An explosion in basic research knowledge, while state of the art and "information rich," has neither advanced patient care options nor delivered on overly optimistic breakthroughs (Mangialasche *et al.* 2010).

10. The continued inability to effectively treat these diseases, both with respect to their increasing incidence and their impact on societal and individual well-being, will have dire consequences for healthcare provision in the near future.

In highlighting these concerns, it is apparent that the translational paradigm in neurodegenerative diseases, like that in psychiatric diseases (see Chapter 1), is far from optimal for facilitating the development of novel therapeutics, especially given the length and complexity of human trials in the area of neurodegeneration. The role of mitochondrial DNA (mtDNA) in the genesis of PD (Keane *et al.* 2011; Schapira 2007) represents a novel approach, especially as mtDNA is more prone to point mutations than DNA and can accumulate somatic mutations, making age an important contribution to neurodegeneration. High levels of mtDNA deletions are also associated with decreased cytochrome oxidase, a key enzyme in electron transport chain (ETC) function, and mitochondrial respiratory chain dysfunction in both older individuals and those with PD (Bender *et al.* 2006).

Gene-based drug discovery in neurodegenerative diseases

A large number of candidate genes and loci identified for neurodegenerative diseases, for example, in excess of 120 for AD with numerous others for PD, MS, HD, and ALS have potentially provided a rich source of new targets for drug discovery. However, for many of these genes, their functions are unknown; for others, their putative function seriously challenges the current hypotheses of disease causality that are being used to drive discovery efforts. Gene-based drug discovery, as already noted, is a concept still very much in its infancy that is perhaps not given sufficient priority, appropriate insights, and time to assure success. For instance, the fact that the considerable efforts addressed to finding both effective palliative and disease-modifying treatments for HD after the discovery of the causal mutation (Huntington's Disease Collaborative Research Group 1993) have yet to yield substantive advances in therapeutics after nearly 20 years is a chilling reminder of the overwhelming challenges associated with this approach. How does gene causality or association translate to a tractable drug target? How do new findings effectively impact the status quo in ongoing research activities?

As AD research continues to focus on modulating the postulated causal effects of amyloid plaques and tau hyperphosphorylation, how do common factors of neurodegeneration such as heat shock proteins (Luo *et al.* 2010), autophagy (Wong and Cuervo 2010), inflammation (Appel *et al.* 2009; Glass *et al.* 2010), oxidative stress (Lin and Beal 2006; Rodrigues *et al.* 2010), the ubiquitin-proteasome system (Chechanover and Brundin 2003; Huang and Figueiredo-Pereira 2009; Rogers *et al.* 2010), and mitochondrial dysfunction (Choi *et al.* 2011; Correia *et al.* 2011; Johri *et al.* 2011; Keane *et al.* 2011; Mounsey and Teismann 2011; Readnower *et al.* 2011; Schapira 2007; Schon *et al.* 2010; Tranah 2011; Yang *et al.* 2008) become focal points and priorities for efforts in objectively searching for alternative approaches to therapeutic options? If the drugs based on these novel mechanisms do not work, are the associations and mechanisms identified rendered invalid?

Future translational aspects

The need for a better understanding of the many genes and proteins that appear to be genetically causal to neurodegeneration (Maltsev *et al.* 2011; Van Broeckhoven 2010), improved animal models (Jucker 2010; Nestler and Hyman 2010), validated biomarkers (Flood *et al.* 2011; Olsson *et al.* 2011), more pragmatic initiatives in improving and facilitating the translational process (Finkbeiner 2010), and a paradigm shift in clinical trial execution (Lang 2010) have all been highlighted as critical elements in improving success in drug discovery in the field of neurodegenerative diseases. For example, the dire predictions for AD (Thies 2011) will certainly become a self-fulfilling prophecy unless research in the area becomes more objective, less exclusionary to new hypotheses, and more focused on the goal of providing therapy via the "programmatic science" that was used so effectively in the Manhattan project (Mukherjee 2010).

Acknowledgments

MW would like to acknowledge the late Mark Smith for his provocative views on AD causality that provided a much-needed call for objectivity in ongoing research in the area and Kevin Mullane for helpful discussions on the topics of translational research and deficits in drug discovery productivity.

References

Aisen PS, Schafer KA, Grundman M *et al.* 2003. Effects of rofecoxib or naproxen vs placebo on Alzheimer disease progression: a randomized controlled trial. *J Am Med Assoc* **289**:2819–2828.

Aizenstein HJ, Nebes RD, Saxton, JA *et al.* 2008. Frequent amyloid deposition without significant cognitive impairment among the elderly. *Arch Neurol* **65**:1509–1517.

Albert MS, DeKosky ST, Dickson D *et al.* 2011. The diagnosis of mild cognitive impairment due to Alzheimer's disease: recommendations from the National Institute on Aging and Alzheimer's Association workgroup. *Alzheimer's Dement*, in press.

Appel SH, Beers DR, Henkel JS. 2009. T-cell microglia dialogue in Parkinson's disease and amyotrophic lateral sclerosis: are we listening? *Trends Immunol* **31**:7–17.

Artemiadis AK, Anagnostouli MC, Alexopoulos EC. 2011. Stress as a risk factor for multiple sclerosis onset or relapse: a systematic review. *Neuroepidemiology* **36**:109–120.

Ascherio A, Munger KL. 2007. Environmental risk factors for multiple sclerosis. Part II: Noninfectious factors. *Ann Neurol* **61**:504–513.

Ascherio A, Munger KL. 2010. Epstein–Barr virus infection and multiple sclerosis: a review *J Neuroimmune Pharmacol* **5**:271–277.

Atwal JK, Chen Y, Chiu C *et al.* 2011. A therapeutic antibody targeting BACE1 inhibits amyloid-beta production in vivo. *Sci Transl Med* **3**:84r43.

Baker LD, Cross DJ, Minoshima S *et al.* 2011. Insulin resistance and Alzheimer-like reductions in regional cerebral glucose metabolism for cognitively normal adults with prediabetes or early type 2 diabetes. *Arch Neurol* **68**:51–57.

Bartus RT. 2000. On neurodegenerative diseases, models and treatment strategies: lessons learned and lessons forgotten a generation following the cholinergic hypothesis. *Exp Neurol* **163**:495–529.

Beal MF. 2005. Mitochondria take center stage in aging and

neurodegeneration. *Ann Neurol* **58**:495–505.

Benabid AL, Chabardes S, Mitrofanis J, Pollak P. 2009. Deep brain stimulation of the subthalamic nucleus for the treatment of Parkinson's disease *Lancet Neurol* **8**:67–81.

Bender A, Krishnan KJ, Morris CM et al. 2006. High levels of mitochondrial DNA deletions in substantia nigra neurons in aging and Parkinson disease. *Nat Genet* **38**:515–517.

Bensimon G, Ludoplh A, Agid Y et al. 2009. Riluzole treatment, survival and diagnostic criteria in Parkinson plus disorders: the NNIPPS study. *Brain* **132**:156–171.

Bertram L, McQueen MB, Mullin K, Blacker D, Tanzi RE. 2007. Systematic meta-analyses of Alzheimer disease genetic association studies: the AlzGene database. *Nat Genet* **39**:17–23.

Billia F, Hauck L, Konecny F et al. 2011. PTEN-inducible kinase 1 (PINK1)/Park6 is indispensable for normal heart function. *Proc Natl Acad Sci USA* **108**:9572–9577.

Bjorklund A, Bjorklund T. 2011. Gene therapy for Parkinson's disease shows promise. *Sci Transl Med* **3**:79ed1.

Blum CA, Ellis JL, Loh C et al. 2011. SIRT1 modulation as a novel approach to the treatment of diseases of aging. *J Med Chem* **54**:417–432.

Bousquet M, Calon F, Cicchetti F. 2011. Impact of omega-3-fatty acids in Parkinson's disease. *Ageing Res Rev* **10**:453–463.

Braskie MN, Jahnshad N, Stein JL et al. 2011. Common Alzheimer's disease risk variant within the *CLU* gene affects white matter microstructure in young adults. *J Neurosci* **31**: 6764–6770.

Brinkmann V, Billich A, Baumruker T et al. 2010. Fingolimod (FTY720): discovery and development of an oral drug to treat multiple sclerosis. *Nat Rev Drug Discov* **9**:883–897.

Brunden KR, Trojanowski JQ, Lee VMY. 2009. Advances in tau-focused drug discovery for Alzheimer's disease and related tauopathies. *Nat Rev Drug Discov* **8**:783–793.

Bueler H. 2009. Impaired mitochondrial dynamics and function in the pathogenesis of Parkinson's disease. *Exp Neurol* **218**:235–246.

Castellani RJ, Lee H-G, Zhu X et al. 2006. Neuropathology of Alzheimer disease: pathognomonic but not pathogenic. *Acta Neuropathol* **111**:503–509.

Castellani RJ, Lee H-G, Zhu X, Perry G, Smith MA. 2008. Alzheimer disease pathology as a host response. *J Neuropathol Exp Neurol* **67**:523–531.

Castellano JM, Kim J, Stewart FR et al. 2011. Human apoE isoforms differentially regulate brain amyloid-beta peptide clearance. *Sci Translat Med* **3**:89ra57.

Chao J, Yu MS, Ho YS, Wang M, Chang RCC. 2008. Dietary oxyresveratrol prevents parkinsonian mimetic 6-hydroxydopamine neurotoxicity. *Free Radical Biol Med* **45**:1019–1026.

Chechanover A, Brundin P. 2003. The ubiquitin-proteasome system in neurodegenerative disorders: sometimes the chicken, sometimes the egg. *Neuron* **40**:427–446.

Chen J-F, Chern Y. 2011. Impacts of methylxanthines and adenosine receptors on neurodegeneration: human and experimental studies. *Handb Exp Pharmacol* **200**:267–310.

Choi WS, Palmiter RD, Xia Z. 2011. Loss of mitochondrial complex I activity potentiates dopamine neuron death induced by microtubule dysfunction in a Parkinson's disease model. *J Cell Biol* **192**:873–882.

Chu J, Pratico D. 2011. 5-Lipoxygenase as an endogenous modulator of amyloid β formation in vivo. *Ann Neurol* **69**:34–46.

Citron M. 2010. Alzheimer's disease: strategies for disease modification *Nat Rev Drug Discov* **9**:387–398.

Compston A, Coles A. 2008. Multiple sclerosis. *Lancet* **372**:1502–1517.

Coppede F, Migliore L. 2010. Evidence linking genetics, environment, and epigenetics to impaired DNA repair in Alzheimer's disease. *J Alzheimer's Dis* **20**:953–966.

Correia SC, Santos RX, Perry G et al. 2011. Insulin-resistant brain state: the culprit in sporadic Alzheimer's disease? *Ageing Res Rev* **10**:264–273.

Coyle JT, Price DL, DeLong MR. 1983. Alzheimer's disease: a disorder of cortical cholinergic innervation. *Science* **219**:1184–1190.

Cummings J. 2010. What can be inferred from the interruption of the semagacestat trial for treatment of Alzheimer's disease? *Biol Psychiatry* **68**:876–878.

de Jong D, Jansen R, Hoefnagels W et al. 2008. No effect of one-year treatment with indomethacin on Alzheimer's disease progression: a randomized controlled trial. *PLoS ONE* **3**:**e1475**.

DeKosky ST, Carrillo MC, Phelps C et al. 2011. Revision of the criteria for Alzheimer's disease: a symposium. *Alzheimer's Dement* **7**:e1–e12.

de la Monte SM, Tong M, Lester-Coll N, Plater M Jr, Wands JR. 2006. Therapeutic rescue of neurodegeneration in experimental type 3 diabetes: relevance to Alzheimer's disease. *J Alzheimer's Dis* **10**:89–109.

De Meyer G, Shapiro F, Vanderstichele H et al. for the Alzheimer's Disease Neuroimaging Initiative 2010. Diagnosis-independent Alzheimer disease biomarker signature in cognitively normal elderly people. *Arch Neurol* 67:949–956.

Deng T, Li B, Liu Y et al. 2009. Dysregulation of insulin signaling, glucose transporters, O-GlcNAcylation and phosphorylation of tau and neurofilaments: relevance to Alzheimer's disease. *Am J Pathol* 175:2089–2098.

Deng X, Dzamk N, Prescott A et al. 2011. Characterization of a selective inhibitor of the Parkinson's disease kinase LRRK2. *Nat Chem Biol* 7:203–205.

DeTaboada L, Yu J, El-Amouri S et al. 2011. Transcranial laser therapy attenuates amyloid-beta peptide neuropathology in amyloid-beta protein precursor transgenic mice. *J Alzheimer's Dis* 23:521–535.

Diniz BS, Pinto JA Jr, Forlenz OV. 2008. Do CSF total tau, phosphorylated tau, and β-amyloid 42 help to predict progression of mild cognitive impairment to Alzheimer's disease? A systematic review and meta-analysis of the literature. *World J Biol Psychiatry* 9:172–182.

Donmez G, Wang D, Cohen DE, Guarente L. 2010. SIRT1 suppresses β-amyloid production by activating the α-secretase gene ADAM10. *Cell* 142:320–332.

Doody RS, Coleb PE, Millerc DS et al. 2011. Global issues in drug development for Alzheimer's disease. *Alzheimer's Dement* 7:197–207.

Doody RS, Gavrilova SI, Sano M et al. 2008. Effect of dimebon on cognition, activities of daily living, behaviour, and global function in patients with mild-to-moderate Alzheimer's disease: a randomised, double-blind, placebo-controlled study. *Lancet* 372:207–215.

Doody RS, Pavlik V, Massman P et al. 2010. Predicting progression of Alzheimer's disease. *Alzheimer's Res Ther* 2:2.

Dubois B, Feldman HH, Jacova J et al. 2010. Revising the definition of Alzheimer's disease: a new lexicon. *Lancet Neurol* 9:1118–1124.

ECNP Summit Report 2011. ECNP Summit on the future of CNS drug research in Europe 2011: report prepared for ECNP by David Nutt and Guy Goodwin. *Eur Neuropsychopharmacol* 21:495–499.

Elbaz A, Ross OA, Ioannidis JPA et al. 2011. Independent and joint effects of the *MAPT* and *SNCA* genes in Parkinson disease. *Ann Neurol* 69:778–792.

Extance A. 2010. Alzheimer's failure raises questions about disease-modifying strategies. *Nat Rev Drug Discov* 9:749–751.

Fagan AM, Mintun MA, Shah AR, Alde P, Roe CM. 2009. Cerebrospinal fluid tau and ptau$_{181}$ increase with cortical amyloid deposition in cognitively normal individuals: implications for future clinical trials of Alzheimer's disease. *EMBO Mol Med* 1:371–380.

Feany MB. 2010. New approaches to the pathology and genetics of neurodegeneration. *Am J Pathol* 176:2058–2066.

Fernandez HH, Greeley DR, Zweig RM et al. for the 6002-US-051 Study Group 2010. Istradefylline as monotherapy for Parkinson disease: results of the 6002-US 051 trial. *Parkinsonism Relat Disord* 16:16–20.

Feulner TM, Laes SM, Friedrich P et al. 2010. Examination of the current top candidate genes for AD in a genome-wide association study. *Mol Psychiatry* 15:756–766.

Finkbeiner S. 2010. Bridging the valley of death of therapeutics for neurodegeneration. *Nat Med* 16:1227–1232.

Flood DG, Marek GJ, Williams M. 2011. Developing predictive CSF biomarkers – a challenge critical to success in Alzheimer's disease and neuropsychiatric translational medicine. *Biochem Pharmacol* 81:1422–1434.

Gao HM, Hong JS. 2011. Gene–environment interactions: key to unraveling the mystery of Parkinson's disease. *Prog Neurobiol* 94:1–19.

Gao X, Chen H, Schwarzschild M, Ascherio A. 2011. Use of ibuprofen and risk of Parkinson's disease. *Neurology* 76:863–869.

Gasser T. 2010. Identifying PD-causing genes and genetic susceptibility factors: current approaches and future prospects. *Prog Brain Res* 183:2–20.

Geser F, Lee VM, Trojanowski JQ. 2010. Amyotrophic lateral sclerosis and frontotemporal lobar degeneration: a spectrum of TDP-43 proteinopathies. *Neuropathology* 30:103–112.

Geser F, Martinez-Lage M, Trojanowski JQ et al. 2009. Amyotrophic lateral sclerosis, frontotemporal dementia and beyond: the TDP-43 diseases. *J Neurol* 256:1205–1214.

Glass CK, Saijo K, Winner B, Marchetto MC, Gage FH. 2010. Mechanisms underlying inflammation in neurodegeneration. *Cell* 10:918–934.

Green RC, Schneider LS, Amato DA et al. 2009. Effect of tarenflurbil on cognitive decline and activities of daily living in patients with mild Alzheimer disease. *J Am Med Assoc* 302:2557–2564.

Haley RW. 2003. Excess incidence of ALS in young Gulf War veterans. *Neurology* 61:750–756.

Hardy J. 2009. The amyloid hypothesis for Alzheimer's disease: a critical reappraisal. *J Neurochem* 110:1129–1134.

Harford T. 2011. Positive Black Swans: How to fund research so that it generates insanely great ideas, not pretty good ones. *Slate*, May 17, 2011. Available at: www.slate.com/id/2293699/pagenum/all/#p2. Accessed August 5, 2011.

Hauser RA, Cantillon M, Pourcher E et al. 2011. Preladenant in patients with Parkinson's disease and motor fluctuations: a phase 2, double-blind, randomised trial. Lancet Neurol **10**:221–229.

Hirsch EC, Hunot S. 2009. Neuroinflammation in Parkinson's disease: a target for neuroprotection? Lancet Neurol **8**:382–397.

Hollingworth P, Harold D, Sims R et al. 2011. Common variants at ABCA7, MS4A6A/MS4A4E, EPHA1, CD33 and CD2AP are associated with Alzheimer's disease. Nat Genet **43**:429–435.

Holmes C, Boche D, Wilkinson D et al. 2008. Long-term effects of Aβ immunisation in Alzheimer's disease: follow-up of a randomised, placebo-controlled phase I trial. Lancet **372**:216–223.

Holtzman DM, Morris JC, Goate AM. 2011. Alzheimer's disease: the challenge of the second century. Sci Transl Med **3**:77sr1/.

Hoyer S. 2004. Glucose metabolism and insulin receptor signal transduction in Alzheimer disease. Eur J Pharmacol **490**:115–125.

Huang Q, Figueiredo-Pereira ME. 2009. Ubiquitin/proteasome pathway impairment in neurodegeneration: therapeutic implications. Apoptosis **15**:1292–1311.

Hunt CE, Turner AJ. 2009. Cell biology, regulation and inhibition of beta-secretase (BACE-1). FEBS J **276**:1854–1859.

Huntington's Disease Collaborative Research Group 1993. A novel gene containing a trinucleotide repeat that is expanded and unstable on Huntington's disease chromosomes. Cell **72**:971–983.

Hynd MR, Scott HL, Dodd PR. 2004. Glutamate-mediated excitotoxicity and neurodegeneration in Alzheimer's disease. Neurochem Int **45**:583–595.

Iadecola C. 2004. Neurovascular regulation in the normal brain and Alzheimer's disease. Nat Rev Neurosci **5**:347–360.

Ilijic E, Guzman JN, Surmeier DJ. 2011. The L-type channel antagonist isradipine is neuroprotective in a mouse model of Parkinson's disease. Neurobiol Dis **43**:364–371.

Imbimbo BP, Giardina GA. 2011. γ-Secretase inhibitors and modulators for the treatment of Alzheimer's disease: disappointments and hopes. Curr Top Med Chem **11**:1555–1570.

Ioannidis JPA, Panagiotou OA. 2011. Comparison of effect sizes associated with biomarkers reported in highly cited individual articles and in subsequent meta-analyses. J Am Med Assoc **305**:2200–2210.

Ittner LM, Gotz J. 2011. Amyloid-β and tau – a toxic *pas de deux* in Alzheimer's disease. Nat Rev Neurosci **12**:65–72.

Jack CR Jr, Albert MS, Knopman DS et al. 2011. Introduction to the recommendations from the National Institute on Aging–Alzheimer's Association workgroups on diagnostic guidelines for Alzheimer's disease. Alzheimer's Dement **7**:257–262.

Jack CR Jr, Wiste HJ, Vemuri P et al. 2010. Brain beta-amyloid measures and magnetic resonance imaging atrophy both predict time-to-progression from mild cognitive impairment to Alzheimer's disease. Brain **133**:3336–3348.

Jankovic J. 2008. Are adenosine antagonists, such as istradefylline, caffeine, and chocolate, useful in the treatment of Parkinson's disease? Ann Neurol **63**:267–269.

Jarraya B, Boulet S, Ralph SG et al. 2009. Dopamine gene therapy for Parkinson's disease in a nonhuman primate without associated dyskinesia. Sci Transl Med **1**:2ra4.

Johri A, Chaturvedi, RK, Beal MF. 2011. Hugging tight in Huntington's. Nat Med **17**:245–246.

Jucker M. 2010. The benefits and limitations of animal models for translational research in neurodegenerative diseases. Nat Med **16**:1210–1214.

Kaduszkiewicz H, Zimmermann T, Beck-Bornholdt H-P, van den Bussche H. 2005. Cholinesterase inhibitors for patients with Alzheimer's disease: systematic review of randomised clinical trials. Br Med J **331**:321.

Keane PC, Kurzawa M, Blain PG, Morris CM. 2011. Mitochondrial dysfunction in Parkinson's disease. Parkinsons Dis **2011**: art.716871.

Khoshnan A, Patterson PH. 2011. The role of IκB kinase complex in the neurobiology of Huntington's disease. Neurobiol Dis **43**:305–311.

Kiernan, MC, Vucic S, Cheah BC et al. 2011. Amyotrophic lateral sclerosis. Lancet **377**:942–955.

Kleinschnitz C, Grund H, Wingler K et al. 2010. Post-stroke inhibition of induced NADPH oxidase type 4 prevents oxidative stress and neurodegeneration. PLoS Biol **8**: e1000479.

Koch G. 2010. rTMS effects on levodopa-induced dyskinesias in Parkinson's disease patients: searching for effective cortical targets. Restor Neurol Neurosci **28**:561–568.

Kolata G. 2010. Years later, no magic bullet against Alzheimer's disease. New York Times, August 28, 2010. Available at: http://www.nytimes.com/2010/08/29/health/research/29prevent.html. Accessed August 5, 2011.

Kurtzke JF, Gudmundsson KR, Bergmann S. 1982. Multiple sclerosis in Iceland: I. Evidence of a postwar epidemic. Neurology **32**:143–150.

Kurz A, Perneczky R. 2011. Amyloid clearance as a treatment target against Alzheimer's disease. J Alzheimer's Dis **24**(Suppl. 2): 61–73.

Lai BC, Marion SA, Teschke K, Tsui JK. 2002. Occupational and environmental risk factors in Parkinson's disease. *Parkinsonism Relat Disord* **8**:297–309.

Lang AE. 2010. Clinical trials of disease-modifying therapies for neurodegenerative diseases: the challenges and the future. *Nat Med* **16**:1223–1226.

Lee H-G, Zhu X, Castellani RJ et al. 2007. Amyloid-β in Alzheimer disease: the null versus the alternate hypotheses. *J Pharmacol Exp Ther* **321**:823–829.

Lemere CA, Masliah E. 2010. Can Alzheimer disease be prevented by amyloid-β immunotherapy? *Nat Rev Neurol* **6**:108–119.

Lesage S, Brice A. 2009. Parkinson's disease: from monogenic forms to genetic susceptibility factors. *Hum Mol Genet* **18**:R48–R59.

LeWitt PA, Rezai AR, Leehey MA et al. 2011. AAV2-GAD gene therapy for advanced Parkinson's disease: a double-blind, sham-surgery controlled, randomised trial. *Lancet Neurol* **10**:309–319.

Lill CM, Roehr JT, McQueen MB et al. 2011. The PD Gene Database. *Alzheimer Research Forum*. http://www.pdgene.org/. Accessed August 5, 2011.

Lin MT, Beal MF. 2006. Mitochondrial dysfunction and oxidative stress in neurodegenerative diseases. *Nature* **443**:787–795.

Liu F, Iqbal K, Grundke-Iqbal I, Hart GW, Gong C-X. 2004. O-GlcNAcylation regulates phosphorylation of tau: a mechanism involved in Alzheimer's disease. *Proc Natl Acad Sci USA* **101**:10804–10809.

Liu W, Vives-Bauza C, Acın-Perez R et al. 2009. PINK1 defect causes mitochondrial dysfunction, proteasomal deficit and a-synuclein aggregation in cell culture models of Parkinson's disease. *PLoS ONE* **4**: e4597.

Lovestone S. 2010. Searching for biomarkers in neurodegeneration. *Nat Med* **16**:1371–1372.

Luo W, Sun W, Taldone T, Rodina A, Chiosis G. 2010. Heat shock protein 90 in neurodegenerative diseases. *Mol Neurodegener* **5**:24.

Maher PA, Schubert DR. 2009. Metabolic links between diabetes and Alzheimer's disease. *Expert Rev Neurother* **9**:617–630.

Maltsev AV, Bystryak S, Galzitskaya OV. 2011. The role of β-amyloid peptide in neurodegenerative diseases. *Ageing Res Rev.* **10**:440–452.

Mangialasche F, Solomon A, Winblad B, Mecocci P, Kivipelto M. 2010. Alzheimer's disease: clinical trials and drug development. *Lancet Neurol* **9**:702–716.

Maragakis N, Rothstein JD. 2011. New treatments in amyotrophic lateral sclerosis. *Neuropsychopharmacology* **36**:370–372.

Marks WJ, Bartus RT, Siffert J et al. 2010. Gene delivery of AAV2-neurturin for Parkinson's disease: a double blind, randomised, controlled trial. *Lancet Neurol* **9**:1164–1172.

Marks WJ, Ostrem JL, Verhagen L et al. 2008. Safety and tolerability of intraputaminal delivery of CERE-120 (adeno-associated virus serotype 2pneurturin) to patients with idiopathic Parkinson's disease: an open-label, phase I trial. *Lancet Neurol* **7**:400–408.

Marrie RA. 2004. Environmental risk factors in multiple sclerosis aetiology. *Lancet Neurol* **3**:709–718.

Mattsson N, Zetterberg H, Hansson O et al. 2009. CSF biomarkers and incipient Alzheimer disease in patients with mild cognitive impairment. *J Am Med Assoc* **302**:385–393.

Maynard CJ, Bush AI, Masters CL, Cappai R, Li QX. 2005. Metals and amyloid-beta in Alzheimer's disease. *Int J Exp Pathol* **86**:147–159.

McAlpine FE, Lee JK, Harms AS et al. 2009. Inhibition of soluble TNF signaling in a mouse model of Alzheimer's disease prevents pre-plaque amyloid-associated neuropathology. *Neurobiol Dis* **34**:163–177.

McElroy JP, Oksenberg JR. 2008. Multiple sclerosis genetics. *Curr Topics Microbiol Immunol* **318**:45–72.

McGeer PL, McGeer EG. 2006. NSAIDs and Alzheimer disease: epidemiological, animal model and clinical studies. *Neurobiol Aging* **28**:639–647.

McGeer PL, Rogers J, McGeer EG. 2006. Inflammation, anti-inflammatory agents and Alzheimer disease: The last 12 years. *J Alzheimer's Dis* **9**(Suppl. 3): 271–276.

McGeer PL, Steele JC. 2011. The ALS/PDC syndrome of Guam: potential biomarkers for an enigmatic disorder. *Prog Neurobiol* **95**:663–669.

McKhann GM, Drachman D, Folstein M et al. 1984. Clinical diagnosis of Alzheimer's disease: report of the NINCDS-ADRDA Work Group under the auspices of Department of Health and Human Services Task Force on Alzheimer's Disease. *Neurology* **34**:939–944.

McKhann GM, Knopman DS, Chertkow H et al. 2011. The diagnosis of dementia due to Alzheimer's disease: recommendations from the National Institute on Aging and the Alzheimer's Association workgroup. *Alzheimer's Dement* **7**:263–269.

McNaught KSP, Olanow CW, Halliwell B, Isacson O, Jenner P. 2001. Failure of the ubiquitin proteasome system in Parkinson's disease. *Nat Rev Neurosci* **2**:589–594.

Meissner WG, Frasier M, Gasser T et al. 2011. Priorities in Parkinson's disease research. *Nat Rev Drug Discov* **10**:377–393.

Mestre L, Docagne F, Correa F et al. 2009. A cannabinoid agonist interferes with the progression of a chronic model of multiple sclerosis by downregulating adhesion molecules. *Mol Cell Neurosci* **40**:258–266.

Migliore L, Coppede F. 2009. Genetics, environmental factors and the emerging role of epigenetics in neurodegenerative diseases. *Mutat Res/Fund Mol Mechanisms Mutagenesis* **667**:82–97.

Mihaescu R, Detmar SB, Cornel MC et al. 2010. Translational research in genomics of Alzheimer's disease: a review of current practice and future perspectives. *J Alzheimer's Dis* **20**:967–980.

Miller G. 2009. Alzheimer's biomarker initiative hits its stride. *Science* **326**:386–389.

Miners JS, Baig S, Tayler H, Kehoe PG, Love S. 2009. Neprilysin and insulin-degrading enzyme levels are increased in Alzheimer disease in relation to disease severity. *J Neuropathol Exp Neurol* **68**:902–914.

Mitchell AJ. 2009. A meta-analysis of the accuracy of the mini-mental state examination in the detection of dementia and mild cognitive impairment. *J Psychiatr Res* **43**:411–431.

Mitchell JD. 2000. Amyotrophic lateral sclerosis: toxins and environment. *Amyotroph Lateral Scler Other Motor Neuron Disord* **1**:235–250.

Mitsumoto Y. 2007. Mitochondrial nutrition as a strategy for neuroprotection in Parkinson's disease – research focus in the Department of Alternative Medicine and Experimental Therapeutics at Hokuriku University. *Evid Based Complement Alternat Med* **4**:263–265.

Moreira PI, Santos MS, Seica R, Oliveria CR. 2007. Brain mitochondrial dysfunction as a link between Alzheimer's disease and diabetes. *J Neurol Sci* **257**:206–214.

Morgan D. 2011. Immunotherapy for Alzheimer's disease. *J Intern Med* **269**:54–63.

Morris JC, Price JL. 2001. Pathologic correlates of non demented aging, mild cognitive impairment, and early-stage Alzheimer's disease. *J Mol Neurosci* **17**:101–118.

Morrissette DA, Parachikova A, Green KN, LaFerla FM. 2009. Relevance of transgenic mouse models to human Alzheimer disease. *J Biol Chem* **284**:6033–6037.

Mounsey RB, Teismann P. 2011. Mitochondrial dysfunction in Parkinson's disease: pathogenesis and neuroprotection. *Parkinson's Dis* doi:10.4061/2011/617472.

Mukherjee, S. 2010. *The Emperor of All Maladies*. New York: Scribner, pp. 119–122.

Naj AC, Jun G, Beecham GW et al. 2011. Common variants at MS4A4/MS4A6E, CD2AP, CD33 and EPHA1 are associated with late-onset Alzheimer's disease. *Nat Genet* **43**:436–441.

Nestler EJ, Hyman SE. 2010. Animal models of neuropsychiatric disorders. *Nat Neurosci* **13**:1161–1169.

Obeso JA, Rodriguez-Oroz MC, Goetz CG et al. 2010. Missing pieces in the Parkinson's disease puzzle. *Nat Med* **16**: 653–661.

Obinu MC, Reibaud M, Blanchard V, Moussaoui S, Imperato A. 2002. Neuroprotective effect of riluzole in a primate model of Parkinson's disease: behavioral and histological evidence. *Mov Disord* **17**:3–19.

Oehlrich D, Berthelot DJ, Gijsen HJ. 2011. Gamma-secretase modulators as potential disease modifying anti-Alzheimer's drugs. *J Med Chem* **54**:669–698.

Olanow CW, Pruisner SB. 2009. Is Parkinson's disease a prion disorder? *Proc Natl Acad Sci USA* **106**:12571–12572.

Olanow CW, Schapira AHV, LeWitt PA et al. 2006. TCH346 as a neuroprotective drug in Parkinson's disease: a double-blind, randomised, controlled trial. *Lancet Neurol* **5**:1013–1020.

Olanow CW, Stern MB, Sethi K. 2009. The scientific and clinical basis for the treatment of Parkinson disease. *Neurology* **72**:S1–S132.

Olson L, Humpel C. 2010. Growth factors and cytokines/chemokines as surrogate biomarkers in cerebrospinal fluid and blood for diagnosing Alzheimer's disease and mild cognitive impairment. *Exp Gerentol* **45**:41–46.

Olsson B, Zetterberg H, Hampel H, Blennow K. 2011. Biomarker-based dissection of neurodegenerative diseases. *Prog Neurobiol* **95**: 520–534.

O'Sullivan SS, Williams DR, Gallagher DA et al. 2008. Nonmotor symptoms as presenting complaints in Parkinson's disease: a clinicopathological study. *Mov Disord* **23**:101–106.

Palop JJ, Mucke L. 2010. Amyloid-beta-induced neuronal dysfunction in Alzheimer's disease: from synapses toward neural networks. *Nat Neurosci* **13**:812–818.

Panza F, Frisardi V, Imbimbo BP et al. 2010. Bapineuzumab: anti-β-amyloid monoclonal antibodies for the treatment of Alzheimer's disease. *Immunotherapy* **2**: 767–782.

Parkinson Study Group PRECEPT Investigators 2007. Mixed lineage kinase inhibitor CEP-1347 fails to delay disability in early Parkinson disease. *Neurology* **69**:1480–1490.

Pertwee RG. 2002. Cannabinoids and multiple sclerosis. *Pharmacol Ther* **95**:165–174.

Peterson LK, Fujinami RS. 2007. Inflammation, demyelination, neurodegeneration and neuroprotection in the pathogenesis of multiple sclerosis. *J Neuroimmunol* **184**:37–44.

Popper K. 2002. *The Logic of Scientific Discovery*. London: Routledge.

Powers KM, Kay DM, Factor SA et al. 2008. Combined effects of smoking, coffee, and NSAIDs on Parkinson's disease risk. *Mov Disord* **23**:88–95.

Prokesch S. 2011. The reluctant social entrepreneur. *Harvard Business Rev* June, 2011. [Prod. #:BR1106-MAG-ENG.]

Ptolemy AS, Rifai N. 2010. What is a biomarker? Research investments and lack of clinical integration necessitate a review of biomarker terminology and validation schema. *Scan J Clin Lab Invest* **70**(Suppl. 242):6–14.

Querfurth HW, LaFerla FM. 2010. Alzheimer's disease. *N Engl J Med* **362**:329–344.

Qui WQ, Folstein MF. 2006. Insulin, insulin-degrading enzyme and amyloid-β peptide in Alzheimer's disease: review and hypothesis. *Neurobiol Aging* **27**:190–198.

Rabinovici GD, Furst AJ, Neil JP et al. 2007. ^{11}C-PIB PET imaging in Alzheimer disease and frontotemporal lobar degeneration. *Neurology* **68**:1205–1212.

Rabinovici G, Miller B. 2010. Frontotemporal lobar degeneration: epidemiology, pathophysiology, diagnosis and management. *CNS Drugs* **24**:375–398.

Raina P, Santaguida P, Ismaila A et al. 2008. Effectiveness of cholinesterase inhibitors and memantine for treating dementia: evidence review for a clinical practice guideline. *Ann Intern Med* **148**:379–397.

Rascol O, Blin O, Thalamas C et al. 1999. ABT-431, a D1 receptor agonist prodrug, has efficacy in Parkinson's disease. *Ann Neurol* **45**:736–741.

Rascol O, Fitzer-Attas CJ, Hauser R et al. 2011. A double-blind, delayed-start trial of rasagiline in Parkinson's disease (the ADAGIO study): pre-specified and post-hoc analyses of the need for additional therapies, changes in UPDRS scores, and non-motor outcomes. *Lancet Neurol* **10**:415–423.

Rascol O, Nutt JG, Blin O et al. 2001. Induction by dopamine D_1 receptor agonist ABT-431 of dyskinesia similar to levodopa in patients with Parkinson disease. *Arch Neurol* **58**:249–254.

Readnower RD, Sauerbeck AD, Sullivan PG. 2011. Mitochondria, amyloid β, and Alzheimer's disease. *Int J Alzheimer's Dis* **22**: art.104545.

Reichling DB, Levine JD. 2011. Pain and death: neurodegenerative disease mechanism in the nociceptor. *Ann Neurol* **69**:13–21.

Reines SA, Block GA, Morris JC et al. 2004. Rofecoxib: no effect on Alzheimer's disease in a 1-year, randomized, blinded, controlled study. *Neurology* **62**:66–71.

Richardson PJ, Kase H, Jenner PG. 1997. Adenosine A_{2A} receptor antagonists as new agents for the treatment of Parkinson's disease. *Trends Pharmacol Sci* **18**:338–344.

Richardson RM, Kells AP, Rosenbluth KH et al. 2011. Interventional MRI-guided putaminal delivery of AAV2-GDNF for a planned clinical trial in Parkinson's disease. *Mol Ther* doi:10.1038/mt.2011.11.

Rodrigues R, Bonda DJ, Perry G et al. 2010. Oxidative stress and neurodegeneration: an inevitable consequence of aging? Implications for therapy. In *Brain Protection in Schizophrenia, Mood and Cognitive Disorders*. Ritsner MS, ed. New York: Springer, pp. 305–323.

Rogers J, Kirby LC, Hempelman SR et al. 1993. Clinical trial of indomethacin in Alzheimer's disease. *Neurology* **43**:1609–1611.

Rogers N, Paine S, Bedford L, Layfield R. 2010. The ubiquitin-proteasome system: contributions to cell death or survival in neurodegeneration. *Neuropathol Appl Neurobiol* **36**:113–124.

Ross GW, Abbott RD, Petrovitch H et al. 2000. Association of coffee and caffeine intake with the risk of Parkinson disease. *J Am Med Assoc* **283**:2674–2679.

Sabbagh MN, Berk C. 2010. Latrepirdine for Alzheimer's disease: trials and tribulations. *Fut Neurol* **5**:645–665.

Saporito MS, Hudkin RL, Maroney A. 2002. Discovery of CEP-1347/KT-7515, an inhibitor of the JNK/SAPK pathway for the treatment of neurodegenerative diseases. *Prog Med Chem* **40**:23–62.

Sastre M, Gentleman SM. 2010. NSAIDs: how they work and the prospects as therapeutics in Alzheimer's disease. *Front Aging Neurosci* **2**:20.

Satake W, Nakabayashi Y, Mizuta I et al. 2009. Genome-wide association study identifies common variants at four loci as genetic risk factors for Parkinson's disease. *Nat Genet* **41**:1303–1307.

Schapira AHV. 2007. Mitochondrial dysfunction in Parkinson's disease. *Cell Death Differ* **14**:1261–1266.

Schapira AHV. 2010. Neuroprotection in Parkinson's disease. *Blue Books Neurol* **34**:301–320.

Schernhammer E, Hansen J, Rugbjerg K, Wermuth L, Ritz B. 2011. Diabetes and the risk of developing Parkinson's disease in Denmark. *Diabetes Care* doi: 10.2337.

Schneider SA, Bhatia KP, Hardy J. 2009. Complicated recessive dystonia parkinsonism syndromes. *Mov Disord* **24**:490–499.

Schon EA, DiMauro S, Hirano M, Gilkerson RW. 2010. Therapeutic prospects for mitochondrial disease. *Trends Mol Med* **16**:268–276.

Schor NF. 2011. What the halted phase III γ-secretase inhibitor trial may (or may not) be telling us. *Ann Neurol* **69**:237–239.

Shults CW, Oakes D, Kieburtz K et al. 2002. Effects of coenzyme Q$_{10}$ in early Parkinson disease: evidence of slowing of the functional decline. *Arch Neurol* **59**:1541–1550.

Schwarzschild MA, Agnati L, Fuxe K, Chen J-F, Morelli M. 2006. Targeting adenosine A$_{2A}$ receptors in Parkinson's disease. *Trends Neurosci* **29**:647–654.

Selkoe D. 2011. Dennis Selkoe on the amyloid hypothesis of Alzheimer's disease. *Science Watch*. March, 2011. Available at: http://sciencewatch.com/ana/st/alz2/11marSTAlz2Selk1/. Accessed August 5, 2011.

Serafini B, Severa M, Columba-Cabezas S et al. 2010. Epstein-Barr virus latent infection and BAFF expression in B cells in the multiple sclerosis brain: implications for viral persistence and intrathecal B-cell activation. *J Neuropathol Exp Neurol* **69**:677–693.

Shaw LM, Vanderstichele H, Knapik-Czajka M et al. 2009. Cerebrospinal fluid biomarker signature in Alzheimer's disease neuroimaging initiative studies. *Ann Neurol* **65**:403–413.

Sherer TB. 2011. Biomarkers for Parkinson's disease. *Sci Transl Med* **3**:79ps14.

Shi JQ, Shen W, Chen J et al. 2011*a*. Anti-TNF-alpha reduces amyloid plaques and tau phosphorylation and induces CD11c-positive dendritic-like cell in the APP/PS1 transgenic mouse brains. *Brain Res* **1368**:239–247.

Shi M, Bradner J, Hancock AM et al. 2011*b*. Cerebrospinal fluid biomarkers for Parkinson disease diagnosis and progression. *Ann Neurol* **69**:570–580.

Simón-Sánchez J, Schulte C, Bras JM et al. 2009. Genome-wide association study reveals genetic risk underlying Parkinson's disease. *Nat Genet* **41**: 1308–1312.

Soininen H, West C, Robbins J, Niculescu L. 2007. Long-term efficacy and safety of celecoxib in Alzheimer's disease. *Dement Geriatr Cogn Disord* **23**:8–21.

Soscia SJ, Kirby JE, Washicosky KJ et al. 2010. The Alzheimer's disease-associated amyloid beta-protein is an antimicrobial peptide. *PLoS One* **3**:e9505.

Sperling RA, Aisen PS, Beckett LA et al. 2011. Toward defining the preclinical stages of Alzheimer's disease: recommendations from the National Institute on Aging and the Alzheimer's Association Workgroup. *Alzheimer's Dement* **7**:280–292.

Stacy M, Silver D, Mendis T et al. 2008. A 12-week, placebo-controlled study (6002-US-006) of istradefylline in Parkinson disease. *Neurology* **70**:2233–2240.

Steen E, Terry BM, Rivera EJ et al. 2005. Impaired insulin and insulin-like growth factor expression and signaling mechanisms in Alzheimer's disease – is this type 3 diabetes? *J Alzheimer's Dis* **7**:63–80.

Swardfager W, Lanctot K, Rothenburg L et al. 2010. A meta-analysis of cytokines in Alzheimer's disease. *Biol Psychiatry* **68**:930–941.

Takeda S, Sato N, Uchio-Yamada K et al. 2010. Diabetes-accelerated memory dysfunction via cerebrovascular inflammation and Aβ deposition in an Alzheimer mouse model with diabetes. *Proc Natl Acad Sci USA* **107**:7036–7041.

Thacker EL, O'Reilly EJ, Weisskopf MG et al. 2007. Temporal relationship between cigarette smoking and risk of Parkinson disease. *Neurology* **68**:764–768.

Thies W. 2011. Stopping a thief and killer – Alzheimer's disease crisis demands greater commitment to research. *Alzheimer's Dement* **7**:175–176.

Thies W, Bleiler L. 2011. Alzheimer's Association Report: 2011 Alzheimer's disease facts and figures. *Alzheimer's Dement* **7**:208–244.

Tobinick EL, Gross H. 2008*a*. Rapid improvement in verbal fluency and aphasia following perispinal etanercept in Alzheimer's disease. *BMC Neurol* **8**:27.

Tobinick EL, Gross H. 2008*b*. Rapid cognitive improvement in Alzheimer's disease following perispinal etanercept administration. *J Neuroinflammation* **5**:2.

Toulouse A, Sullivan AM. 2008. Progress in Parkinson's disease – where do we stand? *Prog Neurobiol* **85**:376–392.

Tranah GJ. 2011. Mitochondrial-nuclear epistasis: implications for human aging and longevity. *Ageing Res Rev* **10**:238–252.

Trist DG. 2011. Scientific process, pharmacology and drug discovery. *Curr Opin Pharmacol.* **11**: 528–537.

U.S.–Venezuela Collaborative Research Project, Wexler NS. 2004. Venezuelan kindreds reveal that genetic and environmental factors modulate Huntington's disease age of onset. *Proc Natl Acad Sci USA* **101**:3498–3503.

Van Broeckhoven C. 2010. The future of genetic research on neurodegeneration. *Nat Med* **16**:1215–1217.

Volonte C, Amadio S, Cavaliere F et al. 2003. Extracellular ATP and neurodegeneration. *Curr Drug Target CNS Neurol Disord* **2**:403–412.

Waldmeier P, Bozyczko-Coyne D, Williams M, Vaught JL. 2006. Recent clinical failures in Parkinson's disease with apoptosis inhibitors underline the need for a paradigm shift in drug discovery for neurodegenerative diseases. *Biochem Pharmacol* **72**:1197–1206.

Waldmeier P, Spooren WP, Hengerer B. 2000. CGP 3466 protects dopaminergic neurons in lesion models of Parkinson's disease. *Naunyn-Schmideber's Arch Pharmacol* **362**:526–537.

Weksler ME, Gouras G, Relkin NR, Szabo P. 2005. The immune system, amyloid-beta peptide, and Alzheimer's disease. *Immunol Rev* **205**:244–256.

Weydt P, Soyal SM, Gellera C et al. 2009. The gene coding for PGC-1α modifies age at onset in Huntington's Disease. *Mol Neurodegener* **4**:3.

Wijesekera LC, Leigh PN. 2009. Amyotrophic lateral sclerosis. *Orphanet J Rare Dis* **4**:3.

Wilcock GK. 2010. Bapineuzumab in Alzheimer's disease: where now? *Lancet Neurol* **9**:134–136.

Williams M. 2009. Progress in Alzheimer's disease drug discovery: an update. *Curr Opin Invest Drugs* **10**:23–34.

Wischik CM, Wischik DJ, Storey JMD, Harrington CR. 2010. Rationale for tau aggregation inhibitor therapy in Alzheimer's disease and other taopathies. In *Emerging Drugs and Targets for Alzheimer's Disease, Vol. 1, Beta-Amyloid, Tau Protein, and Glucose Metabolism.* Martinez A, ed. *RSC Drug Discovery Series.* Cambridge: Royal Chemical Society, pp. 210–232.

Wong E, Cuervo AM. 2010. Autophagy gone awry in neurodegenerative diseases. *Nat Neurosci* **13**:805–811.

World Alzheimer Report 2009. London, UK: Alzheimer's Disease International. Available at: http://www.alz.co.uk/research/files/WorldAlzheimerReport.pdf. Accessed August 5, 2011.

Wu Y, Le W, Jankovic J. 2011. Preclinical biomarkers of Parkinson disease. *Arch Neurol* **68**:22–30.

Xu K, Bastia E, Schwarzschild M. 2005. Therapeutic potential of adenosine A_{2A} receptor antagonists in Parkinson's disease. *Pharmacol Ther* **105**:267–310.

Yang J-L, Weissman L, Bohr VA, Mattson MP. 2008. Mitochondrial DNA damage and repair in neurodegenerative disorders. *DNA Repair* **7**:1110–1120.

Yu TJ, Zhang Y, Kenricj M et al. 2011. Boosting brain uptake of a therapeutic antibody by reducing its affinity for a transcytosis target. *Sci Transl Med* **3**:84ra44.

Zajicek JP, Apostu VI. 2011. Role of cannabinoids in multiple sclerosis. *CNS Drugs* **25**:187–201.

Zetterberg Z, Mattsson N, Blennow K, Olsson B. 2010. Use of theragnostic markers to select drugs for phase II/III trials for Alzheimer disease. *Alzheimer's Res Ther* **2**:32.

Zhao L, Teter B, Morihara T. 2004. Insulin-degrading enzyme as a downstream target of insulin receptor signaling cascade: implications for Alzheimer's disease intervention. *J Neurosci* **24**:11120–11126.

Zheng B, Liao Z, Locascio JJ et al. 2010. PGC-1alpha, a potential therapeutic target for early intervention in Parkinson's disease. *Sci Transl Med* **2**:52ra73.

Zhou Q, Sumbria R, Hui EK-A et al. 2011. Neuroprotection with a brain-penetrating biologic tumor necrosis factor inhibitor. *J Pharmacol Exp Ther* **339**:618–623.

Zuccato C, Valenza M, Cattaneo C. 2010. Molecular mechanisms and potential therapeutical targets in Huntington's disease. *Physiol Rev* **90**:905–981.

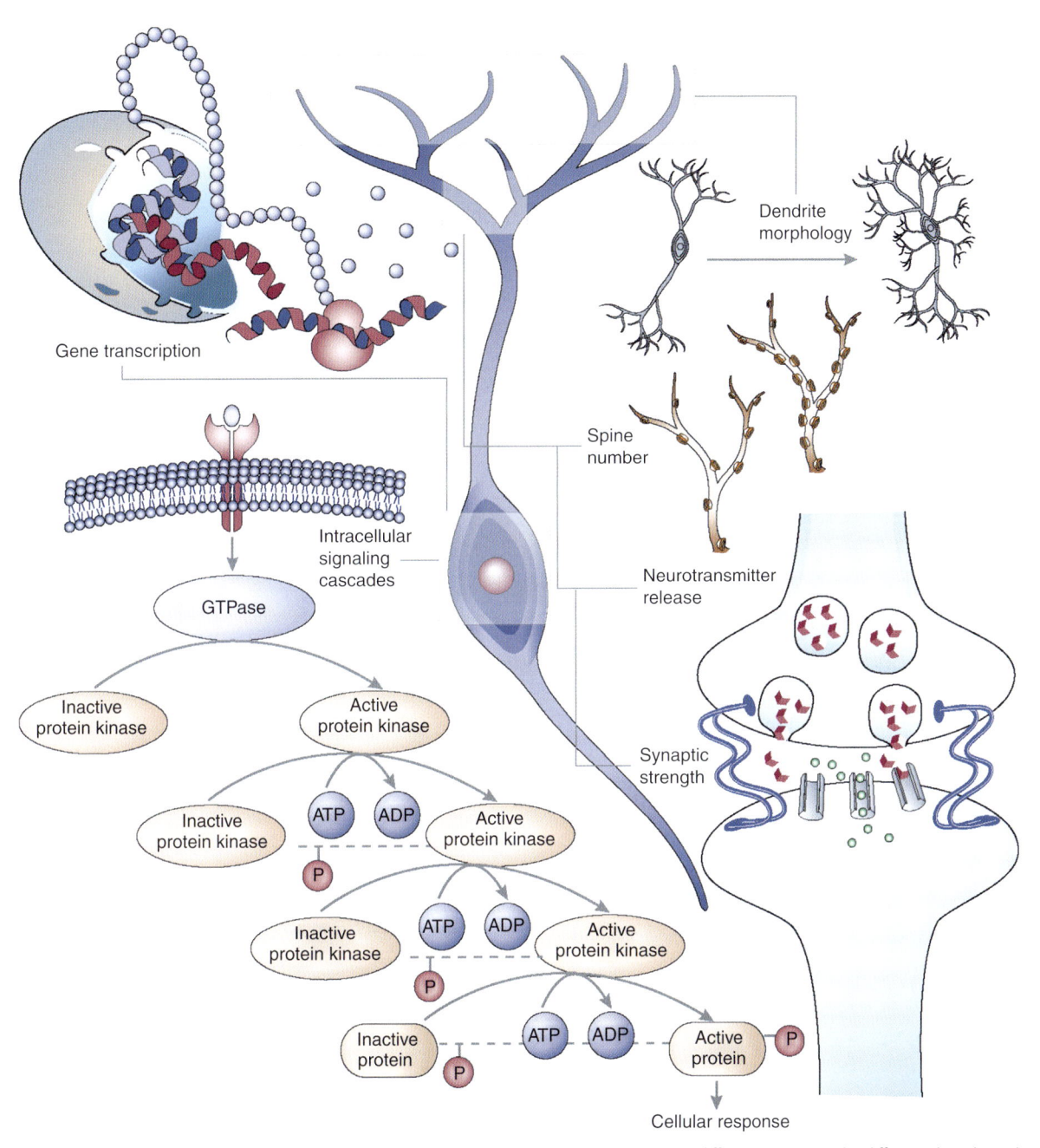

Figure 3.1. A true understanding of the pathophysiology of bipolar disorder must encompass different systems at the different physiological levels at which the disease manifests itself: molecular, cellular, and behavioral. Reprinted with permission from *Neuropsychopharmacology*, Vol. 33, Schloesser RJ, Huang J, Klein PS, Manji HK. Cellular plasticity cascades in the pathophysiology and treatment of bipolar disorder, pp. 110–133, copyright 2008.

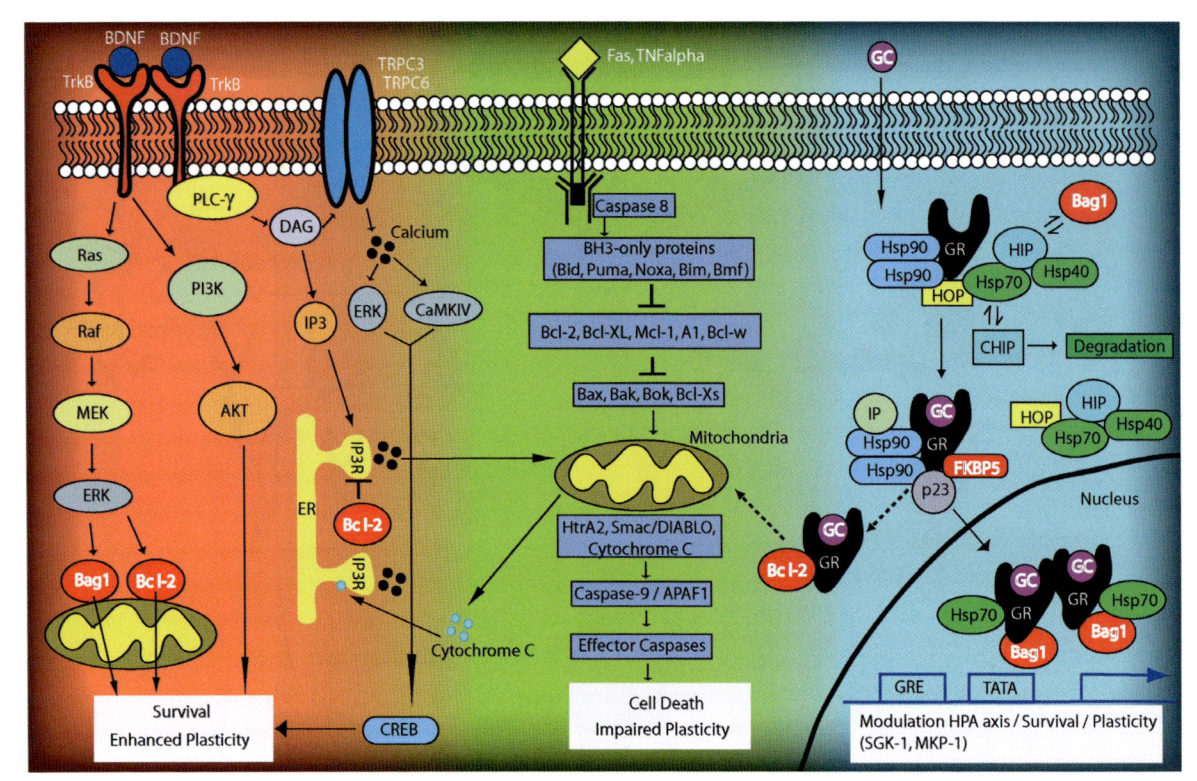

Figure 3.2. Cellular resiliency signaling pathways. (1) Neurotrophic factor signaling (left). BDNF activates its receptor, TrkB; phosphorylation can then activate either the ERK signaling cascade, PI3K, or PLC-γ. Ultimately, these independent pathways converge to enhance plasticity and cell survival. (2) Antiapoptotic signaling (center). Following activation of procaspases (e.g., caspase 8), proapoptotic factors are activated (BH3-only proteins), which in turn inhibit antiapoptotic proteins such as Bcl-2. This step enables proapoptotic members to form pores on the outer mitochondrial membrane, ultimately leading to the release of cytochrome C, activation of effector caspases (e.g., caspase 3) and, eventually, impaired plasticity and cell death. (3) GR signaling. Following a stress response, GCs are released and downregulate the HPA axis, eventually turning off the stress response. At the cellular level, GCs bind to their receptors, whereby different co-chaperones can modulate GR nuclear trafficking. FKBP5 and BAG-1 are two such co-chaperones that have opposing roles in either attenuating or enhancing GR nuclear trafficking, respectively. Once inside the nucleus, GRs bind to GREs and turn on downstream gene targets (e.g., SGK-1 and MKP-1), leading to enhanced survival and plasticity mechanisms. Alternatively, the GR can associate with Bcl-2 (dashed line) following acute doses of corticosterone. This complex translocates (dotted line) to the mitochondria to enhance survival, leading to enhanced cellular plasticity and resiliency. BDNF, brain-derived neurotrophic factor; CREB, cAMP response element binding protein; ERK, extracellular response kinase; GC, glucocorticoid; GR, glucocorticoid receptor; GRE, glucocorticoid response element; HPA, hypothalamic-pituitary-adrenal; TNF, tumor necrosis factor; TrkB, tyrosine kinase B. Reprinted from Brain Research, Vol. 1293, Hunsberger JG, Austin DR, Chen G, Manji HK. Cellular mechanisms underlying affective resiliency: the role of glucocorticoid receptor- and mitochondrially-mediated plasticity, pp. 76–84, copyright 2009, with permission from Elsevier.

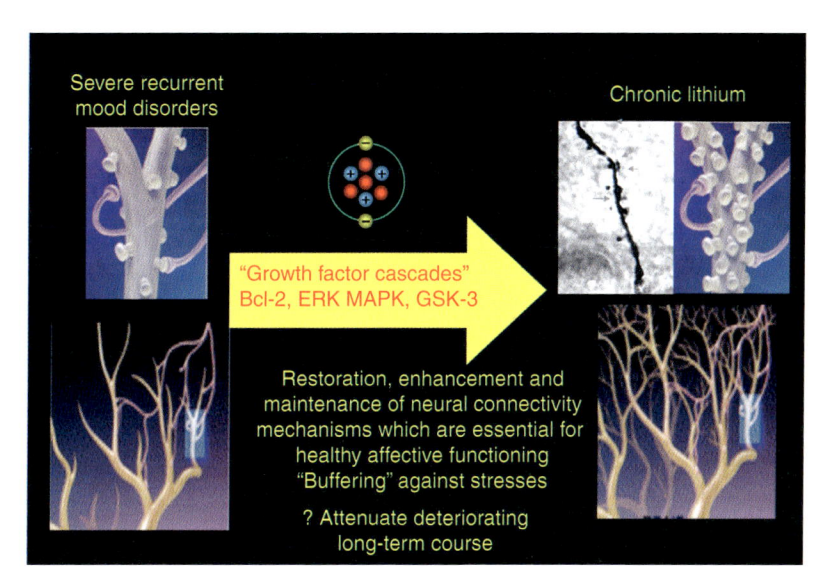

Figure 3.3. Potential impact of the neurotrophic effects of lithium. Many patients with severe mood disorders exhibit volumetric reductions in critical brain areas. However, the available data suggest that – in contrast to traditional neurodegenerative diseases like Alzheimer's disease – severe mood disorders are associated with regional atrophic changes rather than widespread degenerative changes. This figure depicts (left) the reduced neuronal branches and reductions in spine density. It is our contention that these structural impairments contribute to the neural circuitry abnormalities observed in patients (because the dendritic spines represent the processes on which one neuron synapses onto another, the atrophy of dendritic spines results in impaired synaptic connectivity). Lithium exerts major effects on a number of neurotrophic pathways, most notably via inhibition of GSK-3, activation of ERK MAP kinases, and upregulation of neurotrophic members of the Bcl-2 family. Lithium, via these cellular effects, is thought to reverse the illness-related atrophic changes, thereby restoring the synaptic and neural circuitry mediating affective, cognitive, motoric, and neurovegetative functions. These effects would also serve to "buffer" against stresses and likely play a role in attenuating long-term deterioration. GSK-3, glycogen synthase kinase 3. Adapted from *Neuron*, Vol. 34, Nestler EJ, Barrot M, DiLeone RJ, Eisch AJ, Gold SJ, Monteggia LM. Neurobiology of depression, pp. 13–25, copyright 2002, with permission from Elsevier.

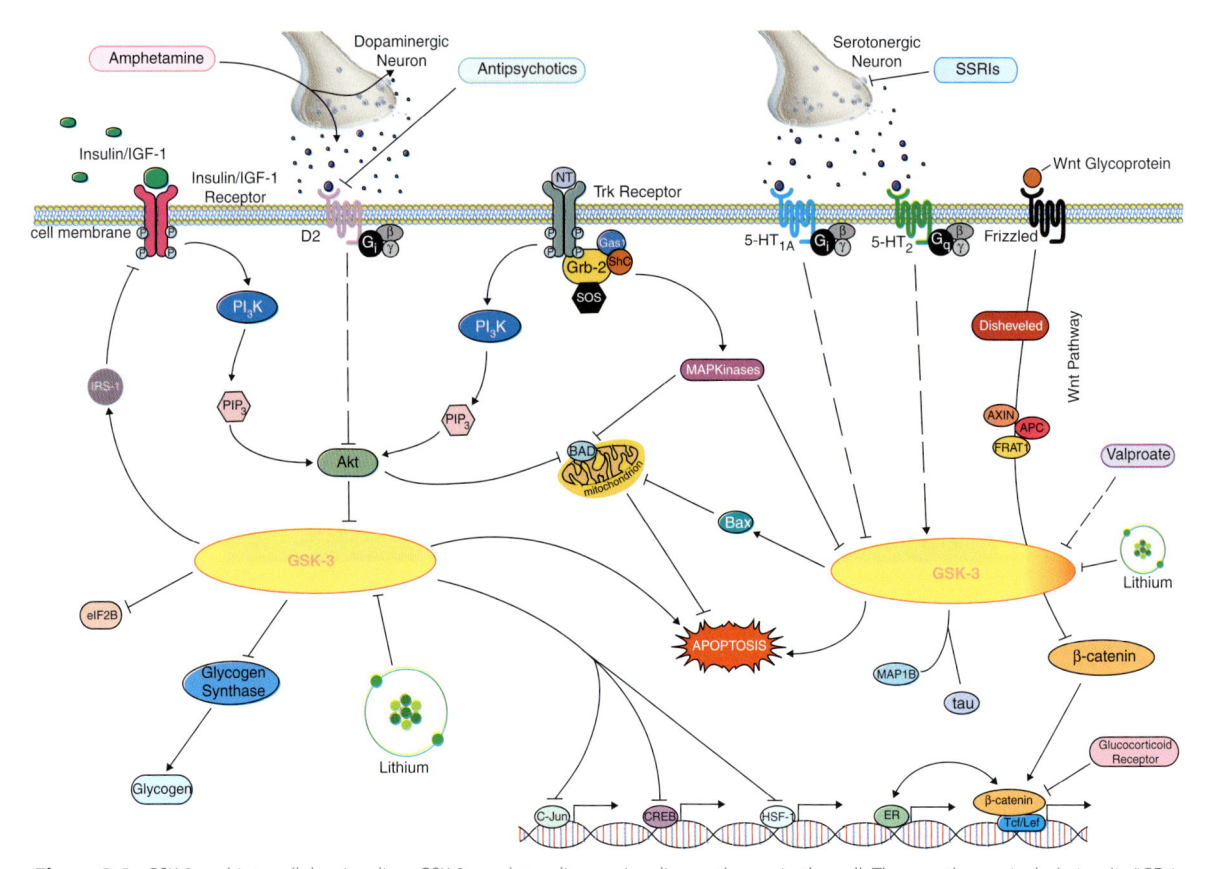

Figure 3.4. GSK-3 and intracellular signaling. GSK-3 regulates diverse signaling pathways in the cell. These pathways include insulin/IGF-1 signaling, neurotrophic factor signaling, and Wnt signaling. Insulin signaling through its Trk receptor activates PI3K-mediated signaling, resulting in GSK-3 inhibition. GSK-3 inhibition activates glycogen synthase and eIF2B while inhibiting IRS-1, an inhibitor of the insulin receptor. Insulin is generally thought to minimally affect central nervous system (CNS) neurons; however, IGF-1 interacting with its cognate receptor appears to have similar functions. NTs act through Trk receptors A, B, and C to activate PI3K and Akt and to inhibit GSK-3. Many effectors have been implicated in the neurotrophic effects of GSK-3 including transcription factors (e.g., HSF-1, C-Jun, and CREB) and BAX, a proapoptotic member of the Bcl-2 family. In the Wnt signaling pathway, secreted Wnt glycoproteins interact with the Frizzled family of receptors and, through disheveled-mediated signaling, inhibit GSK-3. Stability of this process requires the scaffolding proteins AXIN and APC. Normally active GSK-3 phosphorylates β-catenin, leading to its ubiquitin-dependent degradation. However, when GSK-3 is inhibited in the Wnt pathway, β-catenin is not degraded, allowing for its interaction with TCF to act as a transcription factor. β-catenin activity is modulated by the intracellular ER, which also affects transcription of an independent set of genes. As shown in the figure, medications used to treat mood disorders have both direct and indirect effects on GSK-3 and GSK-3-regulated cell signaling pathways, including the direct effects of lithium and indirect effects of antipsychotics, amphetamine, and SSRIs. These distinct pathways have convergent effects on cellular processes such as bioenergetics (energy metabolism), neuroplasticity, neurogenesis, resilience, and survival. Thus, lithium (and other medications) may act by enhancing these processes via GSK-3 inhibition. However, as detailed in the text, GSK-3 modulates a number of signaling pathways not shown in the figure. It remains to be determined which pathway(s) are most relevant to the actions of lithium in the treatment of bipolar disorder and major depressive disorder. G_i refers to G_i/G_o; G_q refers to G_q/G_{11}. APC, adenomatous polyposis coli; CREB, cyclic AMP response element binding protein; eIF2B, eukaryotic initiation factor 2B; ER, estrogen receptor; GSK-3, glycogen synthase kinase 3; HSF-1, heat shock factor-1; insulin-like growth factor 1; IRS-1, insulin receptor substrate-1; NT, neurotrophin; Tcf, T cell-specific transcription factor; Trk, tyrosine receptor kinase. Reprinted from *Current Drug Targets,* Vol. 7, Gould TD, Picchini AM, Einat H, Manji HK. Targeting glycogen synthase kinase-3 in the CNS: implications for the development of new treatments for mood disorders, pp. 1399–1409, copyright 2006, with permission from Bentham Science Publishers.

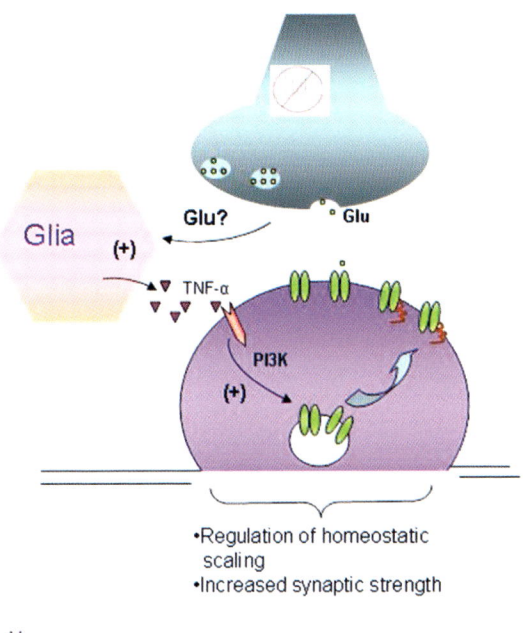

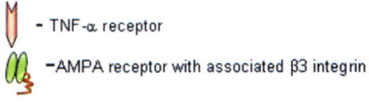

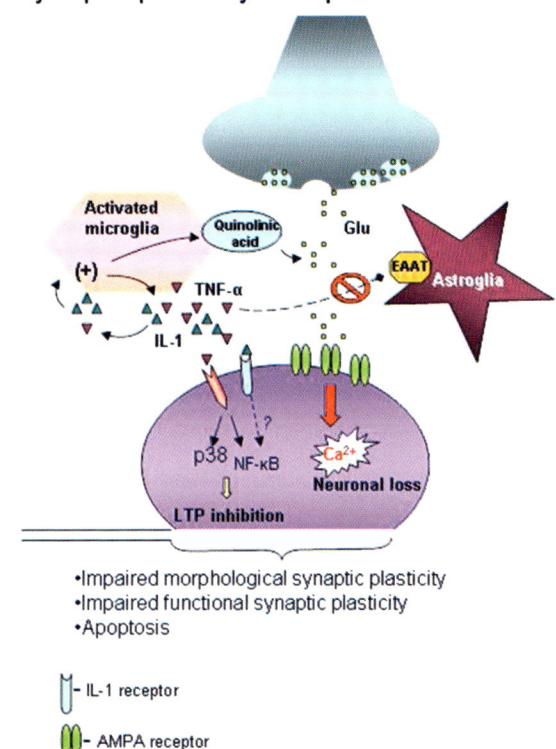

Figure 3.5. Dual role of proinflammatory cytokines in regulating synaptic plasticity. The diagram on the left depicts the critical role of constitutively expressed TNF-alpha in regulating homeostatic synaptic plasticity in the normal brain. Decreased neuronal activity and consequently reduced glutamate release from axons is sensed by glia, which trigger release of TNF-alpha. TNF-alpha activates neuronal TNF-alpha receptor type I (TNFR1), leading to activation of the phosphoinositide-3 kinase (PI3K) pathway and upregulation of the specific adhesion molecule-β3 integrin; this step in turn triggers AMPA receptor insertion to the membrane and increases synaptic strength. The diagram on the right depicts the various signaling cascades initiated by high pathophysiological levels of proinflammatory cytokines in the brain by activated microglia, which might underlie at least some aspects of the pathophysiology of depression. (1) TNF-alpha and IL-1 trigger production of quinolinic acid and release of glutamate by microglia; (2) TNF-alpha and IL-1 inhibit glutamate removal by astrocytes, leading to excess extracellular glutamate and neurotoxicity; (3) TNF-alpha acts via TNFR1 to upregulate membrane expression of calcium-permeable AMPA receptor subunits, thus leading to increased calcium influx and neuronal death; (4) TNFR1 activation coupled to activation of p38 and NF-κB pathways inhibits the early and late phases of LTP. These effects of pathophysiological levels of proinflammatory cytokines on synaptic plasticity at both morphological and functional levels might underlie the cognitive disturbances and memory impairments seen in patients with depression. AMPA, alpha-amino-3-hydroxy-5-methyl-4-isoxazolepropionic acid; Glu, glutamate; TNF, tumor necrosis factor. Reproduced from *International Journal of Neuropsychopharmacology*, Vol. 12, Khairova R, Machado-Vieira R, Du J, Manji HK. A potential role for pro-inflammatory cytokines in regulating synaptic plasticity in major depressive disorder, pp. 561–578, copyright 2009, with permission from Cambridge University Press.

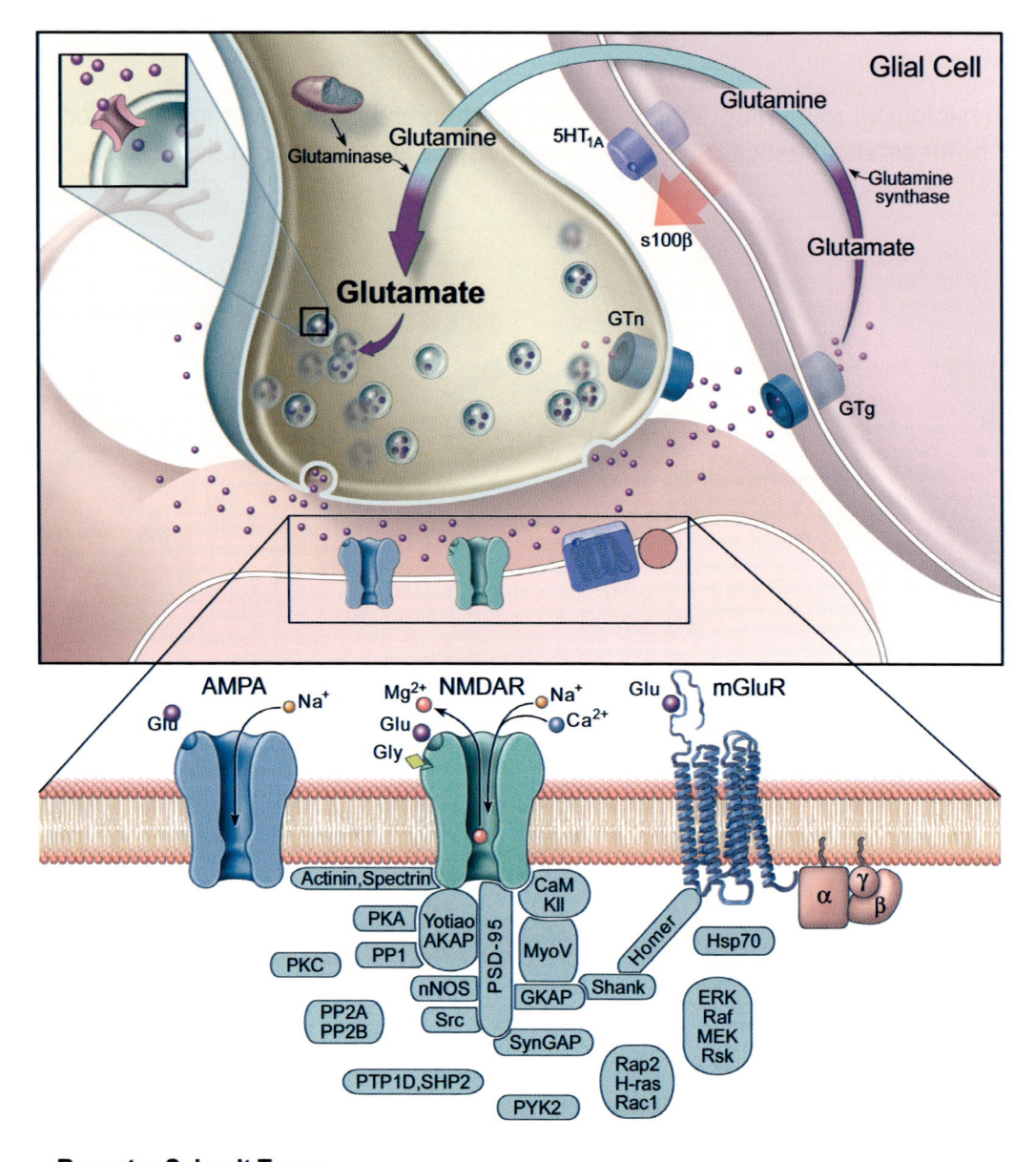

Receptor Subunit Types

Ionotropic			Metabotropic		
NMDA	AMPA	Kainate	Group I	Group II	Group III
NR1	GluR 1	GluR 5	mGlu 1 a-b-c-d	mGlu 2	mGlu 4 a-b
NR2 A-B-C-D	GluR 2	GluR 6	mGlu 5 a-b	mGlu 3	mGlu 6
NR3 A-B	GluR 3	GluR 7			mGlu 7 a-b
	GluR 4	KA 1			mGlu 8 a-b
		KA 2			

Figure 3.6. This figure depicts the various regulatory processes involved in glutamatergic neurotransmission. The biosynthetic pathway for glutamate involves synthesis from glucose and the transamination of a-ketoglutarate; however, a small proportion of glutamate is formed more directly from glutamine by glutamine synthetase. The latter is actually synthesized in glia and, via an active process (requiring ATP), is transported to neurons where, in the mitochondria, glutaminase is able to convert this precursor to glutamate. Furthermore, in astrocytes, glutamine can undergo oxidation to yield a-ketoglutarate, which can also be transported to neurons and participate in glutamate synthesis. Glutamate is either metabolized or sequestered and stored in secretory vesicles by VGluTs. Glutamate can then be released by a calcium-dependent excitotoxic process. Once released from the presynaptic terminal, glutamate binds to numerous excitatory amino acid (EAA) receptors, including ionotropic receptors (e.g., NMDA and mGluRs). Presynaptic regulation of glutamate release occurs through mGluR$_2$ and mGluR$_3$, which subserve the function of autoreceptors; however, these receptors are also located on the postsynaptic element. Glutamate has its action terminated in the synapse by reuptake mechanisms using distinct glutamate transporters (labeled VGT in the figure) that exist

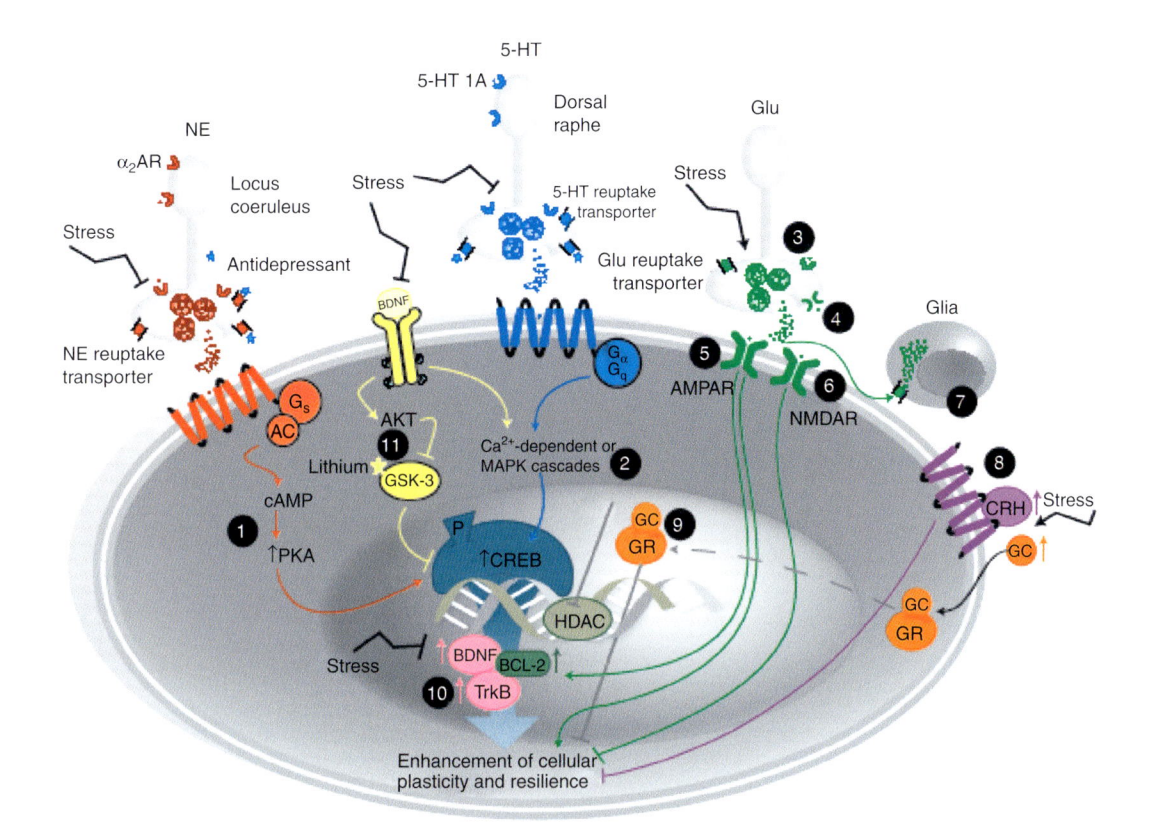

Figure 3.7. Enhancing cellular plasticity and resilience in the development of novel agents for the treatment of severe mood disorders. This figure depicts the multiple targets through which cellular plasticity and resilience may potentially be regulated in the treatment of severe mood disorders. Genetic/neurodevelopmental factors, repeated affective episodes (and likely elevations of glucocorticoids), and illness progression may all contribute to the impaired cellular resilience, volumetric reductions, and cell death and atrophy observed in mood disorders. Bcl-2 attenuates apoptosis by sequestering pro-forms of death-driving cysteine proteases (called caspases), by preventing the release of mitochondrial apoptogenic factors such as calcium, cytochrome c, and AIF into the cytoplasm, and by enhancing mitochondrial calcium uptake. Antidepressants regulate the expression of BDNF, and its receptor TrkB. Both TrkA and TrkB use the PI3K/Akt and ERK MAP kinase pathways to bring about their neurotrophic effects. The ERK MAP kinase cascade also increases the expression of Bcl-2 via its effects on CREB. (1) Phosphodiesterase inhibitors increase the levels of pCREB; (2) MAP kinase modulators increase Bcl-2 expression; (3) mGluR II/III agonists modulate the release of excessive levels of glutamate; (4) drugs such as lamotrigine and riluzole act on sodium channels to attenuate glutamate release; (5) AMPA potentiators upregulate the expression of BDNF; (6) NMDA antagonists such as ketamine enhance plasticity and cell survival; (7) novel drugs to enhance glial release of trophic factors and clear excessive glutamate may be useful for treating mood disorders; (8) CRH and (9) glucocorticoid antagonists attenuate the deleterious effects of hypercortisolemia, and CRH antagonists may exert other beneficial effects in the treatment of depression through non-HPA mechanisms; (10) agents that upregulate Bcl-2 (e.g., lithium, valproate, or pramipexole) could be useful in treating severe mood disorders as well as other disorders associated with atrophic changes; (11) GSK-3 inhibition may prevent apoptosis while also playing a role in synaptic plasticity. AIF, apoptosis-inducing factor; AMPA, alpha-amino-3-hydroxy-5-methyl-4-isoxazolepropionic acid; Bcl-2, B-cell lymphoma 2; BDNF, brain-derived neurotrophic factor; CREB, cAMP response element binding protein; CRH, corticotropin-releasing hormone; Glu, glutamate; HT, hydroxytryptophan; NE, norepinephrine; NMDA, N-methyl-D-aspartate; pCREB, phosphorylated-CREB. Reprinted from *Science Signaling STKE*, Vol. 2004, Issue 225, 2004. Charney DS, Manji HK. Life stress, genes, and depression: multiple pathways lead to increased risk and new opportunities for intervention, p. re5.

Figure 3.6. (cont.)
on not only presynaptic nerve terminals but also astrocytes; indeed, current data suggest that astrocytic glutamate uptake may be more important for clearing excess glutamate, raising the possibility that astrocytic loss (as has been documented in mood disorders) may contribute to deleterious glutamate signaling, but more so by astrocytes. It is now known that a number of important intracellular proteins are able to alter the function of glutamate receptors (see figure). Also, growth factors such as glial-derived neurotrophic factor (GDNF) and S100b secreted from glia exert a tremendous influence on glutamatergic neurons and synapse formation. Notably, serotonin$_{1A}$ (5-HT$_{1A}$) receptors are regulated by antidepressant agents; this receptor is also able to modulate the release of S100b. Modified from Szabo et al. 2004. AKAP, A kinase anchoring protein; CaMKII, Ca^{2+}/calmodulin–dependent protein kinase II; ERK, extracellular response kinase; GKAP, guanylate kinase-associated protein; Glu, glutamate; Gly, glycine; GTg, glutamate transporter glial; GTn, glutamate transporter neuronal; Hsp70, heat shock protein 70; MEK, mitogen-activated protein kinase/ERK; mGluR, metabotropic glutamate receptor; MyoV, myosin V; NMDAR, NMDA receptor; nNOS, neuronal nitric oxide synthase; PKA, protein kinase A; PKC, protein kinase C; PP-1, PP-2A, PP-2B, protein phosphatases; RSK, ribosomal S6 kinase; SHP2, src homology 2 domain–containing tyrosine phosphatase; vGluTs, vesicle glutamate transporters. Reprinted from Szabo S, Gould TD, Manji HK. Neurotransmitters, receptors, signal transduction pathways and second messengers, pp. 3–52, *American Psychiatric Publishing Textbook of Psychopharmacology*, copyright © 2004, with permission from the American Psychiatric Association.

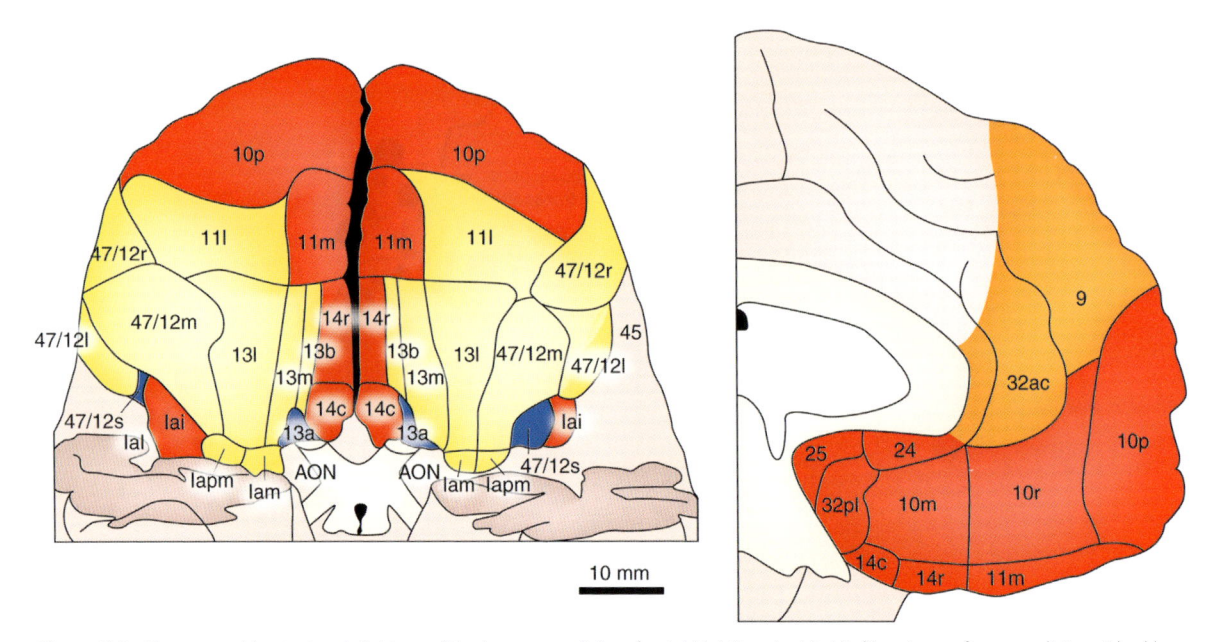

Figure 3.8. The cytoarchitectonic subdivisions of the human medial prefrontal (right) and orbital (left) cortex surfaces are distinguished here as being predominantly in the medial (red) and orbital (yellow) prefrontal networks. The orange areas are part of the dorsal prefrontal system. Modified from *Journal of Comparative Neurology*, Vol. 460, Ongur D, Ferry AT, Price JL. Architectonic subdivision of the human orbital and medial prefrontal cortex, pp. 425–449, copyright 2003, with permission from John Wiley and Sons.

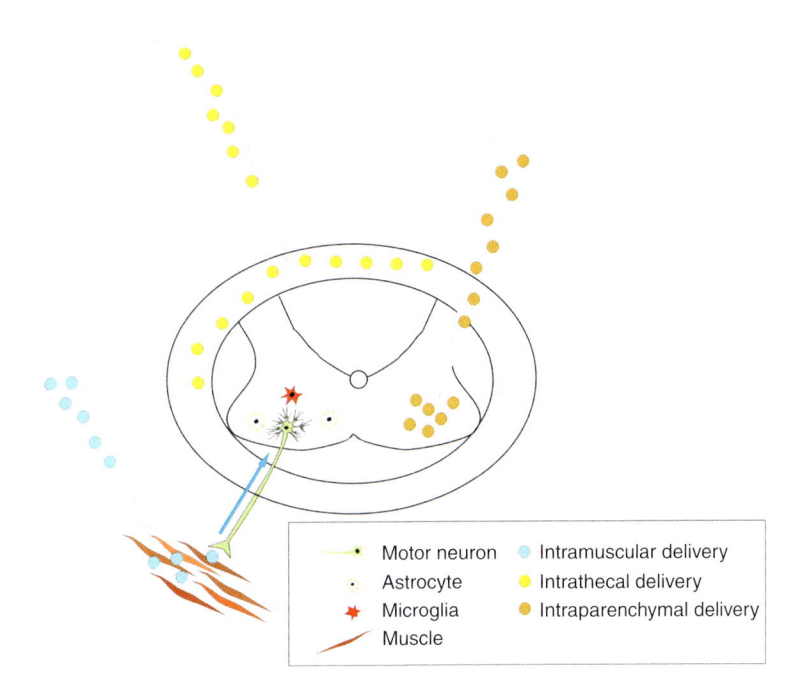

Figure 12.1. Gene therapy applications. Previous studies in animal models and humans with ALS included intraparenchymal spinal cord delivery of viral vectors with genes encoding for growth factors and antiapoptotics (orange circles). Intramuscular injection of viral vectors or transcription factors activating endogenous growth factors (blue circles) result in retrograde transport to the host motor neurons and spinal cord (blue arrow). Ex vivo polymer capsules containing hamster kidney cells expressing CNTF were injected into the CSF space (yellow circles).

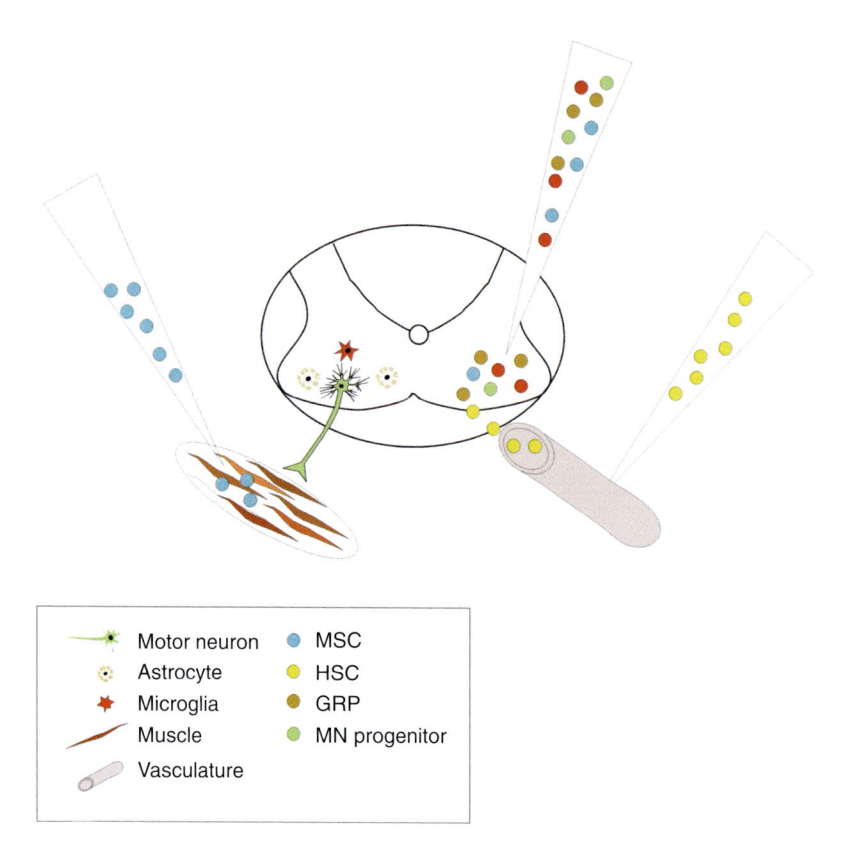

Figure 12.2. Cell transplantation approaches. Potential strategies for cell replacement include direct intraparenchymal delivery of motor neuron, astrocyte, or microglial progenitor cells (red, orange, green circles). Intraparenchymal or muscle delivery of mesenchymal stem cells could provide trophic support to host motor neurons (blue circles). Hematopoietic stem-cell delivery via bone marrow transplantation and delivery of cells into the vasculature offer benefits of lower surgical risk and widespread distribution (yellow circles). MSC, mesenchymal stem cells; HSC, hematopoietic stem cells; GRP, glial restricted precursors; MN, motor neuron progenitors.

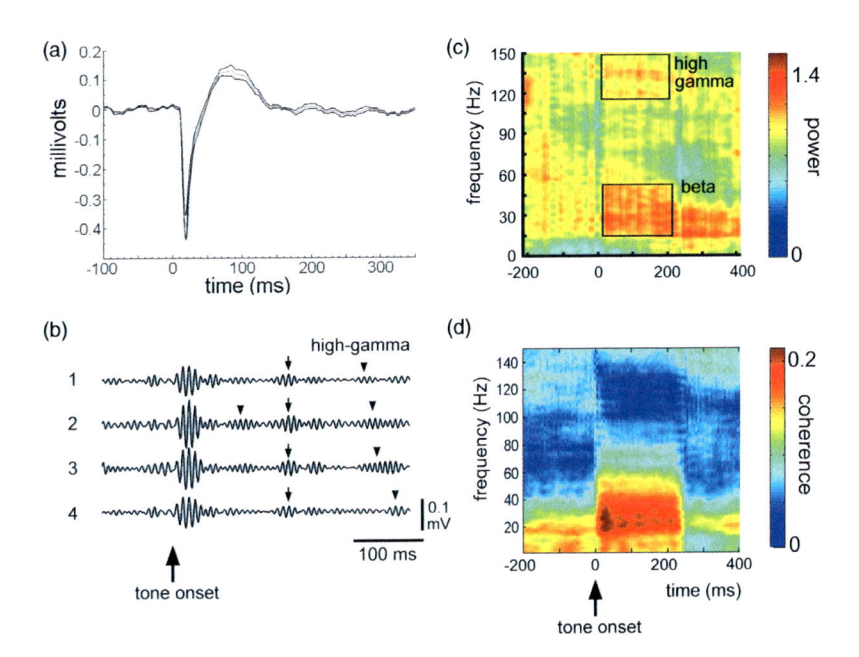

Figure 16.4. Gamma (30–140 Hz) oscillation and coherence within primary auditory cortex (A1) during listening in the awake rat. (A) Wideband local field potential. (B) Gamma oscillations in four simultaneously recorded sites triggered by tone onset. (C) Peristimulus time spectrogram of a characteristic multispike unit recorded from A1 during passive listening. (D) Mean peristimulus time coherogram of single neuron spiking with simultaneously recorded local field potentials during passive listening. Modified from *European Journal of Neuroscience*, Vol. 33, Vianney-Rodrigues P, Iancu OD, Welsh JP. Gamma oscillations in the auditory cortex of awake rats, pp. 119–129, copyright 2011, with permission from John Wiley and Sons.

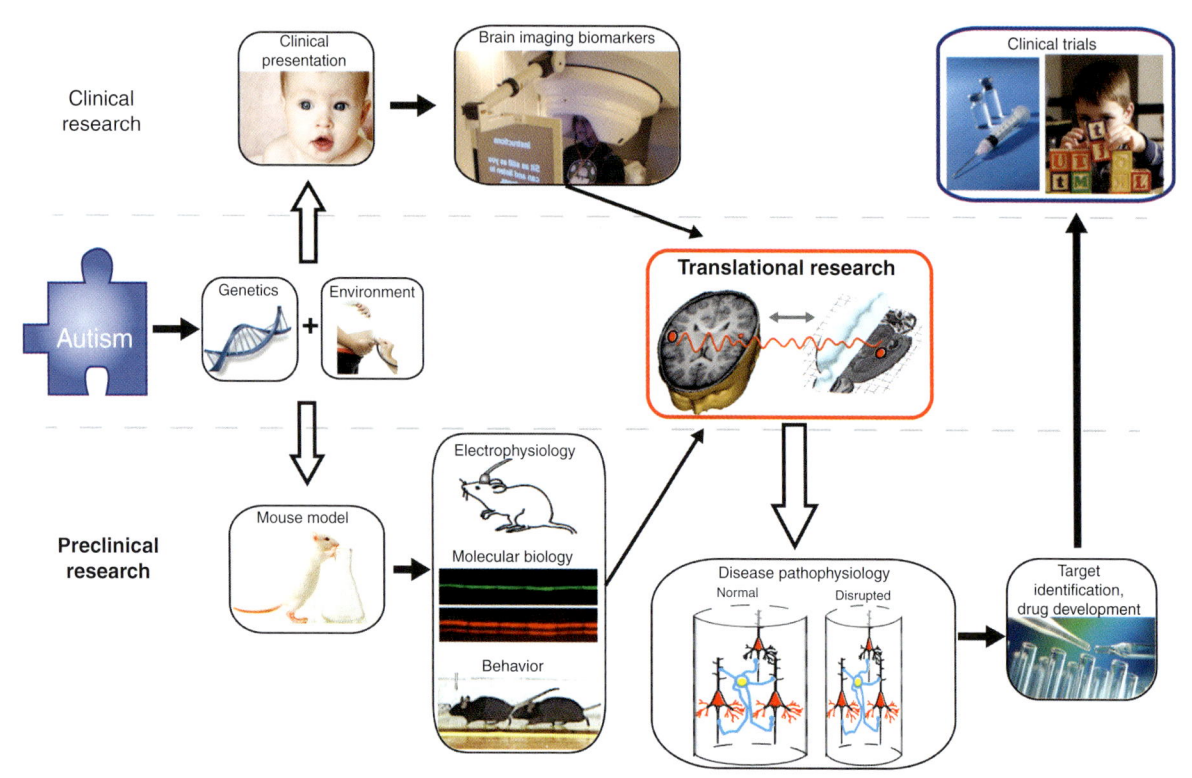

Figure 16.5. Approach to translational research in autism spectrum disorders. Clinical epidemiological studies have identified several autism candidate genes and environmental risk factors. Preclinical mouse models are being developed to recreate these genetic perturbations or environmental exposures. Such rodent models can then be investigated for alterations in molecular and cellular biology, behavior, and electrophysiology. Clinical studies, in particular those involving brain imaging and electrophysiology, are being done to identify autism endophenotypes. These heritable, quantitative metrics are more closely related to the abnormal brain dynamics of autism spectrum disorders than are the behavioral criteria and can help dissect gene–brain–behavior relationships in a complex genetic disorder. Endophenotypes can often be measured directly in preclinical models to help provide insight into the pathophysiology of disease and to provide new targets for preclinical therapeutic development.

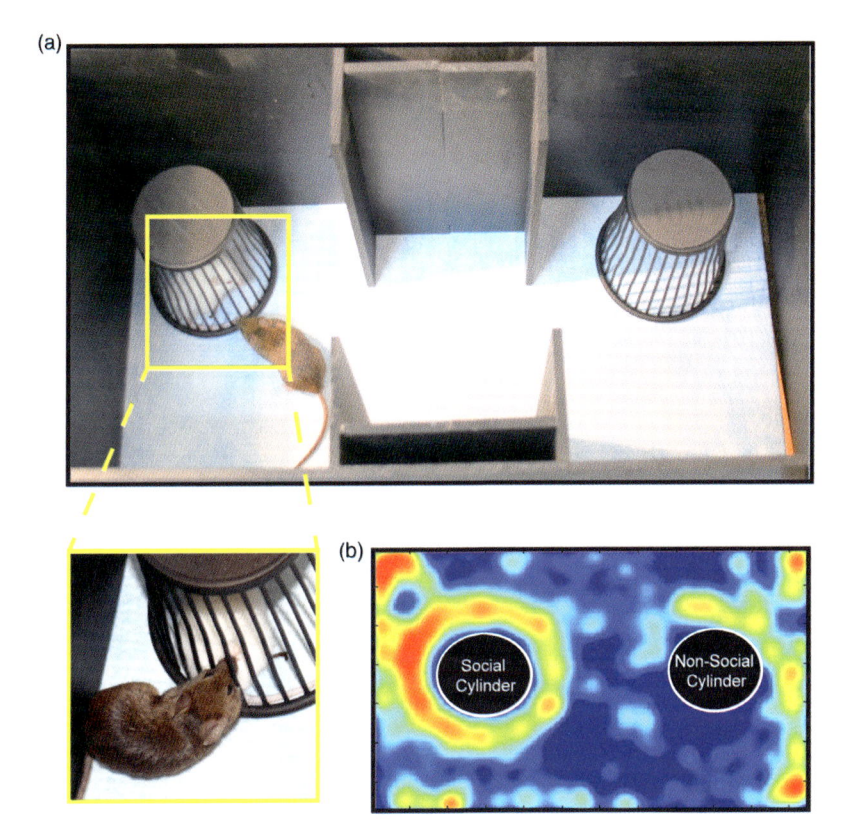

Figure 16.6. Social choice testing in rodents measures affiliative approach-and-avoidance behaviors. (A) A three-chambered social approach/avoidance apparatus is shown with an immobile (white) stimulus mouse and a freely moving (brown) test mouse. A video camera above (not shown) tracks the movements and the sniffing behavior of the test mouse. (Inset) The test mouse can engage in olfactory, auditory, and visual investigation of the stimulus mouse. (B) A heat map indicates where the test mouse is located during a 10-minute session. As shown, the test mouse spends significantly more time investigating the social cylinder than the nonsocial cylinder.

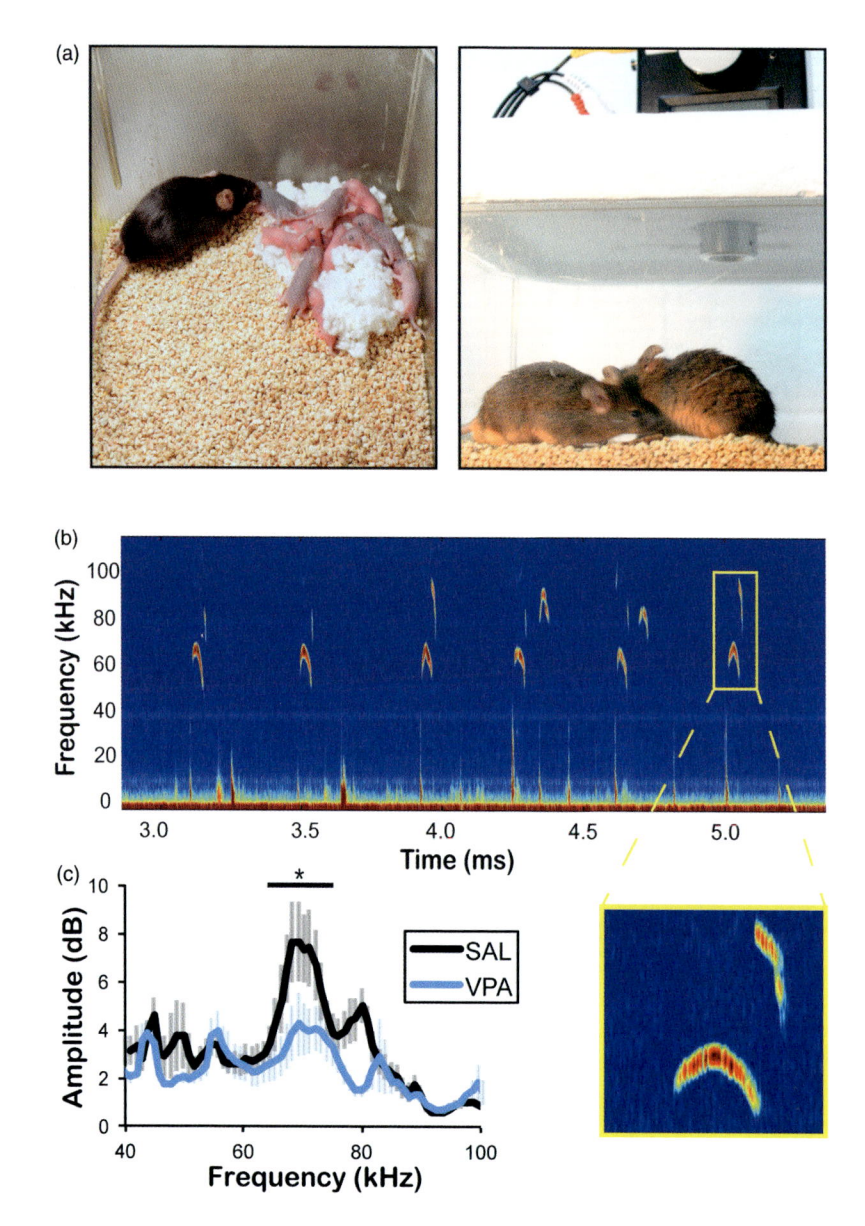

Figure 16.7. Rodent ultrasonic vocalizations are used as a measure of communicative function in preclinical models of autism. (A) In mice, ultrasonic vocalizations are generally investigated in two types of paradigms (Messeri et al. 1975). Neonatal "distress" vocalizations are elicited by temporarily removing a single mouse pup from the litter. Ultrasonic calls emitted by the isolated infant serve as a signal for the dam to come retrieve the pup (Szatmari et al. 2007). Adult same-sex mice will emit ultrasonic vocalizations when paired together after several days of social isolation. In addition, male mice will emit characteristic 70-kHz premating vocalizations and 40-kHz mating vocalizations when paired with a receptive female. (B) Sonogram demonstrating the time and frequency characteristics of mouse vocalizations. Calls can be characterized by density, duration, frequency, intensity, and spectral shape (e.g., prosody). (C) A spectrogram of adult male premating vocalizations recorded from male mice exposed to prenatal valproic acid (VPA) or saline (SAL) when paired with a wild-type receptive female mouse. SAL-exposed mice demonstrate a characteristic peak at 70 kHz that is notably absent in the group exposed to VPA. Modified from *Biological Psychiatry*, Vol. 68, Gandal MJ, Edgar JC, Ehrlichman RS, Mehta M, Roberts TP, Siegel SJ. Validating gamma oscillations and delayed auditory responses as translational biomarkers of autism, pp. 1100–1106, copyright 2010, with permission from Elsevier.

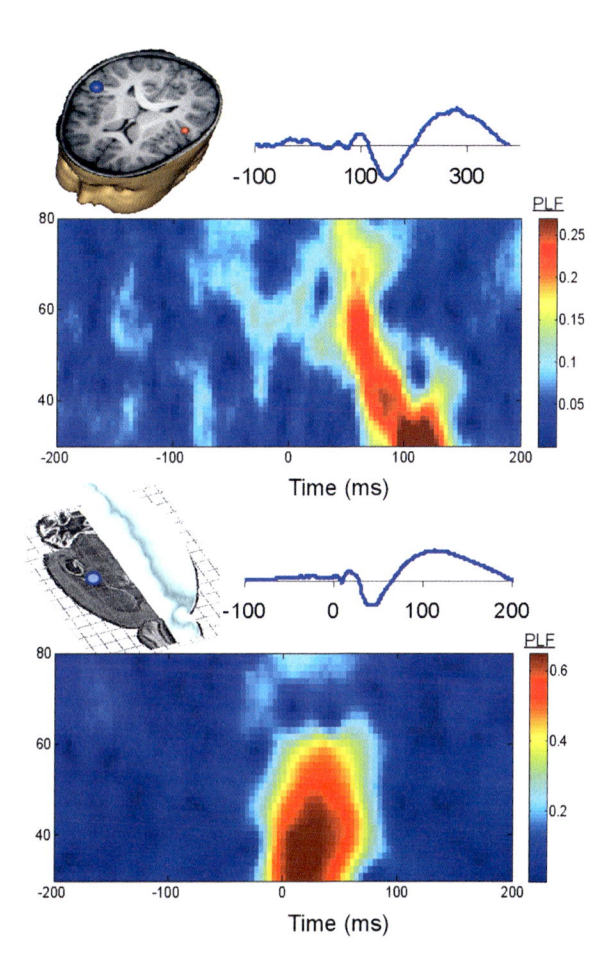

Figure 16.9. Pure-tone auditory evoked responses recorded around the auditory cortex are demonstrated in humans (top) using magnetoencephalography and in mice (bottom) using intracranial electrodes. Top plots show time-domain grand averages of auditory evoked responses, which demonstrate corresponding P1/M50 and N1/M100 peaks. Bottom plots show transient gamma-band phase-locking, with peak responses in both groups occurring at ~40 Hz. Modified from *Biological Psychiatry*, Vol. 68, Gandal MJ, Edgar JC, Ehrlichman RS, Mehta M, Roberts TP, Siegel SJ. Validating gamma oscillations and delayed auditory responses as translational biomarkers of autism, pp. 1100–1106, copyright 2010, with permission from Elsevier.

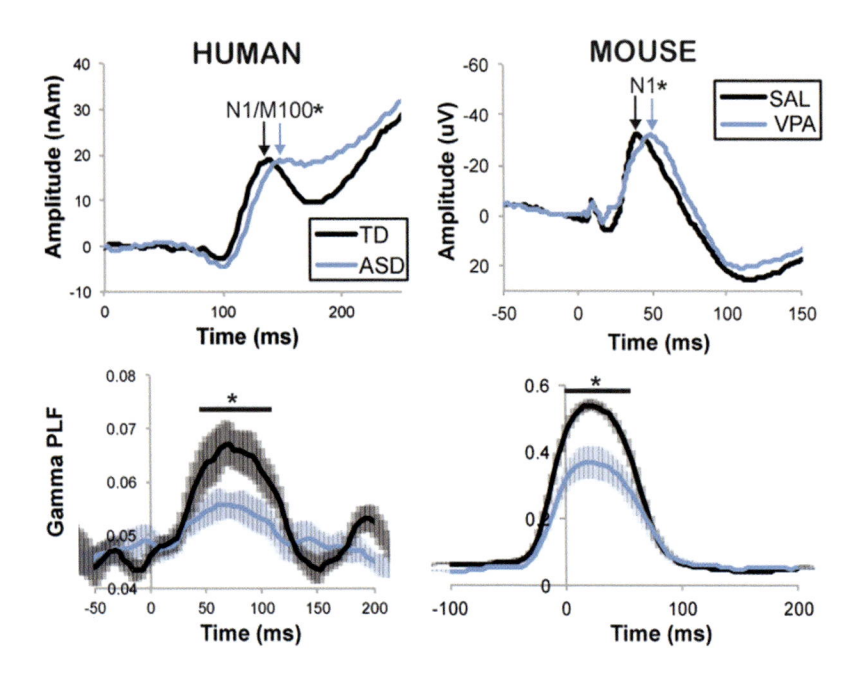

Figure 16.10. The translational potential of auditory evoked-response endophenotypes is demonstrated. (Left column) Pure-tone auditory evoked responses were recorded in children with autism (ASD) and in typically developing (TD) controls. (Right column) Auditory evoked potentials were recorded using analogous methods in the prenatal valproic acid (VPA)-mouse model of autism and in saline (SAL)-treated controls. (Top row) Children with autism and VPA-exposed mice show a significant, ~10% delay in the latency of the N1/M100 auditory evoked response, indicating similar deficits in the temporal precision of auditory stimulus encoding. (Bottom row) Children with autism and VPA-treated mice demonstrate deficits in the transient auditory gamma-band response, suggesting deficient excitatory–inhibitory balance. Modified from *Biological Psychiatry*, Vol. 68, Gandal MJ, Edgar JC, Ehrlichman RS, Mehta M, Roberts TP, Siegel SJ. Validating gamma oscillations and delayed auditory responses as translational biomarkers of autism, pp. 1100–1106, copyright 2010, with permission from Elsevier.

Chapter 8

Alzheimer's disease

Donald L. Price, Alena V. Savonenko, Tong Li, and Philip C. Wong

Over the past two decades, we have seen extraordinary progress in clinical discovery and preclinical research in the field of neurodegenerative disorders (Price *et al.* 2008). These investigations, including studies of animal models (Price *et al.* 2008), have provided important new directions for translation to the benefit of many patients with these illnesses. Studies of Alzheimer's disease (AD), the most common of these diseases of the central nervous system (CNS), illustrate the complementary contributions of advances in both clinical and basic research.

Effective therapies for AD are a major unmet medical need because of its demographics (incidence/prevalence); morbidity/mortality rates; healthcare costs; paucity of mechanism-based treatments; and impact on affected individuals, caregivers, and society at large (Bishop *et al.* 2010; Blennow *et al.* 2006; Perrin *et al.* 2009; Querfurth and LaFerla 2010; Price *et al.* 2008). The clinical syndrome (i.e., cognitive and memory disturbances progressing to dementia in elderly persons) results from the dysfunction and death of neurons in specific brain regions and circuits critical for memory and cognition (Blennow *et al.* 2006; Buckner *et al.* 2008). The neuropathology of AD (Braak *et al.* 2006; Markesbery *et al.* 2006) includes the accumulation of extracellular β-pleated amyloid beta (Aβ) 42 peptides, which, as toxic oligomeric assemblies and/or aggregates (Cai *et al.* 2001; Price *et al.* 2008; Shankar *et al.* 2008; Wong *et al.* 2008), are at the cores of amyloid plaques (surrounded by swollen neurites). As described below, Aβ 42 is neurotoxic, particularly at synapses, and the plaques, at some level, represent sites of synaptic disconnection in the forebrain (Liu *et al.* 2008; Price *et al.* 2008). Within affected neurons, neurofibrillary tangles (NFT) are accumulations of misfolded tau (a microtubule-associated protein), the assembly of which into paired helical filaments (PHF) and, ultimately, into NFT (Ballatore *et al.* 2007; Goedert and Spillantini 2006; Mandkelkow *et al.* 2007), may be driven by the presence of β-sheet fragments of tau generated by cleavages in the microtubule binding domains of tau (Mocanu *et al.* 2008; Wang *et al.* 2007). At present, some investigators have hypothesized a fundamental pathogenic cascade that includes Aβ-mediated damage to synapses; alterations in the neuronal cytoskeleton; "dying back" of axons; and dysfunction of nerve cells (Liu *et al.* 2008). Eventually, those neurons exhibiting tau pathology die (Braak *et al.* 2006; de Calignon *et al.* 2010). The links between the amyloid/Aβ and NFT/tau abnormalities are not yet well defined. Moreover, the roles of microglial cells and astrocytes in pathogenesis and repair require further clarification (Grathwohl *et al.* 2009; Konigsknecht-Talboo *et al.* 2008; Weiner and Frenkel 2006).

As detailed below, this age-associated illness is influenced by genetic risk factors, with a minority of cases having inherited autosomal dominant mutations (*APP*, *PS1*, and *PS2*), and, rarely, duplications of *APP* (Hardy 2006). More commonly, putative sporadic cases are influenced by a variety of susceptibility genes (especially, in a dose-dependent fashion, by *ApoE4*) and possibly by other less well-defined factors (Bertram and Tanzi 2008; Blennow *et al.* 2006; Lambert *et al.* 2009; Perrin *et al.* 2009; Price *et al.* 2008). Symptomatic treatments are available, but, at present, efficacious and safe mechanism-based therapies are not yet available (Aisen 2009; Blennow *et al.* 2006; Perrin *et al.* 2009).

We describe the scientific progress that has led to an understanding of this illness and to the design of new therapeutic approaches targeting disease mechanisms. We emphasize clinical and preclinical studies,

---

Translational Neuroscience, ed. James E. Barrett, Joseph T. Coyle and Michael Williams. Published by Cambridge University Press. © Cambridge University Press 2012.

including advances in assessments of biomarkers, brain imaging, genetics, neuropathological techniques, biochemistry (involves amyloid peptide precursor [APP], Aβ, tau), synaptic biology, and the development of genetically engineered animal models (McGowan *et al.* 2006; Price *et al.* 2008). These animal models have been used in studies of pathogenic mechanisms and in approaches to identify therapeutic targets. Moreover, they have proved valuable for testing a variety of experimental treatments (Ballatore *et al.* 2007; Blennow *et al.* 2006; Brody and Holtzman 2008; Chiti and Dobson 2006; Cohen and Kelly 2003; Goedert and Spillantini 2006; Price *et al.* 2008; Wong *et al.* 2008).

We first describe the syndromes of mild cognitive impairment (MCI) and AD (Blennow *et al.* 2006; Wong *et al.* 2008); the utility of diagnostic tests (Perrin *et al.* 2009), including findings from a variety of brain-imaging studies (Buckner *et al.* 2008; Klunk *et al.* 2004; Villemagne *et al.* 2010); the results of measurements of biomarkers in serum and cerebrospinal fluid (CSF) (Bateman *et al.* 2006, 2009; Fagan *et al.* 2005; Graff-Radford *et al.* 2007; Perrin *et al.* 2009); and the neuropathological and biochemical nature of the disease (Blennow *et al.* 2006; Fagan *et al.* 2005; Graff-Radford *et al.* 2007; Klunk *et al.* 2004). Subsequently, we focus on identified causative and risk genes (Blennow *et al.* 2006; Lambert *et al.* 2009) and information derived from the outcomes of transgenic and gene targeting strategies (Price *et al.* 2008) that have been used to create disease models (i.e., mice expressing AD-linked mutant transgenes) and to identify potential therapeutic opportunities (targeting of genes encoding proteins implicated in disease pathways) (Price *et al.* 2008). Our goal is to show how investigations of model systems have delineated the efficacies and, on some occasions, potential toxicities related to manipulation of therapeutic targets (Price *et al.* 2008). In animal models, documentation of beneficial outcomes and clarification of safety issues are critical for design of the new therapeutic approaches that are beginning to enter human trials. As this science is translated to the bedside, clinical, imaging, and biomarker studies, which are proving to be of value for early and accurate diagnosis of AD, will be critical for assessing the outcomes of these human trials. In our view, these new disease-modifying therapies, applied in the earliest stages of disease, even in borderline or symptomatic individuals with abnormalities in biomarker profiles (decrease in β and increase in τ in CSF or β burden documented on PIB), will have a major impact on the lives of elderly individuals worldwide.

Clinical and laboratory features of individuals with MCI and AD

The index case of AD, a middle-aged woman with behavioral disturbances and dementia, was described, along with the pathological features of AD, more than 100 years ago (Blennow *et al.* 2006; Perrin *et al.* 2009; Price *et al.* 2008). AD affects more than 4 million individuals in the USA and is characterized by progressive impairment in memory and cognitive processes, leading ultimately to dementia (Blennow *et al.* 2006; Perrin *et al.* 2009; Wong *et al.* 2008). Many elderly persons exhibit MCI, characterized by memory complaints and mild abnormalities of performance on formal tests, associated with intact general cognition and preserved activities of daily living (Andrews-Hanna *et al.* 2007; Bishop *et al.* 2010; Blennow *et al.* 2006; Perrin *et al.* 2009; Querfurth and LaFerla 2010). Although not all individuals with MCI progress to AD, this syndrome, particularly the amnestic form (aMCI), is regarded as a transitional stage between normal aging and early AD or as an initial manifestation of AD (Blennow *et al.* 2006; Markesbery *et al.* 2006; Perrin *et al.* 2009). As the illness advances, patients with AD develop progressive difficulties with memory and performances in a variety of cognitive functions (Blennow *et al.* 2006; Buckner *et al.* 2008; Perrin *et al.* 2009). In the late stages, affected individuals become profoundly demented.

In the early stages of the disease, physicians rely for diagnosis on histories, on physical, neurological, and psychiatric examinations, and on the results of neuropsychological tests (Blennow *et al.* 2006; Perrin *et al.* 2009). More recently, studies of biomarkers in body fluids and imaging of the brain offer great promise for early diagnosis and for assessing outcomes of anti-amyloid treatments (Bateman *et al.* 2006, 2009; Fagan *et al.* 2005; Graff-Radford *et al.* 2007; Klunk *et al.* 2004; Perrin *et al.* 2009; Querfurth and LaFerla 2010; Villemagne *et al.* 2010). One recent study demonstrated the association of low plasma Aβ 42/40 ratios with elevated risk for MCI and AD (Graff-Radford *et al.* 2007). Another investigation suggested that levels of blood-borne Aβ dimers correlated with levels of clinical markers (Villemagne *et al.* 2010). In cases of AD, the levels of Aβ peptides in CSF are often low and the levels of tau in CSF are elevated compared with controls (Perrin *et al.* 2009; Sunderland *et al.* 2003). Using a novel in vivo approach, investigators showed that the production and turnover of Aβ in CSF is rapid (Bateman *et al.* 2006; Perrin *et al.* 2009). Imaging studies of value (Buckner *et al.* 2008; Matthews *et al.* 2006; Perrin *et al.* 2009; Sperling *et al.* 2009) include: magnetic resonance imaging, which discloses progressive atrophy of specific regions of the brain, particularly the hippocampus and entorhinal cortex; functional magnetic resonance imaging, which allows assessment of blood flow and synaptic activity (Matthews *et al.* 2006; Perrin *et al.* 2009); and 18F deoxyglucose positron emission tomography (PET) or single photon emission computerized tomography (SPECT), which detects decreased glucose utilization and reductions in regional blood flow, usually in the parietal and temporal lobes (Blennow *et al.* 2006; Klunk *et al.* 2004; Perrin *et al.* 2009). Moreover, inverse relationships may exist between the amyloid load in the brain (as assessed by PET amyloid imaging) and levels (low) of Aβ in CSF. The uptake in the brain of C11-labeled Pittsburgh compound B (PIB), a labeled ligand that binds to Aβ, can be assessed by PET. In individuals with AD (Buckner *et al.* 2008; Klunk *et al.* 2004; Perrin *et al.* 2009), PIB is retained in brain regions commonly associated with amyloid deposition, presumably reflecting the time course of amyloidosis and its relationship to the clinical and pathological stages of disease. It has been suggested that (18F)FDDNP may be retained by NFT, but to date agents that selectively bind to aggregates of tau have not been validated (Perrin *et al.* 2009).

Over the past decade, Raichle and colleagues described the default mode network (DMN) (Zhang and Raichle 2010), an anatomically defined system of interacting brain circuits that are preferentially active when persons are not focused on the external environment. This network exhibits greatest activity when individuals are engaged in internal modes of thought, including retrieval of personal memories, attempts to envision the future, and efforts to appreciate the perspectives of others (Buckner *et al.* 2008; Zhang and Raichle 2010). In these circuits, the medial temporal lobe provides information from prior experiences in the form of memories and associations that are the building blocks of mental simulation, whereas the medial prefrontal subsystem engages in the flexible use of this information during the generation of mental simulations relevant to self (Buckner *et al.* 2008). In turn, this system provides information to integrative nodes, including those in the posterior cingulate and retrosplenial cortex. Thus the DMN uses past experiences to plan for the future, navigate social interactions, and maximize the utility of activities when individuals are not otherwise engaged by the external world (Buckner *et al.* 2008; Zhang and Raichle 2010). Significantly, the high levels of activities exhibited by the DMN require much of the metabolic demand of the brain. Recent studies (Buckner *et al.* 2008; Sperling *et al.* 2009) suggest that abnormalities in the activities of this network may be associated with the manifestations of a variety of mental disorders including AD, autism, and schizophrenia. For example, Sperling and coworkers (2009) used amyloid imaging to demonstrate that amyloid deposition is associated with altered activity of this DMN as measured by functional magnetic resonance imaging in asymptomatic and minimally impaired older individuals; these latter subjects exhibit patterns of dysfunction similar to those occurring in individuals developing AD. These findings are interpreted as evidence for the hypothesis that cognitively intact older individuals with amyloid in the brain may be in the early stages of AD. Moreover, the hypometabolism seen in cases of AD involves regions of the DMN. Significantly, the production of Aβ appears to be closely linked to synaptic activity (Kamenetz *et al.* 2003; Perrin *et al.* 2009). It has been hypothesized that the DMN, because of its high levels of activity over many years, may be particularly vulnerable to increased production of Aβ and, ultimately, to formation of AD plaques (Buckner *et al.* 2008; Perrin *et al.* 2009).

Biomarker and imaging studies should promote more accurate diagnosis of AD in its early stages and presumably will lead to accurate assessments of the efficacies of new antiamyloid therapeutics (Bateman *et al.* 2006, 2009).

Clinical features, neuropathology, and biochemistry

The clinical manifestations of AD arise from abnormalities involving brain regions and neural circuits composed of populations of neurons that are essential for memory, learning, and cognitive performance (Bishop *et al.* 2010; Braak *et al.* 2006; Buckner *et al.* 2008; Markesbery *et al.* 2006; Price *et al.* 2008; Querfurth and LaFerla 2010). Damaged neural systems include: basal forebrain cholinergic neurons; circuits in the amygdala and hippocampus; and, predominantly, glutamatergic nerve cells in the entorhinal and limbic cortices and in the neocortex (Blennow et al. 2006; Braak et al. 2006; Coyle et al. 1983; Markesbery et al. 2006; Whitehouse et al. 1982). In general, the character, distributions, and abundance of abnormalities (i.e., levels of Aβ burden and the presence of neuritic Aβ plaques and NFT [Blennow et al. 2006; Braak et al. 2006], the reductions in neurotransmitter markers [Blennow et al. 2006; Sze et al. 1997], and the degeneration of synapses and nerve cells) are thought to correlate with the clinical states documented in individual cases. In several cognitively characterized cohorts, cases of early AD and cases of aMCI showed significant increases in the numbers of tangles in the ventral medial temporal lobe regions compared with age-matched controls (Markesbery et al. 2006).

The nature, evolution, and possible mechanisms of spread of pathology are the subjects of experimental studies described below. It is thought that aMCI reflects a transitional state in the evolution of AD. Memory deficits appear to correlate most closely with the abundance of NFT in CA1 of the hippocampus and in the entorhinal cortex, suggesting that NFTs, particularly in the medial temporal lobe, may be particularly significant during the progression from normal state to MCI to early AD (Markesbery et al. 2006). It is hypothesized that the spread of NFT beyond the medial temporal lobe (i.e., to areas of neocortex) is closely linked to impairments in cognition and, eventually, to dementia. Abnormalities within affected regions include the presence of conformationally altered isoforms of tau assembled into paired helical filaments (PHFs) in NFT (within neuronal cell bodies and dendrites, in swollen neurites, and in neuropil threads) (Ballatore et al. 2007; Blennow et al. 2006; Mandkelkow et al. 2007; Wang et al. 2007). Aβ-containing neuritic plaques, associated with both astroglial and microglial responses in the local surroundings, are thought to represent sites of synaptic disconnection in regions receiving inputs from disease-vulnerable populations of neurons. In primates and rodents, neuritic swellings represent degenerating axons and terminals and, possibly, dendrites (Martin et al. 1994), whereas axonal varicosities are hypothesized to represent focal perturbations of axonal transport (Mandkelkow et al. 2007; Martin et al. 1994). In the target fields of damaged nerve cells, generic and neurotransmitter-specific synaptic markers are reduced (Coyle et al. 1983; Sze et al. 1997). The mechanisms of synaptic damage, the initial sites of injury (pre- and/or postsynaptic), and the molecular pathways involved in these abnormalities, which appear to be closely linked to Aβ toxicity, are important areas of current research (described below). The mechanisms whereby disease may spread from cell to cell, circuit to circuit, and region to region are uncertain.

Thus, the clinical manifestations of aMCI and AD are attributed to impairments in synaptic communication within subsets of neural circuits, followed, as demonstrated in model systems (Liu et al. 2008), by the "dying back" degeneration of axons and, eventually, by the death of neurons. The presence of toxic Aβ42 peptides in terminal synaptic fields is hypothesized to be linked, in ways still uncertain, to the development of the abnormalities of tau (or tau fragments) in PHF accumulating in both neurites and cell bodies. One hypothesized scenario is as follows: Aβ42 species, liberated at synapses, oligomerize to form extracellular Aβ assemblies or Aβ-derived diffusible ligands (ADDLs) (Klein et al. 2001; Lesne et al. 2006; Liu et al. 2008; Shankar et al. 2008), which impact on pre- and postsynaptic targets, including glutamate receptors and other less well characterized targets possibly including involvement of glutamate transporters (Li 2009), leading to synaptic dysfunction and, eventually, to disconnection of terminals from postsynaptic targets (Lesne et al. 2006; Liu et al. 2008; Martin et al. 1994; Masliah et al. 2005; Selkoe 2002; Wong et al. 2008). Subsequently, a postulated retrograde signal (of uncertain nature), which originates in proximity to damaged terminals, activates ill-defined proteases, which serially cleave tau within the microtubule binding domains (generating self-assembling tau fragments) (Mocanu et al. 2008; Wang et al. 2007), and also presumably activating kinases (or inhibiting phosphatases) leading to hyperphosphorylation of P-tau in cell bodies and dendrites. Pleated β-sheet tau peptide species can bind to full-length tau and lead to well-established conformational changes in this protein and to the formation of PHF, followed by the destabilization of microtubules (Ballatore et al. 2007; Frost et al. 2009a, 2009b; Mandkelkow et al. 2007). Moreover, disturbances of the cytoskeleton are presumably associated with alterations in axonal transport that may influence amyloidogenesis (Goldsbury et al. 2006; Lazarov et al. 2005; Pigino et al. 2009; Price et al. 2008; Wong et al. 2008), which can, in turn, compromise the functions and viabilities of neurons. It is not known whether the tau-related dysfunction, thought to be associated with β-pleated sheet tau fragments, represents a loss of function (altered tubulin stability), the gain of an adverse property (tau sequestered in PHF impacting on axonal transport), or the mixture of these influences on neurons (Ballatore *et al.* 2007). Some of the differences in outcomes described in the literature may reflect the differences in the nature of the studies including: studies in in vitro versus in vivo model systems; different experimental designs; and in the difficulties of identifying specific pathogenic effects linked to different forms of the toxic proteins and their responsive target. The analyses of the character, participants, time courses, and contributions of these events in AD are difficult when investigators must rely on postmortem human tissue alone, and these issues are best examined in animal model systems (see below). Eventually, damaged nerve cells die by an uncertain mechanism (de Calignon *et al.* 2010), and extracellular "tombstone" tangles (Blennow *et al.* 2006; Braak *et al.* 2006) and neuritic amyloid plaques, surrounded by glial cells (Koenigsknecht-Talboo *et al.* 2008), represent the remains of the ravages of the disease.

Current treatment

Early information about the involvement of neurotransmitter-specific circuits damaged by the disease led to the design of early therapies for AD (Blennow *et al.* 2006), which were, in part, patterned on the treatments of Parkinson's disease with L-DOPA. For example, the discovery of cholinergic deficits in the cortex and hippocampus (Coyle *et al.* 1983) and of the degeneration of basal forebrain cholinergic neurons led to the introduction of cholinesterase inhibitors for treatment of patients. Evidence of involvement in glutamate systems in hippocampal and cortical circuits in AD, coupled with information about glutamate excitotoxicity (mediated, in part, by N-methyl-D-aspartate receptor [NMDA-R]), led to trials of memantine, an NMDA-R antagonist (Lipton 2007). This drug is designed to block excitotoxicity and, although not adversely influencing normal functions, is hypothesized to act as a neuroprotective agent in this setting. Both of these strategies may be associated with modest and transient symptomatic benefits in some patients, but neither class of drugs appears to impact directly on pathogenic mechanisms. Clearly, new therapies are needed.

Amyloidogenesis, APP, and amyloid precursor-like proteins (APLPs)

The members of the *APP* gene family (*APP* and *APLP1* and *2*) (Walsh *et al.* 2007) encode type I transmembrane proteins, but the neurobiological functions of these proteins are not clearly understood (Cao and Sudhof 2001; Heber *et al.* 2000; Kamenetz *et al.* 2003; Walsh *et al.* 2007; Wong *et al.* 2008). APP is abundant in the nervous system, is enriched in neurons, and is rapidly transported anterograde, along with components of the secretases, in axons to terminals (Buxbaum *et al.* 1998; Lazarov *et al.* 2005; Sisodia *et al.* 1993). Members of the APP family, APLP1 and 2, discovered by genetic searches, exhibit both similarities and differences compared with APP (Walsh *et al.* 2007). All possess single-pass transmembrane domains and conserved NPXY clathrin internalization signals in the conserved cytoplasmic domain. The APLPs lack the Aβ sequence of APP such that only cleavage of APP forms Aβ (Walsh *et al.* 2007). All three family members undergo shedding of the ectodomain and cleavage by γ-secretase and release of C-terminal intracellular domain fragments, which can mediate signaling functions. Gene targeting studies are consistent with the idea that some redundancies exist in the APP family: selective knockouts of single genes are associated with mild differences in phenotype, but $APLP2^{-/-}/APLP1^{-/-}$ and $APLP2^{-/-}/APP^{-/-}$ mice do not survive, whereas $APP^{-/-}/APLP1^{-/-}$ mice appear relatively normal (Heber *et al.* 2000).

As mentioned above, in the CNS, APP and the pro-amyloidogenic secretases are present in neurons and are carried anterograde by fast axonal transport (Buxbaum *et al.* 1998; Lazarov *et al.* 2005; Sisodia *et al.* 1993). At nerve terminals, Aβ peptides are generated by sequential endoproteolytic cleavages by BACE1 (at the Aβ +1 and +11 sites) to generate APP-β carboxyl terminal fragments (Buxbaum *et al.* 1998; Cai *et al.* 2001) and by the γ-secretase complex to form a variety of Aβ peptides (Iwata *et al.* 2004; Iwatsubo 2004; Jack *et al.* 2004; Kamenetz *et al.* 2003; Klunk *et al.* 2004; Klyubin *et al.* 2005; Ma *et al.* 2005). Moreover, the intramembranous cleavage of APP-β carboxyl terminal fragments by γ-secretase releases an APP intracellular domain (AICD) (Cao and Sudhof 2001), which can form a complex with Fe65, a nuclear adaptor protein (Cao and Sudhof 2001). Cao and Sudhof proposed that Fe65 and AICD or Fe65 alone (in a novel conformation) can gain access to the nucleus to influence gene transcription, a signaling mechanism analogous to that occurring in the pathway to generate the Notch1 intracellular domain (NICD). AICD signaling may play a role in learning and memory.

All three members of the APP family, which are cleaved by BACE1 to shed APP ectodomains (APPs) and are cleaved by γ-secretase to release C-terminal intracellular domain fragments, can serve signaling functions. BACE1 cleaves at the +1 and +11 sites of Aβ (see below) producing C-terminal peptides and a secreted ectodomain (APPs). Within endocytic compartments, γ-secretase cleavages generate the C-termini of Aβ peptides and short C-terminal fragments including an AICD (Cai et al. 2001; Laird et al. 2005; Li et al. 2003; Ma et al. 2005; Selkoe 2002; Vassar et al. 1999). Opinions differ as to the compartmental location of these biochemical events within neurons: One view holds that most of the Aβ is produced in presynaptic endosomes and is released at synapses; another school argues that Aβ peptides accumulate within neurons (Laferla et al. 2007).

BACE1 and BACE2

A transmembrane aspartyl protease, BACE1, is directly involved in the cleavage of APP at the +11 and +1 sites of Aβ in APP (Cai et al. 2001; Laird et al. 2005; Vassar et al. 1999). In the CNS, BACE1 is demonstrable in a variety of presynaptic terminals (Laird et al. 2005). Brain cells from *BACE1-/-* mice (Cai et al. 2001; Laird et al. 2005; Luo et al. 2001) do not produce Aβ1–40/42 and Aβ11–40/42, indicating that BACE1 is the neuronal β secretase (Cai et al. 2001; Laird et al. 2005). Compared with wild-type APP, *APPswe* is cleaved more efficiently than at the +1 site, resulting in an increase in BACE1 cleavage products (elevating all Aβ species).

BACE2 is not a pro-amyloidogenic enzyme in that it cleaves APP between residues 19 and 20 and 20 and 21 of the Aβ sequence. Although BACE2 appears in several populations of neurons in the CNS, its distribution is different from that of BACE1.

γ-Secretase

This multiprotein complex includes: presenilin (PS) 1 and PS2; nicastrin (Nct), a type I transmembrane glycoprotein; and Aph-1 and Pen-2, two multipass transmembrane proteins (De Strooper et al. 1998, 1999; Li et al. 2003; Selkoe 2003; Shen and Kelleher 2007; Wolfe 2006; Wolfe et al. 1999; Wong et al. 2008). This complex is essential for the regulated intramembranous proteolysis of a variety of transmembrane proteins, including APP and Notch (Li et al. 2003; Ma et al. 2005; Selkoe 2003; Shen and Kelleher 2007). PS1 and PS2 are two highly homologous 43- to 50-kD multipass transmembrane proteins (Selkoe 2003; Wolfe et al. 1999). PS contains two aspartyl residues that play roles in intramembranous cleavage at D257 in TM 6 and at D385 in TM 7; substitutions of these residues reduce secretion of Aβ and cleavage of Notch1 in vitro (Wolfe 2006; Wolfe et al. 1999). The functions of the various γ-secretase proteins and their interactions in the complex are not yet fully defined, but it has been suggested that the ectodomain of Nct may be important in substrate recognition and binding of amino-terminal stubs (of APP and other transmembrane proteins) generated by a sheddase (i.e., BACE1 for APP). In one model, Aph-1 and Nct form a precomplex that interacts with PS; subsequently, Pen-2 enters the complex, apparently conferring "preseninilase" activity, which cleaves PS to form an N-terminal ~28-kDa fragment and a C-terminal ~18-kDa fragment, both of which are critical components of the γ-secretase complex (Wolfe 2006; Wolfe et al. 1999; Wong et al. 2008). As mentioned below, nearly 50% of early-onset cases of familial AD (FAD) are linked to more than 100 different mutations in *PS1* (Hardy 2006; Price et al. 2008; Wong et al. 2008). A relatively small number of *PS2* mutations can also cause autosomal dominant FAD. The majority of abnormalities in *PS* genes are missense mutations that alter γ-secretase activities to increase the level of the Aβ42/Aβ40 ratio.

α-Secretase

The enzyme responsible for the α-cleavage site (+17) in the CNS is TACE (TNF alpha converting enzyme), also known as ADAM10. However, it is expressed at low levels in neurons of the CNS. In other cells in other organs, APP is predominantly cleaved endoproteolytically within the Aβ sequence via alternative, nonamyloidogenic pathways. For example, ADAM10 cleaves between Aβ residues 16 and 17 (Sisodia et al. 1990). The cleavage by α-secretase, which occurs predominantly in non-neural tissues, precludes the formation of Aβ peptides and serves to protect these cells and organs from Aβ amyloidosis (Wong et al. 2001).

Genetics
FAD and influences of risk factors

The genetics of AD are complex, often influencing phenotype in an age-dependent manner. Rare early-onset FAD mutations in *APP* and *PS* genes are inherited as autosomal dominant disorders; late-onset cases of AD without clear familial association reflect the influences of a variety of risk factors (Bertram and Tanzi 2008; Hardy 2006; Wong *et al.* 2008). FAD-causing mutations, occurring in three different genes, *APP* (chromosome 21), *PS1* (chromosome 14), or *PS2* (chromosome 1), located on three different chromosomes, increase the production of Aβ, leading to an overabundance of the Aβ42 species. *PS1*, the most frequently mutated gene, accounts for the majority of early-onset cases. The role of *APP* gene dosage has been documented in families with *APP* duplications and in individuals with Down syndrome (trisomy 21) who have an extra copy of *APP* (Hardy 2006). Moreover, the presence of specific alleles of other genes, including ApoE4, is a risk factor for putative sporadic disease (Bertram and Tanzi 2008; Hardy 2006; Price *et al.* 2008; Wong *et al.* 2008) (see below).

Autosomal dominant mutations usually manifest signs earlier than in sporadic cases, with the majority of mutations in *APP*, *PS1*, and *PS2* influencing BACE1 or γ-secretase cleavages of APP to increase the levels of all Aβ species or the relative amounts of toxic Aβ42. Individuals with duplications of *APP* (Rovelet-Lecrux *et al.* 2006) or with trisomy 21 (Hardy 2006) have an additional copy of *APP* and develop pathological signs of AD relatively early in life. Cases with autosomal dominant duplications of *APP* often show evidence of abundant vascular and parenchymal amyloid (Rovelet-Lecrux *et al.* 2006). The *APPswe* mutation enhances BACE1 cleavage at the +1 site N-terminus of Aβ, resulting in significant increases in the levels of all Aβ peptides. The *APP717* mutations promote γ-secretase cleavages to increase secretion of Aβ42, the most toxic Aβ peptide. Whereas these *APP* mutations alter the processing of APP and increase the production of Aβ peptides or the amounts of the more toxic Aβ42, other *APP* mutations enhance local fibril formation and some appear to promote vascular amyloidosis (congophilic angiopathy).

The *Apoε4* allele of the *apolipoprotein E* gene (chromosome 19q13) has been consistently demonstrated to be a major dose-dependent risk factor in a large number of studies across many ethnic groups (Bu 2009; Kim *et al.* 2009). *ApoE4* is a confirmed susceptibility allele, whereas *ApoE2*, a low-frequency allele, exhibits a weak protective effect. *ApoE4* is neither necessary nor sufficient to cause AD but appears to operate as a genetic risk modifier by reducing the age of onset in a gene dose-dependent manner. The biochemical consequences of the presence of *ApoE4* in the pathogenesis of AD are not yet fully understood, but this variant has been hypothesized to influence Aβ metabolism and Aβ aggregation, degradation, and particularly clearance (Bu 2009; DeMattos *et al.* 2004; Holtzman *et al.* 2000; Kim *et al.* 2009). ApoE isoforms also appear to differentially facilitate Aβ degradation by two metalloproteases, neprilysin and insulin degrading enzyme. In respect to Aβ disposition/clearance, ApoE4 appears to be the least effective ApoE variant. More recently, with regard to clearance of Aβ, new gene variants linked to late-onset AD cases are being identified. It should be emphasized that *APP*, *PS1* and *2*, and *ApoE* account for less than 50% of the genetic variants of AD (Wong *et al.* 2008).

Other risk genes

Recent research has identified gene variants encoding ubiquilin1 (*UBQLN1*) (Bertram *et al.* 2005) and sortilin1 (*SORL1*) (Rogaeva *et al.* 2007) as risk factors that may act by influencing ubiquilin-mediated proteosomal degradation and trafficking in endosomal pathways, respectively (Bertram *et al.* 2005; Rogaeva *et al.* 2007). The inherited variants of SORL1 are thought to influence levels of expression of the protein, a part of the retromer complex that plays an important role in APP trafficking and pathways of recycling such that reduced expression increases entry of APP into compartments generating Aβ (Rogaeva *et al.* 2007). Genome-wide association studies (GWAS) have shown that variants of *CLU* and *PICALM* or *CRI* genes are associated with AD (Harold *et al.* 2009; Lambert *et al.* 2009). It is unclear how many of the newly recognized susceptibility loci uncovered by systematic meta-analyses (Bertram and Tanzi 2008) will prove to be significant risk factors. To date, hundreds of independent association studies have not identified a single gene that contributes a risk approaching the same degree of consistency as *APOE4*.

Transgenic models of Aβ amyloidosis and tauopathies

In the autosomal dominant forms of this disorder (Hardy 2006), the misfolded proteins (tau) and peptides (Aβ) acquire properties that have direct or indirect impacts on the functions and viabilities of neural cells. Results of genetic investigations have led researchers to express mutant FAD genes in mice to model the disease (Borchelt et al. 1997; Jankowsky et al. 2005; Koenigsknecht-Talboo et al. 2008; LaFerla et al. 2007; Lesne et al. 2006; McGowan et al. 2006; Mocanu et al. 2008; Oddo et al. 2003; Price et al. 2008; Querfurth and LaFerla 2010; Savonenko et al. 2006; Wong et al. 2008; Yan et al. 2009) and to ablate genes in the disease pathways in efforts to define the molecular participants critical to pathogenesis (Cai et al. 2001; Chow et al. 2010; Laird et al. 2005; Lesne et al. 2006; Li et al. 2007b, 2009; Luo et al. 2001; McGowan et al. 2006; Price et al. 2008; Savonenko et al. 2006; Selkoe and Schenk 2003; Wong et al. 2008). Models of this disease have provided new insights into how these altered proteins contribute to pathogenic mechanisms (gains of adverse properties, loss of functions), particularly with regard to the roles of abnormal conformations of p-tau/tau fragments or cleavage-generated Aβ peptides (Borchelt et al. 1997; Frost and Diamond 2010; Lesne et al. 2006; McGowan et al. 2006; Serneels et al. 2009; Wong et al. 2008). Moreover, these models have been useful in identifying potential targets for therapy and in assessing new treatments and strategies (Brody and Holtzman 2008; Chow et al. 2010; Perrin et al. 2009; Wong et al. 2008).

Models of Aβ amyloidosis

Investigators have used genetic information to produce transgenic mouse models of amyloidosis (McGowan et al. 2006; Price et al. 2008; Querfurth and LaFerla 2010; Savonenko et al. 2006). Mice expressing *APPswe* or *APP717* (with or without mutant *PS1*) develop Aβ amyloidosis in the CNS (Borchelt et al. 1997; Chishti et al. 2001; Lesne et al. 2006; Liu et al. 2008; McGowan et al. 2006; Savonenko et al. 2005; Yan et al. 2009). Mutant *APP* + *PS1* mice develop an accelerated amyloidosis secondary to increased levels of Aβ (particularly Aβ42). In this model, diffuse deposits of Aβ and neuritic plaques have been associated with local glial responses in the hippocampus and cortex (McGowan et al. 2006). With age, levels of Aβ peptides, particularly Aβ42, increase significantly in the brain (Borchelt et al. 1997; Savonenko et al. 2005), and oligomeric species, variously termed Aβ-derived diffusible ligands (ADDLs), Aβ*56, etc., appear in the CNS (Klein et al. 2001; Klyubin et al. 2005; Lesne et al. 2006; Walsh et al. 2002; Wong et al. 2008). In part, depending on the nature of the mouse strain, transgene construct, types of mutations, and levels of expression, lines of mice show various degrees of amyloid deposition in vessels. In forebrain regions, the density of synaptic terminals is decreased (Liu et al. 2008), and axons show that retrograde degeneration (Liu et al. 2008; Savonenko et al. 2005) and levels of transmitter markers can be modestly reduced. In some settings, alterations occur in synaptic transmission, and, in some lines of mice, there is evidence of degeneration of subsets of neurons (Liu et al. 2008). In a series of experiments by Borchelt et al. (1997), *APPswe/ind* mice, whose transgene is regulated by doxycycline, showed high levels of transgene expression and exhibited amyloidosis in the brain (Jankowsky et al. 2005). After administration of doxycycline, levels of transgene expression were decreased (95%), accompanied by a decrease in Aβ production levels to those seen in nontransgenic animals. However, clearance of amyloid plaques appears to have been slow, and that strain of mice continues to exhibit significant Aβ burden after 6 months of treatment with doxycycline.

A variety of imaging approaches have been used to examine abnormalities in lines of mutant mice (Higuchi et al. 2005; Jack et al. 2004; Maeda et al. 2007; Meyer-Luehmann et al. 2008). Two recent studies are noteworthy: In one study, 11-carbon Pittsburgh compound B was interpreted to demonstrate significant retention of label in regions containing amyloid (Maeda et al. 2007); in a second investigation, a two-photon image of labeled compounds disclosed the rapid appearance of amyloid deposits associated with the appearance of dysmorphic neurites and the subsequent recruitment of microglia (Konigsknecht-Talboo et al. 2008; Meyer-Luehmann et al. 2008).

Behavioral studies of these lines of mice, including those generated by Savonenko et al. (2005, 2006), disclose deficits in spatial reference memory (Morris Water Maze task) and episodic-like memory (Repeated Reversal and Radial Water Maze tasks). Although *APPswe/PS1dE9* mice develop plaques at 6 months of age, at this stage, the performance of these mice on cognitive tests is indistinguishable from that of wild-type mice. However, by 18 months of age, *APPswe/PS1dE9* mice are impaired on all cognitive tasks. Relationships exist between deficits in episodic-like memory tasks and total loads of Aβ in the brain (Savonenko *et al.* 2005, 2006). In concert, these studies of *APPswe/PS1dE9* mice suggest that some form of Aβ (ultimately associated with amyloid deposition) disrupts circuits critical for memory, with episodic-like memory being the most sensitive to the toxic effects of Aβ.

In a recently published investigation (Liu *et al.* 2008), we asked whether the *APPswe/PS1_E9* mouse model recapitulates the progressive monoaminergic (MAergic) degeneration occurring in AD. In the model, the progressive increase of deposition of Aβ in the forebrain was associated with a reduction of the MAergic afferents in the hippocampus and cortex. Significantly, this degeneration was associated with some atrophy of cell bodies and, eventually, led to significant (50%) loss of subcortical MAergic neurons. Degeneration of these neurons occurred without obvious local Aβ or tau abnormalities of neurons at the subcortical sites. These results demonstrate that the mutant mice with Aβ abnormalities developed progressive MAergic neurodegeneration, thereby sharing some features with those pathologies occurring in cases of AD (Liu *et al.* 2008).

The site(s) of early appearance of Aβ neurotoxicity, involving terminal axons, presynaptic and postsynaptic components, and the molecular interactions that trigger synaptic disconnection and axonal degeneration, remain to be defined (Klein *et al.* 2001; Klyubin *et al.* 2005; Lesne *et al.* 2006; Li *et al.* 2009; Meyer-Luehmann *et al.* 2003). Behavioral, physiological, and structural synaptic abnormalities have been linked to the presence of Aβ oligomers (Lesne *et al.* 2006; Li *et al.* 2009; Shankar *et al.* 2008). Studies of T_S2576 mice suggest that extracellular accumulations of 56KD-soluble amyloid assemblies (termed Aβ*56), purified from the brains of memory-impaired mice, interfere with memory when delivered to young rats (Lesne *et al.* 2006). A variety of Aβ42 species, ranging from monomers, oligomers, structural assemblies, and fibrillar amyloid deposits in neuritic plaques, have been suggested to contribute to the impairment of synaptic communication at synapses. These ideas have been tested by experimental manipulations. For example, in one study, an Aβ peptide (naturally secreted in vitro) was injected into the ventricular system of rats and shown to inhibit long-term potentiation in the hippocampus (Klyubin *et al.* 2005). The adverse activity of this peptide was blocked by the injection of a monoclonal Aβ antibody; active immunization was less effective in rescuing functions (Klyubin *et al.* 2005). These observations and others are consistent with the concept that oligomeric species are synaptic toxins in the brain (Klyubin *et al.* 2005; Li *et al.* 2009) and that these peptides are both are necessary and sufficient to perturb learning and memory. Moreover, some of these abnormalities can be reversed by antibody-mediated reductions of levels of Aβ in the brain (Klyubin *et al.* 2005; Lesne *et al.* 2006). Although these transgenic lines do not reproduce the full phenotype of AD (including NFT and death of neurons), these studies demonstrate that the mutant mice are useful subjects for research designed to link behavior and Aβ amyloidosis, to delineate disease mechanisms and targets for treatment, and to test novel therapies including combinations of different approaches (Brody and Holtzman 2008; Chow *et al.* 2010; Jiang *et al.* 2008; Lesne *et al.* 2006; Li *et al.* 2009; McGowan *et al.* 2006; Price *et al.* 2008; Savonenko *et al.* 2005, 2006, 2008).

Models of tauopathies

Tau, a low-molecular-weight, microtubule-associated protein, is a key cytoskeletal protein important in protein trafficking and is important especially in axonal transport (Ballatore *et al.* 2007; Frost *et al.* 2009a, 2009b; Goedert and Spillantini 2006; Mandkelkow *et al.* 2007; Mocanu *et al.* 2008; Wang *et al.* 2002, 2007). Early efforts to express *tau* transgenes in mice did not lead to striking clinical phenotypes or abnormalities (Ballatore *et al.* 2007; McGowan *et al.* 2006). The absence of tau abnormalities in lines of mutant *APP* and *PS* mice (with Aβ burdens) may be related to differences in the tau isoforms expressed in mice. When neuronal-specific promoters were used to drive expression of *tau* P301L (a mutation linked to autosomal dominant frontotemporal dementia with parkinsonism), some brain and spinal cord neurons developed tangles (Ballatore *et al.* 2007; Oddo *et al.* 2003; Querfurth and LaFerla 2010). In *tauP301L* mice, injection of Aβ42 fibrils into specific regions of the brain increased the number of tangles in the neurons, which projected to sites of Aβ injections (Gotz *et al.* 2001; Gotz and Ittner 2008). Moreover, mice expressing *APPswe/tau*P301L exhibited enhanced tangle-like abnormalities in the limbic system and olfactory cortex (Lewis *et al.* 2001), an observation consistent with the hypothesis that the presence of Aβ in proximity to terminals is, in unknown ways, able to promote the formation of tangles in cell bodies of those neurons whose axons project to target fields containing Aβ and that are genetically predisposed to form NFT.

A triple transgenic mouse, created by microinjecting *APPswe* and *tau P301L* into single cells derived from monozygous *PS1M146V* knockin mice, developed age-related plaques and tangles as well as deficits in long-term potentiation that appeared to antedate overt abnormalities (Oddo *et al.* 2003). Conditional *P301L Tau* mice exhibited expression restricted to the forebrain. They manifested behavioral impairments and showed NFT and loss of neurons in the forebrain. After lowering of tau expression by administration of doxycycline, which suppresses the expression of the gene, memory functions recovered, and the numbers of neurons stabilized, but NFT continued to accumulate. The authors suggested that, in this model, NFT are not sufficient to cause cognitive decline or neuron death. Finally, recent studies (Clavaguera *et al.* 2009; Frost *et al.* 2009*a*, 2009*b*) suggested that the misfolded tau (or tau peptides) can pass from cell to cell and propagate "informational" abnormalities related to the conformational state. Some of the spread is thought to occur via conformational alterations related to tau β-sheet fragments (Frost and Diamond 2010; Wang *et al.* 2007) as described for transmission of prion diseases (Aguzzi and Rajendran 2009; Frost and Diamond 2010).

To understand the functions of some of the proteins thought to play roles in pathology resembling that described in AD, investigators have targeted a variety of genes including APP, APLP, and family members, *BACE1*, *PS1*, *Nct*, and *Aph-1*.

B*ACE1-/-* mice

BACE1-/- mice are fertile and exhibit no obvious abnormalities (Cai *et al.* 2001; Laird *et al.* 2005). *BACE1-/-* neurons do not cleave APP at the +1 and +11 sites of Aβ, and the production of Aβ peptides is abolished (Cai *et al.* 2001; Laird *et al.* 2005). These findings indicate that BACE1 is the neuronal β-secretase required to generate the N-termini of Aβ. However, *BACE1-/-*mice show altered performance on some tests of cognition and emotion (Laird *et al.* 2005; Savonenko *et al.* 2008). *BACE1* null mice manifest alterations in both hippocampal synaptic plasticity and in performance on tests of cognition and emotion (Laird *et al.* 2005); some of the memory deficits (but not emotional alterations) in *BACE1-/-* mice are prevented by co-expression of *APPswe/PS1ΔE9* transgenes, suggesting that APP processing influences cognition and memory and that the other potential substrates of BACE1 may play roles in neural circuits related to emotion. More recently, two studies (Hu *et al.* 2006; Willem *et al.* 2006) demonstrated that genetic deletion of *BACE1* is associated with a delay in myelination, reduced thickness of myelin sheaths, increased g-ratios, and decreased myelin markers. These abnormalities reflect alterations in the biology of neuregulin (NRG), which is known to be a signal by which axons communicate with ensheathing glial cells and influence myelination during development. BACE1 cleaves NRG, and processed NRG regulates myelination by phosphorylation of Akt. In *BACE1-/-*mice, NRG cleavage products are decreased and full-length NRG is increased; levels of phosphorylated Akt are diminished (Hu *et al.* 2006). In concert, these investigations of *BACE1*-targeted mice suggest that BACE1 and APP/NRG processing pathways are critical for cognitive, emotional, and synaptic functions and for myelination during development of the PNS and CNS.

PS1-/- mice

*PS1-/-*embryos develop severe abnormalities of the axial skeleton, ribs, and spinal ganglia; this lethal outcome resembles a partial *Notch 1-/-* phenotype (Wong *et al.* 1997). *PS1-/-* cells secrete decreased levels of Aβ (De Strooper *et al.* 1998, 1999; Saura *et al.* 2004) because PS1 (along with PS2, Nct, Aph-1, and Pen-2) is a component of the γ-secretase complex that also carries out the S3 intramembranous cleavage of Notch1 (De Strooper *et al.* 1999; Li *et al.* 2003). Without γ-secretase activity, cleavage of the NEXT (Notch extracellular truncation) to Notch1 intracellular domain (NICD) does not occur; the NICD is not released from the plasma membrane and cannot reach the nucleus to provide a signal to initiate transcriptional processes essential for cell fate decisions. Significantly, conditional *PS1/2* targeted mice show impairments in memory and in hippocampal synaptic plasticity (Saura *et al.* 2004), raising important questions as to the roles of loss of PS functions in neurodegeneration and in AD (Shen and Kelleher 2007).

Nct-/- mice

Nct-/- mice embryos die early and exhibit several patterning defects (Li *et al.* 2003), including abnormal segmentation of somites, a phenotype closely resembling that occurring in *Notch1-/-* and *PS 1/2-/-* embryos. Importantly, *Nct-/-* cells do not secrete Aβ peptides, whereas *Nct+/-* cells show reductions of ~50% (Li *et al.* 2003). The failure of *Nct-/-* cells to generate Aβ peptides is accompanied by accumulation of APP C-terminal fragments. Importantly, *Nct +/-* mice develop tumors of the skin, a phenotype accelerated by reducing PS1 and P53, both of which manipulations exacerbate the tumor phenotype (Li *et al.* 2007a). The formation of these tumors appears to reflect decreased γ-secretase activities and reduced activity of Notch1, a tumor suppressor in the skin.

Aph-1-/- mice

Aph-1a, *Aph-1b*, and *Aph-1c* encode four distinct Aph-1 isoforms: Aph-1aL and Aph-1aS (derived from differential splicing of Aph-1a, Aph-1b, and Aph-1c [Ma *et al.* 2005]). *Aph-1a-/-* embryos have patterning defects that resemble, but are not identical to, those of *Notch1*, *Nct*, or *PS1* null embryos (Ma *et al.* 2005; Serneels *et al.* 2009). Moreover, in *Aph-1a-/-* derived cells, the levels of Nct, PS fragments, and Pen-2 are decreased, and one sees a concomitant reduction in levels of the high-molecular-weight γ-secretase complex and a decrease in secretion of Aβ (Ma *et al.* 2005). In *Aph-1a-/-* cells, other mammalian Aph-1 isoforms can restore the levels of Nct, PS, and Pen-2 (Ma *et al.* 2005).

Experimental manipulations and potential therapeutic strategies

Models relevant to amyloidogenesis provide an opportunity to test the influence of ablations or knockdowns of specific genes; to modulate cleavage patterns influencing generation of neurotoxic peptides; and to enhance clearance and/or degradation of Aβ (Ghosh *et al.* 2008; Klyubin *et al.* 2005; Laird *et al.* 2005; Lesne *et al.* 2006; Li *et al.* 2003; Price *et al.* 2008; Savonenko *et al.* 2006; Wong *et al.* 2008). New approaches using conditional expression systems, RNAi silencing, or manipulations of transcription will allow investigators to examine the roles of specific proteins in the pathogenesis of AD and to assess the degrees of reversibility of the disease processes (Laird *et al.* 2005; Singer *et al.* 2005). The results of these approaches, along with the development of brain-penetrant inhibitors or modulators of enzyme activity and immunotherapy (Brody and Holtzman, 2008), can be tested in clinical trials. We will now review selected experimental studies focusing on specific therapeutic targets that hold promise for development of mechanism-based therapeutics to benefit patients with AD (Chow *et al.* 2010; Savonenko *et al.* 2006; Laird *et al.* 2005).

BACE1

BACE1-/-/APPswe/PS1ΔE9 mice do not develop Aβ deposits or age-associated abnormalities in memory that occur in the *APPswe/PS1ΔE9* model of Aβ amyloidosis (Laird *et al.* 2005). Moreover, Aβ deposits are sensitive to BACE1 dosage and can be efficiently cleared from regions of the CNS when BACE1 is silenced (Laird *et al.* 2005; Singer *et al.* 2005). Although BACE1 is an attractive therapeutic target (Citron 2004; Ghosh *et al.* 2008; Laird *et al.* 2005), several potential problems exist with this approach. First, the BACE1 catalytic site is large, and it is not yet known whether it is possible to achieve adequate brain penetration of a compound of sufficient size to be active in vivo. We believe that this issue will be solved by medicinal chemists. Second, existing BACE1 inhibitors are transported out of the brain by a p-glycoprotein, potentially an issue in trying to maintain adequate concentrations of inhibitors in the brain. In a study, an inhibitor of this process was used with some success to increase the levels of a BACE1 inhibitor in the CNS (Hussain *et al.* 2007). Third, BACE1 null mice manifest alterations in both hippocampal synaptic plasticity and performance on tests of cognition and emotion (Laird *et al.* 2005). Fourth, as described above, genetic deletion of BACE1 causes hypomyelination in the developing PNS and CNS (Hu *et al.* 2006; Willem *et al.* 2006), a phenotype that likely reflects alterations in the NRG–Akt pathway. Thus, although inhibition of β-secretase activity represents an exciting therapeutic opportunity, additional studies are needed to assess possible mechanism-based side effects that may occur with strong inhibition of BACE1 (Laird *et al.* 2005; Savonenko *et al.* 2006; Wong *et al.* 2008). It is more likely that dialing down secretase activities in combination with other treatment strategies (Brody and Holtzman 2008; Chow *et al.* 2010) will promote an effective and safe approach (see below).

γ-Secretase

Both genetic and pharmaceutical reductions of γ-secretase activity decrease production of Aβ peptides in cell-free and cell-based systems and reduce levels of Aβ in mutant mice with Aβ amyloidosis, indicating that γ-secretase activity is a significant target for therapy (Li *et al.* 2003; Ma *et al.* 2005; Saura *et al.* 2004; Wolfe *et al.* 1999; Wong *et al.* 2008). However, γ-secretase activity is also essential for processing Notch and a variety of other transmembrane proteins that are critical for many properties of cells including lineage specification and cell growth during embryonic development (Li *et al.* 2003; Ma *et al.* 2005; Saura *et al.* 2004; Wong *et al.* 2008). Significantly, one inhibitor of γ-secretase (LY– 411,575) reduces production of Aβ, but it also has profound effects on T- and B-cell development and on the appearance of intestinal mucosa (Barten *et al.* 2005). Although *Nct+/-APPswe/PS1ΔE9* mice show reduced levels of Aβ and amyloid plaques (Li *et al.* 2010), these mice also develop skin tumors, presumably, in part, due to reduction of γ-secretase activity and the role of Notch as a tumor suppressor in skin (Li *et al.* 2010). The mechanism whereby decrements in activity of γ-secretase lead to squamous cell tumors is not fully understood, but it appears to be related to tumor-suppressing activity of the enzyme in the epithelium. In *Nct+/-* animals, Notch signaling is reduced and the epidermal growth factor receptor is activated; levels of the receptor are inversely correlated with proliferative activity in the cells of the skin (Li *et al.* 2010). During trials of inhibitors, it will be necessary to be alert to potential adverse events. Indeed, the recent discontinuation of semagacestat (LY 450139) in phase III trials due to a lack of efficacy (a worsening of cognitive symptoms) and to the development of skin cancer raises some concern about this approach, but further studies with different compounds and with γ-modulators are warranted before concluding that this target has too many liabilities (Extance 2010).

Gamma-secretase (modulators)

Retrospective epidemiological studies suggested that significant exposure to NSAIDs reduced the risk of AD, an outcome initially interpreted as related to the impact of NSAIDs on an inflammatory process occurring in the brains of patients with AD (Weggen *et al.* 2001). However, in vitro studies indicated that a subset of NSAIDs modulated γ-secretase cleavages to form shorter, less toxic Aβ species without altering the processing of Notch or other transmembrane proteins (Weggen *et al.* 2001). Biochemical studies are beginning to clarify the actions of γ-secretase modulators. Short-term treatment of mutant mice appears to have some benefit in terms of lowering levels of Aβ and the number of plaques (Lim *et al.* 2000). Unfortunately, a phase III clinical trial of one putative γ-secretase modulator failed because of poor brain penetration of the agent.

Aβ Immunotherapy

To date, the most exciting findings regarding clearance of Aβ are derived from studies using active and passive Aβ immunotherapy (Brody and Holtzman 2008; Golde *et al.* 2009; Hock *et al.* 2003; Monsonego and Weiner 2003; Savonenko *et al.* 2006; Selkoe and Schenk 2003; Sudol *et al.* 2009; Weiner and Frenkel 2006). In treatment trials in mutant mice, both Aβ immunization (with Freund's adjuvant) and passive transfer (anti-Aβ antibodies) reduced levels of Aβ and plaque burden (Bard *et al.* 2000; Brody and Holtzman 2008; Dodart *et al.* 2002; Klyubin *et al.* 2005; Monsonego and Weiner 2003; Oddo *et al.* 2004; Zamora *et al.* 2006). The mechanisms whereby immunotherapy enhances clearance are not completely understood (Brody and Holtzman 2008; Bu 2009; Price *et al.* 2008; Wong *et al.* 2008). Investigators have proposed several not mutually exclusive hypotheses including (1) a small amount of Aβ antibody enters the brain, binds to Aβ peptides, promotes the disassembly of fibrils, and, via the Fc antibody domain, encourages activated microglia to enter the affected regions and to remove Aβ; and (2) serum antibodies serve as a "sink" for the amyloid peptides (derived from neuronal APP) that enter the circulation, thus changing the equilibrium of Aβ in different compartments and promoting removal of Aβ from the CNS (Brody and Holtzman 2008; Cirrito *et al.* 2003; Dodart *et al.* 2002). Several published studies have assessed the roles of microglia in disease. In PD APP mice, investigators (Koenigsknecht-Talboo *et al.* 2008) have shown that treatment with anti-Aβ antibody is associated with increased numbers of microglia around plaques. In a different experiment, Grathwohl and colleagues (2009) used mutant APP mice mated to a line of mice in which microglia were almost completely ablated; neither amyloid deposition nor dystrophy appeared to require the presence of microglia. Whatever the mechanisms of cell damage and the responses to Aβ immunotherapy are in mutant mice, immunotherapy appears to be successful in partially clearing Aβ, in attenuating learning and behavioral deficits in several different models of mutant *APP* or *APP/PS1* mice, and in partially reducing tau abnormalities in the triple transgenic mice (Dodart *et al.* 2002; Oddo *et al.* 2003; Savonenko *et al.* 2006).

Unfortunately, several problems have been associated with Aβ immunotherapy. In the presence of congophilic angiopathy, brain hemorrhages may be exacerbated by immunotherapy (Pfeifer *et al.* 2002), perhaps because the presence of amyloid in vessels can weaken vascular walls. Immunotherapeutic removal of some intramural vascular amyloid could contribute to rupture of damaged vessels and to local bleeding. More significant, in the first part of the vaccination trial, a subset of patients receiving Aβ vaccination with certain adjuvants developed meningoencephalitis (Brody and Holtzman 2008).

To illustrate the challenges of extrapolating outcomes in mice to trials with humans, it is useful to discuss recent problems with Aβ immunotherapy. In preclinical trials, both Aβ immunization (with Freund's adjuvant) and passive transfer of Aβ antibodies reduced levels of Aβ and plaque burden in mutant APP transgenic mice (Brody and Holtzman 2008; Savonenko *et al.* 2006). Thus immunotherapy in transgenic mice was successful in clearing some of the Aβ and in attenuating learning and behavioral deficits in at least two cohorts of mutant *APP* mice. However, patients receiving vaccinations with preaggregated Aβ and an adjuvant (followed by a booster) developed antibodies that recognized Aβ in the brain and vessels (Brody and Holtzman 2008). Although phase I vaccination trials with Aβ peptide and adjuvant were not associated with any adverse events, phase II trials were associated with meningoencephalitis in a subset of patients and were suspended (Brody and Holtzman 2008; Masliah *et al.* 2005; Monsonego and Weiner 2003; Nicoll *et al.* 2003). During the trial, some changes were made in adjuvant and/or formulation. The abnormalities in the index case showing this outcome were consistent with T-cell meningitis (Nicoll *et al.* 2003). Data were interpreted to show some clearance of Aβ deposits, but some regions contained a relatively high density of tangles, neuropil threads, and vascular amyloid (Nicoll *et al.* 2003). Aβ immunoreactivity was sometimes associated with microglia. T cells were conspicuous in the subarachnoid space and around some vessels (Nicoll *et al.* 2003). In another case, there was significant reduction in amyloid deposits in the absence of clinical evidence of encephalitis (Masliah *et al.* 2005). Although the trial was stopped because of these events, assessment of cognitive functions in a small subset of patients who received vaccination and booster immunizations disclosed that patients who successfully generated Aβ antibodies (as measured by a new assay) appeared to have a slower decline in several functional measures. Significantly, in a long-term follow-up study of another cohort of patients who were immunized, it appeared that the immunization protocol had little clinical benefit; although treatment resulted in reduction of Aβ plaques in the brain, the effect was not sufficient to prevent progressive neurodegeneration (Holmes *et al.* 2008). However, the problem with this study may have been that the disease was too far advanced at the initiation of treatment. Several of these observations illustrate the challenges of extrapolating outcomes in mutant mice to human trials. Moreover, in concert with new combination treatments tested in mutant mice, many investigators have suggested that a combination approach (reduced Aβ production and enhanced Aβ clearance) is a more attractive strategy for the future (Chow *et al.* 2010). Moreover, it will be important to start therapy early in the course of the disease. Ultimately, preventive and early interventional approaches will be necessary.

Combination therapies

In our discussions of the effects, positive and negative, of lowering secretase levels, we have emphasized the need for safe and effective mechanism-based therapies for AD. New treatments will probably require combinatorial approaches (Brody and Holtzman 2008; Chow *et al.* 2010). Although γ-secretase and BACE1 are well-recognized therapeutic targets for AD, untoward side effects associated with major inhibition in activity of these proteases have raised concerns regarding their therapeutic potential. Although moderate decreases of either γ-secretase or BACE1 are not associated with mechanism-based toxicities, they provide only modest benefits in reducing Aβ in the brains of *APPswe/PS1DE9* mice. Because the processing of APP to generate Aβ requires both BACE1 and γ-secretase, we hypothesize that moderate reductions of both enzymes would provide additive, significant protection against Aβ amyloidosis. In a recent study (Chow *et al.* 2010), we tested this hypothesis using a novel antiamyloid combination therapy in mutant

APP + PS1 mice. Genetic reductions in the levels of both BACE1 and γ-secretase activity additively attenuated the amyloid burden and ameliorated cognitive deficits occurring in aged *APPswe/PS1DE9* animals. We observed no evidence of mechanism-based toxicities associated with decreases in both enzymes. Thus, we propose that reducing both γ-secretase and BACE1, eventually in concert with immunotherapy to promote clearance of Aβ (Brody and Holtzman 2008) or other approaches, may prove to be an effective and safe treatment strategy for AD.

Conclusions

Over the past two decades, great progress has been made in understanding AD. The features of MCI and early AD have been defined, and diagnostic and outcome measures, using biomarkers and imaging, have been developed. The stages of the pathological and biochemical processes have been characterized and correlated with the clinical features of MCI, early AD, and progressive phases of AD. Genetic studies have provided information regarding the roles of autosomal-dominant mutations in *APP* and *PS* genes and the dose-dependent risks of the *ApoE4* alleles and other loci of risk. Parallel studies of AD and of genetically engineered models of Aβ amyloidosis and, more recently, of the tauopathies have greatly increased our understanding of pathogenic mechanisms, of possible therapeutic targets, and of the ways mechanism-based treatments can be designed to benefit patients with AD. Decreasing production and assembly of misfolded proteins (Aβ and tau) and promoting degradation and clearance of neurotoxic peptides are central to many of these strategies. This field is now on the threshold of implementing novel treatments based on an understanding of the neurobiological, neuropathological, and biochemical characteristics of this illness. Over the next few years, this information will be vital in the design of new mechanism-based therapies that can be tested in vitro and in animal models. These approaches, if beneficial and safe, will be initiated early in the course of the disease in order to benefit patients with this devastating illness.

Acknowledgments

The authors wish to thank the many colleagues with whom they have worked at Johns Hopkins Medical School, including Drs. Sangram Sisodia, David Borchelt, Fiona Laird, Ying Liu, Marilyn Albert, Juan Troncoso, Huaibin Cai, Lee Martin, Micheal Lee, Vivian Chow, Mohamed Farah, and Gopal Thinakaran, as well as collaborators at other institutions, for their contributions to much of the original work cited in this review. In writing this review, we have drawn information from several earlier manuscripts in press or recently published including Dumoulin (2010), Price *et al.* (2010), and Wong *et al.* (2008). Aspects of this work were supported by grants from the US Public Health Service (P50 AGO05146, R01 NS041438, P01 NS047308, R01 NS045150) as well as the Adler Foundation, the Ellison Medical Foundation, the Alzheimer's Association, Wallace Foundation, CART Foundation, and private gifts.

References

Aguzzi A, Rajendran L. 2009. The transcellular spread of cytosolic amyloids, prions, and prionoids. *Neuron* 64:783–790.

Aisen PS. 2009. Alzheimer's disease therapeutic research: the path forward. *Alzheimer's Res Ther* 1:1–6.

Andrews-Hanna JR, Snyder AZ, Vincent JL et al. 2007. Disruption of large-scale brain systems in advanced aging. *Neuron* 56:924–935.

Ballatore C, Lee VMY, Trojanowski JQ. 2007. Tau-mediated neurodegeneration in Alzheimer's disease and related disorders. *Nat Rev Neurosci* 8:663–672.

Bard F, Cannon C, Barbour R et al. 2000. Peripherally administered antibodies against amyloid beta-peptide enter the central nervous system and reduce pathology in a mouse model of Alzheimer disease. *Nat Med* 6:916–919.

Barten DM, Guss VL, Corsa JA et al. 2005. Dynamics of {beta}-amyloid reductions in brain, cerebrospinal fluid, and plasma of {beta}-amyloid precursor protein transgenic mice treated with a γ-secretase inhibitor. *J Pharmacol Exp Ther* 312:635–643.

Bateman RJ, Munsell LY, Morris JC et al. 2006. Human amyloid-beta synthesis and clearance rates as measured in cerebrospinal fluid in vivo. *Nat Med* 12:856–861.

Bateman RJ, Siemers ER, Mawuenyega KG et al. 2009. A gamma-secretase inhibitor decreases amyloid-beta production in the central nervous system. *Ann Neurol* 66:48–54.

Bertram L, Hiltunen M, Parkman M et al. 2005. Family-based association between Alzheimer's disease and variants in UBQLN1. *N Engl J Med* 352:884–894.

Bertram L, Tanzi RE. 2008. Thirty years of Alzheimer's disease genetics: the implications of systematic meta-analyses. *Nat Rev Neurosci* **9**:768–778.

Bishop NA, Lu T, Yankner BA. 2010. Neural mechanisms of ageing and cognitive decline. *Nature* **464**:529–535.

Blennow K, de Leon MJ, Zetterberg H. 2006. Alzheimer's disease. *Lancet* **368**:387–403.

Borchelt DR, Ratovitski T, Van Lare J et al. 1997. Accelerated amyloid deposition in the brains of transgenic mice coexpressing mutant presenilin 1 and amyloid precursor proteins. *Neuron* **19**:939–945.

Braak H, Alafuzoff I, Arzberger T et al. 2006. Staging of Alzheimer disease-associated neurofibrillary pathology using paraffin sections and immunocytochemistry. *Acta Neuropathol* **112**:389–404.

Brody DL, Holtzman DM. 2008. Active and passive immunotherapy for neurodegenerative disorders. *Annu Rev Neurosci* **31**:175–193.

Bu G. 2009. Apolipoprotein E and its receptors in Alzheimer's disease: pathways, pathogenesis and therapy 1. *Nat Rev Neurosci* **10**:333–344.

Buckner RL, Andrews-Hanna JR, Schacter DL. 2008. The brain's default network: anatomy, function, and relevance to disease. *Ann N Y Acad Sci* **1124**:1–38.

Buxbaum JD, Thinakaran G, Koliatsos V et al. 1998. Alzheimer amyloid protein precursor in the rat hippocampus: transport and processing through the perforant path. *J Neurosci* **18**:9629–9637.

Cai H, Wang Y, McCarthy D et al. 2001. BACE1 is the major beta-secretase for generation of Abeta peptides by neurons. *Nat Neurosci* **4**:233–234.

Cao X, Sudhof TC. 2001. A transcriptionally (correction of transcriptively) active complex of APP with Fe65 and histone acetyltransferase Tip60. *Science* **293**:115–120.

Chishti MA, Yang DS, Janus C et al. 2001. Early-onset amyloid deposition and cognitive deficits in transgenic mice expressing a double mutant form of amyloid precursor protein 695. *J Biol Chem* **276**:21562–21570.

Chiti F, Dobson CM. 2006. Protein misfolding, functional amyloid, and human disease. *Annu Rev Biochem* **75**:333–366.

Chow VW, Savonenko AV, Melnikova T et al. 2010. Modeling an anti-amyloid combination therapy for Alzheimer's disease. *Sci Transl Med* **2**:13ra1.

Cirrito JR, May PC, O'Dell MA et al. 2003. In vivo assessment of brain interstitial fluid with microdialysis reveals plaque-associated changes in amyloid-beta metabolism and half-life. *J Neurosci* **23**:8844–8853.

Citron M. 2004. (beta)-Secretase inhibition for the treatment of Alzheimer's disease – promise and challenge. *Trends Pharmacol Sci* **25**:92–97.

Clavaguera F, Bolmont T, Crowther RA et al. 2009. Transmission and spreading of tauopathy in transgenic mouse brain. *Nat Cell Biol* **11**:909–913.

Cohen FE, Kelly JW. 2003. Therapeutic approaches to protein-misfolding diseases. *Nature* **426**:905–909.

Coyle JT, Price DL, DeLong MR. 1983. Alzheimer's disease: a disorder of cortical cholinergic innervation. *Science* **219**:1184–1190.

de Calignon A, Fox LM, Pitstick R et al. 2010. Caspase activation precedes and leads to tangles. *Nature* **464**:1201–1204.

De Strooper B, Annaert WG, Cupers P et al. 1999. A presenilin-1-dependent gamma-secretase-like protease mediates release of Notch intracellular domain. *Nature* **398**:518–522.

De Strooper B, Saftig P, Craessaerts K et al. 1998. Deficiency of presenilin-1 inhibits the normal cleavage of amyloid precursor protein. *Nature* **391**:387–390.

DeMattos RB, Cirrito JR, Parsadanian M et al. 2004. ApoE and clusterin cooperatively suppress Abeta levels and deposition: evidence that ApoE regulates extracellular Abeta metabolism in vivo. *Neuron* **41**:193–202.

Dodart JC, Bales KR, Gannon KS et al. 2002. Immunization reverses memory deficits without reducing brain Abeta burden in Alzheimer's disease model. *Nat Neurosci* **5**:452–457.

Dumoulin, M. 2010. Familial amyloidosis caused by lysozyme mutations. In *Protein Misfolding Diseases: Current and Emerging Principles and Therapies*. Ramirez-Alvarado M, Kelly JW, Dobson CM, eds. Hoboken, NJ: John Wiley & Sons, pp. 867–884.

Extance A. 2010. Alzheimer's failure raises questions about disease-modifying strategies. *Nat Rev Drug Discovery* **9**:749–751.

Fagan AM, Mintun MA, Mach RH et al. 2005. Inverse relation between in vivo amyloid imaging load and cerebrospinal fluid Abeta42 in humans. *Ann Neurol* **59**:512–519.

Frost B, Diamond MI. 2010. Prion-like mechanisms in neurodegenerative diseases. *Nat Rev Neurosci* **11**:155–159.

Frost B, Jacks RL, Diamond MI. 2009a. Propagation of tau misfolding from the outside to the inside of a cell 1. *J Biol Chem* **284**:12845–12852.

Frost B, Ollesch J, Wille H, Diamond MI. 2009b. Conformational diversity of wild-type Tau fibrils specified by templated conformation change. *J Biol Chem* **284**:3546–3551.

Ghosh AK, Gemma S, Tang J. 2008. Beta-secretase as a therapeutic target for Alzheimer's disease. *Neurotherapeutics* **5**:399–408.

Goedert M, Spillantini MG. 2006. A century of Alzheimer's disease. *Science* **314**:777–781.

Golde TE, Das P, Levites Y. 2009. Quantitative and mechanistic studies of Abeta immunotherapy. *CNS Neurol Disord Drug Targets* **8**:31–49.

Goldsbury C, Mocanu MM, Thies E et al. 2006. Inhibition of APP trafficking by tau protein does not increase the generation of amyloid-beta peptides. *Traffic* **7**:873–888.

Gotz J, Chen F, Van Dorpe J, Nitsch RM. 2001. Formation of neurofibrillary tangles in P3011 tau transgenic mice induced by Abeta fibrils. *Science* **293**:1491–1495.

Gotz J, Ittner LM. 2008. Animal models of Alzheimer's disease and frontotemporal dementia. *Nat Rev Neurosci* **9**:532–544.

Graff-Radford NR, Crook JE, Lucas J et al. 2007. Association of low plasma Abeta42/Abeta40 ratios with increased imminent risk for mild cognitive impairment and Alzheimer disease. *Arch Neurol* **64**:354–362.

Grathwohl SA, Kalin RE, Bolmont T et al. 2009. Formation and maintenance of Alzheimer's disease beta-amyloid plaques in the absence of microglia. *Nat Neurosci* **12**:1361–1363.

Hardy J. 2006. Amyloid double trouble. *Nat Genet* **38**:11–12.

Harold D, Abraham R, Hollingworth P et al. 2009. Genome-wide association study identifies variants at CLU and PICALM associated with Alzheimer's disease. *Nat Genet* **41**:1088–1093.

Heber S, Herms J, Gajic V et al. 2000. Mice with combined gene knock-outs reveal essential and partially redundant functions of amyloid precursor protein family members. *J Neurosci* **20**:7951–7963.

Higuchi M, Iwata N, Matsuba Y et al. 2005. F and H MRI detection of amyloid beta plaques in vivo. *Nat Neurosci* **8**:527–533.

Hock C, Konietzko U, Streffer JR et al. 2003. Antibodies against beta-amyloid slow cognitive decline in Alzheimer's disease. *Neuron* **38**:547–554.

Holmes C, Boche D, Wilkinson D et al. 2008. Long-term effects of Abeta42 immunisation in Alzheimer's disease: follow-up of a randomised, placebo-controlled phase I trial. *Lancet* **372**:216–223.

Holtzman DM, Bales KR, Tenkova T et al. 2000. Apolipoprotein E isoform-dependent amyloid deposition and neuritic degeneration in a mouse model of Alzheimer's disease. *Proc Natl Acad Sci USA* **97**:2892–2897.

Hu X, Hicks CW, He W et al. 2006. Bace1 modulates myelination in the central and peripheral nervous system. *Nat Neurosci* **9**:1520–1525.

Hussain I, Hawkins J, Harrison D et al. 2007. Oral administration of a potent and selective non-peptidic BACE-1 inhibitor decreases beta-cleavage of amyloid precursor protein and amyloid-beta production in vivo. *J Neurochem* **100**:802–809.

Iwata N, Mizukami H, Shirotani K et al. 2004. Presynaptic localization of neprilysin contributes to efficient clearance of amyloid-beta peptide in mouse brain. *J Neurosci* **24**:991–998.

Iwatsubo T. 2004. The gamma-secretase complex: machinery for intramembrane proteolysis. *Curr Opin Neurobiol* **14**:379–383.

Jack CR Jr, Garwood M, Wengenack TM et al. 2004. In vivo visualization of Alzheimer's amyloid plaques by magnetic resonance imaging in transgenic mice without a contrast agent. *Magn Reson Med* **52**:1263–1271.

Jankowsky JL, Slunt HH, Gonzales V et al. 2005. Persistent amyloidosis following suppression of Aβ production in a transgenic model of Alzheimer disease. *PLoS Med* **2**(12): e355.

Jiang Q, Lee CY, Mandrekar S et al. 2008. ApoE promotes the proteolytic degradation of Abeta. *Neuron* **58**:681–693.

Kamenetz F, Tomita T, Hsieh H et al. 2003. APP processing and synaptic function. *Neuron* **37**:925–937.

Kim J, Basak JM, Holtzman DM. 2009. The role of apolipoprotein E in Alzheimer's disease. *Neuron* **63**:287–303.

Klein WL, Krafft GA, Finch CE. 2001. Targeting small Aβ oligomers: the solution to an Alzheimer's disease conundrum? *Trends Neurosci* **24**:219–223.

Klunk WE, Engler H, Nordberg A et al. 2004. Imaging brain amyloid in Alzheimer's disease using the novel positron emission tomography tracer, Pittsburgh compound-B. *Ann Neurol* **55**:1–14.

Klyubin I, Walsh DM, Lemere CA et al. 2005. Amyloid beta protein immunotherapy neutralizes Abeta oligomers that disrupt synaptic plasticity in vivo. *Nat Med* **11**:556–561.

Koenigsknecht-Talboo J, Meyer-Luehmann M, Parsadanian M et al. 2008. Rapid microglial response around amyloid pathology after systemic anti-Abeta antibody administration in PDAPP mice. *J Neurosci* **28**:14156–14164.

Laferla FM, Green KN, Oddo S. 2007. Intracellular amyloid-beta in Alzheimer's disease. *Nat Rev Neurosci* **8**:499–509.

Laird FM, Cai H, Savonenko AV et al. 2005. BACE1, a major determinant of selective vulnerability of the brain to Aß amyloidogenesis is essential for cognitive, emotional and synaptic functions. *J Neurosci* **25**:11693–11709.

Lambert J-C, Heath S, Even G et al. 2009. Genome-wide association study identifies variants at CLU and CR1 associated with Alzheimer's disease. *Nat Genet* **41**:1094–1099.

Lazarov O, Morfini GA, Lee EB et al. 2005. Axonal transport, amyloid precursor protein, kinesin-1, and the processing apparatus: revisited. *J Neurosci* **25**:2386–2395.

Lesne S, Koh MT, Kotilinek L et al. 2006. A specific amyloid-(beta) protein assembly in the brain impairs memory. *Nature* **440**:352–357.

Lewis J, Dickson DW, Lin WL et al. 2001. Enhanced neurofibrillary degeneration in transgenic mice expressing mutant tau and APP. *Science* **293**:1487–1491.

Li S, Hong S, Shepardson NE et al. 2009. Soluble oligomers of amyloid Beta protein facilitate hippocampal long-term depression by disrupting neuronal glutamate uptake. *Neuron* **62**:788–801.

Li T, Ma G, Cai H, Price DL, Wong PC. 2003. Nicastrin is required for assembly of presenilin/gamma-secretase complexes to mediate Notch signaling and for processing and trafficking of beta-amyloid precursor protein in mammals. *J Neurosci* **23**:3272–3277.

Li T, Wen H, Brayton C et al. 2007a. Epidermal growth factor receptor and Notch pathways participate in the tumor suppressor function of gamma-secretase. *J Biol Chem* **282**:32264–32273.

Li T, Wen H, Brayton C et al. 2007b. Moderate reduction of gamma-secretase attenuates amyloid burden and limits mechanism-based liabilities. *J Neurosci* **27**:10849–10859.

Lim GP, Yang F, Chu T et al. 2000. Ibuprofen suppresses plaque pathology and inflammation in a mouse model for Alzheimer's disease. *J Neurosci* **20**:5709–5714.

Lipton SA. 2007. Pathologically activated therapeutics for neuroprotection. *Nat Rev Neurosci* **8**:803–808.

Liu Y, Yoo MJ, Savonenko A et al. 2008. Amyloid pathology is associated with progressive monoaminergic neurodegeneration in a transgenic mouse model of Alzheimer's disease. *J Neurosci* **28**:13805–13814.

Luo Y, Bolon B, Kahn S et al. 2001. Mice deficient in BACE1, the Alzheimer's beta-secretase, have normal phenotype and abolished beta-amyloid generation. *Nat Neurosci* **4**:231–232.

Ma G, Li T, Price DL, Wong PC. 2005. APH-1a is the principal mammalian APH-1 isoform present in gamma-secretase complexes during embryonic development. *J Neurosci* **25**:192–198.

Maeda J, Ji B, Irie T et al. 2007. Longitudinal, quantitative assessment of amyloid, neuroinflammation, and anti-amyloid treatment in a living mouse model of Alzheimer's disease enabled by positron emission tomography. *J Neurosci* **27**:10957–10968.

Mandkelkow EM, Thies E, Mandelkow E. 2007. Tau and axonal transport in Alzheimer's Disease. In *Alzheimer's Disease: Advances in Genetics, Molecular and Cellular Biology*. New York: Springer, pp. 237–256.

Markesbery WR, Schmitt FA, Kryscio RJ et al. 2006. Neuropathologic substrate of mild cognitive impairment. *Arch Neurol* **63**:38–46.

Martin LJ, Pardo CA, Cork LC, Price DL. 1994. Synaptic pathology and glial responses to neuronal injury precede the formation of senile plaques and amyloid deposits in the aging cerebral cortex. *Am J Pathol* **145**:1358–1381.

Masliah E, Hansen L, Adame A et al. 2005. A{beta} vaccination effects on plaque pathology in the absence of encephalitis in Alzheimer disease. *Neurology* **64**:129–131.

Matthews PM, Honey GD, Bullmore ET. 2006. Applications of fMRI in translational medicine and clinical practice. *Nat Rev Neurosci* **7**:732–744.

McGowan E, Eriksen J, Hutton M. 2006. A decade of modeling Alzheimer's disease in transgenic mice. *Trends Genet* **22**:281–289.

Meyer-Luehmann M, Spires-Jones TL, Prada C et al. 2008. Rapid appearance and local toxicity of amyloid-beta plaques in a mouse model of Alzheimer's disease. *Nature* **451**:720–724.

Meyer-Luehmann M, Stalder M, Herzig MC et al. 2003. Extracellular amyloid formation and associated pathology in neural grafts. *Nat Neurosci* **6**:370–377.

Mocanu MM, Nissen A, Eckermann K et al. 2008. The potential for beta-structure in the repeat domain of Tau protein determines aggregation, synaptic decay, neuronal loss, and coassembly with endogenous Tau in inducible mouse models of tauopathy. *J Neurosci* **28**:737–748.

Monsonego A, Weiner HL. 2003. Immunotherapeutic approaches to Alzheimer's disease. *Science* **302**:834–838.

Nicoll JA, Wilkinson D, Holmes C et al. 2003. Neuropathology of human Alzheimer disease after immunization with amyloid-beta peptide: a case report. *Nat Med* **9**:448–452.

Oddo S, Billings L, Kesslak JP, Cribbs DH, LaFerla FM. 2004. Abeta immunotherapy leads to clearance of early, but not late, hyperphosphorylated tau aggregates via the proteasome. *Neuron* **43**:321–332.

Oddo S, Caccamo A, Shepherd JD et al. 2003. Triple-transgenic model of Alzheimer's disease with plaques and tangles: intracellular Abeta and synaptic dysfunction. *Neuron* **39**:409–421.

Perrin RJ, Fagan AM, Holtzman DM. 2009. Multimodal techniques for diagnosis and prognosis of Alzheimer's disease. *Nature* **461**:916–922.

Pfeifer M, Boncristiano S, Bondolfi L et al. 2002. Cerebral hemorrhage after passive anti-Abeta immunotherapy. *Science* **298**:1379.

Pigino G, Morfini G, Atagi Y et al. 2009. Disruption of fast axonal transport is a pathogenic mechanism for intraneuronal amyloid beta. *Proc Natl Acad Sci USA* **106**:5907–5912.

Price DL, Martin LJ, Savonenko AV et al. 2008. Selected genetically engineered models relevant to human neurodegenerative disease. In *The Molecular and Genetic Basis of Neurologic and Psychiatric Disease*, 4th edn. Rosenberg RN, DiMauro S, Paulson HL, Ptácek L, Nestler EJ, eds. Philadelphia, PA: Lippincott Williams and Wilkins, pp. 35–62.

Price D, Savonenko AV, Li T, Lee MK, Wong P. 2010. Alzheimer disease: protein misfolding, model systems, and experimental therapeutics. In *Protein Misfolding Diseases*. Ramirez-Alvarado M, Kelly JW, Dobson CM, eds. Hoboken, NJ: John Wiley & Sons, pp. 233–258.

Querfurth HW, LaFerla FM. 2010. Alzheimer's disease. *N Engl J Med* **362**:329–344.

Rogaeva E, Meng Y, Lee JH et al. 2007. The neuronal sortilin-related receptor SORL1 is genetically associated with Alzheimer's disease. *Nat Genet* **39**:168–177.

Rovelet-Lecrux A, Hannequin D, Raux G et al. 2006. APP locus duplication causes autosomal dominant early-onset Alzheimer disease with cerebral amyloid angiopathy. *Nat Genet* **38**:24–26.

Saura CA, Choi SY, Beglopoulos V et al. 2004. Loss of presenilin function causes impairments of memory and synaptic plasticity followed by age-dependent neurodegeneration. *Neuron* **42**:23–36.

Savonenko AV, Laird FM, Troncoso JC, Wong PC, Price DL. 2006. Role of Alzheimer's disease models in designing and testing experimental therapeutics. *Drug Discov Today* **2**:305–312.

Savonenko A, Xu GM, Melnikova T et al. 2005. Episodic-like memory deficits in the APPswe/PS1dE9 mouse model of Alzheimer's disease: relationships to (beta)-amyloid deposition and neurotransmitter abnormalities. *Neurobiol Dis* **18**:602–617.

Savonenko AV, Melnikova T, Laird FM et al. 2008. Alteration of BACE1-dependent NRG1/ErbB4 signaling and schizophrenia-like phenotypes in BACE1-null mice. *Proc Nat Acad Sci USA* **105**:5585–5590.

Selkoe DJ. 2002. Alzheimer's disease is a synaptic failure. *Science* **298**:789–791.

Selkoe DJ, Schenk D. 2003. Alzheimer's disease: molecular understanding predicts amyloid-based therapeutics. *Annu Rev Pharmacol Toxicol* **43**:545–584.

Serneels L, Van Biervliet J, Craessaerts K et al. 2009. Gamma-secretase heterogeneity in the Aph1 subunit: relevance for Alzheimer's disease. *Science* **324**:639–642.

Shankar GM, Li S, Mehta TH et al. 2008. Amyloid-beta protein dimers isolated directly from Alzheimer's brains impair synaptic plasticity and memory. *Nat Med* **14**:837–842.

Shen J, Kelleher RJ III. 2007. The presenilin hypothesis of Alzheimer's disease: evidence for a loss-of-function pathogenic mechanism. *Proc Natl Acad Sci USA* **104**:403–409.

Singer O, Marr RA, Rockenstein E et al. 2005. Targeting BACE1 with siRNAs ameliorates Alzheimer disease neuropathology in a transgenic model. *Nat Neurosci* **8**:1343–1349.

Sisodia SS, Koo EH, Beyreuther KT, Unterbeck A, Price DL. 1990. Evidence that ß-amyloid protein in Alzheimer's disease is not derived by normal processing. *Science* **248**:492–495.

Sisodia SS, Koo EH, Hoffman PN, Perry G, Price DL. 1993. Identification and transport of full-length amyloid precursor proteins in rat peripheral nervous system. *J Neurosci* **13**: 3136–3142.

Sperling RA, Laviolette PS, O'Keefe K et al. 2009. Amyloid deposition is associated with impaired default network function in older persons without dementia. *Neuron* **63**:178–188.

Sudol KL, Mastrangelo MA, Narrow WC et al. 2009. Generating differentially targeted amyloid-beta specific intrabodies as a passive vaccination strategy for Alzheimer's disease. *Mol Ther* **17**:2031–2040.

Sunderland T, Linker G, Mirza N et al. 2003. Decreased beta-amyloid1–42 and increased tau levels in cerebrospinal fluid of patients with Alzheimer disease. *J Am Med Assoc* **289**:2094–2103.

Sze CI, Troncoso JC, Kawas CH et al. 1997. Loss of the presynaptic vesicle protein synaptophysin in hippocampus correlates with early cognitive decline in aged humans. *J Neuropathol Exp Neurol* **56**:933–944.

Vassar R, Bennett BD, Babu-Khan S et al. 1999. ß-secretase cleavage of Alzheimer's amyloid precursor protein by the transmembrane aspartic protease BACE. *Science* **286**:735–741.

Villemagne VL, Perez KA, Pike KE et al. 2010. Blood-borne amyloid-beta dimer correlates with clinical markers of Alzheimer's disease. *J Neurosci* **30**:6315–6322.

Walsh DM, Klyubin I, Faden AI et al. 2002. Naturally secreted oligomers of amyloid ß-protein potently inhibit hippocampal LTP in vivo. *Nature* **416**:535–539.

Walsh DM, Minogue AM, Sala Frigerio C et al. 2007. The APP family of proteins: similarities and differences. *Biochem Soc Trans* **35**:416–420.

Wang HW, Pasternak JF, Kuo H et al. 2002. Soluble oligomers of beta amyloid (1–42) inhibit long-term potentiation but not long-term depression in rat dentate gyrus. *Brain Res* **924**:133–140.

Wang YP, Biernat J, Pickhardt M, Mandelkow E, Mandelkow EM.

2007. Stepwise proteolysis liberates tau fragments that nucleate the Alzheimer-like aggregation of full-length tau in a neuronal cell model. *Proc Natl Acad Sci USA* **104**:10252–10257.

Weggen S, Eriksen JL, Das P et al. 2001. A subset of NSAIDs lower amyloidogenic Aß42 independently of cyclooxygenase activity. *Nature* **414**:212–216.

Weiner HL, Frenkel D. 2006. Immunology and immunotherapy of Alzheimer's disease. *Nat Rev Immunol* **6**:404–416.

Whitehouse PJ, Price DL, Struble RG et al. 1982. Alzheimer's disease and senile dementia: loss of neurons in the basal forebrain. *Science* **215**:1237–1239.

Willem M, Garratt AN, Novak B et al. 2006. Control of peripheral nerve myelination by the beta-secretase BACE1. *Science* **314**:664–666.

Wolfe MS. 2006. Shutting down Alzheimer's. *Sci Am* **294**:72–79.

Wolfe MS, Xia W, Ostaszewski BL et al. 1999. Two transmembrane aspartates in presenilin-1 required for presenilin endoproteolysis and gamma-secretase activity. *Nature* **398**:513–517.

Wong PC, Price DL, Bertram L, Tanzi RE. 2008. Alzheimer's disease: Genetics, pathogenesis, models, and experimental therapeutics. In *Molecular Biology of Aging* (Cold Spring Harbor Monograph Series 51). Guarente LP, Partridge L, Wallace DC, eds. New York, NY: Cold Spring Harbor Laboratory Press, pp. 371–407.

Wong PC, Price DL, Cai H. 2001. The brain's susceptibility to amyloid plaques. *Science* **293**:1434–1435.

Wong PC, Zheng H, Chen H et al. 1997. Presenilin 1 is required for Notch1 and DII1 expression in the paraxial mesoderm. *Nature* **387**:288–292.

Yan P, Bero AW, Cirrito JR et al. 2009. Characterizing the appearance and growth of amyloid plaques in APP/PS1 mice. *J Neurosci* **29**:10706–10714.

Zamora E, Handisurya A, Shafti-Keramat S et al. 2006. Papillomavirus-like particles are an effective platform for amyloid-beta immunization in rabbits and transgenic mice. *J Immunol* **177**:2662–2670.

Zhang D, Raichle ME. 2010. Disease and the brain's dark energy. *Nat Rev Neurol* **6**:15–28.

Chapter 9

Pain therapeutics

Anthony W. Bannon

Pain is a defensive or protective mechanism that allows an organism to survive. The pain pathway consists of sensory nerve endings that respond to noxious stimuli and transmit this information to the spinal cord and then to supraspinal levels where the processing of this sensory information occurs. Basic research has increased our understanding of the molecular and cellular components along this pathway that ultimately can be used as targets for the development of therapeutic agents for pain. Given the number of putative targets that have been identified, however, the relative number of novel pharmacological treatments that have been successfully developed and made available to patients remains relatively low. As in other fields of drug discovery, in the research and development of pain drugs translational medicine is being emphasized with the goal of improving the successful development of therapeutic agents. This chapter provides background information for understanding the current use and limitations of translational research as it applies to the discovery and development of novel therapeutic agents for pain.

Overview of pain states

Clinical pain states are often categorized based on duration in the broad categories of acute and chronic pain (e.g., pain lasting > 6 months). Acute pain is associated with cuts, incisions, ischemia, broken bones, and burns. Chronic pain is associated with conditions such as arthritis and nerve injury like that associated with neuropathies (e.g., diabetes; chemotherapy) or mechanical injury (e.g., amputations, spinal cord injury). Clinically, chronic pain states are often further characterized as inflammatory or neuropathic. These descriptors help associate pain with its presumed primary source and guide the selection of therapeutics to treat the pain. Basic research has provided insight into distinct underlying mechanisms associated with the various types of pain and concurrently helped to identify numerous targets for the development of therapeutic agents.

Acute pain may be considered as nociceptive pain, as recently described by Costigan *et al.* (2009). This type of pain is the natural response to help protect against injury and help avoid noxious stimuli that can cause injury or damage. Technically, nociceptive pain is terminated once the noxious stimulus is removed. Where there is tissue damage, however, other mechanisms such as inflammation may contribute to ongoing nociceptive pain. Specific neuronal fibers involved in transmitting nociceptive pain include high-threshold unmyelinated C fibers and thinly myelinated Aδ fibers that send signals to the spinal cord and then to supraspinal sites involved in pain processing (Woolf and Ma 2007).

Inflammatory pain is associated with tissue injury and the subsequent release of inflammatory mediators from multiple cell types that help drive the pain response. In inflammatory pain, persistent drive from the various inflammatory mediators can sensitize the neurons in the pain pathways that in turn help underlie the symptoms such as painful responses to normally nonpainful stimuli (allodynia) and exaggerated responses to noxious stimuli (hyperalgesia) (Juhl *et al.* 2008). For example, following a cut or incision that causes acute pain, increased sensitivity to touch or pressure around the cut or incision may persist for days. This change in sensitivity is thought to result from tissue damage that in turn results in release of inflammatory mediators and subsequent change in response neurons in the pain pathway.

A third general category of pain is neuropathic pain, defined as pain associated with damage to the

---

Translational Neuroscience, ed. James E. Barrett, Joseph T. Coyle and Michael Williams. Published by Cambridge University Press. © Cambridge University Press 2012.

somatosensory system (Treede *et al.* 2008). This damage may be caused by a variety of mechanisms including trauma, metabolic disorders, toxic agents (e.g., chemotherapeutics), infections, or tumors. As with inflammatory pain, plastic changes in pain pathways and supraspinal sites result in abnormal processing of sensory and pain transmission (Costigan *et al.* 2009). Neuropathic pain is unique in that, unlike nociceptive pain and inflammatory pain, which have protective functions, neuropathic pain has no specific purpose for the injured individual and is often chronic. Clinical conditions such as fibromyalgia share many of the features of neuropathic pain but the original source or cause is unknown. Multiple mechanisms can be involved in neuropathic pain, including continuous ectopic firing from injured afferents, structural changes at the level of the spinal cord, an expanding receptive field, and involvement of low-threshold Aβ fibers that normally carry nonnoxious sensory information (e.g., touch) (Kinloch and Cox 2005). All of these mechanisms can contribute to an increased sensitivity at the level of the spinal cord that is also referred to as central sensitization. Evidence also shows that neuroimmune responses may be involved (Moalem and Tracey 2006; Thacker *et al.* 2007). Symptoms reported in patients with neuropathic pain include spontaneous pain, allodynia, and hyperalgesia.

Although specific classification of pain states can help guide therapeutic approaches, often clinical pain states are complex and involve multiple mechanisms. Pain states such as low back pain or pain related to osteoarthritis may involve multiple mechanisms such as sensitization of primary afferents as well as central sensitization. In clinical situations the affective and emotional components of pain also impact an individual's response to pain. All of these factors contribute to the difficulty encountered in treating human pain conditions.

Current pharmacological approaches to pain management

Nociceptive pain

The choice of drug treatment for acute pain is typically a function of the severity of the pain (Krenzischek *et al.* 2008). For example, treatment of moderate to severe pain following a major surgical procedure typically involves the use of potent opioid agonists such as fentanyl, morphine, oxycodone, and oxymorphone. For less severe pain, less potent opioids such as codeine may be prescribed, often in combination with nonsteroidal anti-inflammatory drugs (NSAIDs) such as ibuprofen or acetaminophen. Obviously, nonprescription forms of many NSAIDs are available to the consumer to treat minor aches and pains.

Inflammatory pain

The treatment of inflammatory pain typically focuses on reducing the inflammation. Drugs such as NSAIDs are most often used (Herndon *et al.* 2008). Selective cyclooxygenase-2 (COX-2) inhibitors were developed to treat inflammatory pain and are less likely than nonselective COX inhibitors to produce injury to the gastrointestinal tract (e.g., bleeding). However, only one of these drugs, celecoxib (Celebrex®; Pfizer, New York, NY) remains on the market today. Other COX-2 inhibitors were removed from the market after an increased incidence of cardiovascular events (i.e., heart attacks, stroke) was found to be associated with their use (Farkouh and Greenberg 2009).

Neuropathic pain

Unlike inflammatory pain, the current approved treatments for neuropathic pain focus on treating the symptoms and not necessarily the underlying causes (O'Connor and Dworkin 2009). Drugs used to treat neuropathic pain fall into diverse categories of pharmacological mechanisms and include tricyclic antidepressants, antiepileptics, and anesthetics. Approved drugs for the treatment of neuropathic pain conditions in the USA are shown in Table 9.1. Interestingly, all of these approved treatments for neuropathic pain were initially developed for other conditions. Gabapentin, for example, was originally approved as an adjunctive treatment for partial seizures (McLean 1995) and duloxetine was originally developed and approved for the treatment of depression (Mallinckrodt *et al.* 2004). Although the lidocaine patch was developed for the treatment of pain, the active ingredient lidocaine was first used as an anesthetic agent.

Research and development in pain therapeutics

To better understand the role of translational medicine in the development of pain treatments, it is useful

Chapter 9: Pain therapeutics

Table 9.1. Drugs approved in the USA to treat neuropathic pain conditions and fibromyalgia.

Generic name	Marketed name in the USA	Approved label
Gabapentin	Neurontin® (Pfizer, New York, NY)	Postherpetic neuralgia
Pregabalin	Lyrica® (Pfizer, New York, NY)	Diabetic neuropathy; postherpetic neuralgia; fibromyalgia
5% Lidocaine patch	Lidoderm® (Endo Pharmaceuticals, Newark, DE)	Postherpetic neuralgia
Duloxetine	Cymbalta® (Lilly USA, Indianapolis, IN)	Diabetic neuropathy; fibromyalgia
Milnacipran	Savella® (Forest Laboratories, New York, NY)	Fibromyalgia

to have a general understanding of the drug discovery process for pain drugs with particular emphasis on the use of animal models that currently play a major role in identifying candidate molecules for clinical trials. These preclinical models have also played a major role in advancing our understanding of the mechanisms and pathways involved in pain, which in turn has helped identify targets for drug discovery.

The drug discovery process typically involves identifying a target of interest. Targets are typically selected based on some type of validation such as genetic information. For example, mutations of the sodium channel gene, *Nav1.7*, impact pain in humans. Mutations that increase the function of this channel are associated with a specific pain syndrome (Fischer *et al.* 2009; Nilsen *et al.* 2009; Yang *et al.* 2004), whereas mutations that lead to diminished activity of this channel have been shown to decrease response to pain (Goldberg *et al.* 2007). These types of data in humans provide a strong basis for developing pain drugs that block this channel. More often, the validation data initially come from data generated in preclinical species such as genetically modified animals, anatomical findings (i.e., distribution of a specific gene in pain pathways), or even pharmacological validation in preclinical animal models.

Based on validation data of a specific target, typically a high-throughput screen is conducted to identify compounds that interact in the desired manner with the target (e.g., blockers of specific ion channels; agonist of a specific G protein-coupled receptor). The complexities of finding drug-like molecules are beyond the scope of this chapter, but a primary goal of this effort is to identify candidate molecules that can be tested in animal models of pain (Negus *et al.* 2006).

Animal models of pain

Similar to the clinical classification of pain, animal models have been developed to address acute, inflammatory, and neuropathic pain.

Acute or nociceptive pain models

Models of acute pain in animals use noxious stimuli to elicit a response. A classic example of this type of model is the hot plate assay (D'Amour and Smith 1941). This model uses a plate heated to a temperature that is noxious to the animal and elicits a response such as licking or jumping. Once this response occurs, the animal is removed from the hot plate and the latency to the response is recorded. Similar models have been described using cold as a stimulus (Bennett and Xie 1988). Other methods allow more discrete application of the noxious stimulus such as to a single paw; the original method was published by Hargreaves *et al.* (1988). Another type of nociceptive pain model is visceral pain such as colonic distension (Ness and Gebhart 1988). This method uses noxious pressure to elicit a response and has been developed to mimic deep tissue/organ pain. In all of these animal models of nociceptive pain, hypersensitivity can be induced by a variety of methods (inflammatory and neuropathic insults).

Inflammatory pain models

The most common models of inflammatory pain in rodents involve the administration of an insult that results in an inflammatory response (Sandkuhler 2009). Injection of inflammatory agents is often local such as into the paw of a rodent. Commonly used agents included complete Freund's adjuvant or carrageenan, although there are many others. Injection of agents such as monoiodoacetic acid or kaolin into the joints is another method used to produce inflammatory pain. As with injection into the paw, symptoms are usually limited to the single paw or joint. One advantage of these discrete injuries is that they allow use of the contralateral side as a control.

The behavioral end points used in rodent models of inflammatory pain include evoked responses as well as functional responses (e.g., weight bearing). Common evoked responses include the measurement of mechanical hyperalgesia, tactile allodynia, or thermal hyperalgesia. Mechanical hyperalgesia (paw pressure) is typically measured using a Randall–Selitto apparatus and variations of this (Randall and Selitto 1957). This end point measures the threshold to withdrawal in response to increasing pressure (i.e., on the paw or joint). The inflammatory insult decreases the paw withdrawal threshold (i.e., animal responds to a lower pressure) relative to the contralateral side or to the response in sham-treated animals. In the drug discovery scenario, blockade or reversal of the mechanical hyperalgesia by the test agent is the desired effect. This end point may be considered to be analogous to the increased sensitivity to pressure experienced at and around the site of tissue injury in clinical pain states. Measurement of weight bearing (Zhu et al. 2008) is based on the idea that a normal animal will distribute its body weight evenly across its paws (e.g., 50/50 hindpaw weight distribution). If the animal is given an inflammatory insult in a single paw, then it may put less weight on the injured paw. In the drug-testing scenario, normalization of the weight distribution is the desired effect. This end point has the face validity of being a functional measure, meaning a response does not have to be elicited.

Tactile allodynia is most commonly measured using calibrated fibers called Von Frey filaments. Animal models include various methods of using these fibers; one of the most common is the determination of a response threshold (Chaplan et al. 1994). As for mechanical hyperalgesia, inflammatory insults can lower the response threshold to nonnoxious tactile stimuli relative to the noninflamed condition; a beneficial treatment is one that restores the threshold to noninflamed levels. This end point may be considered analogous to increased sensitivity to normally nonnoxious touch that can occur at or around the site of tissue injury.

In inflammatory pain models some end points are more functional in nature. Weight bearing on the hindpaws, for example, has been used as an end point to assess the effects of putative antinociceptive agents. This model works on the premise that a normal animal will evenly distribute its weight across its back paws. Injury to one limb can cause the animal to favor the uninjured limb and thus put more weight on the noninjured limb and less weight on the injured limb. Agents effective in reducing the nociception associated with this injury can normalize the weight bearing back towards even distribution of the weight. Other models attempt to measure disruption of gait as a consequence of an inflammatory insult (Boettger et al. 2009). Few reports thus far describe use of this end point, perhaps because of the relatively high cost of equipment (e.g., video tracking) and the time-consuming methodology.

Neuropathic pain models

The development of animal models of neuropathic pain over the past couple of decades has played a significant role in driving basic science and associated drug discovery in neuropathic pain. Several recently published reviews describe the numerous animal models of neuropathic pain (Jarvis and Boyce-Rustay 2009; Mogil 2009; Negus et al. 2006). Neuropathic pain models in animals involve damage to specific nerves. The primary species used for this research are rodents. Damage to the nerves can be produced by a variety of methods including cutting the nerve, surgery, chemical-induced damage (e.g., chemotherapy agents), and damage as a consequence of an induced-disease state. These models are used in the drug discovery setting to provide evidence of efficacy for agents in neuropathic pain conditions.

Surgically induced models involve targeting specific nerves or a specific nerve. Common surgical models include the chronic constriction injury model (Bennett and Xie 1988); partial sciatic nerve ligation (Seltzer et al. 1990); the spinal nerve ligation model (SNL) (Kim and Chung 1992); and the spared nerve injury model (Decosterd and Woolf 2000). Common to all of these models are hyperalgesia and allodynia, but the duration and sensitivity to specific stimuli (e.g., heat, cold, touch) vary. The development of hyperalgesia and allodynia in these models gives them face validity with regards to clinical neuropathic pain conditions in which these symptoms may be present.

Animal models of neuropathic pain have also been developed to mimic the human conditions in which neuropathic pain is observed. Examples include chemotherapy-induced neuropathic pain, virus-induced neuropathic pain, and neuropathic pain associated with disease such as diabetes (Jarvis and Boyce-Rustay 2009). As with the surgical models, these models produce the clinically relevant symptoms of hyperalgesia and allodynia but the duration and sensitivity to various stimuli vary.

Cancer pain

Cancer pain models have been developed in animals (Medhurst *et al.* 2002). These models are relatively new and as with human cancer pain they have components across the domains of pain, such as nociceptive pain and neuropathic pain, and may thus prove useful in identifying agents to treat cancer pain (Mantyh, 2006).

Animal models of pain: are they translational models?

Animal models are used in drug discovery as a means to predict efficacy of novel agents in human conditions. Typically, the criteria for pharmacological validation of an animal model involve showing efficacy in the animal model of known agents used to treat human pain. As Mogil (2009) notes, this is backward validation, meaning that efficacy of the agent was first demonstrated in humans, then in the animal model. Thus, the ability of animal models of pain to predict efficacy of unproven mechanisms in humans is a constant concern. Is this concern valid?

One case that fueled this concern was the development of neurokinin-1 (substance P) receptor antagonists for the treatment of pain. Extensive data in animal models of pain did not translate once tested in controlled trials in humans. This case as well as others brings into question the ability of animal models to predict effects of novel mechanisms in humans. However, with neuropathic models such as the SNL, it is interesting that thus far, all Food and Drug Administration-approved drugs for the treatment of human neuropathic pain show efficacy in the related animal models. These drugs involve a diverse set of pharmacological mechanisms. Whiteside *et al.* (2008) have shown that for some known treatments for neuropathic pain, exposure levels in the SNL model seem to predict levels required to see efficacy in humans. Thus, at least for this domain of pain the animal models of neuropathic pain appear to detect a variety of mechanisms, making it plausible that novel mechanisms may be predicted.

Another valid concern regarding the use of animal models is that across the various domains of human pain, spontaneous pain is frequently reported (Arning and Baron 2009; La Montagna *et al.* 1997). In animal models of pain, it is not clear whether there is ongoing spontaneous pain comparable with that observed in human pain conditions, particularly chronic pain conditions. Behavioral effects such as flinching or biting in animals may be interpreted as spontaneous pain, but these effects are typically transient, unlike the spontaneous pain found in chronic pain conditions in humans. Examples of these animal models include the flinching and biting that occur following injection of formalin (e.g., 1%–5% formalin) as well as other alogenic agents such as capsaicin, mustard oil, and bradykinin.

Most of the pain models routinely used for drug discovery were developed as disease models, attempting to mimic aspects of human pain conditions. These models may all be considered translational in that they are used to predict efficacy in human pain states. However, the number of new medications brought to market for the treatment of pain has been relatively low given the effort and resources expended by pharmaceutical companies in this endeavor. Obviously, compounds fail to advance for many reasons, such as toxicological findings or inadequate pharmacokinetic properties in humans. However, the lack of efficacy of novel treatments in humans can call into question the translational or predictive value of the preclinical models of pain. The pharmaceutical industry is thus studying novel paradigms to minimize clinical failures due to lack of efficacy, an issue at the fore of translational medicine.

Use of translational medicine for the discovery of novel treatments of pain

Translational medicine can be defined as the bridging of effects in animals to effects in humans. In the recent past, in pharmaceutical companies communication was minimal between scientists responsible for the initial discovery and characterization of potential new therapies and scientists involved in the clinical development of these therapies. Preclinical scientists had little understanding of the methods used by clinical scientists, and conversely the clinical scientists lacked understanding of the basic science and methods used by preclinical researchers. In recent years that knowledge gap has begun to close as communication has increased between these two groups and both increasingly appreciate the potential value of this improved understanding in developing new therapeutic agents.

Preclinical researchers have increased their awareness of how pain is measured in humans and how drug exposure levels and efficacy are determined. Both of these factors may be helpful in advancing compounds to become marketed products as well as stopping advancement of ineffective compounds at earlier stages of clinical development, in turn reducing failures in late-stage clinical trials.

Experimental pain models in humans

For our purposes, experimental pain models in humans are defined as models conducted in normal individuals (i.e., not patients with specific pain conditions). In drug development these models may be used in normal volunteers in the earliest stages of drug testing in humans (i.e., phase I). As with animal models, a variety of models and techniques are associated with experimental models in humans (Schmelz 2009). Initially, simple acute pain models were used to test analgesic agents but overall these models proved to be of little value in identifying analgesic agents in humans (Chapman *et al.* 1965). As understanding of pain mechanisms advanced, more sophisticated models of human pain were developed that are thought to incorporate specific aspects of various pain states such as peripheral sensitization associated with inflammatory pain or central sensitization involved in neuropathic pain states (e.g., capsaicin-induced secondary hyperalgesia). One limitation of many of the experimental models in humans is that the models have no clear correlates in preclinical species; thus they are not true translational models.

Two models that are starting to be utilized in the drug discovery process as translational models are the ultraviolet model (Bishop *et al.* 2007; Eissenberg *et al.* 2000; Koppert *et al.* 1999; Seifert *et al.* 2008) and the capsaicin model (Hughes *et al.* 2002; Scanlon *et al.* 2006; Wang *et al.* 2008). The human ultraviolet model is a model of inflammatory pain that has the properties of hyperalgesia and has been validated with drugs known to be effective in treating pain associated with inflammation such as NSAIDs and selective COX-2 inhibitors (Maihofner *et al.* 2007; Sycha *et al.* 2005). Currently, reports are limited regarding the ultraviolet model in preclinical species (Bishop *et al.* 2007; Gougat *et al.* 2004), but in the pharmaceutical industry interest is growing in using this preclinical model in the early stages of clinical development (personal observation).

The capsaicin model (Petersen and Rowbotham 1999) has been brought to the forefront in the development of transient receptor potential cation channel, subfamily V (TRPV1) antagonists for the treatment of pain (Broad *et al.* 2008; Gunthorpe and Chizh 2009). Capsaicin is an agonist for TRPV1; thus the capsaicin model can be used preclinically as well as clinically as a pharmacodynamic model for this particular target. The capsaicin model in rodents and humans has also been described as a model of central sensitization (LaMotte *et al.* 1991; Treede *et al.* 1992). This model may be useful for testing any pharmacological mechanism believed to impact central sensitization. Further, because neuropathic pain conditions involve central sensitization, the capsaicin model may be useful for identifying compounds that will be effective in neuropathic pain. To date, data with known analgesic drugs in the human model are equivocal (Dirks *et al.* 2002; Gottrup *et al.* 2004; Wallace *et al.* 2002a, 2002b, 2004; Wallace and Schulteis 2008). In the rat capsaicin model, compounds with diverse pharmacological mechanisms are active (Bingham *et al.* 2005; Jarvis *et al.* 2007; Jones *et al.* 2006; Medhurst *et al.* 2007; Piu *et al.* 2008; Yao *et al.* 2009). However, no published data in humans thus far confirm whether the rat model is predictive of human efficacy. Thus, as with the ultraviolet model it is likely too early to determine the value of the capsaicin model as a translational model.

Neuroimaging

Neuroimaging in translational medicine pain therapeutics is an emerging field that holds tremendous potential for facilitating the identification of novel agents. Imaging techniques have the advantages of being noninvasive and providing objective end points. In pain research the most commonly used neuroimaging techniques are functional magnetic resonance imaging (fMRI) and positron emission tomography (PET). Readers should refer to recent reviews for more in-depth information (Bingel and Tracey 2008; Lawrence and Mackey 2008; Neugebauer et al. 2009; Stephenson and Arneric 2008; Tracey 2007; Wartolowska and Tracey 2009). In translational medicine and pain research these techniques have been more thoroughly explored in human subjects than in preclinical species.

Techniques such as fMRI have been used to help elucidate the brain structures or regions that respond to painful stimuli in normal individuals as well as to characterize the responses of these structures in clinical pain states. fMRI studies have identified a complex of neuronal structures involved in processing pain signals referred to as the pain matrix (May 2007). Neuronal structures outside of the pain matrix, however, such as the amygdala, caudate, and parahippocampal area can also impact pain perception (Seifert and Maihofner 2009). Lawrence and Mackey (2008) note that the ultimate goal is to define the neuronal map that underlies responses to pain. Such a map could be used as an objective end point to assess the impact of drug treatments in pain conditions. Given the complexities of human pain conditions, which involve cognitive as well as affective influences, however, defining a simple neuronal map will be difficult.

Positron emission tomography is another functional neuroimaging technique used to study pain processing. PET has been used to identify neural correlates involved in pain processing for both evoked responses in normal individuals as well as neuronal correlates in various pain conditions (Stephenson and Arneric 2008). PET has also been used to investigate the role of various drugs using labeled compounds as well as the role of specific neurotransmitters.

To date neuroimaging techniques such as fMRI are not used routinely for defining efficacy of novel pain therapeutics. More common may be the use of PET to characterize target coverage of specific drugs (i.e., interaction of a compound with a specific molecular entity), but this approach depends on the ability to generate the appropriate ligand for this type of study. Interest in neuroimaging is high in both academia and industry and these techniques will likely become commonplace in drug discovery and development.

Conclusions

The use of translational medicine in the development of pain therapeutics is an emerging paradigm with only a limited number of preclinical (i.e., nonhuman) models with direct human model correlates. Basic research is helping drive the understanding of underlying mechanisms of various types of pain, and improved communication between basic and clinical scientists is facilitating the development of additional models and methods for use in translational medicine. Further technological developments in areas such as neuroimaging will likely bring additional options for translational medicine that will be used to improve the successful development of new pain treatments.

References

Arning K, Baron R. 2009. Evaluation of symptom heterogeneity in neuropathic pain using assessments of sensory functions. *Neurotherapeutics* **6**:738–748.

Bennett GJ, Xie YK. 1988. A peripheral mononeuropathy in rat that produces disorders of pain sensation like those seen in man. *Pain* **33**:87–107.

Bingel U, Tracey I. 2008. Imaging CNS modulation of pain in humans. *Physiology (Bethesda)* **23**:371–380.

Bingham S, Beswick PJ, Bountra C et al. 2005. The cyclooxygenase-2 inhibitor GW406381X [2-(4-ethoxyphenyl)-3-[4-(methylsulfonyl)phenyl]-pyrazolo [1,5-b]pyridazine] is effective in animal models of neuropathic pain and central sensitization. *J Pharmacol Exp Ther* **312**:1161–1169.

Bishop T, Hewson DW, Yip PK et al. 2007. Characterisation of ultraviolet-B-induced inflammation as a model of hyperalgesia in the rat. *Pain* **131**:70–82.

Boettger MK, Weber K, Schmidt M et al. 2009. Gait abnormalities differentially indicate pain or structural joint damage in monoarticular antigen-induced arthritis. *Pain* **145**:142–150.

Broad LM, Keding SJ, Blanco MJ. 2008. Recent progress in the development of selective TRPV1 antagonists for pain. *Curr Top Med Chem* **8**:1431–1441.

Chaplan SR, Bach FW, Pogrel JW, Chung JM, Yaksh TL. 1994. Quantitative assessment of tactile allodynia in the rat paw. *J Neurosci Methods* **53**:55–63.

Chapman LF, Dingman HF, Ginzberg SP. 1965. Failure of systemic analgesic agents to alter the absolute sensory threshold for the simple detection of pain. *Brain* **88**:1011–1022.

Costigan M, Scholz J, Woolf CJ. 2009. Neuropathic pain: a maladaptive response of the nervous system to damage. *Annu Rev Neurosci* **32**:1–32.

D'Amour F, Smith D. 1941. A method for determining loss of pain sensation. *J Pharmacol Exp Ther* **72**:74–79.

Decosterd I, Woolf CJ. 2000. Spared nerve injury: an animal model of persistent peripheral neuropathic pain. *Pain* **87**:149–158.

Dirks J, Petersen KL, Rowbotham MC, Dahl JB. 2002. Gabapentin suppresses cutaneous hyperalgesia following heat-capsaicin sensitization. *Anesthesiology* **97**:102–107.

Eissenberg T, Riggins EC 3rd, Harkins SW, Weaver MF. 2000. A clinical laboratory model for direct assessment of medication-induced antihyperalgesia and subjective effects: initial validation study. *Exp Clin Psychopharmacol* **8**:47–60.

Farkouh ME, Greenberg BP. 2009. An evidence-based review of the cardiovascular risks of nonsteroidal anti-inflammatory drugs. *Am J Cardiol* **103**:1227–1237.

Fischer TZ, Gilmore ES, Estacion M et al. 2009. A novel Nav1.7 mutation producing carbamazepine-responsive erythromelalgia. *Ann Neurol* **65**:733–741.

Goldberg YP, MacFarlane J, MacDonald ML et al. 2007. Loss-of-function mutations in the Nav1.7 gene underlie congenital indifference to pain in multiple human populations. *Clin Genet* **71**:311–319.

Gottrup H, Juhl G, Kristensen AD et al. 2004. Chronic oral gabapentin reduces elements of central sensitization in human experimental hyperalgesia. *Anesthesiology* **101**:1400–1408.

Gougat J, Ferrari B, Sarran L et al. 2004. SSR240612 [(2R)-2-[((3R)-3-(1,3-benzodioxol-5-yl)-3-[[(6-methoxy-2-naphthyl)sulfonyl]amino]propanoyl)amino]-3-(4-[[2R,6S)-2,6-dimethylpiperidinyl]methyl]pheny l)-N-isopropyl-N-methylpropanamide hydrochloride], a new nonpeptide antagonist of the bradykinin B1 receptor: biochemical and pharmacological characterization. *J Pharmacol Exp Ther* **309**:661–669.

Gunthorpe MJ, Chizh BA. 2009. Clinical development of TRPV1 antagonists: targeting a pivotal point in the pain pathway. *Drug Discov Today* **14**:56–67.

Hargreaves KM, Dubner R, Brown F, Flores C, Joris J. 1988. A new and sensitive method for measuring thermal nociception in cutaneous hyperalgesia. *Pain* **32**:77–88.

Herndon CM, Hutchison RW, Berdine HJ et al. 2008. Management of chronic nonmalignant pain with nonsteroidal antiinflammatory drugs. Joint opinion statement of the Ambulatory Care, Cardiology, and Pain and Palliative Care Practice and Research Networks of the American College of Clinical Pharmacy. *Pharmacotherapy* **28**:788–805.

Hughes A, Macleod A, Growcott J, Thomas I. 2002. Assessment of the reproducibility of intradermal administration of capsaicin as a model for inducing human pain. *Pain* **99**:323–331.

Jarvis MF, Boyce-Rustay JM. 2009. Neuropathic pain: models and mechanisms. *Curr Pharm Des* **15**:1711–1716.

Jarvis MF, Honore P, Shieh CC et al. 2007. A-803467, a potent and selective Nav1.8 sodium channel blocker, attenuates neuropathic and inflammatory pain in the rat. *Proc Natl Acad Sci USA* **104**:8520–8525.

Jones CK, Alt A, Ogden AM et al. 2006. Antiallodynic and antihyperalgesic effects of selective competitive GLUK5 (GluR5) ionotropic glutamate receptor antagonists in the capsaicin and carrageenan models in rats. *J Pharmacol Exp Ther* **319**:396–404.

Juhl GI, Jensen TS, Norholt SE, Svensson P. 2008. Central sensitization phenomena after third molar surgery: a quantitative sensory testing study. *Eur J Pain* **12**:116–127.

Kim SH, Chung JM. 1992. An experimental model for peripheral neuropathy produced by segmental spinal nerve ligation in the rat. *Pain* **50**:355–363.

Kinloch RA, Cox PJ. 2005. New targets for neuropathic pain therapeutics. *Expert Opin Ther Targets* **9**:685–698.

Koppert W, Likar R, Geisslinger G et al. 1999. Peripheral antihyperalgesic effect of morphine to heat, but not mechanical, stimulation in healthy volunteers after ultraviolet-B irradiation. *Anesth Analg* **88**:117–122.

Krenzischek DA, Dunwoody CJ, Polomano RC, Rathmell JP. 2008. Pharmacotherapy for acute pain: implications for practice. *J Perianesth Nurs* **23**(1 Suppl.):S28–S42.

La Montagna G, Tirri R, Baruffo A, Preti B, Viaggi S. 1997. Clinical pattern of pain in rheumatoid arthritis. *Clin Exp Rheumatol* **15**:481–485.

LaMotte RH, Shain CN, Simone DA, Tsai EF. 1991. Neurogenic hyperalgesia: psychophysical studies of underlying mechanisms. *J Neurophysiol* **66**:190–211.

Lawrence J, Mackey SC. 2008. Role of neuroimaging in analgesic drug development. *Drugs R D* **9**:323–334.

Maihofner C, Ringler R, Herrndobler F, Koppert W. 2007. Brain imaging of analgesic and antihyperalgesic effects of cyclooxygenase inhibition in an experimental human pain model: a functional MRI study. *Eur J Neurosci* **26**:1344–1356.

Mallinckrodt CH, Raskin J, Wohlreich MM, Watkin JG, Detke MJ. 2004. The efficacy of duloxetine: a comprehensive summary of results from MMRM and LOCF_ANCOVA in eight clinical trials. *BMC Psychiatry* **4**:26.

Mantyh P. 2006. Cancer pain and its impact on diagnosis, survival and quality of life. *Nat Rev Neurosci* **7**:797–808.

May A. 2007. Neuroimaging: visualising the brain in pain. *Neurol Sci* **28**(Suppl. 2):S101–S107.

McLean MJ. 1995. Gabapentin. *Epilepsia* **36**(Suppl. 2):S73–S86.

Medhurst AD, Briggs MA, Bruton G et al. 2007. Structurally novel histamine H3 receptor antagonists GSK207040 and GSK334429 improve scopolamine-induced memory impairment and capsaicin-induced secondary allodynia in rats. *Biochem Pharmacol* **73**:1182–1194.

Medhurst SJ, Walker K, Bowes M et al. 2002. A rat model of bone cancer pain. *Pain* **96**:129–140.

Moalem G, Tracey DJ. 2006. Immune and inflammatory mechanisms in neuropathic pain. *Brain Res Rev* **51**:240–264.

Mogil JS. 2009. Animal models of pain: progress and challenges. *Nat Rev Neurosci* **10**:283–294.

Negus SS, Vanderah TW, Brandt MR et al. 2006. Preclinical assessment of candidate analgesic drugs: recent advances and future challenges. *J Pharmacol Exp Ther* **319**:507–514.

Ness TJ, Gebhart GF. 1988. Colorectal distension as a noxious visceral stimulus: physiologic and pharmacologic characterization of pseudaffective reflexes in the rat. *Brain Res* **450**:153–169.

Neugebauer V, Galhardo V, Maione S, Mackey SC. 2009. Forebrain pain mechanisms. *Brain Res Rev* **60**:226–242.

Nilsen KB, Nicholas AK, Woods CG et al. 2009. Two novel SCN9A mutations causing insensitivity to pain. *Pain* **143**:155–158.

O'Connor AB, Dworkin RH. 2009. Treatment of neuropathic pain: an overview of recent guidelines. *Am J Med* **122**(10 Suppl.):S22–S32.

Petersen KL, Rowbotham MC. 1999. A new human experimental pain model: the heat/capsaicin sensitization model. *Neuroreport* **10**:1511–1516.

Piu F, Cheevers C, Hyldtoft L et al. 2008. Broad modulation of neuropathic pain states by a selective estrogen receptor beta agonist. *Eur J Pharmacol* **590**:423–429.

Randall LO, Selitto JJ. 1957. A method for measurement of analgesic activity on inflamed tissue. *Arch Int Pharmacodyn Ther* **111**:409–419.

Sandkuhler J. 2009. Models and mechanisms of hyperalgesia and allodynia. *Physiol Rev* **89**:707–758.

Scanlon GC, Wallace MS, Ispirescu JS, Schulteis G. 2006. Intradermal capsaicin causes dose-dependent pain, allodynia, and hyperalgesia in humans. *J Investig Med* **54**:238–244.

Schmelz M. 2009. Translating nociceptive processing into human pain models. *Exp Brain Res* **196**:173–178.

Seifert F, Jungfer I, Schmelz M, Maihöfner C. 2008. Representation of UV-B-induced thermal and mechanical hyperalgesia in the human brain: a functional MRI study. *Hum Brain Mapp* **29**:1327–1342.

Seifert F, Maihofner C. 2009. Central mechanisms of experimental and chronic neuropathic pain: findings from functional imaging studies. *Cell Mol Life Sci* **66**:375–390.

Seltzer Z, Dubner R, Shir Y. 1990. A novel behavioral model of neuropathic pain disorders produced in rats by partial sciatic nerve injury. *Pain* **43**:205–218.

Stephenson DT, Arneric SP. 2008. Neuroimaging of pain: advances and future prospects. *J Pain* **9**:567–679.

Sycha T, Anzenhofer S, Lehr S et al. 2005. Rofecoxib attenuates both primary and secondary inflammatory hyperalgesia: a randomized, double blinded, placebo controlled crossover trial in the UV-B pain model. *Pain* **113**:316–322.

Thacker MA, Clark AK, Marchand F, McMahon SB. 2007. Pathophysiology of peripheral neuropathic pain: immune cells and molecules. *Anesth Analg* **105**:838–847.

Tracey I. 2007. Neuroimaging of pain mechanisms. *Curr Opin Support Palliat Care* **1**:109–116.

Treede RD, Jensen TS, Campbell JN et al. 2008. Neuropathic pain: redefinition and a grading system for clinical and research purposes. *Neurology* **70**:1630–1635.

Treede RD, Meyer RA, Raja SN, Campbell JN. 1992. Peripheral and central mechanisms of cutaneous hyperalgesia. *Prog Neurobiol* **38**:397–421.

Wallace MS, Barger D, Schulteis G. 2002a. The effect of chronic oral desipramine on capsaicin-induced allodynia and hyperalgesia: a double-blinded, placebo-controlled, crossover study. *Anesth Analg* **95**:973–978.

Wallace MS, Quessy S, Schulteis G. 2004. Lack of effect of two oral sodium channel antagonists, lamotrigine and 4030W92, on intradermal capsaicin-induced hyperalgesia model. *Pharmacol Biochem Behav* **78**:349–355.

Wallace MS, Ridgeway B 3rd, Leung A, Schulteis G, Yaksh TL. 2002b. Concentration-effect relationships for intravenous alfentanil and ketamine infusions in human volunteers: effects on acute thresholds and capsaicin-evoked hyperpathia. *J Clin Pharmacol* **42**:70–80.

Wallace MS, Schulteis G. 2008. Effect of chronic oral gabapentin on capsaicin-induced pain and hyperalgesia: a double-blind, placebo-controlled, crossover study. *Clin J Pain* **24**:544–549.

Wang H, Bolognese J, Calder N et al. 2008. Effect of morphine and pregabalin compared with diphenhydramine hydrochloride and placebo on hyperalgesia and allodynia induced by intradermal capsaicin in healthy male subjects. *J Pain* **9**:1088–1095.

Wartolowska K, Tracey I. 2009. Neuroimaging as a tool for pain diagnosis and analgesic development. *Neurotherapeutics* **6**:755–760.

Whiteside GT, Adedoyin A, Leventhal L. 2008. Predictive validity of animal pain models? A comparison of the pharmacokinetic-pharmacodynamic relationship for pain drugs in rats and humans. *Neuropharmacology* **54**:767–775.

Woolf CJ, Ma Q. 2007. Nociceptors – noxious stimulus detectors. *Neuron* **55**:353–364.

Yang Y, Wang Y, Li S *et al*. 2004. Mutations in SCN9A, encoding a sodium channel alpha subunit, in patients with primary erythermalgia. *J Med Genet* **41**:171–174.

Yao BB, Hsieh G, Daza AV *et al*. 2009. Characterization of a cannabinoid CB2 receptor-selective agonist, A-836339 [2,2,3,3-tetramethyl-cyclopropanecarboxylic acid [3-(2-methoxy-ethyl)-4,5-dimethyl-3H-thiazol-(2Z)-ylidene]-amide], using in vitro pharmacological assays, in vivo pain models, and pharmacological magnetic resonance imaging. *J Pharmacol Exp Ther* **328**:141–151.

Zhu CZ, Baker S, EI-Kouhen O *et al*. 2008. Analgesic activity of metabotropic glutamate receptor 1 antagonists on spontaneous post-operative pain in rats. *Eur J Pharmacol* **580**: 314–321.

Chapter 10

Multiple sclerosis

Alfred W. Sandrock, Jr and Richard A. Rudick

Translational medicine, the discipline that transforms advances in laboratory-based basic research into human therapeutics, is beginning to be successfully applied in multiple sclerosis (MS), heralded by the introduction of the first disease-modifying therapies for relapsing MS in the early 1990s. Moreover, biological, imaging, and clinical measurements used in patients with MS treated with these disease-modifying therapies have greatly increased our understanding of MS pathogenesis – a demonstration of "reverse" translational medicine. The overall aim of this chapter is to review how advances in our understanding of MS and our ability to measure MS are contributing to the application of translational medicine in this disorder. These past advances will undoubtedly expedite the development of new therapies for MS.

A historical perspective on the evolution of disease-modifying treatments

Interferon beta (IFNβ), the first effective disease-modifying therapy to become available for MS, was tested in this disease based on the hypothesis that it may have a viral etiology. Early work by Tourtellotte and colleagues (1984) found that the antibody response in the cerebrospinal fluid (CSF) of patients with MS was similar to that seen in patients with a viral infection, such as subacute sclerosing panencephalitis caused by the measles virus. In addition, endogenous interferon production by lymphocytes was deficient in patients with MS (Neighbour et al. 1981). Human interferons α, β, and γ were tested in clinical trials, but only IFNβ provided sustained benefit on relapse rates (Jacobs and Johnson 1994; Jacobs et al. 1981, 1982, 1986; Panitch et al. 1987). In the randomized controlled studies of natural IFNβ performed by Jacobs and colleagues in the 1980s (Jacobs et al. 1981, 1982, 1986), intrathecally administered IFNβ reduced relapse rates in patients with MS. These studies enrolled homogeneous groups of patients with relapsing-remitting MS (RRMS) who were followed for a relatively long time (2 years) (Jacobs et al. 1986). The failure to identify a causative virus led to the modified view that MS may be a chronic autoimmune disease initiated by possible early infection. It was hypothesized that anti-inflammatory agents such as corticosteroids may suppress the immune responses responsible for the disease (Herndon et al. 1983). Unfortunately, many of the early corticosteroid trials produced inconclusive results because of suboptimal designs: some were not randomized or controlled; others did not have uniform inclusion criteria (Perkin 1987). However, one multicenter, placebo-controlled trial of adrenocorticotropic hormone (ACTH) stood out. It used a double-blind, randomized design, and patients were preevaluated for relapse rates. Several outcome measures, including a clinical estimate of neurological impairment, disability scoring, and tabulation of subjective symptoms, were used to assess the efficacy of treatment (Rose et al. 1970). Although this study failed to demonstrate substantial benefits for patients with MS attributable to ACTH, it laid the groundwork for future well-designed clinical trials.

In addition to immunomodulation, immunological "desensitization" or "tolerance" to potential antigens such as myelin basic protein was also hypothesized to specifically inhibit the immune response that leads to development of MS lesions (Herndon et al. 1983). Glatiramer acetate (GA), a random polymer that simulates myelin basic protein but is not encephalitogenic, was tested in a double-blind, randomized, placebo-controlled pilot trial. GA exhibited beneficial effects on relapse rates over placebo in patients with RRMS (Bornstein et al. 1987).

Translational Neuroscience, ed. James E. Barrett, Joseph T. Coyle and Michael Williams. Published by Cambridge University Press. © Cambridge University Press 2012.

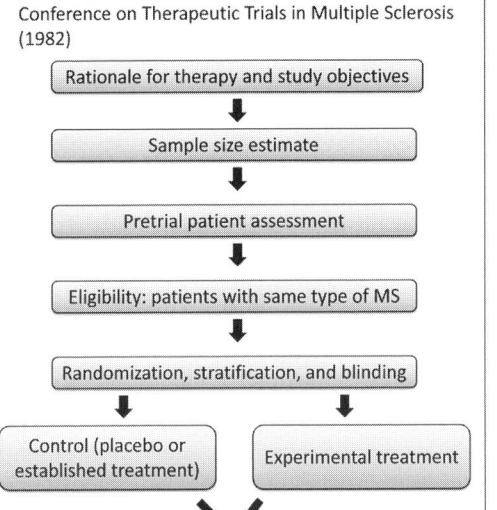

Figure 10.1. Design considerations for multiple sclerosis clinical trials.

Working protocol proposed at the first International Conference on Therapeutic Trials in Multiple Sclerosis (1982)

- Rationale for therapy and study objectives
- Sample size estimate
- Pretrial patient assessment
- Eligibility: patients with same type of MS
- Randomization, stratification, and blinding
- Control (placebo or established treatment) / Experimental treatment
- Clinical outcomes

Revisions proposed by an international workshop on MS trials in a new therapeutic era (2004)

Alternative study design to reduce or eliminate the use of placebo for RRMS; "selective weeding" or "add on" design for progressive forms of MS

Validated novel clinical outcomes and validated surrogate outcomes

---

These early studies on IFNβ (Jacobs *et al.* 1981, 1982, 1986), ACTH (Rose *et al.* 1970), and GA (Bornstein *et al.* 1987) provided the impetus for the modern clinical trials that soon followed. The development of IFNβ and GA was in a very early stage when groups convened to agree on the important factors that need to be considered for proper design of definitive trials in MS therapy. These considerations were summarized after the first International Conference on Therapeutic Trials in Multiple Sclerosis in 1982 (Herndon *et al.* 1983) and later by Weiss *et al.* (1988). The protocol for trials in MS should start with a clearly stated rationale for therapy and goals of treatment or study end points (relapses and/or measures of disability), depending on the stage of MS being treated. It was recommended that patients enrolled in the study have the same type of MS for a clearer demonstration of efficacy and safety and that pretrial patient assessments ensure the inclusion of patients who were most likely to be sensitive to treatment effects (excluding patients in extended periods of remission). In addition, a placebo control group was recommended, and randomization, stratification, and blinding as well as other ways of reducing bias were felt to be crucial to the precision of the trial. Finally, the sample size, determined by the expected effect of therapy, must be statistically appropriate and sufficient to address the proposed study objectives (Fig. 10.1). These recommendations remain appropriate to this day for the design of MS clinical trials.

Potential therapies originating from a biological hypothesis can be directly tested in clinical trials in humans, as in the case of IFNβ, but more often these candidate therapies are first tested in an animal model. GA was successfully evaluated in the animal model of MS, experimental autoimmune encephalomyelitis (EAE), before being studied in clinical trials (Steinman and Zamvil 2006). However, drugs such as IFNγ and antitumor necrosis factor antibody were effective in the EAE model but worsened clinical and/or magnetic resonance imaging (MRI) outcomes in MS in clinical trials (Sriram and Steiner 2005), highlighting the pitfalls of overreliance on the EAE model for proof of principle (see section on "The appropriate use of animal models of disease" below).

Use of MRI measures as potential markers to monitor the response to therapy also contributed to the rapid advances in clinical trials in MS. MRI was adopted early as an outcome measure in IFNβ studies (IFNB Multiple Sclerosis Study Group and the University of British Columbia MS/MRI Analysis Group 1995; Jacobs *et al.* 1996; PRISMS Study Group 1998); its use was recommended early on by the US National MS Society Task Force (Miller *et al.* 1996). MRI has become particularly useful as the primary end point in proof-of-concept (phase II) trials in RRMS (Cohen and Rudick 2007). Novel imaging techniques are being explored in progressive forms of the disease as well (see section on "The availability of imaging surrogate biomarkers of disease activity in proof-of-concept trials" below).

The development of disease-modifying therapies in MS was spurred by existing hypotheses of MS pathogenesis and the presumed mechanism of action of available candidate drugs. Whether these early hypotheses were correct is a matter of debate, but the emergence of disease-modifying therapies would not have been possible without the appropriate use of accepted clinical outcome measures in well-designed, well-controlled clinical trials that enrolled active, relatively homogeneous patient populations. These factors not only were fundamental to the early pioneering studies but also will continue to contribute to the rational development of disease-modifying therapies in the future.

Pathogenesis

Whereas the success of clinical trials need not rely on a thorough understanding of human pathogenesis, the efficiency of translational activities undoubtedly improves with an increased appreciation of molecular pathophysiology. MS is a chronic inflammatory disease of the CNS. The autoimmune hypothesis is supported by many studies linking cellular and humoral immune responses against CNS myelin antigens to demyelinating lesions in patients with MS (Raine 1994; Trapp *et al.* 1998). Arguably, the best evidence that MS is caused by autoimmunity comes from the success of immunomodulatory and immune cell-depleting therapies as well as the finding that MS disease-susceptibility genes encode proteins involved in immune regulation, such as major histocompatibility complex, class II, DR beta 1, also known as HLA-DRB1; the interleukin-2 receptor α (IL2RA); or the interleukin-7 receptor α (IL7RA). The role of the HLA-DR2 haplotype (*DRB1*1501-DQB1*0602*) in increasing the risk of MS in whites has been known for many years (Sawcer *et al.* 2005), but the fact that a unique haplotype of an older African origin (*DRB1*15*, independent of *DQB1*0602*) increases the risk of MS in African-Americans (Oksenberg *et al.* 2004) makes an autoimmune pathogenesis even more likely. Whether autoimmunity is a primary pathogenic event or whether it is secondary to a primary neurodegenerative process has not been determined,

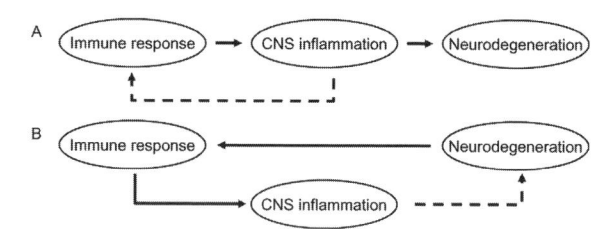

Figure 10.2. Models of disease pathogenesis in multiple sclerosis. MS is commonly regarded as a chronic inflammatory disease of the central nervous system (CNS). The traditional neuropathological view of multiple sclerosis (A) highlights the neurodegeneration as a consequence of an autoimmune response. An alternative hypothesis (B) proposes that the autoimmunity observed may be secondary to a primary neurodegenerative process. Reprinted from *Neuron*, Vol. 52, Hauser SL, Oksenberg JR. The neurobiology of multiple sclerosis: genes, inflammation, and neurodegeneration, pp. 61–76, copyright 2006, with permission from Elsevier.

despite extensive recent discussion (Fig. 10.2) (Hohlfeld and Wekerle 2004).

The etiology of MS is largely unknown; it has been hypothesized that the autoimmune process may be triggered by microbial infections or other environmental factors. Epstein–Barr virus (EBV) was suggested as a causal agent in the early 1980s (Warner and Carp 1981). The B lymphocyte is susceptible to EBV infection, which could provide the virus access to the CNS during the insult to the brain or spinal cord. Ascherio and colleagues (2001) recently provided epidemiological evidence suggesting an association between infection with EBV and risk of MS: They found significant elevations in serum anti-EBV antibody titers before onset of MS. If more proof of causality were demonstrated, this finding might suggest that antiviral approaches may one day be useful in treating MS or, perhaps more likely, in preventing MS in at-risk individuals.

The autoimmune model of MS provided the rationale for developing immunotherapies, first anti-inflammatory drugs and more recently agents that selectively target components of the immune response (Feldmann and Steinman 2005; Hohlfeld and Wekerle 2004; Noseworthy 2003). However, immunotherapy is more effective during the early relapsing-remitting phase (including the earliest phase of the disease, called clinically isolated syndrome) than the subsequent secondary progressive phase of MS (SPMS) (Frohman *et al.* 2006) (Fig. 10.3), which suggests that the disease processes that drive disability progression during these two phases of the disease may be different (Frohman *et al.* 2006). In addition to RRMS and

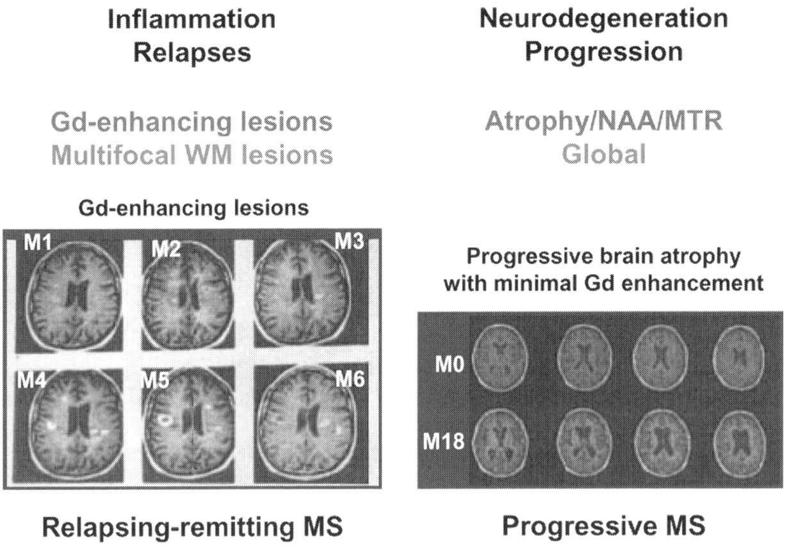

Figure 10.3. Clinical course of multiple sclerosis (MS) and associated magnetic resonance imaging (MRI) image changes. The early phase of MS, relapsing-remitting MS, is predominated by multifocal inflammation and relapses; the later phase, secondary progressive MS, is characterized by progressive neuroaxonal loss and increasing disability. Gd, gadolinium; MTR, magnetization transfer ratio; NAA, N-acetylaspartate; WM, white matter. Reprinted from *NeuroRx*, Vol. 1, Miller DH. Biomarkers and surrogate outcomes in neurodegenerative disease: lessons from multiple sclerosis, pp. 284–294, copyright 2004, with permission from Elsevier.

SPMS, other clinical manifestations of MS include primary progressive MS (PPMS), which is characterized by continuous neurological deterioration from disease onset without relapses, and progressive relapsing MS (PRMS), which is characterized by neurological progression from onset superimposed with relapses (Lublin and Reingold 1996). These different clinical manifestations suggest that the underlying disease mechanisms might also differ for these less common types of the disease. For example, a less common form of optic-spinal MS called Devic's disease, which more commonly affects Asians than whites and has recently been associated with antibodies to aquaporin-4 (Lennon *et al.* 2005), appears not to respond well to therapies effective in RRMS and may respond better to therapies that affect humoral factors, such as plasmapheresis (Keegan *et al.* 2005). The heterogeneity of MS, even when classified by relatively straightforward clinical phenotypes, serves to underscore the crucial importance of enrolling well-defined, homogeneous patient populations in clinical trials of MS, depending on the presumed mechanism of action of the drug being tested.

Lucchinetti and colleagues (2000) have called attention to the heterogeneity in MS lesions based on the systematic histopathological examination of a large number of biopsy and autopsy specimens from patients with MS and have proposed four distinct patterns of demyelinating lesions. All four types are associated with T-lymphocyte- and macrophage-dominated inflammation but with different major features: macrophage-mediated demyelination in type I, antibody-mediated demyelination in type II, distal oligodendrogliopathy in type III, and demyelination secondary to nonapoptotic oligodendrocyte degeneration in type IV. The patterns of demyelination were observed to differ from patient to patient but were homogeneous within multiple active lesions from the same patient, suggesting that MS may be several diseases with distinct pathological processes. If true, this patient-to-patient heterogeneity has important therapeutic implications: it suggests that optimal MS therapeutics may require targeting specific drugs for specific groups of patients with one type of lesion. A retrospective study of 19 patients with Devic's disease treated with therapeutic plasma exchange (TPE) provided evidence to support this concept. Therapeutic plasma exchange was used to treat severe relapses unresponsive to corticosteroids. In this study, 10 patients responded favorably to TPE, but nine did not. All patients with a favorable response had type II lesions, whereas the nine who did not respond had type I or III lesions (Keegan *et al.* 2005). The different responses to TPE, therefore, seem to correlate with variations in the pathology of the disease. This report has not been confirmed, probably because lesion biopsies are not generally obtained in patients with MS and because MRI signatures of these lesion types have not been developed.

However, Barnett and Prineas (2004) demonstrated that active lesions from the same patient may have features of more than one category of lesions as defined by Lucchinetti and colleagues. For example, lesions with extensive oligodendrocyte apoptosis (one of the features of type III lesions) exhibited complement activation (one of the features of type II lesions) but no infiltrating lymphocytes or macrophages. This observation suggests that the four types of lesions described by Lucchinetti and colleagues (2000) merely reflect lesions at various stages of evolution. Regardless of which explanation is correct, these findings indicate a need for updating the pathological classification of MS, perhaps by employing biological or imaging measures that reflect the predominant underlying demyelinating lesion type in a given patient. A modern biologically based disease classification may improve the power of clinical trials by allowing for the enrollment of patients more likely to respond to certain targeted therapies or, at the very least, allow for personalized approaches to MS therapies.

In addition to inflammatory demyelination, axonal damage has been described early in actively demyelinating lesions (Trapp *et al.* 1998); damaged axons, devoid of myelin, may have difficulty surviving for long periods and are thus prone to degenerate. This situation is likely in peripheral demyelinating diseases such as Charcot–Marie–Tooth disease, type I (Krajewski *et al.* 2000). Cumulative axonal loss is thought to ultimately determine the irreversible disability that occurs during SPMS (Frohman *et al.* 2006).

Axons can be damaged by T-lymphocyte-mediated immune responses, but the B-cell immune response is also relevant. Lymphoid follicle-like structures were recently detected in the cerebral meninges of patients with SPMS (Magliozzi *et al.* 2007; Serafini *et al.* 2004). These ectopic B-cell follicles with germinal centers may sustain B-cell maturation locally within the CNS, contributing to the compartmentalization of the disease and local amplification of the chronic humoral autoimmune response (Magliozzi *et al.* 2007). The ectopic lymphoid tissue formation was found to be associated with an early onset of disease, irreversible disability and death, and more severe cortical damage (Magliozzi *et al.* 2007). The clonal expansion of B cells in the CSF, the high prevalence of CSF oligoclonal bands in MS, and the recent work by Obermeier and colleagues (2008) that demonstrated the B-cell clones isolated from the CSF are the source of these oligoclonal bands, strongly suggest that at least some of the autoimmunity in MS is driven by processes on the CNS side of the blood–brain barrier (and ultimately independently of immune cells in the periphery). To fully arrest the autoimmunity in MS, especially in SPMS, therefore, may require drugs capable of crossing the blood–brain barrier to disrupt the formation or maturation of ectopic lymphoid follicles, inhibit B-cell clonal expansion, or suppress the secretion of cytokines and/or immunoglobulins from cells resident in the CNS. Of note, approaches that deplete peripheral immune cells, such as bone marrow transplantation (Burt *et al.* 1998, 2009) or rituximab treatment (Hauser *et al.* 2008), which are effective in suppressing inflammation in relapsing forms of MS, have less dramatic effects in progressive forms of MS (Burt *et al.* 2003; Hawker *et al.* 2009) and have limited effects on depleting activated CSF B cells (Mondria *et al.* 2008; Monson *et al.* 2005).

Considerable progress has been made in understanding the pathogenesis of MS, which undoubtedly contributes to designing targeted therapies. However, MS is a complicated disease, and our understanding of its pathogenesis is still incomplete. Recent evidence suggests that pathogenic mechanisms of MS change over the course of the disease. When Fisher and colleagues (2008) studied the MRI correlates of gray matter atrophy in patients with RRMS and SPMS, they found several MRI measures related to MS lesions and normal-appearing white matter that correlated with gray matter atrophy over the next 4 years in patients with RRMS, but none of the measures were related to subsequent gray matter atrophy in patients with SPMS. These results imply that pathogenic mechanisms driving gray matter atrophy change with the progression of the disease, which further implies that therapeutic targets may change as the disease advances. This idea is of course consistent with the observations that currently approved disease-modifying drugs have maximal benefit during the RRMS stage of disease and appear ineffective in patients with purely progressive forms of the disease. Continued research into the underlying disease mechanisms is needed to facilitate the development of novel therapeutic interventions in MS, which may in turn shed light on the processes that mediate disease progression at various stages.

Table 10.1. Factors that improve the efficiency of translational medicine in multiple sclerosis.

The identification of drug targets within well-validated biological pathways

The use of pharmocodynamic markers, especially in early proof-of-concept and dose-ranging clinical trials

The appropriate use of animal models of disease

The availability of imaging surrogate markers of disease activity in proof-of-concept clinical trials

The use of validated clinical outcome measures that confirm clinically meaningful treatment effects

Factors that improve the efficiency of translational medicine

Successful application of translational medicine in MS has resulted in it becoming a treatable disease. Based on our accumulated experience, five factors that improve the efficiency of translational medicine in MS have been identified. These factors include (1) the identification of drug targets within well-validated biological pathways; (2) the use of pharmacodynamic markers, especially in early proof-of-concept and dose-ranging clinical trials; (3) the appropriate use of animal models of disease; (4) the availability of imaging surrogate biomarkers of disease activity in proof-of-concept clinical trials; and (5) the use of validated clinical outcome measures that confirm clinically meaningful treatment effects so as to gain widespread regulatory approval and adoption by treating neurologists (Table 10.1).

The identification of drug targets within well-validated biological pathways

The modern pharmaceutical sciences are adept at producing drug candidates (both small molecules and biologics) against certain "targets" (e.g., intracellular enzymes, cell surface receptors). The ultimate success of these drug candidates depends, at least in part, on whether these drug targets exist in biological pathways that play a crucial role in the initiation or progression of disease. Identifying these pathways is one of the goals of translational medicine. How is this achieved?

A biological pathway may be considered to have achieved a high level of validation when a drug that targets a constituent of the pathway is confirmed to show clinically meaningful efficacy in a well-designed clinical trial. However, even in this situation some caution is warranted because the full repertoire of the biological activities of a given drug is seldom known. In the case of MS, the first disease-modifying drugs were so pleiotropic that no clear drug targets could be immediately identified. For example, by binding cell surface receptors that are present on a diversity of cell types, IFNβ induces a cascade of events inside cells resulting in changes in the expression of hundreds of genes. These gene products in turn induce a further cascade of biological effects. Which of these events (or, more likely, combination of events) leads to the efficacy observed in MS clinical trials is difficult to discern. More recent drugs, such as natalizumab, which selectively blocks α_4 integrins (Rudick and Sandrock 2004), and rituximab, which selectively depletes CD20-bearing cells (Hauser et al. 2008), provide more specificity as to the biological pathways and cell types that are important for disease activity in relapsing MS. Thus, the α_4 subunit of integrins can be considered a validated drug target, and other drugs that functionally inhibit its biological activities are likely to be efficacious in relapsing MS. Another cell surface receptor that has been validated is the sphingosine-1-phosphate (S1P) receptor, of which there are five known subtypes (Young and Van Brocklyn 2006); functional inhibitors of the S1P1 receptor subtype, such as fingolimod, cause lymphopenia and reduce relapses and gadolinium-enhancing lesions on MRI scans in patients with relapsing MS (Kappos et al. 2006). Careful examination of the biological pathways "upstream" and "downstream" of such validated targets may also lead to novel drugs that offer different benefits and risks for patients and may improve the ease of drug administration for patients. Agents that deplete circulating lymphocytes, such as rituximab (Hauser et al. 2008), alemtuzumab (Hirst et al. 2008), and cladribine (Beutler 1992; Sipe 2005) as well as bone marrow depletion with stem-cell rescue (Burt et al. 1998, 2009), have also been shown to decrease relapse rates, decrease gadolinium-enhancing lesions, or improve neurological symptoms in relapsing MS;

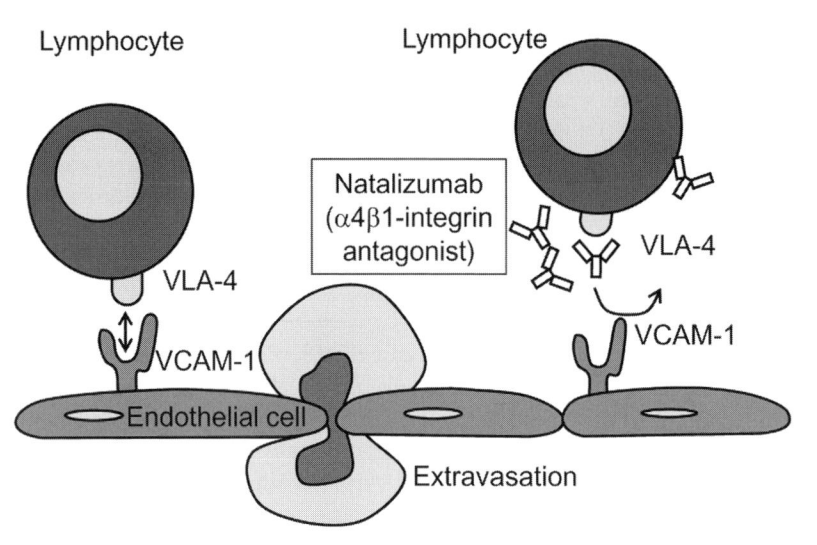

Figure 10.4. The proposed mechanism of action of natalizumab. $\alpha_4\beta_1$ integrin is expressed on the surface of lymphocytes and required for the migration of these cells across the blood–brain barrier. Natalizumab, a recombinant humanized α_4 integrin antibody, blocks the movement of lymphocytes from the periphery into the central nervous system. VCAM-1, vascular adhesion molecule 1; VLA, $\alpha_4\beta_1$ integrin very late activation antigen. Reprinted from *CNS Drugs*, Vol. **19**, Sheremata WA, Minagar A, Alexander JS, Vollmer T. The role of alpha-4 integrin in the aetiology of multiple sclerosis: current knowledge and therapeutic implications, pp. 909–922, copyright 2005, with permission from Wolters Kluwer Health.

however, the long-term safety of lymphocyte depletion remains unknown.

When no clinical trial data are available to direct drug development toward a specific biological pathway or cell type, one is left to generate drug candidates against targets based on indirect evidence. A therapeutic hypothesis is formed, guided by what is known of the human biology of the disease. Observations from human cells and tissues that are consistent with the therapeutic hypothesis increase the confidence that the drug will be successful. Is the drug target expressed by the appropriate cells in the tissue of interest in humans with the disease? Are the pattern and timing of expression consistent with a causative role of the drug target in disease activity and progression? Can any ex vivo studies with human cells or tissues be done to further address the role of the drug target in disease causation? It may be illustrative to review the indirect evidence in humans with MS that led to the enthusiasm for developing natalizumab, a recombinant humanized antibody that binds to α_4 integrins.

Active MS lesions were known to be characterized by the perivascular infiltration of mononuclear lymphocytes (Katz *et al.* 1993). Animal studies of lymphocyte trafficking into inflamed tissues pointed to the importance of α_4 integrins (Lobb and Hemler 1994), especially $\alpha_4\beta_1$ integrins, in CNS inflammation (Engelhardt *et al.* 1998; Yednock *et al.* 1992). Vora and colleagues (1996) showed that in patients with MS, circulating peripheral blood mononuclear cells exhibited increased adhesion to endothelial cell monolayers treated with proinflammatory cytokines and that the increase in adhesion was, at least in part, explained by cell surface $\alpha_4\beta_1$ integrins and temporally related to disease activity (relapse). The expression of $\alpha_4\beta_1$ integrin and one of its ligands, vascular cell adhesion molecule-1, was further shown to be increased in histological studies of active MS lesions (Cannella and Raine 1995). Increased vascular cell adhesion molecule-1 expression on microvessels (Washington *et al.* 1994), pericytes (Verbeek *et al.* 1995), and perivascular macrophages/microglia (Peterson *et al.* 2002) of MS lesions was also reported. The importance of the role of $\alpha_4\beta_1$ integrin on the surface of lymphocytes and monocytes that migrate across the blood–brain barrier into the active MS lesions had thus received substantial support from studies in tissues and cells from humans with MS (Fig. 10.4). These observations provided a strong rationale for testing natalizumab in patients with relapsing MS.

Phase 1 clinical trials, in conjunction with the standard preliminary assessment of the relationship between the administered dose and the safety and pharmacokinetics of the drug candidate, may provide an opportunity to assess target engagement in the tissue of interest by the drug candidate. For natalizumab, peripheral blood mononuclear cells were examined ex vivo for the degree of α_4 integrin saturation by the antibody (European Medicines Agency 2006). For many drugs whose target is in the CNS, this process will pose a significant challenge in humans, although inferences may be drawn from studies of drug concentration or target engagement in CSF. Another potential way to assess receptor occupancy is to perform positron emission tomography, if positron emission tomographic ligands are available.

Ideas for rational design of novel targeted drugs can also come from human genetic studies. It is widely known that genetic predisposition contributes to the pathogenesis of MS: genes may influence disease susceptibility (Hauser and Oksenberg 2006), disease severity, clinical course, or other aspects of the clinical phenotype in patients with MS (Barcellos et al. 2002; Brassat et al. 1999; GAMES and the Transatlantic Multiple Sclerosis Genetics Cooperative 2003). Genetic studies could help to identify biological pathways that are linked, directly or indirectly, to the underlying cause of MS. Genes that are associated with disease risk (i.e., disease-susceptibility genes) likely point to biological pathways that lead to initiation of disease, and genes that are associated with disease course or severity (i.e., disease-modifying genes) likely point to biological pathways that lead to disease progression. Drugs that successfully target either of these biological pathways are likely to benefit patients with MS.

Many human genetic studies, including genome-wide linkage scans in families, association studies in sporadic cases, and microarray expression analyses, have been conducted to identify susceptibility loci and candidate genes that predispose people to MS. These studies consistently identified the major histocompatibility complex mapping to chromosome 6p21.3 as the genomic region harboring MS susceptibility genes (Fernald et al. 2005; Kantarci et al. 2002). The HLA-DR2 haplotype contained in the region is the strongest genetic factor identified so far influencing susceptibility to MS (Hauser and Oksenberg 2006), which again points to the importance of autoimmunity in MS pathogenesis.

Other predisposing genes within the major histocompatibility complex region and other disease-susceptibility loci also exist. A recent large-scale, genome-wide association study by the International MS Genetics Consortium led to the identification of additional alleles that were strongly associated with MS: two single nucleotide polymorphisms (SNPs) within the IL2RA gene, a nonsynonymous SNP in the IL7RA gene, and multiple SNPs in the HLA-DRA locus (Hafler et al. 2007). These findings indicate that genes related to immune regulation are important factors in MS, which add indirectly to the evidence for an immunological basis for MS. When disrupted in mice, the interleukin-2 gene can lead to an autoimmune disease characterized by the dysfunction of regulatory T cells expressing CD4 and CD25 (Bayer et al. 2007; Yu and Malek 2006); compromised function of CD4+CD25+ T cells has been reported in patients with MS (Haas et al. 2005; Viglietta et al. 2004). Interleukin-7 may be important for the expansion of autoreactive T lymphocytes from memory T cells (Bielekova et al. 1999) and for the development of gamma delta T cells observed early in acute MS lesions (Bielekova et al. 1999; He and Malek 1996; Wucherpfennig et al. 1992). These studies support the idea that the SNPs within IL2RA and IL7RA genes could be linked to the pathogenic events that result in MS and therefore are worthy targets of further investigation and drug development. It is intriguing to note that an anti-interleukin-2 receptor monoclonal antibody has been developed and that its clinical efficacy in MS has been demonstrated in two phase II studies (Bielekova et al. 2004; Montalban et al. 2007; Rose et al. 2004).

Identification of disease-modifying genes is equally if not more important for the discovery of biological pathways that affect disease progression, but it has relied heavily on population association studies, which are easily confounded by ethnic variation or other population variables. As a result, although several disease-modifying genes with probable importance have been identified, such as HLA class II, apolipoprotein E, interleukin-1β (IL-1β), and IL-1 receptor antagonist, their biological effects on MS clinical phenotypes are less clear (GAMES and the Transatlantic Multiple Sclerosis Genetics Cooperative 2003). Inconsistent analysis of disease phenotype in the different studies has also contributed to the discrepant reports on how these genes affect the clinical course of MS. Further studies are needed to confirm the involvement of these genes in the course of MS and its severity.

Since the introduction of disease-modifying treatments for MS, it has become abundantly clear from the clinical trial data as well as the day-to-day experience of clinical practice that some patients respond better to a given therapy than others (Keegan et al. 2005; Waubant et al. 2003). As we improve our understanding of how to define, characterize, and classify responders and nonresponders (Rudick and Polman 2009), we predict that in the future we will determine methods for tailoring the right drug for the right patient with MS at a given stage of the disease. Such "personalized medicine" approaches will ensure that drugs and drug combinations are optimized for each patient.

The use of pharmacodynamic markers, especially in early proof-of-concept and dose-ranging clinical trials

Pharmacodynamic markers can be measured in humans as an indication of whether the biological pathway of interest has been engaged (blocked or activated) in the appropriate tissue. Many treatment-related biomarkers have been identified for the current standard therapies of MS, including IFNβ, natalizumab, and GA. Interferon-stimulated gene products – neopterin or the antiviral protein MxA – were used as biological response markers for IFNβ (Alam et al. 1997; Pachner et al. 2003). Natalizumab, through inhibition of leukocyte migration out of the vascular space (Fig. 10.4), increases the number of circulating lymphocytes, monocytes, eosinophils, and basophils (but not neutrophils) in peripheral blood (data on file; Biogen Idec, Inc., Cambridge, MA, USA). Lymphocytosis was therefore used as a pharmacodynamic marker for natalizumab treatment in clinical trials (Tubridy et al. 1999). Regarding GA, a shift of the T helper cells from proinflammatory (Th1) to immunomodulatory (Th2), or the ratio of TH1 to Th2 cytokines, has been proposed as a marker for responsiveness to GA therapy, but its validity needs to be confirmed in prospective trials (Cohen and Rudick 2007).

Identification of pharmacodynamic markers is of great interest because they are not only useful in verifying the proposed mechanism of action of a drug but also valuable in interpreting the outcomes of clinical trials, especially unsuccessful proof-of-concept trials. The absence of pharmacodynamic markers may leave open the question of whether the therapeutic hypothesis was adequately tested, for example, whether the dose was inadequate or whether the drug failed to reach the intended tissue compartment to engage its target. Under these circumstances, it is difficult to ascertain whether a pathway should be tested again using a different drug or another dose of the same drug, hampering progress in translational medicine. Conversely, in the face of an adequate pharmacodynamic response, failure of a well-conducted clinical trial may be a major contribution to the field because a relevant pathological role for the targeted pathway can be more confidently excluded.

The appropriate use of animal models of disease

Animal models are important tools for understanding the pathogenesis of human diseases and for testing therapeutic approaches that either improve symptoms or modify the course of a disease. Validated, predictive animal models can make important contributions to the process of translational medicine. Parkinson's disease was the first neurological disease to be successfully modeled, which subsequently led to the development of neurotransmitter replacement therapy (Betarbet et al. 2002). Whereas the current Parkinson's disease models may be useful for screening drugs that might provide symptomatic relief for patients with the disease, they may be less useful in testing potentially disease-modifying drugs.

Unlike the situation with Parkinson's disease, it is difficult to model some symptoms of MS in animals (e.g., fatigue, pain, and spasticity). EAE, the primary animal model for MS induced by the major known CNS antigens that elicit the autoimmune response in humans, has been used mainly for testing disease-modifying therapies (in addition to studying disease mechanisms). However, positive effects of a drug in the EAE model do not always predict clinical efficacy in MS (Table 10.2). Some drugs that produced promising results in EAE have proven to be of little value in humans. For example, anti-TNF antibody reverses EAE, but worsens MS in humans; IFNγ can either ameliorate or worsen EAE depending on route of administration, but it worsens MS (Panitch et al. 1987; Sriram and Steiner 2005). In other cases, treatments with demonstrated efficacy in humans showed contradictory results in the initial animal model testing. For example, IFNβ decreases relapse rates and disability progression in patients with relapsing MS, but it has variable effects in EAE and can worsen EAE if given after immunization (Sriram and Steiner 2005). Similarly, natalizumab is an effective disease-modifying treatment in humans with relapsing MS, but it has discordant effects before and after onset of relapsing EAE (Theien et al. 2001). Examples of success do exist: GA and mitoxantrone were both developed for treatment of MS after promising results in the EAE model (Table 10.2) (Steinman and Zamvil 2006).

Table 10.2. Effects of multiple sclerosis treatments and potential treatments in the EAE animal model and in patients with MS.

Immunotherapy	Effects in EAE	Effects in patients with MS
Anti-TNF antibody	Reverses EAE	Worsens MS
Interferon-γ	Worsens or ameliorates EAE depending on route of administration	Increases relapse rates
Interferon-β	Variable; can worsen EAE if given after immunization	Decreases relapse and slows disability progression
Natalizumab	Has discordant effects before and after onset of relapsing EAE	Reduces relapses and improves disability
Glatiramer acetate	Suppresses the induction of acute EAE and blocks relapsing EAE	Reduces relapses and improves disability
Mitoxantrone	Reverses ongoing paralysis and reduces the number and extent of perivascular brain lesions	Reduces frequency of relapses and slows clinical progression

EAE, experimental allergic encephalomyelitis; MS, multiple sclerosis.
Reprinted from *Annals of Neurology*, Vol. 58, Sriram S, Steiner I. Experimental allergic encephalomyelitis: a misleading model of multiple sclerosis, pp. 939–945, copyright 2005, with permission from John Wiley and Sons.

EAE has been used as an animal model for MS for almost 80 years. Our current understanding of the pathogenesis of MS, especially with respect to the "effector" side of immunopathogenesis, may benefit from research in EAE, but it is important to recognize its limited value in identifying drug targets or for screening for safe and effective drugs in MS. We prefer to view animal models such as EAE not as models of the human disease per se but as models with certain pathophysiological features of the human disease.

The availability of imaging surrogate biomarkers of disease activity in proof-of-concept trials

Whereas EAE may be of limited use in MS research, the ability to efficiently conduct well-controlled proof-of-concept clinical trials in humans has allowed for much of the success in translational research that we see today. McFarland was among the first to recognize the value of MRI assessment in obtaining proof of concept for new treatments that affect inflammation in MS (Fig. 10.3) (McFarland et al. 1992). A recent meta-analysis of all randomized trials in RRMS reporting MRI variables and relapses demonstrated that treatment effects on MRI lesions correlated well with treatment effects on relapse rates (Sormani et al. 2009), strongly supporting the use of MRI parameters as end points in phase II trials. Widespread use of MRI as a surrogate for relapse in RRMS proof-of-concept trials has played a major role in the development of new treatments. However, its use as a primary end point in pivotal trials is still not accepted by regulatory authorities.

Unfortunately, indices of disease activity in RRMS are not readily transferable to progressive forms of MS, which are characterized by gradual neurological degeneration and irreversible disability rather than the periodic inflammatory attacks and relapses that characterize RRMS. Currently, no consensus exists on optimal measures for use in proof-of-concept trials in progressive forms of MS. Conventional MRI measures such as T2-weighted imaging are considered to reflect overall lesion burden, but correlate poorly with physical disability. This finding potentially could be attributed to a lack of ability to differentiate between inflammation, edema, demyelination, axonal degeneration, and axonal loss (Zivadinov and Bakshi 2004). Fisher and colleagues (2007) studied the correlations between MRI and pathological characteristics in a rapid autopsy program and found that only 55% of T2 lesions were demyelinated, compared with 83% of demyelinated lesions that were bright on T2-weighted images, were dark on T1-weighted images, and showed low magnetization transfer ratios (MTR) (Fisher et al. 2007). This finding directly demonstrated that almost half of all lesions defined by T2 hyperintensity are nondestructive, explaining one reason for low correlations between T2 lesions and disability. In approximately the past decade, newer MRI techniques have been introduced to better monitor the destructive pathological expression of MS lesions. Increased lesion hypointensity on T1-weighted images ("black holes") (Loevner et al. 1995), reduced MTR (Loevner et al. 1995), abnormal water diffusion on diffusion tensor imaging (Werring et al. 1999), and reduced neuronal marker N-acetyl aspartate on magnetic resonance spectroscopy (Husted et al. 1994; Matthews et al. 1996; Narayanan et al. 1997) are all expected to better reflect tissue damage and loss. Because MS lesions occur not only in white matter but also in gray matter (Geurts et al. 2005), diffusion tensor imaging, magnetic resonance spectroscopy, and other emerging imaging techniques are also being developed to assess tissue damage in gray matter (Barkhof et al. 2009; Sastre-Garriga et al. 2005).

In addition to lesion-based measures, whole-brain volume change over time on serial MRI is receiving increased attention as one of the best-studied methods for quantifying neurodegeneration in MS (Barkhof et al. 2009). Global brain atrophy can be measured with precision and is sensitive to change over time. Most importantly, it seems to correlate with measures of disability. Sample-size estimates for detecting treatment effects on brain atrophy suggest that it can be used as an outcome measure in phase II trials for SPMS. Nevertheless, whole-brain atrophy is not without its drawbacks, one of which is the lack of specificity for location- and tissue-specific processes. For example, "pseudoatrophy" has been noted to occur with agents that reduce inflammation – the rapid resolution of edema from an inflamed brain may be mistakenly interpreted as worsening brain atrophy (Hardmeier et al. 2005). Another drawback is the potentially slow responsiveness to therapeutic interventions that requires trial durations of at least 1 year. More advanced imaging techniques may be needed to detect early signs of neurodegeneration before they become irreversible (Cohen and Rudick 2007).

Brain imaging techniques provide sensitive means of tracking treatment effects on pathological processes and have proven to be useful for efficient testing of immunotherapies in RRMS. Whereas a cogent argument could be made that surrogacy of gadolinium-enhancing lesions for relapse rates in RRMS has been well established, no imaging outcome measure has yet been determined to be predictive of treatment effects on the progression of disability in SPMS. Until that time comes, it is probably wise to assume that beneficial treatment effects in SPMS can only be determined by measuring functional impairment or disability. As discussed in the next section, the Multiple Sclerosis Functional Composite (MSFC) measure may prove to be a more clinically relevant measure of impairment and disability than the more widely used Expanded Disability Status Scale (EDSS). Other tests that may be useful in proof-of-concept studies are in development, including tests of ambulation, cognitive function, and visual function.

The use of validated clinical outcome measures that confirm clinically meaningful treatment effects

Traditional outcome measures for clinical trials in MS are relapse-related measures and impairment/disability ratings. Relapses were defined by Schumacker and colleagues (1965) as neurological symptoms attributable to dysfunction of the CNS, lasting more than 24 hours and separated by at least a month of clinical stability, confirmed by objective abnormalities on neurological examination, and not explained by some other disease processes (e.g., fever). Relapse-related measures include the annualized relapse rate, the number of relapse-free patients, and the time to first relapse under treatment. Although conceptually clear, care must be taken to ensure that relapses are properly measured in clinical trials. Relapse assessment necessarily includes a subjective component: the patient must believe a relapse is occurring and report it to the clinical trial site. Moreover, the patient must be seen by a neurologist before objective changes in the neurological examination have subsided, and the investigator must in turn report the findings at an unscheduled clinic visit in an objective manner. Thus, relapse assessments are subject to the frequency of study visits and to the specific definitions and methods used in a particular trial and may be subject to expectation bias (on the part of both the patient and the clinical investigator) if the trial is not effectively blinded. Relapse-related measures are useful in controlled trials; the best protection against bias is double blinding. If a double-blind design is not feasible, the neurological assessment must be performed by a neurologist who is masked to treatment assignment.

The main goal of treatment for patients with MS is reducing disability or slowing its progression. Development of the EDSS enabled the measurement of treatment effects on disability progression in clinical trials. The EDSS (Kurtzke 1983) in use today comprises 19 steps between 0 and 10, each separated by 0.5 points except the step between 0 and 1. The score is derived from a standard neurological examination of eight functional systems (pyramidal, cerebellar, brainstem, sensory, bowel and bladder, visual, cerebral, and other) and an evaluation of ambulation abilities. Increasing EDSS scores indicate increasing disability, which conveniently categorizes patients according to their disease severity. The EDSS is the most frequently used scale for disability rating in MS and the only one accepted by the US Food and Drug Administration and the European Medicines Agency (D'Souza et al. 2008). Despite its popularity, the EDSS has several well-known shortcomings (Whitaker et al. 1995): it is an ordinal (not metric) scale, lacks linearity, has poor inter-rater reliability, relies heavily on ambulation with poor assessment of upper limb function (especially between the scores of 4.0 and 6.5), and is insensitive to cognitive decline. At the low end of the scale, the EDSS may change because of clinically insignificant changes on certain functional system scales (e.g., bladder) or because of imprecision in defining the functional system scores; at the middle range, the EDSS reflects only ambulation, and the scale is insensitive to change over time. Concerns about the biological correlates of EDSS progression were raised by a recent report that demonstrated sustained EDSS worsening failed to correlate with gray matter atrophy in a longitudinal study, whereas sustained worsening on the MSFC correlated well (Rudick et al. 2009b). These shortcomings of the EDSS impair its ability to measure treatment effects on neurological functions; more reliable and sensitive clinical outcome measures are needed to allow better assessment of impairment and disability in MS.

The MSFC was developed to address the limitations of the EDSS. The MSFC (Rudick et al. 1997) comprises the timed 25-foot walk for evaluating ambulation and leg function; the nine-hole peg test for measuring arm function; and the 3-second version of the Paced Auditory Serial Addition Test (PASAT) for testing neuropsychological function. Individual component scores are transformed to z scores based on the mean and standard deviation of a reference population, and the individual z scores are combined to create a summary z score. In contrast to the EDSS, the MSFC captures information on cognitive function and upper limb function and, as a metric scale, is potentially more sensitive to change over time. The MSFC relies on well-standardized procedures, which increase the inter- and intrarater reliability. Currently, the MSFC does not include a measure of visual function, but this measure could be added as a fourth parameter to improve its overall value (Balcer et al. 2003). Another shortcoming of the current MSFC is that the PASAT test is subject to a marked learning effect; therefore, it does not often worsen in the time frame of a clinical trial. This test needs further refinement to be a sensitive cognitive measure.

The MSFC has been validated against other measures of MS in a number of studies. It has shown correlations with the EDSS (Cohen et al. 2001; Cutter et al. 1999; Hoogervorst et al. 2002; Kalkers et al. 2000; Miller et al. 2000), with patient-reported outcomes and quality of life (Hoogervorst et al. 2001; Miller et al. 2000), and with disease phenotype and disability status (Kalkers et al. 2000). When compared to the EDSS, the MSFC correlated more strongly with MRI lesion loads, whole-brain atrophy, and long-term disability status (Fisher et al. 2000; Kalkers et al. 2001; Rudick et al. 2001). The phase III trial, the International MS Secondary Progressive Avonex Controlled Trial (IMPACT), used the MSFC as the primary clinical outcome measure and confirmed that the MSFC is more sensitive to neurological change over time than the EDSS (Table 10.3) (Cohen et al. 2002). The two pivotal trials of natalizumab, the Natalizumab Safety and Efficacy in Relapsing-Remitting Multiple Sclerosis (AFFIRM) study and the Safety and Efficacy of Natalizumab in Combination with Interferon Beta-1a in Patients with Relapsing-Remitting Multiple Sclerosis (SENTINEL) study, included the MSFC as a secondary measure. Both studies showed consistent benefits of natalizumab on quality of life, the EDSS, the MSFC, and relapse (Rudick et al. 2007). Although the MSFC has demonstrated more favorable performance characteristics than the EDSS, it has not been accepted by regulatory authorities as a primary outcome measure in pivotal trials. Ongoing development of the MSFC aims to identify clinically meaningful changes in the individual components of this instrument, a better understanding of which might

Table 10.3. Mean change from baseline to month 24 in MSFC and component z scores and EDSS scores in IMPACT.

Test	Placebo (n = 219)	Interferon β-1a (n = 217)	P Value
MSFC	−0.495	−0.362	0.033[a]
T25FW	−1.191	−0.979	0.378[a]
9HPT	−0.290	−0.202	0.024[a]
PASAT3	−0.004	+0.094	0.061[a]

Test	Placebo (n = 193)	Interferon β-1a (n = 186)	P Value
EDSS	0.272	0.258	0.362[a]
Stable	59.1%	64.0%	
Worse	33.7%	28.5%	
Better	7.3%	7.5%	0.56[b]

[a] Analysis of covariance on ranks;
[b] Fisher exact test.
EDSS, Expanded Disability Status Scale; IMPACT, International MS Secondary Progressive Avonex Controlled Trial; MSFC, Multiple Sclerosis Functional Composite; 9HPT, nine-hole peg test; PASAT3, Paced Auditory Serial Addition Test with a 3-second interstimulus interval; T25FW, timed 25-foot walk.
Reprinted from *Neurology*, Vol. 59, Cohen JA, Cutter GR, Fischer JS et al., Benefit of interferon beta-1a on MSFC progression in secondary progressive MS, pp. 679–687, copyright 2002, with permission from Wolters Kluwer Health.

positively affect its acceptance by regulators. A recent post hoc analysis of data from the natalizumab studies (AFFIRM and SENTINEL) (Rudick et al. 2009a) has defined an MSFC disability event as a 20% worsening from baseline in any of the MSFC components, persisting for at least 3 months. With this definition of clinical meaning, MSFC disability progression correlated well with other disease severity measures; with self-reported quality of life measures; and was sensitive to treatment effects with natalizumab. Further development of this approach, particularly with refinement of the cognitive measure PASAT and inclusion of a visual measure, is likely to result in a significantly improved clinical outcome measure for future MS trials.

Other clinical outcome measures have been proposed, including the short and graphic assessment scale, the MS Impairment Scale, and a modified version of the EDSS known as the Multiple Sclerosis Severity Score. However, these instruments are not yet sufficiently well validated for use in clinical trials as primary outcomes (D'Souza et al. 2008).

In addition to the traditional objective clinical outcome measures, patient-reported outcome measures increasingly are being accepted as important instruments for assessing the impact of MS from the patients' perspective. The Guy's Neurological Disability Scale and the Multiple Sclerosis Quality of Life Inventory recently have been introduced and used in MS clinical trials to assess patient-perceived disability and response to treatment (Miller et al. 2000; Hoogervorst et al. 2001). However, these scales have not undergone extensive validity testing, nor have they received consensus as the standard measures for patient-reported outcomes. The lack of a universally accepted subjective outcome measure makes it difficult to compare the relative benefits of one therapy versus another. The Neuro-QOL project, a National Institute of Neurological Disorders and Stroke-funded project to develop a health-related quality of life assessment tool for patients with common neurological disorders (including MS), could potentially address the issue (National Institutes of Health 2009). Neuro-QOL uses the Item Response Theory tool, recently proposed by the National Institutes of Health Patient-Reported Outcomes Measurement Information System (Fries et al. 2005), to develop core item banks that are universal to patients with chronic neurological disease and supplemental item banks that are specific to particular groups of patients with a given condition. Scoring these item banks will be standardized so that the results are interpretable across the field. Neuro-QOL is an ongoing project; the tools developed by this project, once they are completed, should facilitate the comparison of treatment effects across clinical trials in different neurological diseases, including MS.

Selection of outcome measures in MS clinical trials depends on the expected mechanism of action of the drug. For example, neuroprotective therapies may not alter relapse-related measures. Multiple clinical outcomes or combined outcomes as secondary outcome measures may be used to compensate for the shortcomings of individual outcome measures.

The future of disease-modifying therapies

With the tremendous progress that has been made in understanding the pathogenesis of MS, many novel disease-modifying treatments for relapsing forms of MS and, more recently, agents aimed at neuroprotection and neurorepair are being explored in clinical trials. The development of novel imaging outcomes and new clinical outcomes will facilitate more comprehensive evaluations of these new therapeutic interventions than has previously been possible. However, acceptance of these novel measures as valid outcomes for use in MS clinical trials is proceeding slowly.

A particular concern with the testing of potential treatments for relapsing forms of MS is the use of placebo controls. Since the first International Conference on Therapeutic Trials in Multiple Sclerosis in 1982 (Herndon *et al.* 1983), six drugs have been approved for the management of RRMS. The availability of these treatments raises the question of whether it can be considered ethical to include a placebo control group in RRMS clinical trials. From the practical point of view, it is becoming increasingly difficult to recruit patients for placebo-controlled trials, and these trials do not include comparisons between the study treatment and other available agents. Innovative trial designs have been proposed to help solve this issue either by reducing the duration or the number of patients exposed to placebo treatments or completely eliminating placebo controls (McFarland and Reingold 2005). Replacing a placebo arm or part of the placebo arm with an arm using the lowest dose of the study drug, unbalanced randomization (more patients randomized to the active agent than the placebo), and deferred randomization (monitoring patients prior to randomization to select the most sensitive cohort) are expected to reduce the number of patients treated with placebo. Deferred treatment design (a short-term placebo treatment followed by crossover to the active treatment) and use of surrogate end points may shorten the duration of placebo treatments. Add-on study design (which compares the effect of adding a new drug or adding placebo to an established drug), active treatment comparisons, and modeling of data from virtual or historic placebo controls may completely eliminate the use of placebo controls in RRMS clinical trials. Active treatment comparisons can theoretically be designed and powered for superiority of one drug over another or for noninferiority or equivalence. However, it is important to note that most of these novel alternative trial designs will be more useful for phase II proof-of-concept studies than for phase III pivotal studies, with the possible exception of add-on study design and active treatment comparisons.

For novel agents targeting neurodegeneration, there is concern over how these agents may be appropriately tested in humans. Because patients who are candidates for such treatments most likely have been treated with disease-modifying therapies to reduce inflammation, the add-on study design or the use of neuroprotection and neurorepair agents as adjuncts to previous therapies might be most appropriate for both phase 2 and phase 3 trials. The immediate need though is to develop proof-of-concept trials that can be performed rapidly and efficiently. A group of MS researchers recently convened to discuss designs of proof-of-concept studies for tissue-protective treatments in MS. The favored design from the panel discussion was a "randomized, double-blind, parallel-group study of active treatment versus placebo focusing on changes in brain volume from a post-baseline scan (3–6 months after starting treatment) to the final visit 1 year later" (Mehta *et al.* 2009). Identification of surrogate biological markers for a particular agent or development of reliable imaging markers certainly will shorten study durations, but, as discussed previously, successful validation of these markers is essential before they can be used as informative outcome measures. Use of "selective weeding" to establish "lead drugs" is another aspect of study design that may be valuable for phase II proof-of-concept trials. The advantage of this approach is that several agents can be compared simultaneously, allowing rapid determination of the best candidates for further study (McFarland and Reingold 2005).

Conclusions

The application of translational medicine concepts to MS is relatively well advanced. We examined five factors that contribute to the continuum of transforming advances in laboratory-based research into clinically meaningful human therapeutics as it pertains to MS. Gaps in the flow of discovery need to be filled, particularly with regard to making the best outcome measurements at the different stages of drug development. However, the continuing rapid accumulation of knowledge and understanding of MS undoubtedly will help to accelerate the process of developing novel therapies for MS. The broad range of MS therapies currently in the late stages of clinical development is a testament to the principles of translational medicine in practice.

References

Alam J, Goelz S, Rioux P et al. 1997. Comparative pharmacokinetics and pharmacodynamics of two recombinant human interferon beta-1a (IFN beta-1 a) products administered intramuscularly in healthy male and female volunteers. *Pharm Res* **14**:546–549.

Ascherio A, Munger KL, Lennette ET et al. 2001. Epstein-Barr virus antibodies and risk of multiple sclerosis: a prospective study. *J Am Med Assoc* **286**:3083–3088.

Balcer LJ, Baier ML, Cohen JA et al. 2003. Contrast letter acuity as a visual component for the Multiple Sclerosis Functional Composite. *Neurology* **61**:1367–1373.

Barcellos LF, Oksenberg JR, Green AJ et al. 2002. Genetic basis for clinical expression in multiple sclerosis. *Brain* **125**:150–158.

Barkhof F, Calabresi PA, Miller DH, Reingold SC. 2009. Imaging outcomes for neuroprotection and repair in multiple sclerosis trials. *Nat Rev Neurol* **5**:256–266.

Barnett MH, Prineas JW. 2004. Relapsing and remitting multiple sclerosis: pathology of the newly forming lesion. *Ann Neurol* **55**:458–468.

Bayer AL, Yu A, Malek TR. 2007. Function of the IL-2R for thymic and peripheral CD4+CD25+ Foxp3 + T regulatory cells. *J Immunol* **178**:4062–4071.

Betarbet R, Sherer TB, Greenamyre JT. 2002. Animal models of Parkinson's disease. *Bioessays* **24**:308–318.

Beutler E. 1992. Cladribine (2-chlorodeoxyadenosine). *Lancet* **340**:952–956.

Bielekova B, Muraro PA, Golestaneh L et al. 1999. Preferential expansion of autoreactive T lymphocytes from the memory T-cell pool by IL-7. *J Neuroimmunol* **100**:115–123.

Bielekova B, Richert N, Howard T et al. 2004. Humanized anti-CD25 (daclizumab) inhibits disease activity in multiple sclerosis patients failing to respond to interferon beta. *Proc Nat Acad Sci USA* **101**:8705–8708.

Bornstein MB, Miller A, Slagle S. 1987. A pilot trial of Cop 1 in exacerbating-remitting multiple sclerosis. *N Engl J Med* **317**:408–414.

Brassat D, Azais-Vuillemin C, Yaouanq J et al. 1999. Familial factors influence disability in MS multiplex families. French Multiple Sclerosis Genetics Group. *Neurology* **52**:1632–1636.

Burt RK, Cohen BA, Russell E. 2003. Hematopoietic stem cell transplantation for progressive multiple sclerosis: failure of a total body irradiation-based conditioning regimen to prevent disease progression in patients with high disability scores. *Blood* **102**:2373–2378.

Burt RK, Loh Y, Cohen B. 2009. Autologous non-myeloablative haemopoietic stem cell transplantation in relapsing-remitting multiple sclerosis: a phase I/II study. *Lancet Neurol* **8**:244–253.

Burt RK, Traynor AE, Cohen B et al. 1998. T cell-depleted autologous hematopoietic stem cell transplantation for multiple sclerosis: report on the first three patients. *Bone Marrow Transplant* **21**:537–541.

Cannella B, Raine CS. 1995. The adhesion molecule and cytokine profile of multiple sclerosis lesions. *Ann Neurol* **37**:424–435.

Cohen JA, Cutter GR, Fischer JS. 2001. Use of the multiple sclerosis functional composite as an outcome measure in a phase 3 clinical trial. *Arch Neurol* **58**:961–967.

Cohen JA, Cutter GR, Fischer JS. 2002. Benefit of interferon beta-1a on MSFC progression in secondary progressive MS. *Neurology* **59**:679–687.

Cohen JA, Rudick RA, eds. 2007. *Multiple Sclerosis Therapeutics*, 3rd edn. London: Informa UK.

Cutter GR, Baier ML, Rudick RA. 1999. Development of a multiple sclerosis functional composite as a clinical trial outcome measure. *Brain* **122**:871–882.

D'Souza M, Kappos L, Czaplinski A. 2008. Reconsidering clinical outcomes in multiple sclerosis: relapses, impairment, disability and beyond. *J Neurol Sci* **274**:76–79.

Engelhardt B, Laschinger M, Schulz M et al. 1998. The development of experimental autoimmune encephalomyelitis in the mouse requires alpha4-integrin but not alpha4beta7-integrin. *J Clin Invest* **102**:2096–2105.

European Medicines Agency 2006. *European Public Assessment Report: Tysabri INN-Natalizumab*. Rep. no. H-603-en6.

Feldmann M, Steinman L. 2005. Design of effective immunotherapy for human autoimmunity. *Nature* **435**:612–619.

Fernald GH, Yeh RF, Hauser L, Oksenberg JR, Baranzini SE. 2005. Mapping gene activity in complex disorders: integration of expression and genomic scans for multiple sclerosis. *J Neuroimmunol* **167**:157–169.

Fisher E, Chang A, Fox RJ. 2007. Imaging correlates of axonal swelling in chronic multiple sclerosis brains. *Ann Neurol* **62**:219–228.

Fisher E, Lee JC, Nakamura K, Rudick RA. 2008. Gray matter atrophy in multiple sclerosis: a longitudinal study. *Ann Neurol* **64**:255–265.

Fisher E, Rudick RA, Cutter G. 2000. Relationship between brain atrophy and disability: an 8-year follow-up study of multiple sclerosis patients. *Mult Scler* **6**:373–377.

Fries JF, Bruce B, Cella D. 2005. The promise of PROMIS: using item response theory to improve assessment of patient-reported outcomes. *Clin Exp Rheumatol* **23**:S53–S57.

Frohman EM, Racke MK, Raine CS. 2006. Multiple sclerosis – the plaque and its pathogenesis. *N Engl J Med* **354**:942–955.

GAMES and the Transatlantic Multiple Sclerosis Genetics Cooperative 2003. A meta-analysis of whole genome linkage screens in multiple sclerosis. *J Neuroimmunol* **143**:39–46.

Geurts JJ, Bo L, Pouwels PJ *et al*. 2005. Cortical lesions in multiple sclerosis: combined postmortem MR imaging and histopathology. *Am J Neuroradiol* **26**:572–577.

Haas J, Hug A, Viehover A *et al*. 2005. Reduced suppressive effect of CD4 +CD25 high regulatory T cells on the T cell immune response against myelin oligodendrocyte glycoprotein in patients with multiple sclerosis. *Eur J Immunol* **35**:3343–3352.

Hafler DA, Compston A, Sawcer S. 2007. Risk alleles for multiple sclerosis identified by a genomewide study. *N Engl J Med* **357**:851–862.

Hardmeier M, Wagenpfeil S, Freitag P. 2005. Rate of brain atrophy in relapsing MS decreases during treatment with IFNbeta-1a. *Neurology* **64**:236–240.

Hauser SL, Oksenberg JR. 2006. The neurobiology of multiple sclerosis: genes, inflammation, and neurodegeneration. *Neuron* **52**:61–76.

Hauser SL, Waubant E, Arnold DL. 2008. B-cell depletion with rituximab in relapsing-remitting multiple sclerosis. *N Engl J Med* **358**:676–688.

Hawker K, O'Connor P, Freedman M. 2009. Efficacy and safety of rituximab in patients with primary progressive multiple sclerosis (PPMS): results of a randomized double-blind placebo-controlled multicenter trial. *Neurology* **72** (Suppl):A254. Abstract S21.003.

He YW, Malek TR. 1996. Interleukin-7 receptor alpha is essential for the development of gamma delta + T cells, but not natural killer cells. *J Exp Med* **184**:289–293.

Herndon RM, Murray TJ, Multiple Sclerosis Society of Canada, National Multiple Sclerosis Society (U.S.) 1983. Multiple sclerosis. Proceedings of the International Conference on Therapeutic Trials in Multiple Sclerosis. Grand Island, NY, April 23–24, 1982. *Arch Neurol* **40**:663–710.

Hirst CL, Pace A, Pickersgill TP. 2008. Campath 1-H treatment in patients with aggressive relapsing remitting multiple sclerosis. *J Neurol* **255**: 231–238.

Hohlfeld R, Wekerle H. 2004. Autoimmune concepts of multiple sclerosis as a basis for selective immunotherapy: from pipe dreams to (therapeutic) pipelines. *Proc Nat Acad Sci USA* **101**(Suppl. 2):14599–14606.

Hoogervorst EL, Kalkers NF, Uitdehaag BM, Polman CH. 2002. A study validating changes in the multiple sclerosis functional composite. *Arch Neurol* **59**:113–116.

Hoogervorst EL, van Winsen LM, Eikelenboom MJ *et al*. 2001. Comparisons of patient self-report, neurologic examination, and functional impairment in MS. *Neurology* **56**:934–937.

Husted CA, Goodin DS, Hugg JW. 1994. Biochemical alterations in multiple sclerosis lesions and normal-appearing white matter detected by in vivo 31P and 1H spectroscopic imaging. *Ann Neurol* **36**:157–165.

IFNB Multiple Sclerosis Study Group and the University of British Columbia MS/MRI Analysis Group 1995. Interferon beta-1b in the treatment of multiple sclerosis: final outcome of the randomized controlled trial. *Neurology* **45**:1277–1285.

Jacobs L, Johnson KP. 1994. A brief history of the use of interferons as treatment of multiple sclerosis. *Arch Neurol* **51**:1245–1252.

Jacobs L, O'Malley J, Freeman A, Ekes R. 1981. Intrathecal interferon reduces exacerbations of multiple sclerosis. *Science* **214**:1026–1028.

Jacobs L, O'Malley J, Freeman A, Murawski J, Ekes R. 1982. Intrathecal interferon in multiple sclerosis. *Arch Neurol* **39**:609–615.

Jacobs L, Salazar AM, Herndon R. 1986. Multicentre double-blind study of effect of intrathecally administered natural human fibroblast interferon on exacerbations of multiple sclerosis. *Lancet* **2**:1411–1413.

Jacobs LD, Cookfair DL, Rudick RA. 1996. Intramuscular interferon beta-1a for disease progression in relapsing multiple sclerosis. The Multiple Sclerosis Collaborative Research Group (MSCRG). *Ann Neurol* **39**:285–294.

Kalkers NF, Bergers L, de Groot V. 2001. Concurrent validity of the MS Functional Composite using MRI as a biological disease marker. *Neurology* **56**:215–219.

Kalkers NF, de Groot V, Lazeron RH. 2000. MS functional composite: relation to disease phenotype and disability strata. *Neurology* **54**: 1233–1239.

Kantarci OH, de Andrade M, Weinshenker BG. 2002. Identifying disease modifying genes in multiple sclerosis. *J Neuroimmunol* **123**: 144–159.

Kappos L, Antel J, Comi G. 2006. Oral fingolimod (FTY720) for relapsing multiple sclerosis. *N Engl J Med* **355**:1124–1140.

Katz D, Taubenberger JK, Cannella B *et al*. 1993. Correlation between magnetic resonance imaging findings and lesion development in chronic, active multiple sclerosis. *Ann Neurol* **34**:661–669.

Keegan M, Konig F, McClelland R. 2005. Relation between humoral pathological changes in multiple sclerosis and response to therapeutic plasma exchange. *Lancet* **366**:579–582.

Krajewski KM, Lewis RA, Fuerst DR. 2000. Neurological dysfunction and axonal degeneration in Charcot-Marie-Tooth disease type 1A. *Brain* **123**(pt 7):1516–1527.

Kurtzke JF. 1983. Rating neurologic impairment in multiple sclerosis: an expanded disability status scale (EDSS). *Neurology* **33**:1444–1452.

Lennon VA, Kryzer TJ, Pittock SJ, Verkman AS, Hinson SR. 2005. IgG marker of optic-spinal multiple sclerosis binds to the aquaporin-4 water channel. *J Exp Med* **202**:473–477.

Lobb RR, Hemler ME. 1994. The pathophysiologic role of alpha 4 integrins in vivo. *J Clin Invest* **94**:1722–1728.

Loevner LA, Grossman RI, McGowan JC, Ramer KN, Cohen JA. 1995. Characterization of multiple sclerosis plaques with T1-weighted MR and quantitative magnetization transfer. *Am J Neuroradiol* **16**:1473–1479.

Lublin FD, Reingold SC. 1996. Defining the clinical course of multiple sclerosis: results of an international survey. National Multiple Sclerosis Society (USA) Advisory Committee on Clinical Trials of New Agents in Multiple Sclerosis. *Neurology* **46**:907–911.

Lucchinetti C, Bruck W, Parisi J et al. 2000. Heterogeneity of multiple sclerosis lesions: implications for the pathogenesis of demyelination. *Ann Neurol* **47**:707–717.

Magliozzi R, Howell O, Vora A. 2007. Meningeal B-cell follicles in secondary progressive multiple sclerosis associate with early onset of disease and severe cortical pathology. *Brain* **130**:1089–1104.

Matthews PM, Pioro E, Narayanan S. 1996. Assessment of lesion pathology in multiple sclerosis using quantitative MRI morphometry and magnetic resonance spectroscopy. *Brain* **119** (Pt 3):715–722.

McFarland HF, Frank JA, Albert PS. 1992. Using gadolinium-enhanced magnetic resonance imaging lesions to monitor disease activity in multiple sclerosis. *Ann Neurol* **32**:758–766.

McFarland HF, Reingold SC. 2005. The future of multiple sclerosis therapies: redesigning multiple sclerosis clinical trials in a new therapeutic era. *Mult Scler* **11**:669–676.

Mehta LR, Schwid SR, Arnold DL. 2009. Proof of concept studies for tissue-protective agents in multiple sclerosis. *Mult Scler* **15**:542–546.

Miller DH. 2004. Biomarkers and surrogate outcomes in neurodegenerative disease: lessons from multiple sclerosis. *NeuroRx* **1**:284–294.

Miller DH, Albert PS, Barkhof F. 1996. Guidelines for the use of magnetic resonance techniques in monitoring the treatment of multiple sclerosis. US National MS Society Task Force. *Ann Neurol* **39**:6–16.

Miller DM, Rudick RA, Cutter G, Baier M, Fischer JS. 2000. Clinical significance of the multiple sclerosis functional composite: relationship to patient-reported quality of life. *Arch Neurol* **57**:1319–1324.

Mondria T, Lamers CH, te Boekhorst PA, Gratama JW, Hintzen RQ. 2008. Bone-marrow transplantation fails to halt intrathecal lymphocyte activation in multiple sclerosis. *J Neurol Neurosurg Psychiatry* **79**:1013–1015.

Monson NL, Cravens PD, Frohman EM, Hawker K, Racke MK. 2005. Effect of rituximab on the peripheral blood and cerebrospinal fluid B cells in patients with primary progressive multiple sclerosis. *Arch Neurol* **62**:258–264.

Montalban X, Wynn D, Kaufman M. 2007. Daclizumab in patients with active, relapsing multiple sclerosis on concurrent interferon-beta therapy week 24 data-phase II (CHOICE). Oral presentation at the 23rd Congress of the European Committee for the Treatment and Research in Multiple Sclerosis. *Mult Scler* **13**:S18. Abstract 50.

Narayanan S, Fu L, Pioro E. 1997. Imaging of axonal damage in multiple sclerosis: spatial distribution of magnetic resonance imaging lesions. *Ann Neurol* **41**:385–391.

National Institutes of Health, National Institute of Neurological Disorders and Strokes, Evanston Northwestern Healthcare, Center on Outcomes, Research and Education 2009. *Neuro-QOL: Progress Report 2004–2007*. Rep. no. HHS-N265-2004-236-01-C.

Neighbour PA, Miller AE, Bloom BR. 1981. Interferon responses of leukocytes in multiple sclerosis. *Neurology* **31**:561–566.

Noseworthy JH. 2003. Management of multiple sclerosis: current trials and future options. *Curr Opin Neurol* **16**:289–297.

Obermeier B, Mentele R, Malotka J. 2008. Matching of oligoclonal immunoglobulin transcriptomes and proteomes of cerebrospinal fluid in multiple sclerosis. *Nat Med* **14**:688–693.

Oksenberg JR, Barcellos LF, Cree BA. 2004. Mapping multiple sclerosis susceptibility to the HLA-DR locus in African Americans. *Am J Hum Gen* **74**:160–167.

Pachner AR, Bertolotto A, Deisenhammer F. 2003. Measurement of MxA mRNA or protein as a biomarker of IFNbeta bioactivity: detection of antibody-mediated decreased bioactivity (ADB). *Neurology* **61**:S24–S26.

Panitch HS, Hirsch RL, Schindler J, Johnson KP. 1987. Treatment of multiple sclerosis with gamma interferon: exacerbations associated with activation of the immune system. *Neurology* **37**:1097–1102.

Perkin GD. 1987. A critique of steroid trials in multiple sclerosis. *Neuroepidemiology* **6**:40–45.

Peterson JW, Bo L, Mork S et al. 2002. VCAM-1-positive microglia target oligodendrocytes at the border of multiple sclerosis lesions. *J Neuropath Exp Neurol* **61**:539–546.

PRISMS (Prevention of Relapses and Disability by Interferon beta-1a

Subcutaneously in Multiple Sclerosis) Study Group 1998. Randomised double-blind placebo-controlled study of interferon beta-1a in relapsing/remitting multiple sclerosis. *Lancet* 352:1498–1504.

Raine CS. 1994. The Dale E. McFarlin Memorial Lecture: the immunology of the multiple sclerosis lesion. *Ann Neurol* 36 (Suppl.):S61–S72.

Rose AS, Kuzma JW, Kurtzke JF *et al.* 1970. Cooperative study in the evaluation of therapy in multiple sclerosis. ACTH vs. placebo – final report. *Neurology* 20:1–59.

Rose JW, Watt HE, White AT, Carlson NG. 2004. Treatment of multiple sclerosis with an anti-interleukin-2 receptor monoclonal antibody. *Ann Neurol* 56:864–867.

Rudick R, Antel J, Confavreux C. 1997. Recommendations from the National Multiple Sclerosis Society Clinical Outcomes Assessment Task Force. *Ann Neurol* 42:379–382.

Rudick RA, Cutter G, Baier M. 2001. Use of the Multiple Sclerosis Functional Composite to predict disability in relapsing MS. *Neurology* 56:1324–1330.

Rudick RA, Lee JC, Nakamura K, Fisher E. 2009. Gray matter atrophy correlates with MS disability progression measured with MSFC but not EDSS. *J Neurol Sci* 282:106–111.

Rudick RA, Miller D, Hass S. 2007. Health-related quality of life in multiple sclerosis: effects of natalizumab. *Ann Neurol* 62:335–346.

Rudick RA, Polman CH. 2009. Current approaches to the identification and management of breakthrough disease in patients with multiple sclerosis. *Lancet Neurol* 8:545–559.

Rudick R, Polman C, Cohen J. 2009. Assessing disability progression with the Multiple Sclerosis Functional Composite. *Mult Scler* 15:984–997.

Rudick RA, Sandrock A. 2004. Natalizumab: alpha 4-integrin antagonist selective adhesion molecule inhibitors for MS. *Expert Rev Neurother* 4:571–580.

Sastre-Garriga J, Ingle GT, Chard DT. 2005. Metabolite changes in normal-appearing gray and white matter are linked with disability in early primary progressive multiple sclerosis. *Arch Neurol* 62:569–573.

Sawcer S, Ban M, Maranian M. 2005. A high-density screen for linkage in multiple sclerosis. *Am J Hum Gen* 77:454–467.

Schumacker GA, Beebe G, Kibler RF. 1965. Problems of experimental trials of therapy in multiple sclerosis: report by the Panel of the Evaluation of Experimental Trials of Therapy in Multiple Sclerosis. *Ann N Y Acad Sci* 122:552–568.

Serafini B, Rosicarelli B, Magliozzi R, Stigliano E, Aloisi F. 2004. Detection of ectopic B-cell follicles with germinal centers in the meninges of patients with secondary progressive multiple sclerosis. *Brain Pathol* 14:164–174.

Sheremata WA, Minagar A, Alexander JS, Vollmer T. 2005. The role of alpha-4 integrin in the aetiology of multiple sclerosis: current knowledge and therapeutic implications. *CNS Drugs* 19:909–922.

Sipe JC. 2005. Cladribine for multiple sclerosis: review and current status. *Expert Rev Neurother* 5:721–727.

Sormani MP, Bonzano L, Roccatagliata L *et al.* 2009. Magnetic resonance imaging as a potential surrogate for relapses in multiple sclerosis: a meta-analytic approach. *Ann Neurol* 65:268–275.

Sriram S, Steiner I. 2005. Experimental allergic encephalomyelitis: a misleading model of multiple sclerosis. *Ann Neurol* 58:939–945.

Steinman L, Zamvil SS. 2006. How to successfully apply animal studies in experimental allergic encephalomyelitis to research on multiple sclerosis. *Ann Neurol* 60:12–21.

Theien BE, Vanderlugt CL, Eagar TN. 2001. Discordant effects of anti-VLA-4 treatment before and after onset of relapsing experimental autoimmune encephalomyelitis. *J Clin Invest* 107:995–1006.

Tourtellotte WW, Walsh MJ, Baumhefner RW, Staugaitis SM, Shapshak P. 1984. The current status of multiple sclerosis intra-blood-brain-barrier IgG synthesis. *Ann N Y Acad Sci* 436:52–67.

Trapp BD, Peterson J, Ransohoff RM *et al.* 1998. Axonal transection in the lesions of multiple sclerosis. *N Engl J Med* 338:278–285.

Tubridy N, Behan PO, Capildeo R. 1999. The effect of anti-alpha4 integrin antibody on brain lesion activity in MS. The UK Antegren Study Group. *Neurology* 53:466–472.

Verbeek MM, Westphal JR, Ruiter DJ, de Waal RM. 1995. T lymphocyte adhesion to human brain pericytes is mediated via very late antigen-4/vascular cell adhesion molecule-1 interactions. *J Immunol* 154:5876–5884.

Viglietta V, Baecher-Allan C, Weiner HL, Hafler DA. 2004. Loss of functional suppression by CD4+CD25+ regulatory T cells in patients with multiple sclerosis. *J Exp Med* 199:971–979.

Vora AJ, Perkin GD, McCoy T, Dumonde DC, Brown KA. 1996. Enhanced binding of lymphocytes from patients with multiple sclerosis to tumour necrosis factor-alpha (TNF-alpha)-treated endothelial monolayers: associations with clinical relapse and adhesion molecule expression. *Clin Exp Immunol* 105:155–162.

Warner HB, Carp RI. 1981. Multiple sclerosis and Epstein-Barr virus. *Lancet* 2:1290.

Washington R, Burton J, Todd RF III *et al.* 1994. Expression of immunologically relevant endothelial cell activation antigens on isolated central nervous system microvessels from patients with multiple sclerosis. *Ann Neurol* 35:89–97.

Waubant E, Vukusic S, Gignoux L. 2003. Clinical characteristics of responders to interferon therapy for relapsing MS. *Neurology* **61**:184–189.

Weiss W, Bornstein MB, Miller A, Slagle S. 1988. Clinical trial design in multiple sclerosis therapy. *Neurology* **38**:80–81.

Werring DJ, Clark CA, Barker GJ, Thompson AJ, Miller DH. 1999. Diffusion tensor imaging of lesions and normal-appearing white matter in multiple sclerosis. *Neurology* **52**:1626–1632.

Whitaker JN, McFarland HF, Rudge P, Reingold SC. 1995. Outcomes assessment in multiple sclerosis clinical trials: a critical analysis. *Mult Scler* **1**:37–47.

Wucherpfennig KW, Newcombe J, Li H et al. 1992. Gamma delta T-cell receptor repertoire in acute multiple sclerosis lesions. *Proc Nat Acad Sci USA* **89**:4588–4592.

Yednock TA, Cannon C, Fritz LC et al. 1992. Prevention of experimental autoimmune encephalomyelitis by antibodies against alpha 4 beta 1 integrin. *Nature* **356**:63–66.

Young N, Van Brocklyn JR. 2006. Signal transduction of sphingosine-1-phosphate G protein-coupled receptors. *Sci World J* **6**:946–966.

Yu A, Malek TR. 2006. Selective availability of IL-2 is a major determinant controlling the production of CD4+CD25+Foxp3+ T regulatory cells. *J Immunol* **177**:5115–5121.

Zivadinov R, Bakshi R. 2004. Role of MRI in multiple sclerosis. I: inflammation and lesions. *Front Biosci* **9**:665–683.

Chapter 11

Parkinson's disease

Jiang-Fan Chen

Parkinson's disease (PD), first described by James Parkinson in 1817 in his famous "Essay on the shaking palsy," is the second most common neurodegenerative disease in the USA. At age 55 years, the incidence of PD is approximately 20 per 10,000, increasing significantly to 120 per 10,000 at age 70 and affecting more than 1 million people in the USA (Dauer and Przedborski 2003; Lang and Lozano 1998a, 1998b). In about 5% of PD cases, the disease is inherited, but the majority (> 95%) of PD cases are sporadic with unknown cause (Lazzarini et al. 1994; Payami and Zareparsi 1998). Hallmarks of PD pathology are the loss of dopaminergic neurons in the substantia nigra pars compacta (SNpc) of the midbrain and proteinaceous intracellular inclusions (Lewy bodies) (Dauer and Przedborski 2003; Lang and Lozano 1998a, 1998b). As result of dopaminergic neurodegeneration, dopamine levels in the striatum decrease markedly, leading to clinical presentation of the cardinal motor symptoms, including the asymmetrical onset of bradykinesia, rigidity, rest tremor, and postural instability (Dauer and Przedborski 2003; Lang and Lozano 1998a, 1998b). Recognition has increased in recent years that a spectrum of nonmotor manifestations contribute significantly to disease-related disability, including sleep disturbance, autonomic dysfunction, depression, and dementia (O'Sullivan et al. 2008; Shulman et al. 2001; Simuni and Sethi 2008). Based on the pathology of PD, replenishment of striatal dopamine was introduced as a primary therapy 40 years ago and remains the mainstay of PD treatment today (Olanow 2004; Olanow et al. 2004). L-dopa treatment does not modify PD disease course or address nonmotor symptoms of PD, however, and long-term treatment produces many debilitating motor and nonmotor complications (Fahn 1999, 2000; Olanow 2004; Olanow et al. 2004). It is estimated that the number of PD cases will double by 2030, as the population ages and life expectancy increases (Dorsey et al. 2007). Thus, the need is critical for more effective long-term management of PD to maintain quality of life for patients and reduce the socioeconomic burden of this disease.

Clinical and pathological characteristics
Motor symptoms

Parkinson's disease is a progressive disease with a mean age of onset of 55 years and a steady increase in severity, pathology, and mortality. The cardinal motor symptoms were first described more than 100 years ago, including bradykinesia (slowness of movement), rigidity (i.e., the increased resistance and stiffness to passive movement), resting tremor, and postural instability (Dauer and Przedborski 2003; Lang and Lozano 1998a, 1998b; Olanow 2004). Freezing, the inability to initiate a voluntary movement such as walking, is a common symptom of parkinsonism. Preliminary diagnosis may be made on clinical grounds, but definitive diagnosis requires the postmortem identification of both Lewy bodies and loss of dopaminergic neurons. A London Brain Bank study revealed 82% accuracy in diagnoses based on clinical presentation, particularly when responsiveness to l-dopa treatment was required for diagnosis (Daniel and Lees 1993; Hughes et al. 1992a, 1992b). The characteristic motor symptoms result from degeneration of dopaminergic neurons in the SNpc and consequent depletion of dopamine in the striatum (Agid et al. 1989). Dopaminergic neurons in the SNpc have significant amounts of neuromelanin; thus their loss produces the classic gross neuropathological finding of depigmentation of the SNpc. The pattern of SNpc cell loss parallels the reduced expression of dopamine

---

Translational Neuroscience, ed. James E. Barrett, Joseph T. Coyle and Michael Williams. Published by Cambridge University Press. © Cambridge University Press 2012.

transporter (DAT) mRNA and depletion of DA in the caudate-putamen, particularly in the dorsolateral putamen (Dauer and Przedborski 2003). At the onset of motor symptoms, putamenal dopamine is depleted by ~80%, and dopaminergic neurons in the SNpc are reduced by 60%. Notably, the cell bodies of mesolimbic dopaminergic neurons in the ventral tegmental area are much less affected in PD (Fearnley and Lees 1991). As noted in the London Brain Bank study (Daniel and Lees 1993; Hughes *et al.* 1992*a*, 1992*b*), ~20% of cases initially diagnosed as PD are not the result of dopaminergic neurodegeneration but are caused by other neurological disorders that produce striatal DA deficiency, leading to "parkinsonism" with identical motor symptoms (Dauer and Przedborski 2003; Lang and Lozano 1998*a*, 1998*b*).

Nonmotor symptoms

Although PD is traditionally recognized by its motor symptoms, refinement of our clinical and pathological tools has led to increasing recognition that PD also causes significant nonmotor deficits (Langston 2006; O'Sullivan *et al.* 2008; Shulman *et al.* 2001; Simuni and Sethi 2008). Some nonmotor signs and symptoms can precede the clinical appearance of parkinsonism by surprisingly long periods. These include rapid-eye-movement sleep behavioral disorders, olfactory dysfunction, cardiac sympathetic denervation, and constipation (Langston 2006; O'Sullivan *et al.* 2008; Shulman *et al.* 2001; Simuni and Sethi 2008). For example, a large body of evidence indicates that abnormal olfaction is detected in up to 100% of patients with PD (Langston 2006; Muller *et al.* 2002). Similarly, nearly 40% of patients with rapid-eye-movement behavior disorder (RBD) develop parkinsonism an average of ~13 years after RBD diagnosis (Schenck *et al.* 1996). Interestingly, in the prospective Honolulu Heart Program involving 8000 Japanese American men, men who reported less than one bowel movement per day in midlife were more than four times more likely to develop PD in late life than men who reported having two or more bowel movements per day (Abbott *et al.* 2003). The recognition of these nonmotor symptoms is supported by the pathological finding of Lewy bodies in brain structures beyond the nigrostriatal dopaminergic system (Braak *et al.* 2001, 2002; Langston 2006). Neurodegeneration and Lewy body formation are found in noradrenergic (locus ceruleus), serotonergic (raphe), and cholinergic (nucleus basalis of Meynert, dorsal motor nucleus of vagus) systems, as well as in the cerebral cortex (especially cingulated and entorhinal cortices), the olfactory bulb, and the autonomic nervous system. Although degeneration of hippocampal structure and cholinergic cortical inputs is believed to contribute to the high rate of dementia in PD, the clinical correlates of lesions to the serotonergic and noradrenergic pathways have not been clearly characterized. Some researchers argue that these clinical and neurochemical changes in multiple systems are all part of the disease process, regardless of whether parkinsonism is clinically manifest (Langston 2006). Furthermore, experts still debate whether degeneration of these neurochemical systems occurs in early- or late-stage disease. Notably, using newer staining techniques, particularly synuclein histochemistry, to study both non-PD and PD brain, Braak and colleagues (2001, 2002) have provided pathological evidence that PD may begin in the lower brainstem and olfactory bulb, progresses to affect the nigrostriatal system in the midcourse of the disease, and eventually affects neocortical areas in later stages. Further studies are clearly needed to establish the temporal sequence of damage to specific neurochemical systems.

Etiology: environmental and genetic factors

Environmental factors

The cause of sporadic PD is unknown and the relative contributions of environmental toxins and genetic factors to PD pathogenesis remain unclear. For most of the past century, the predominant hypothesis was that PD-related neurodegeneration results from exposure to environmental factors, in particular dopaminergic neurotoxins (Bronstein *et al.* 2009; Dauer and Przedborski 2003). The finding that drug addicts intoxicated with 1-methyl-4-phenyl-1,2,3,6-tetrahydropyridine (MPTP) developed overnight a syndrome nearly identical to PD (Langston *et al.* 1983) provided a powerful example of how the effects of an exogenous toxin can mimic the clinical and pathological features of PD. Importantly, human epidemiological studies have consistently associated residence in a rural environment and related exposure to herbicides and pesticides with an elevated risk of PD (Tanner 1992). For example, neurotoxins such as the herbicide paraquat (structurally similar to the active metabolite of MPTP, MPP+) and the insecticide rotenone are associated with increased risk for PD. Moreover, neurotoxins (i.e., 6-hydroxydopamine [6-OHDA], MPTP, and rotenone) produce selective degeneration of dopaminergic neurons in rodents and nonhuman primates, and neurotoxin-based animal models of PD have provided most insights into the mechanisms underlying dopaminergic neurodegeneration (Dauer and Przedborski 2003). Yet, chronic environmental exposure to MPP+ or rotenone is unlikely to cause PD given that MPP+ is a quaternary ammonium cation with poor blood–brain barrier permeability, and rotenone is unstable in solution, lasting only a few days in lakes (Hisata 2002). So far, no convincing data implicate specific toxins as a cause of sporadic PD. Second, because of the example of postencephalitic PD (as described vividly in the book *Awakenings* by Oliver Sacks), researchers speculate that inflammation may be a contributing factor in PD. However, available epidemiological data show no significant change in incidence of PD over the past century. The possible involvement of neuroinflammation in PD pathogenesis was recently revisited and was supported by the epidemiological finding of inverse correlation between use of nonsteroidal anti-inflammatory drugs and risk for developing PD (Chen et al. 2003), by the demonstration of long-lasting microglial activation in the substantia nigra of postmortem PD brain (Langston et al. 1999; McGeer et al. 1988) and by the neuroprotective effect of anti-inflammatory drugs such as minocycline in animal models of PD (Wu et al. 2002). However, the exact role of neuroinflammation in PD patients is not clear. Third, large prospective studies have firmly established that cigarette smoking and coffee drinking are inversely associated with the risk for development of PD (Hernan et al. 2002) (see section on "Disease-modifying effect of adenosine A_{2A} receptor antagonists" for detailed description of epidemiological studies of caffeine in PD). These findings reinforce the concept that some environmental factors including neurotoxin exposure and dietary factors modify PD susceptibility.

Genetic factors

Although the increased incidence of PD in some families was noted early on, several twin studies clearly demonstrated a low rate of concordance in monozygotic and dizygotic twins, indicative of a lack of genetic susceptibility to PD (Laihinen et al. 2000; Tanner et al. 1999; Ward et al. 1983). These twin studies shifted PD research away from genetics until 1997 when the first PD-associated gene was discovered in a large Greek/Italian family (Polymeropoulos et al. 1997). Genetic studies have since identified eight PD-associated genes (*PARK1–PARK8*) with both dominant and recessive heredity, changing the landscape of PD research (Dauer and Przedborski 2003; Hardy et al. 2006; Moore et al. 2005). The genetics of PD have been extensively and expertly reviewed in recent years (see Gasser 2009; Hardy et al. 2009; Hardy and Orr 2006 for review). Here we describe selected PD genes to illustrate how advances in understanding the genetics of familial PD have shed new light on the pathogenesis of PD and identified novel targets for PD therapy.

Gain-of-function mutations

α-Synuclein is a 140-amino-acid protein with diffuse cellular localization and unknown function. Two missense α-synuclein mutations (*A53T* and *A30P*) cause autosomal dominant PD (Kruger et al. 1998; Polymeropoulos et al. 1997), and these pathogenic mutations are believed to be associated with the formation of protofibrils, which promote neuronal toxicity (Moore et al. 2005). Recent evidence, however, suggests that oligomeric α-synuclein promotes cell death whereas polymeric α-synuclein is protective (Lee and Trojanowski 2006). A critical role of α-synuclein in PD pathogenesis is supported by the finding that duplication or triplication of the wild-type α-synuclein causes autosomal dominant PD (Singleton et al. 2003) and that polymorphisms in the α-synuclein promoter that alter the level of α-synuclein expression are associated with an increased risk for PD (Pals et al. 2004). Consistent with this notion, genetic deletion of α-synuclein protects against the MPTP-induced loss of dopamine neurons (Dauer et al. 2002). Most importantly, α-synuclein is identified as a major component of Lewy bodies and Lewy neuritis, a pathological hallmark of sporadic PD (Spillantini et al. 1997). This finding demonstrates that common molecular events underlie both familial and sporadic forms of PD. Thus, insight into the pathogenesis of familial PD should critically advance our knowledge of sporadic PD and therapeutic targets for familial PD may be applicable to the sporadic PD population at large.

LRRK2 mutations also cause dominantly inherited PD, likely via gain of function (Paisán-Ruiz *et al.* 2004; Zimprich *et al.* 2004). One mutation of *LRRK2*, *G2019S*, is the most common mutant found so far in sporadic cases, with estimated frequencies of more than 2% in the general North American clinical population and English PD Brain Bank specimens (Gilks *et al.* 2005; Nichols *et al.* 2005). Thus, understanding *LRRK2* function and its role in PD pathogenesis will likely benefit a wide spectrum of PD patients. LRRK2 is a 280-kDa protein localized to the cytoplasm, associated with mitochondrial and other cellular membranes (Biskup *et al.* 2006; West *et al.* 2005). LRRK2 belongs to a novel subgroup of the Ras/GTPase superfamily, the ROCO protein family, and has multiple conserved modules, including GTPase, Roco, and kinase domains (Gupta *et al.* 2008). Available data suggest that individual *LRRK2* mutations found in PD families, including the *G2019S* and *I2020T* mutations, show increased intrinsic kinase activity (Ito *et al.* 2007; West *et al.* 2007). Although no definitive LRRK2 phosphorylation substrates have been identified yet, increased or abnormal phosphorylation of critical LRRK2 substrates is postulated to be involved in neurodegeneration induced by mutant *LRRK2* (Gupta *et al.* 2008).

Loss-of-function mutations

Mutations in *UCH-L1* (Leroy *et al.* 1998), *PINK1* (Valente *et al.* 2004), and *DJ-1* (Bonifati *et al.* 2003) cause autosomal recessive PD in a manner consistent with loss of function (Hardy and Orr 2006). UCH-L1 is an E3 ubiquitin ligase that catalyzes the final step of protein ubiquitination for targeting and degradation of damaged proteins by the ubiquitin proteasome system (UPS) (Shimura *et al.* 2000). Thus, due to UPS dysfunction, *UCH-L1* mutation is expected to result in accumulation of abnormal proteins (Leroy *et al.* 1998). However, patients with PD who have the *UCH-L1* mutation do not have greater numbers of Lewy bodies (Gupta *et al.* 2008). The discovery of mutations in *PINK1* and *DJ-1* underscores mitochondrial dysfunction as another critical molecular pathway in the development of PD (Gupta *et al.* 2008; Hardy and Orr 2006; Moore *et al.* 2005). *DJ-1* mutations are rare, but individuals with these mutations develop early onset of PD (Lockhart *et al.* 2004). Experimental evidence suggests that DJ-1 functions as an atypical peroxiredoxin-like peroxidase that scavenges mitochondrial peroxide through oxidation of its cysteine 106 (Andres-Mateos *et al.* 2007). Consistent with loss of mitochondrial function, *DJ-1*-deficient *Drosophila* and mice are more sensitive to oxidative neurotoxins (Menzies *et al.* 2005; Meulener *et al.* 2005; Park *et al.* 2005; Yang *et al.* 2005). PINK is a mitochondrial serine/threonine kinase (Valente *et al.* 2004). Animal models of mutant *PINK1* and inhibition of *PINK1* expression in cultured cells both demonstrate that the *PINK* mutation results in altered mitochondrial structure and function, likely through a loss-of-function mutation (Clark *et al.* 2006; Exner *et al.* 2007; Park *et al.* 2006). It is hypothesized that the loss of phosphorylation of PINK1 substrates leads to mitochondrial dysfunction and triggers or promotes neurodegeneration.

These PD-associated mutations highlight the critical role of protein ubiquitination and mitochondrial dysfunction in PD pathogenesis (Gupta *et al.* 2008; Hardy and Orr 2006; Moore *et al.* 2005). Alterations in UPS and mitochondrial dysfunction are thought to play a role in PD because these defects in the UPS are found in sporadic PD and because extensive evidence from toxin-based PD models supports their roles in PD pathogenesis (Dauer and Przedborski 2003). However, studies in transgenic animal models indicate that these mutations do not explain the relatively selective loss of dopaminergic neurons in PD. It has become increasingly clear that pathogenesis of PD likely involves multiple genetic factors (Bras and Singleton 2009; Langston 2006; Youdim *et al.* 2007). Recent studies with genome-wide association confirm involvement of several genes that are "usual suspects" but also identify many additional genes that associate with PD, including α-synuclein and the *MAPT* locus (Fung *et al.* 2006; Maraganore *et al.* 2005; Pankratz *et al.* 2009; Simon-Sanchez *et al.* 2009).

Current clinical treatment

Three main treatment strategies are currently used to provide motor symptom relief in patients with early PD. l-dopa and dopamine agonists provide the backbone of current PD treatment and yield an excellent response for several years. For long-term management of PD, several strategies have been developed to better control l-dopa-induced motor complications, particularly dyskinesia. These strategies include using dopamine agonists as monotherapy, long-lasting dopamine therapy, and nondopaminergic agents. Finally, surgical intervention, such as deep brain stimulation (DBS), is considered when dyskinesia is difficult to control with medication.

L-dopa and dopamine agonists

Based on the degeneration of the nigrostriatal dopaminergic neurons and consequent profound depletion of striatal dopamine in patients with PD, l-dopa was introduced as a dopamine replacement strategy for PD treatment more than 40 years ago (Agid et al. 1989). Today, l-dopa remains the most effective treatment for improving motor symptoms and is considered the gold standard against which all other antiparkinsonian drugs are compared (Lang and Lozano 1998a, 1998b). For example, the ELLDOPA study, a 42-week randomized, double-blind, placebo-controlled trial involving 361 treatment-naïve patients, demonstrated that carbidopa-levodopa at doses of 37.5–600 mg/kg decreased the severity of parkinsonism (Olanow et al. 2009b). Motor benefit was observed after a 2-week washout period. Dopamine agonists, most of them synthetic nonergot agonists with affinity for the D_2 receptor, have also been used for many years in the treatment of PD. Many well-designed randomized, double-blind, placebo-controlled clinical trials have confirmed the efficacy of dopamine agonists, e.g., pramipexole and ropinirole, as monotherapy for PD. Recently, long-acting preparations of dopamine agonists have been introduced to delay the initiation of l-dopa treatment. In addition, new delivery techniques for dopaminergic drugs have been devised, such as transdermal patches (Watts et al. 2006) and intraduodenal infusions (Nyholm and Aquilonius 2004; Stocchi et al. 2005), but no novel drug class has been introduced into therapy for decades (Johnston and Brotchie 2006). The introduction of dopamine agonists or long-acting dopamine has allowed better control of l-dopa-induced dyskinesia, as confirmed by several randomized, double-blind, placebo-controlled clinical trials (Hauser et al. 2007; Parkinson Study Group 2002, 2003; Stocchi et al. 2008). Thus, l-dopa and dopamine agonists are the primary treatments for PD and are very effective for motor symptoms, particularly at the early stage of PD (first 5 years after diagnosis).

Nondopaminergic treatment strategies

The potential of nondopaminergic approaches for the treatment of PD has been extensively reviewed recently (Bonuccelli and Del Dotto 2006; Johnston and Brotchie 2006; Korczyn and Nussbaum 2002; Wu and Frucht 2005). In addition to dopamine replacement therapy, nondopaminergic treatments have been used, including anticholinergic agents to improve tremor (Olanow et al. 2001), and the weak N-methyl-d-aspartate (NMDA) antagonist amantadine has been used for suppression of dyskinesia (Metman et al. 1999; Olanow et al. 2001). Given the intrinsic relationship between dopamine neurotransmission and the most debilitating motor complication, dyskinesia, there has been great interest over the past 10 years in developing nondopaminergic agents to control l-dopa-induced dyskinesia, including noradrenergic antagonists, serotonergic drugs, and glutamate antagonists. However, these nondopaminergic agents have not been introduced into general clinical practice to date, despite impressive effects in preclinical models of PD. Conversely, with increasing recognition of the nonmotor symptoms of PD and of pathological changes in various brain structures far beyond dopaminergic neurons, the role of nondopaminergic neurotransmission in the pathogenesis of PD has been increasingly appreciated (Braak et al. 2003; Obeso et al. 2000; Obeso et al. 2004). Consequently, nondopaminergic neurotransmitters and receptors have become an attractive target for treatment of some nonmotor symptoms.

Deep brain stimulation for the treatment of L-dopa-induced motor complications

When motor fluctuation and dyskinesia become so debilitating that they cannot be controlled with medication, surgical intervention such as DBS has been shown to provide relief of tremor, bradykinesia, rigidity, "off" time, and in particular, dsykinesia (Lang and Lozano 1998a, 1998b; Olanow 2004). The subthalamic nucleus (STN) is the preferred target of DBS for PD (Limousin et al. 1998; Volkmann et al. 2001), but the globus pallidus has also been considered (Volkmann et al. 1998, 2001). Recent randomized trial studies show that DBS-STN reduces parkinsonian severity as well as l-dopa-induced dyskinesia and "off" time by about 50%, whereas the other best medication reduces parkinsonian symptoms but worsens dyskinesia slightly (Deep-Brain Stimulation for Parkinson's Disease Study Group 2001; Deuschl et al. 2006), a conclusion substantiated by a meta-analysis of 921 patients who underwent DBS-STN

(Kleiner-Fisman *et al.* 2006). A 5-year prospective study of the first 49 consecutive patients treated with DBS-STN showed that motor improvement continued over the baseline in the stimulation on-off medication state (Krack *et al.* 2003). Motor improvement is not better than with medication, however, and thus the main benefit of DBS-STN is better management of l-dopa-induced dyskinesia and other motor complications. Furthermore, PD progression continues and some serious adverse events (including perioperative intracerebral hemorrhage) occur after DBS (Krack *et al.* 2003).

Medical needs not met by current therapies

Life expectancy for patients with PD has remained largely unchanged over the past 40 years: The mortality rate of PD is about three times higher than the mortality rate in the normal age-matched population before the introduction of l-dopa treatment. While l-dopa has revolutionized PD treatment by controlling motor symptoms and improving quality of life, population-based surveys suggest that patients on l-dopa therapy continue to display decreased longevity compared with the general population (Driver *et al.* 2008; Hely *et al.* 1989; Levy *et al.* 2002; Marras *et al.* 2005). Three large studies conducted during different periods – Hoehn and Yahr (1967), the Sydney Multicentre Study in 1989 (Hely *et al.* 1989), and the Physicians' Health Study in 2008 (Driver *et al.* 2008) – showed no significant change in the life expectancy of PD patients over the past 40 years.

Motor and nonmotor complications of long-term l-dopa treatment: Long-term treatment with l-dopa produces debilitating motor complications (Fahn 2000; Bezard *et al.* 2001), including loss of l-dopa effectiveness, the "on" and "off" motor response phenomenon, and involuntary choreic or dystonic movements, namely dyskinesia. These motor complications were observed in ~50% of patients after 5 years of l-dopa treatment. Recently, the incidence of severe dyskinesia has been reduced by early use of dopamine agonists (Olanow 2002), more judicious use of l-dopa (Olanow *et al.* 2004), and the introduction of surgical approaches such as DBS (Lang and Widner 2002). However, motor complications of long-term l-dopa treatment remain the limiting factor in management of the later stages of PD (Fahn 2000).

Nonmotor symptoms result from the degeneration of neuronal fields outside the dopaminergic systems in the substantia nigra: Recent study of postmortem human PD brain has identified additional fields of neurodegeneration outside the striatum and substantia nigra including the locus ceruleus, substantia innominata, the autonomic nervous system, and the cerebral cortex, with noradrenergic, serotonergic, and cholinergic neurons affected (Braak *et al.* 2002; Langston 2006). Degeneration in these systems may be responsible for nonmotor symptoms including cognitive dysfunction, depression, fatigue, balance impairment, sleep disturbance, and autonomic dysfunction, as well as gastrointestinal and genitourinary disturbances. These nonmotor features progress, dominating the later stages of PD. Although the clinical consequences of nondopaminergic neuronal involvement usually become apparent years before diagnosis, the sequence in which PD pathology develops is debated. The distribution of Lewy body formation might include nondopaminergic areas at an early stage; however, it remains to be shown that cell death occurs in these areas before the substantia nigra. Because nonmotor symptoms generally do not respond to dopaminergic medication, alleviation of these symptoms remains a major unmet need in the clinical management of PD (Chaudhuri *et al.* 2006).

Lack of disease-modifying therapy: Despite remarkable advances in our understanding of the molecular and neurochemical basis of PD over the past 50 years, no drug is currently approved for use for disease modification. l-dopa offers no clear benefit in treating the underlying neurodegeneration of dopaminergic neurons. Based primarily on in vitro cell culture studies, concerns have been raised that l-dopa may actually accelerate this process. This concern has prompted many clinicians to avoid prescribing l-dopa early in the course of PD (Melamed *et al.* 1998). Despite clinical trials of several neuroprotective strategies for PD, including monoamine oxidase B (MAO B) inhibitors (selegiline) (Olanow 2004; Shoulson 1998), antioxidants (vitamin E) (Shoulson 1998), excitotoxicity antagonists (e.g. remacemide) (Greenamyre *et al.* 1994), neurotrophic factors (Gash *et al.* 1996; Grondin *et al.* 2002), dopamine agonists (Olanow 2002, 2004; Schapira and Olanow 2003), the mixed-lineage kinase inhibitor, CEP-1347

(Waldmeier *et al.* 2006), and the glyceraldehyde-3-phosphate (GAPDH) ligand, TCH346 (Waldmeier *et al.* 2006), no neuroprotective therapy has yet emerged for the treatment of PD. Thus, the need remains critical to develop effective neuroprotective strategies as well as improved motor-activating antiparkinsonian strategies that may serve as alternatives or adjuvants to standard dopaminergic therapy for PD.

Opportunities for diagnosis and therapeutic biomarkers

To accelerate the development of novel PD therapies, it is essential to identify reliable biomarkers for PD. Biomarkers help identify at-risk individuals before clinical symptoms appear and help monitor PD progression. Despite intensive preclinical and clinical research, no fully validated biomarker is yet available for PD.

Biomarkers for diagnosis

In vivo brain imaging has been tested as a biomarker for diagnosis of at-risk individuals. Two recent studies (the community neurologist-based study and the CUPS study [clinically uncertain parkinsonian syndromes]) directly assessed the accuracy of DAT imaging in subjects with a clinical diagnosis of PD (Catafau and Tolosa 2004; Jennings *et al.* 2004). In these longitudinal studies, DAT imaging was compared with a gold standard clinical diagnosis. A reduction in DAT density was associated with high risk for a clinical diagnosis of PD. These dopamine/DAT image markers, however, cannot distinguish between idiopathic PD and other parkinsonisms such as progressive supranuclear palsy, multiple system atrophy, and diffuse Lewy body disease. Recognition that some nonmotor symptoms of PD precede the cardinal motor symptoms by many years has spurred an effort to identify biomarkers for nondopaminergic early clinical manifestations of PD as well. Nonmotor clinical features of PD are most often associated with pathology in noradrenergic, serotonergic, cholinergic, or other neuronal systems; thus biomarkers for these systems have begun to be evaluated. The presence of early nonmotor clinical manifestations of PD has been combined with imaging and with blood and cerebrospinal fluid biomarkers to identify populations that include many individuals at risk for PD (Ponsen *et al.* 2004; Stiasny-Kolster *et al.* 2005). For example, early dysfunctions in norepinephrine neurotransmission in autonomic neurons were evaluated using cardiac imaging with ^{123}I-MIBG (^{123}I-labeled metaiodobenzylguanidine) uptake to identify patients with PD and individuals at risk for PD (Oka *et al.* 2007; Spiegel *et al.* 2005).

Biomarkers for progression

Brain imaging with F-dopa, VMAT2 (vesicular monoamine transporter 2), DAT (dopamine transporter), B-CIT [(123I) beta-carboxymethyoxy-3-beta-(4-iodophenyl) tropane] and CFT [(11)C-2-B-carbomethoxy-3B-(4-fluorophenyl) tropane], and fluorodeoxyglucose using both positron emission tomography and single-photon emission computed tomography has been used to assay PD progression in clinical trials (Marek *et al.* 2008). Longitudinal studies of PD with these image markers have demonstrated an annual rate of reduction in striatal dopaminergic content of about 4–13% in patients with PD compared with 0–2.5% change in healthy control subjects (Brooks *et al.* 2003; Fahn *et al.* 2004; Marek *et al.* 2001). This finding is consistent with the evidence from studies of patients with hemi-PD in which a 5–10% reduction per year in dopamine image markers is estimated, as patients with hemi-PD become affected bilaterally in 3–6 years (i.e., 25–35% reduction in 3–6 years) (Booij *et al.* 1998; Guttman *et al.* 1997; Innis *et al.* 1993). Caution should be exercised in interpreting imaging data using DAT and dopamine as ligands, however, because dopamine replacement therapy may alter the expression of DAT directly, independent of PD progression. Conversely, recent imaging studies have indicated that biomarkers for neuroinflammation in substantia nigra, such as microglial activation (Gerhard *et al.* 2006) and nigral ultrasound hyperechogenicity (Gaenslen *et al.* 2008), did not correlate with PD progression. Interestingly, two large PD clinical trials have recently shown that in addition to reduced risk for development of PD, increased urate levels may be inversely associated with PD disease progression (Ascherio *et al.* 2009; Schwarzschild *et al.* 2008) and thus urate might merit further study as a potential biomarker.

Recent advances in proteomics, metabolomics, and transcriptomics (Mandel *et al.* 2003, 2007; Riederer *et al.* 2008) *and in vivo brain imaging offer great promise for the identification of PD biomarkers.*

To expedite the discovery of useful markers, a major initiative has been proposed to develop PD progression biomarkers through a consortium of academic centers, government agencies, PD foundations, and pharmaceutical and biotechnology companies (Marek et al. 2008). This consortium would jointly develop a comprehensive, focused, and collaborative strategy to test and validate biomarkers of PD progression utilizing existing and new clinical PD cohorts at different disease stages.

New molecular and therapeutic approaches: a case study of adenosine A$_{2A}$ antagonists

Over the past decade, adenosine A$_{2A}$ receptor antagonists have emerged as leading nondopaminergic drugs for treatment of PD and have undergone large phase II and III clinical trials with proven efficacy of motor relief in patients with advanced PD. The adenosine A$_{2A}$ receptor (A$_{2A}$R) gene belongs to the G protein-coupled adenosine receptor family of which four subtypes (A$_1$, A$_{2A}$, A$_{2B}$, and A$_3$) have been characterized (Fredholm et al. 2001). A$_{2A}$Rs are highly concentrated in the striatum, nucleus accumbens, and olfactory tubercle (Fink et al. 1992; Schiffmann et al. 1991). This unique cellular location of the A$_{2A}$R provides the anatomical basis for the adenosine–dopamine interactions that underlie the motor symptomatic benefit of A$_{2A}$R antagonists in PD.

Preclinical studies

Behavioral studies have demonstrated that the nonspecific adenosine antagonists caffeine and theophylline (Ferre et al. 1992; Fredholm et al. 1999; Ongini and Fredholm 1996) stimulate locomotor activity in normal animals as well as in dopamine-depleted animals. Thus, A$_{2A}$R agonists and antagonists function as dopamine antagonists and agonists, respectively, in modulating motor activity. In rodents, nonspecific adenosine antagonists (such as caffeine) as well as specific A$_{2A}$R antagonists (such as KW6002) increase motor activity in animals depleted of dopamine by MPTP or reserpine and increase contralateral rotation in unilaterally lesioned (hemiparkinsonian) animals (Ferre et al. 1992, 1997; Shiozaki et al. 1999). The ability of A$_{2A}$R antagonists to stimulate motor activity was also documented in MPTP-treated nonhuman primates (Grondin et al. 1999; Kanda et al. 1998). A$_{2A}$R antagonists stimulate motor activity in dopamine-depleted animals either alone or by synergizing with l-dopa and other dopamine agonists. In support of these behavioral findings, neurochemical studies have demonstrated that activation of the A$_{2A}$ receptor counteracts D$_2$ receptor function in the striatum at the level of the intramembrane interaction, G protein coupling, neurotransmitter release, and gene expression. The mechanism of motor enhancement has been attributed to three possible effects of A$_{2A}$ antagonists: (1) a direct receptor–receptor (A$_{2A}$–D$_2$) antagonistic interaction at the membrane level (Ferre et al. 1991; Fuxe et al. 1998); (2) opposing but independent signaling pathways triggered by A$_{2A}$ and D$_2$ receptors (Aoyama et al. 2000; Chen et al. 2001a; Svenningsson et al. 1999); or (3) A$_{2A}$ receptor modulation of γ-aminobutyric acid release in the basal ganglia (Mori et al. 1996; Richardson et al. 1999; Shindou et al. 2001). These preclinical studies set the stage for clinical trials to evaluate the ability of the A$_{2A}$R antagonist KW6002 to relieve motor symptoms in patients with late-stage PD.

Clinical trials with the A2A antagonist istradefylline

In a proof-of-concept study conducted in 15 patients with PD (Bara-Jimenez et al. 2003), the acute effects of istradefylline (KW022) were evaluated using l-dopa infusions for 2 weeks. Istradefylline (40 and 80 mg) alone provided no antiparkinsonian response in patients with moderately advanced PD, in contrast to the normalization of locomotor function that had been observed in primates. However, consistent with the primate studies, coadministration of istradefylline lowered the dose of l-dopa necessary to maintain a good antiparkinsonian response with less dyskinesia. In addition, the prolongation of the efficacy half-time following discontinuation of l-dopa infusion suggested that istradefylline might reduce "off" time in patients with motor fluctuations on levodopa.

In a 12-week, randomized, placebo-controlled, double-blind, exploratory clinical trial (US-001) (Hauser et al. 2003), patients with moderately advanced PD with both motor fluctuations and dyskinesias on l-dopa continued their baseline medication regimens and were randomly assigned to undergo additional treatment with placebo (n = 29), istradefylline up to 20 mg/day (n = 26), or istradefylline up to 40 mg/day (n = 28). Consistent with results from the proof-of-concept study, istradefylline reduced "off" time by 1.7 hours compared with placebo as assessed by home diaries. Notably, istradefylline increased "on" time with dyskinesia by 2.1 hours compared with placebo.

Two large, 12-week, randomized, double-blind, placebo-controlled phase II studies were subsequently conducted in patients on l-dopa with motor fluctuations (with or without dyskinesia) (Lewitt et al. 2008; Stacy et al. 2008). In both studies, patients continued their baseline medication regimens and were randomly assigned to the addition of istradefylline or placebo. In the first study (US-005) (Lewitt et al. 2008), starting at 2 weeks and continuing throughout the remainder of the study, istradefylline 40 mg/day reduced "off" time by 1.2 hours compared with placebo ($P = 0.005$). In the second (US-006) (Stacy et al. 2008), istradefylline 20 and 60 mg/day reduced "off" time by 0.64 and 0.77 hours, respectively. Increases in "on" time with dyskinesia were observed in both studies, but this was principally nontroublesome dyskinesia.

Similar results were observed in a large phase III clinical trial (US-013) (Hauser et al. 2008), in which the addition of istradefylline 20 mg/day decreased "off" time compared with placebo by 0.7 hours ($P = 0.03$). Istradefylline was well tolerated, with dyskinesia, lightheadedness, tremor, constipation, and weight decrease reported more often with istradefylline than placebo. In contrast, another phase III clinical trial that evaluated 10, 20, and 40 mg/day istradefylline in patients with motor fluctuations on l-dopa did not demonstrate a significant reduction in "off" time compared with placebo at any istradefylline dose (Guttman 2006). The reason for this negative result is not known but could be chance or suboptimal clinical trial implementation.

Istradefylline 40 mg/day was recently compared with placebo as monotherapy in early PD in a 12-week, double-blind, randomized, multicenter study involving 176 subjects (Fernandez et al. 2010). Istradefylline provided numerical improvement at the 2-week time point over the placebo in Unified Parkinson Disease Rating Scale (UPDRS) motor scores but did not reach the primary end point (i.e., the difference in the change from baseline to end point across groups was not statistically significant). These results differ from the preclinical animal studies in MPTP-treated primates in which a moderate reversal of motor deficits was demonstrated unambiguously. Together, the results of these clinical trials suggest that further clinical investigation of istradefylline is warranted to understand its full potential as a treatment for PD.

Disease-modifying effect of adenosine A2A receptor antagonists

Epidemiological and animal studies suggest a possible disease-modifying effect of adenosine A_{2A} receptor antagonists. In 2000, Ross and colleagues reported a large prospective study showing that there is an inverse relationship between consumption of the non-selective adenosine antagonist caffeine and the risk of developing PD over a 30-year follow-up study of 8004 Japanese-American men in the Honolulu Heart Program (Ross et al. 2000). The age- and smoking-adjusted risk of PD was five times higher among men who reported no coffee consumption compared with men who reported a daily consumption of 28 oz (150 mg) or more of coffee. This finding was substantiated by a similar inverse relationship between the consumption of caffeinated (but not decaffeinated) coffee and the risk of developing PD in two larger, more ethnically diverse cohorts – the Health Professionals' Follow-Up Study and the Nurses' Health Study – involving 47,351 men and 88,565 women (Ascherio et al. 2001). These studies firmly established a relationship between increased caffeine consumption and decreased risk of developing PD in men. In support of the neuroprotective effect of caffeine in PD, animal studies demonstrated that pharmacological blockade (by caffeine or specific $A_{2A}R$ antagonists) or genetic depletion of the $A_{2A}R$ attenuates dopaminergic neurotoxicity and neurodegeneration in both MPTP and 6-OHDA models of PD (Chen et al. 2001b; Ikeda et al. 2002; Xu et al. 2002). This neuroprotection is seen after acute coadministration as well as following repeated injection of caffeine (Xu et al. 2002). This protection is likely mediated by $A_{2A}Rs$ given that similar results are obtained with various $A_{2A}R$ antagonists and genetic deletion of the $A_{2A}R$, but not with A_1R antagonists (Chen et al. 2001b; Ikeda et al. 2002; Pierri et al. 2005). These studies provide a neurobiological basis for the inverse relationship between increased caffeine consumption and reduced risk of developing PD.

Translation from animal models to the clinic in developing neuroprotective strategies

Relevance of apoptosis pathway to neurodegeneration in Parkinson's disease

Based on the evidence from animal models of PD, two novel chemical entities, CEP-137 and TCH346, were developed and selected to target two key apoptosis pathways, the mixed-lineage kinase family and glyceraldehyde phosphate dehydrogenase (GAPDH), in recent clinical trials of PD. The failure in these PD clinical trials raises questions about the relevance of these apoptosis pathways to PD neurodegeneration. Based on what we know about the disease, PD pathogenesis involves multiple and complex mechanisms such as oxidative stress, nitrative stress, mitochondrial dysfunction, excitotoxicity, and proteasomal dysfunction. Complex interactions among these factors make it impossible to define which events are primary and which are secondary. Thus, we can speculate that effective neuroprotection will require targeting multiple pathways simultaneously.

Animal models do not accurately replicate the chronic neurodegeneration of PD: Many pharmacological agents are effective in animal models of PD but have failed to slow dopaminergic neurodegeneration significantly in PD clinical trials. Thus the extent to which the animal models of PD capture the pathophysiological changes of PD is in question (Dauer and Przedborski 2003; Jenner 2008; Waldmeier *et al.* 2006). The acute toxins model of PD in rodents and nonhuman primates is a model of selective nigral degeneration and is useful in predicting motor responses to antiparkinsonian drugs. However, these acute toxin models of PD fail to capture the progressive nature of clinical PD (Jenner 2008). Conversely, models of PD generated by transgenic overexpression or target gene knockout of the genes associated with PD have failed to produce selective neurodegeneration of dopaminergic neurons (Dauer and Przedborski 2003; Chesselet *et al.* 2008; Harvey *et al.* 2008). These limitations likely contributed to the recent failure of putative disease-modifying drugs to perform as expected in clinical trials (Waldmeier *et al.* 2006).

Lack of good clinical trial design for testing neuroprotective effect: One of the main problems in the design of clinical trials for PD is the difficulty in distinguishing disease-modifying effects of treatment from short-term beneficial effects on symptoms. For example, the early DATATOP study (Shoulson 1998) found that deprenyl (selegiline, an MAO B inhibitor) appeared to delay the need to start l-dopa treatment of PD, an indicator of possible neuroprotective effect, but this interpretation was confounded by a previously underappreciated symptomatic effect of the drug (Shoulson 1998). To address this issue, novel clinical trial designs such as delayed-start design (also called the randomized-start design) have been proposed and employed to evaluate the neuroprotective effect of MAO B inhibitors (D'Agostino 2009; Olanow *et al.* 2009a). This design consists of two phases: In phase I, untreated patients are randomly assigned to initiate therapy with either the study intervention or placebo. In phase II, patients in both treatment groups receive the same active study intervention and are followed for an additional period. At the end of phase I, the possible difference between the two groups would be caused by symptomatic or neuroprotective effects, or both. At the end of phase II, the possible difference between two treatment groups is attributed to a neuroprotective effect. This study design has recently been employed to test the MAO B inhibitor rasagiline in clinical PD trials (Olanow *et al.* 2009a). Other strategies, such as using futility designs, have also been proposed (Tilley *et al.* 2006).

Lack of validated biomarkers for monitoring PD progression: In clinical studies, where it is difficult to separate the effects of the study drug on motor symptoms and dopaminergic neurodegeneration, a fully validated biomarker for assaying PD progression is essential. Available DAT image markers are potentially confounded by their possible direct pharmacological effect on these markers, rather than the assessment of PD progression (Marek *et al.* 2008). The lack of a fully validated biomarker makes it difficult to define effective dose ranges and to guide proper dosing in human studies (Olanow *et al.* 2008).

Difficulty in defining proper agents and proper dose of the study drug in a clinical trial (Waldmeier *et al.* 2006): Traditionally, the doses for clinical trials are selected to produce plasma concentrations similar to those that were effective in animal models. In neuroprotection studies, it is the brain concentration of the study drug that is relevant and this concentration may not mirror plasma concentrations. The doses that were effective in animal studies may still be below the threshold for neuroprotection in clinical trials (Olanow *et al.* 2008).

Conclusions

A major shift in basic science research and clinical management of PD has occurred over the past 10 years. First, genetic studies have not only identified many genetic loci associated with familial PD but also provided critical insights into the molecular pathogenesis of PD. This knowledge of PD genetics has just begun to impact basic science (e.g., new transgenic animal models) and clinical practice (e.g., genetic consultation). Second, with refined research tools and better control of motor symptoms with current therapy, nonmotor symptoms are increasingly recognized as critical components of PD, leading to the concept that PD may be a complex disorder affecting multiple organs, with motor symptoms as the "tip of the iceberg," as revealed by newer α-synuclein immunohistochemistry methods. Third, as dopamine therapy is intrinsically linked to motor complications such as dyskinesia and fails to control nonmotor symptoms, the search for a nondopaminergic therapeutic strategy has become increasingly compelling. This is exemplified by the preclinical and clinical development of the adenosine A_{2A} receptor antagonist KW6002 in patients with advanced PD. Lastly, equipped with new understanding of the molecular basis of PD, efforts are now targeted toward overcoming the major obstacles to developing an effective neuroprotective therapy for PD, including accurate animal models of PD, fully validated biomarkers, and effective clinical trial design.

References

Abbott RD, Ross GW, White LR et al. 2003. Environmental, life-style, and physical precursors of clinical Parkinson's disease: recent findings from the Honolulu-Asia Aging Study. *J Neurol* **250**(Suppl. 3): III30–III39.

Agid Y, Cervera P, Hirsch E et al. 1989. Biochemistry of Parkinson's disease 28 years later: a critical review. *Mov Disord* **4**:S126–S144.

Andres-Mateos E, Perier C, Zhang L et al. 2007. DJ-1 gene deletion reveals that DJ-1 is an atypical peroxiredoxin-like peroxidase. *Proc Natl Acad Sci USA* **104**:14807–14812.

Aoyama S, Kase H, Borrelli E. 2000. Rescue of locomotor impairment in dopamine D2 receptor-deficient mice by an adenosine A2A receptor antagonist. *J Neurosci* **20**:5848–5852.

Ascherio A, LeWitt PA, Xu K et al. 2009. Urate as a predictor of the rate of clinical decline in Parkinson disease. *Arch Neurol* **66**:1460–1468.

Ascherio A, Zhang SM, Hernan MA et al. 2001. Prospective study of caffeine consumption and risk of Parkinson's disease in men and women. *Ann Neurol* **50**:56–63.

Bara-Jimenez W, Sherzai A, Dimitrova T et al. 2003. Adenosine A(2A) receptor antagonist treatment of Parkinson's disease. *Neurology* **61**:293–296.

Bezard E, Brotchie JM, Gross CE. 2001. Pathophysiology of levodopa-induced dyskinesia: potential for new therapies. *Nat Rev Neurosci* **2**:577–588.

Biskup S, Moore DJ, Celsi F et al. 2006. Localization of LRRK2 to membranous and vesicular structures in mammalian brain. *Ann Neurol* **60**:557–569.

Bonifati V, Rizzu P, van Baren MJ et al. 2003. Mutations in the DJ-1 gene associated with autosomal recessive early-onset parkinsonism. *Science* **299**:256–259.

Bonuccelli U, Del Dotto P. 2006. New pharmacologic horizons in the treatment of Parkinson disease. *Neurology* **67**:S30–S38.

Booij J, Habraken JB, Bergmans P et al. 1998. Imaging of dopamine transporters with iodine-123-FP-CIT SPECT in healthy controls and patients with Parkinson's disease. *J Nucl Med* **39**:1879–1884.

Braak H, Del Tredici K, Bratzke H et al. 2002. Staging of the intracerebral inclusion body pathology associated with idiopathic Parkinson's disease (preclinical and clinical stages). *J Neurol* **249**(Suppl. 3):III/1–5.

Braak E, Sandmann-Keil D, Rub U et al. 2001. Alpha-synuclein immunopositive Parkinson's disease-related inclusion bodies in lower brain stem nuclei. *Acta Neuropathol* **101**:195–201.

Braak H, Tredici KD, Rub U et al. 2003. Staging of brain pathology related to sporadic Parkinson's disease. *Neurobiol Aging* **24**:197–211.

Bras JM, Singleton A. 2009. Genetic susceptibility in Parkinson's disease. *Biochim Biophys Acta* **1792**:597–603.

Bronstein J, Carvey P, Chen H et al. 2009. Meeting report: consensus statement – Parkinson's disease and the environment: Collaborative on Health and the Environment and Parkinson's Action Network (CHE PAN) conference 26–28 June 2007. *Environ Health Perspect* **117**:117–121.

Brooks DJ, Frey KA, Marek KL et al. 2003. Assessment of neuroimaging techniques as biomarkers of the progression of Parkinson's disease. *Exp Neurol* **184**(Suppl. 1): S68–S79.

Catafau AM, Tolosa E. 2004. Impact of dopamine transporter SPECT using 123I-Ioflupane on diagnosis and management of patients with clinically uncertain Parkinsonian syndromes. *Mov Disord* **19**:1175–1182.

Chaudhuri KR, Healy DG, Schapira AH. 2006. Non-motor symptoms of Parkinson's disease: diagnosis and management. *Lancet Neurol* **5**:235–245.

Chen JF, Moratalla R, Impagnatiello F et al. 2001a. The role of the D(2) dopamine receptor (D(2)R) in A(2A) adenosine receptor (A(2A)R)-mediated behavioral and cellular responses as revealed by A(2A) and D(2) receptor knockout mice. *Proc Natl Acad Sci USA* **98**:1970–1975.

Chen JF, Xu K, Petzer JP et al. 2001b. Neuroprotection by caffeine and A(2A) adenosine receptor inactivation in a model of Parkinson's disease. *J Neurosci* **21**: RC143.

Chen H, Zhang SM, Hernan MA et al. 2003. Nonsteroidal anti-inflammatory drugs and the risk of Parkinson disease. *Arch Neurol* **60**:1059–1064.

Chesselet MF, Fleming S, Mortazavi F, Meurers B. 2008. Strengths and limitations of genetic mouse models of Parkinson's disease. *Parkinsonism Relat Disord* **14** (Suppl. 2):S84–S87.

Clark IE, Dodson MW, Jiang C et al. 2006. Drosophila pink1 is required for mitochondrial function and interacts genetically with parkin. *Nature* **441**:1162–1166.

D'Agostino RB Sr. 2009. The delayed-start study design. *N Engl J Med* **361**:1304–1306.

Daniel SE, Lees AJ. 1993. Parkinson's Disease Society Brain Bank, London: overview and research. *J Neural Transm Suppl* **39**:165–172.

Dauer W, Kholodilov N, Vila M et al. 2002. Resistance of alpha-synuclein null mice to the parkinsonian neurotoxin MPTP. *Proc Natl Acad Sci USA* **99**:14524–14529.

Dauer W, Przedborski S. 2003. Parkinson's disease: mechanisms and models. *Neuron* **39**:889–909.

Deep-Brain Stimulation for Parkinson's Disease Study Group. 2001. Deep-brain stimulation of the subthalamic nucleus or the pars interna of the globus pallidus in Parkinson's disease. *N Engl J Med* **345**:956–963.

Deuschl G, Schade-Brittinger C, Krack P et al. 2006. A randomized trial of deep-brain stimulation for Parkinson's disease. *N Engl J Med* **355**:896–908.

Dorsey ER, Constantinescu R, Thompson JP et al. 2007. Projected number of people with Parkinson disease in the most populous nations, 2005 through 2030. *Neurology* **68**:384–386.

Driver JA, Kurth T, Buring JE, Gaziano JM, Logroscino G. 2008. Parkinson disease and risk of mortality: a prospective comorbidity-matched cohort study. *Neurology* **70**:1423–1430.

Exner N, Treske B, Paquet D et al. 2007. Loss-of-function of human PINK1 results in mitochondrial pathology and can be rescued by parkin. *J Neurosci* **27**:12413–12418.

Fahn S. 1999. Parkinson disease, the effect of levodopa, and the ELLDOPA trial. Earlier vs Later L-DOPA. *Arch Neurol* **56**:529–535.

Fahn S. 2000. The spectrum of levodopa-induced dyskinesias. *Ann Neurol* **47**:S2–S9; discussion S9–S11.

Fahn S, Oakes D, Shoulson I et al. 2004. Levodopa and the progression of Parkinson's disease. *N Engl J Med* **351**:2498–2508.

Fearnley JM, Lees AJ. 1991. Ageing and Parkinson's disease: substantia nigra regional selectivity. *Brain* **114** (Pt 5):2283–2301.

Fernandez HH, Greeley DR, Zweig RM et al. 6002-US-051 Study Group. 2010. Istradefylline as monotherapy for Parkinson disease: results of the 6002-US-051 trial. *Parkinsonism Relat Disord* **16**:16–20. Epub 2009 Jul 19.

Ferre S, Fredholm BB, Morelli M, Popoli P, Fuxe K. 1997. Adenosine–dopamine receptor–receptor interactions as an integrative mechanism in the basal ganglia. *Trends Neurosci* **20**:482–487.

Ferre S, Fuxe K, von Euler G, Johansson B, Fredholm BB. 1992. Adenosine–dopamine interactions in the brain. *Neuroscience* **51**:501–512.

Ferre S, von Euler G, Johansson B, Fredholm BB, Fuxe K. 1991. Stimulation of high-affinity adenosine A2 receptors decreases the affinity of dopamine D2 receptors in rat striatal membranes. *Proc Natl Acad Sci USA* **88**:7238–7241.

Fink JS, Weaver DR, Rivkees SA et al. 1992. Molecular cloning of the rat A2 adenosine receptor: selective co-expression with D2 dopamine receptors in rat striatum. *Brain Res Mol Brain Res* **14**:186–195.

Fredholm BB, Battig K, Holmen J, Nehlig A, Zvartau EE. 1999. Actions of caffeine in the brain with special reference to factors that contribute to its widespread use. *Pharmacol Rev* **51**:83–133.

Fredholm BB, Ijzerman A, Jacobson KA, Klotz KN, Linden J. 2001. International Union of Pharmacology. XXV. Nomenclature and classification of adenosine receptors. *Pharmacol Rev* **53**:527–552.

Fung HC, Scholz S, Matarin M et al. 2006. Genome-wide genotyping in Parkinson's disease and neurologically normal controls: first stage analysis and public release of data. *Lancet Neurol* **5**:911–916.

Fuxe K, Ferré S, Zoli M, Agnati LF. 1998. Integrated events in central dopamine transmission as analyzed at multiple levels. Evidence for intramembrane adenosine A2A/dopamine D2 and adenosine A1/dopamine D1 receptor interactions in the basal ganglia. *Brain Res Brain Res Rev* **26**:258–273.

Gaenslen A, Unmuth B, Godau J et al. 2008. The specificity and sensitivity of transcranial ultrasound in the differential diagnosis of Parkinson's disease: a prospective blinded study. *Lancet Neurol* **7**:417–424.

Gash DM, Zhang Z, Ovadia A et al. 1996. Functional recovery in parkinsonian monkeys treated with GDNF. *Nature* **380**:252–255.

Gasser T. 2009. Mendelian forms of Parkinson's disease. *Biochim Biophys Acta* **1792**:587–596.

Gerhard A, Pavese N, Hotton G et al. 2006. In vivo imaging of microglial activation with [11C](R)-PK11195 PET in idiopathic Parkinson's disease. *Neurobiol Dis* **21**:404–412.

Gilks WP, Abou-Sleiman PM, Gandhi S et al. 2005. A common LRRK2 mutation in idiopathic Parkinson's disease. *Lancet* **365**:415–416.

Greenamyre JT, Eller RV, Zhang Z et al. 1994. Antiparkinsonian effects of remacemide hydrochloride, a glutamate antagonist, in rodent and primate models of Parkinson's disease. *Ann Neurol* **35**:655–661.

Grondin R, Bedard PJ, Hadj Tahar A et al. 1999. Antiparkinsonian effect of a new selective adenosine A2A receptor antagonist in MPTP-treated monkeys. *Neurology* **52**:1673–1677.

Grondin R, Zhang Z, Yi A et al. 2002. Chronic, controlled GDNF infusion promotes structural and functional recovery in advanced parkinsonian monkeys. *Brain* **125**:2191–2201.

Gupta A, Dawson VL, Dawson TM. 2008. What causes cell death in Parkinson's disease? *Ann Neurol* **64** (Suppl. 2):S3–S15.

Guttman M. 2006. Efficacy of istradefylline in Parkinson's disease patients treated with levodopa with motor response complications: results of the KW-6002 US-018 study. *Mov Disord* **21**(Suppl. 15):S585.

Guttman M, Burkholder J, Kish SJ et al. 1997. [11C]RTI-32 PET studies of the dopamine transporter in early dopa-naive Parkinson's disease: implications for the symptomatic threshold. *Neurology* **48**:1578–1583.

Hardy J, Cai H, Cookson MR, Gwinn-Hardy K, Singleton A. 2006. Genetics of Parkinson's disease and parkinsonism. *Ann Neurol* **60**:389–398.

Hardy J, Lewis P, Revesz T, Lees A, Paisan-Ruiz C. 2009. The genetics of Parkinson's syndromes: a critical review. *Curr Opin Genet Dev* **19**:254–265.

Hardy J, Orr H. 2006. The genetics of neurodegenerative diseases. *J Neurochem* **97**:1690–1699.

Harvey BK, Wang Y, Hoffer BJ. 2008. Transgenic rodent models of Parkinson's disease. *Acta Neurochir Suppl* **101**:89–92.

Hauser R, Shulman LM, Trugman JM et al. 2008. Study of istradefylline in patients with Parkinson's disease on levodopa with motor fluctuations. *Mov Disord* **23**:2177–2185.

Hauser RA, Hubble JP, Truong DD. 2003. Randomized trial of the adenosine A(2A) receptor antagonist istradefylline in advanced PD. *Neurology* **61**:297–303.

Hauser RA, Salin L, Juhel N, Konyago VL. 2007. Randomized trial of the triple monoamine reuptake inhibitor NS 2330 (tesofensine) in early Parkinson's disease. *Mov Disord* **22**:359–365.

Heart Protection Study Collaborative Group 2002. MRC/BHF Heart Protection Study of cholesterol lowering with simvastatin in 20,536 high-risk individuals: a randomised placebo-controlled trial. *Lancet* **360**:7–22.

Hely MA, Morris JG, Rail D et al. 1989. The Sydney Multicentre Study of Parkinson's disease: a report on the first 3 years. *J Neurol Neurosurg Psychiatry* **52**:324–328.

Hernan MA, Takkouche B, Caamano-Isorna F, Gestal-Otero JJ. 2002. A meta-analysis of coffee drinking, cigarette smoking, and the risk of Parkinson's disease. *Ann Neurol* **52**:276–284.

Hisata J. 2002. *Final Supplemental Environmental Impact Statement. Lake and Stream Rehabilitation: Rotenone Use and Health Risks*. Washington, DC: Department of Fish and Wildlife.

Hoehn MM, Yahr MD. 1967. Parkinsonism: onset, progression and mortality. *Neurology* **17**:427–442.

Hughes AJ, Ben-Shlomo Y, Daniel SE, Lees AJ. 1992a. What features improve the accuracy of clinical diagnosis in Parkinson's disease: a clinicopathologic study. *Neurology* **42**:1142–1146.

Hughes AJ, Daniel SE, Kilford L, Lees AJ. 1992b. Accuracy of clinical diagnosis of idiopathic Parkinson's disease: a clinico-pathological study of 100 cases. *J Neurol Neurosurg Psychiatry* **55**:181–184.

Ikeda K, Kurokawa M, Aoyama S, Kuwana Y. 2002. Neuroprotection by adenosine A2A receptor blockade in experimental models of Parkinson's disease. *J Neurochem* **80**:262–270.

Innis RB, Seibyl JP, Scanley BE et al. 1993. Single photon emission computed tomographic imaging demonstrates loss of striatal dopamine transporters in Parkinson disease. *Proc Natl Acad Sci USA* **90**:11965–11969.

Ito G, Okai T, Fujino G et al. 2007. GTP binding is essential to the protein kinase activity of LRRK2, a causative gene product for familial Parkinson's disease. *Biochemistry* **46**:1380–1388.

Jenner P. 2008. Functional models of Parkinson's disease: a valuable tool in the development of novel therapies. *Ann Neurol* **64**(Suppl. 2): S16–S29.

Jennings DL, Seibyl JP, Oakes D et al. 2004. (123I) beta-CIT and single-photon emission computed tomographic imaging vs clinical evaluation in Parkinsonian syndrome: unmasking an early diagnosis. *Arch Neurol* **61**:1224–1229.

Johnston TH, Brotchie JM. 2006. Drugs in development for Parkinson's disease: an update. *Curr Opin Investig Drugs* **7**:25–32.

Kanda T, Tashiro T, Kuwana Y, Jenner P. 1998. Adenosine A2A receptors modify motor function in MPTP-treated common marmosets. *Neuroreport* **9**:2857–2860.

Kleiner-Fisman G, Herzog J, Fisman DN et al. 2006. Subthalamic nucleus deep brain stimulation: summary and meta-analysis of outcomes. *Mov Disord* **21**(Suppl. 14):S290–S304.

Korczyn AD, Nussbaum M. 2002. Emerging therapies in the pharmacological treatment of Parkinson's disease. *Drugs* **62**:775–786.

Krack P, Batir A, Van Blercom N et al. 2003. Five-year follow-up of bilateral stimulation of the subthalamic nucleus in advanced Parkinson's disease. *N Engl J Med* **349**:1925–1934.

Kruger R, Kuhn W, Muller T et al. 1998. Ala30Pro mutation in the gene encoding alpha-synuclein in Parkinson's disease. *Nat Genet* **18**:106–108.

Laihinen A, Ruottinen H, Rinne JO et al. 2000. Risk for Parkinson's disease: twin studies for the detection of asymptomatic subjects using [18F]6-fluorodopa PET. *J Neurol* **247**(Suppl. 2):II110–II113.

Lang AE, Lozano AM. 1998a. Parkinson's disease. First of two parts. *N Engl J Med* **339**:1044–1053.

Lang AE, Lozano AM. 1998b. Parkinson's disease. Second of two parts. *N Engl J Med* **339**:1130–1143.

Lang AE, Widner H. 2002. Deep brain stimulation for Parkinson's disease: patient selection and evaluation. *Mov Disord* **17**(Suppl. 3):S94–S101.

Langston JW. 2006. The Parkinson's complex: parkinsonism is just the tip of the iceberg. *Ann Neurol* **59**:591–596.

Langston JW, Ballard P, Tetrud JW, Irwin I. 1983. Chronic Parkinsonism in humans due to a product of meperidine-analog synthesis. *Science* **219**:979–980.

Langston JW, Forno LS, Tetrud J et al. 1999. Evidence of active nerve cell degeneration in the substantia nigra of humans years after 1-methyl-4-phenyl-1,2,3,6-tetrahydropyridine exposure. *Ann Neurol* **46**:598–605.

Lazzarini AM, Myers RH, Zimmerman TR Jr et al. 1994. A clinical genetic study of Parkinson's disease: evidence for dominant transmission. *Neurology* **44**:499–506.

Lee VM, Trojanowski JQ. 2006. Mechanisms of Parkinson's disease linked to pathological alpha-synuclein: new targets for drug discovery. *Neuron* **52**:33–38.

Leroy E, Boyer R, Auburger G et al. 1998. The ubiquitin pathway in Parkinson's disease. *Nature* **395**:451–452.

Levy G, Tang MX, Louis ED et al. 2002. The association of incident dementia with mortality in PD. *Neurology* **59**:1708–1713.

Lewitt PA, Guttman M, Tetrud JW et al. 2008. Adenosine A(2A) receptor antagonist istradefylline (KW-6002) reduces "off" time in Parkinson's disease: a double-blind, randomized, multicenter clinical trial (6002-US-005). *Ann Neurol* **63**:295–302.

Limousin P, Krack P, Pollak P et al. 1998. Electrical stimulation of the subthalamic nucleus in advanced Parkinson's disease. *N Engl J Med* **339**:1105–1111.

Lockhart PJ, Lincoln S, Hulihan M et al. 2004. DJ-1 mutations are a rare cause of recessively inherited early onset parkinsonism mediated by loss of protein function. *J Med Genet* **41**:e22.

Mandel SA, Fishman T, Youdim MB. 2007. Gene and protein signatures in sporadic Parkinson's disease and a novel genetic model of PD. *Parkinsonism Relat Disord* **13**(Suppl 3):S242–S247.

Mandel S, Weinreb O, Youdim MB. 2003. Using cDNA microarray to assess Parkinson's disease models and the effects of neuroprotective drugs. *Trends Pharmacol Sci* **24**:184–191.

Maraganore DM, de Andrade M, Lesnick TG et al. 2005. High-resolution whole-genome association study of Parkinson disease. *Am J Hum Genet* **77**:685–693.

Marek K, Innis R, van Dyck C et al. 2001. [123I]beta-CIT SPECT imaging assessment of the rate of Parkinson's disease progression. *Neurology* **57**:2089–2094.

Marek K, Jennings D, Tamagnan G, Seibyl J. 2008. Biomarkers for Parkinson's [corrected] disease: tools to assess Parkinson's disease onset and progression. *Ann Neurol* **64**(Suppl. 2):S111–S121.

Marras C, McDermott MP, Rochon PA et al. 2005. Survival in Parkinson disease: thirteen-year follow-up of the DATATOP cohort. *Neurology* **64**:87–93.

McGeer PL, Itagaki S, Boyes BE, McGeer EG. 1988. Reactive microglia are positive for HLA-DR in the substantia nigra of Parkinson's and Alzheimer's disease brains. *Neurology* **38**:1285–1291.

Melamed E, Offen D, Shirvan A et al. 1998. Levodopa toxicity and apoptosis. *Ann Neurol* **44**:S149–S154.

Menzies FM, Yenisetti SC, Min KT. 2005. Roles of *Drosophila* DJ-1 in survival of dopaminergic neurons and oxidative stress. *Curr Biol* **15**:1578–1582.

Metman LV, Del Dotto P, LePoole K et al. 1999. Amantadine for levodopa-induced dyskinesias: a 1-year follow-up study. *Arch Neurol* **56**:1383–1386.

Meulener M, Whitworth AJ, Armstrong-Gold CE et al. 2005. *Drosophila* DJ-1 mutants are selectively sensitive to environmental toxins associated with Parkinson's disease. *Curr Biol* **15**:1572–1577.

Moore DJ, West AB, Dawson VL, Dawson TM. 2005. Molecular pathophysiology of Parkinson's disease. *Annu Rev Neurosci* **28**:57–87.

Mori A, Shindou T, Ichimura M, Nonaka H, Kase H. 1996. The role of adenosine A2a receptors in regulating GABAergic synaptic transmission in striatal medium spiny neurons. *J Neurosci* **16**:605–611.

Muller A, Reichmann H, Livermore A, Hummel T. 2002. Olfactory function in idiopathic Parkinson's disease (IPD): results from cross-sectional studies in IPD patients and long-term follow-up of de-novo IPD patients. *J Neural Transm* **109**:805–811.

Nichols WC, Pankratz N, Hernandez D et al. 2005. Genetic screening for a single common LRRK2 mutation in familial Parkinson's disease. *Lancet* **365**:410–412.

Nyholm D, Aquilonius SM. 2004. Levodopa infusion therapy in Parkinson disease: state of the art in 2004. *Clin Neuropharmacol* **27**:245–256.

Obeso JA, Rodriguez-Oroz M, Marin C et al. 2004. The origin of motor fluctuations in Parkinson's disease: importance of dopaminergic innervation and basal ganglia circuits. *Neurology* **62**:S17–S30.

Obeso JA, Rodriguez-Oroz MC, Rodriguez M et al. 2000. Pathophysiology of the basal ganglia in Parkinson's disease. *Trends Neurosci* **23**:S8–S19.

Oka H, Yoshioka M, Morita M et al. 2007. Reduced cardiac 123I-MIBG uptake reflects cardiac sympathetic dysfunction in Lewy body disease. *Neurology* **69**:1460–1465.

Olanow CW. 2002. The role of dopamine agonists in the treatment of early Parkinson's disease. *Neurology* **58**:S33–S41.

Olanow CW. 2004. The scientific basis for the current treatment of Parkinson's disease. *Annu Rev Med* **55**:41–60.

Olanow CW, Agid Y, Mizuno Y et al. 2004. Levodopa in the treatment of Parkinson's disease: current controversies. *Mov Disord* **19**:997–1005.

Olanow CW, Kieburtz K, Schapira AH. 2008. Why have we failed to achieve neuroprotection in Parkinson's disease? *Ann Neurol* **64**(Suppl. 2):S101–S110.

Olanow CW, Rascol O, Hauser R et al. 2009a. A double-blind, delayed-start trial of rasagiline in Parkinson's disease. *N Engl J Med* **361**:1268–1278.

Olanow CW, Stern MB, Sethi K. 2009b. The scientific and clinical basis for the treatment of Parkinson disease. *Neurology* **72** (21 Suppl. 4):s1–s136.

Olanow CW, Watts RL, Koller WC. 2001. An algorithm (decision tree) for the management of Parkinson's disease (2001): treatment guidelines. *Neurology* **56**:S1–S88.

Ongini E, Fredholm BB. 1996. Pharmacology of adenosine A2A receptors. *Trends Pharmacol Sci* **17**:364–372.

O'Sullivan SS, Williams DR, Gallagher DA et al. 2008. Nonmotor symptoms as presenting complaints in Parkinson's disease: a clinicopathological study. *Mov Disord* **23**:101–106.

Paisán-Ruíz C, Jain S, Evans EW et al. 2004. Cloning of the gene containing mutations that cause PARK8-linked Parkinson's disease. *Neuron* **44**:595–600.

Pals P, Lincoln S, Manning J et al. 2004. Alpha-synuclein promoter confers susceptibility to Parkinson's disease. *Ann Neurol* **56**:591–595.

Pankratz N, Wilk JB, Latourelle JC et al. 2009. Genomewide association study for susceptibility genes contributing to familial Parkinson disease. *Hum Genet* **124**:593–605.

Park J, Kim SY, Cha GH et al. 2005. *Drosophila* DJ-1 mutants show oxidative stress-sensitive locomotive dysfunction. *Gene* **361**:133–139.

Park J, Lee SB, Lee S et al. 2006. Mitochondrial dysfunction in *Drosophila* PINK1 mutants is complemented by parkin. *Nature* **441**:1157–1161.

Parkinson Study Group 2002. Dopamine transporter brain imaging to assess the effects of pramipexole vs levodopa on Parkinson disease progression. *J Am Med Assoc* **287**:1653–1661.

Parkinson Study Group 2003. A controlled trial of rotigotine monotherapy in early Parkinson's disease. *Arch Neurol* **60**:1721–1728.

Payami H, Zareparsi S. 1998. Genetic epidemiology of Parkinson's disease. *J Geriatr Psychiatry Neurol* **11**:98–106.

Pierri M, Vaudano E, Sager T, Englund U. 2005. KW-6002 protects from MPTP-induced dopaminergic toxicity in the mouse. *Neuropharmacology* **48**:517–524.

Polymeropoulos MH, Lavedan C, Leroy E et al. 1997. Mutation in the alpha-synuclein gene identified in families with Parkinson's disease. *Science* **276**:2045–2047.

Ponsen MM, Stoffers D, Booij J et al. 2004. Idiopathic hyposmia as a preclinical sign of Parkinson's disease. *Ann Neurol* **56**:173–181.

Richardson PJ, Gubitz AK, Freeman TC, Dixon AK. 1999. Adenosine receptor antagonists and Parkinson's disease: actions of the A2A receptor in the striatum. *Adv Neurol* **80**:111–119.

Riederer P, Youdim MB, Mandel S, Gerlach M, Grunblatt E. 2008. Genomic aspects of sporadic Parkinson's disease. *Parkinsonism Relat Disord* **14**(Suppl. 2):S88–S91.

Ross GW, Abbott RD, Petrovitch H et al. 2000. Association of coffee and caffeine intake with the risk of Parkinson disease. *J Am Med Assoc* **283**:2674–2679.

Schapira AH, Olanow CW. 2003. Rationale for the use of dopamine agonists as neuroprotective agents in Parkinson's disease. *Ann Neurol* **53**(Suppl. 3):S149–S157; discussion S157–S159.

Schenck CH, Bundlie SR, Mahowald MW. 1996. Delayed emergence of a parkinsonian disorder in 38% of 29 older men initially diagnosed with idiopathic rapid eye movement sleep behaviour disorder. *Neurology* **46**:388–393.

Schiffmann SN, Jacobs O, Vanderhaeghen JJ. 1991. Striatal restricted adenosine A2 receptor (RDC8) is expressed by enkephalin but not by substance P neurons: an in situ hybridization histochemistry study. *J Neurochem* **57**:1062–1067.

Schwarzschild MA, Schwid SR, Marek K et al. 2008. Serum urate as a predictor of clinical and radiographic progression in Parkinson disease. *Arch Neurol* **65**:716–723.

Shimura H, Hattori N, Kubo S et al. 2000. Familial Parkinson disease gene product, parkin, is a ubiquitin-protein ligase. *Nat Genet* **25**:302–305.

Shindou T, Mori A, Kase H, Ichimura M. 2001. Adenosine A(2A) receptor enhances GABA(A)-mediated IPSCs in the rat globus pallidus. *J Physiol* **532**:423–434.

Shiozaki S, Ichikawa S, Nakamura J et al. 1999. Actions of adenosine A2A receptor antagonist KW-6002 on drug-induced catalepsy and hypokinesia caused by reserpine or MPTP. *Psychopharmacology (Berl)* **147**:90–95.

Shoulson I. 1998. DATATOP: a decade of neuroprotective inquiry. Parkinson Study Group. Deprenyl and tocopherol antioxidative therapy of parkinsonism. *Ann Neurol* **44**:S160–S166.

Shulman LM, Taback RL, Bean J, Weiner WJ. 2001. Comorbidity of the nonmotor symptoms of Parkinson's disease. *Mov Disord* **16**:507–510.

Simon-Sanchez J, Schulte C, Bras JM et al. 2009. Genome-wide association study reveals genetic risk underlying Parkinson's disease. *Nat Genet* **41**:1308–1312.

Simuni T, Sethi K. 2008. Nonmotor manifestations of Parkinson's disease. *Ann Neurol* **64**(Suppl. 2):S65–S80.

Singleton AB, Farrer M, Johnson J et al. 2003. Alpha-synuclein locus triplication causes Parkinson's disease. *Science* **302**:841.

Spiegel J, Mollers MO, Jost WH et al. 2005. FP-CIT and MIBG scintigraphy in early Parkinson's disease. *Mov Disord* **20**:552–561.

Spillantini MG, Schmidt ML, Lee VM et al. 1997. Alpha-synuclein in Lewy bodies. *Nature* **388**:839–840.

Stacy M, Silver D, Mendis T et al. 2008. A 12-week, placebo-controlled study (6002-US-006) of istradefylline in Parkinson disease. *Neurology* **70**:2233–2240.

Stiasny-Kolster K, Doerr Y, Moller JC et al. 2005. Combination of 'idiopathic' REM sleep behaviour disorder and olfactory dysfunction as possible indicator for alpha-synucleinopathy demonstrated by dopamine transporter FP-CIT-SPECT. *Brain* **128**:126–137.

Stocchi F, Hersh BP, Scott BL, Nausieda PA, Giorgi L. 2008. Ropinirole 24-hour prolonged release and ropinirole immediate release in early Parkinson's disease: a randomized, double-blind, non-inferiority crossover study. *Curr Med Res Opin* **24**:2883–2895.

Stocchi F, Vacca L, Ruggieri S, Olanow CW. 2005. Intermittent vs continuous levodopa administration in patients with advanced Parkinson disease: a clinical and pharmacokinetic study. *Arch Neurol* **62**:905–910.

Svenningsson P, Le Moine C, Fisone G, Fredholm BB. 1999. Distribution, biochemistry and function of striatal adenosine A2A receptors. *Prog Neurobiol* **59**:355–396.

Tanner CM. 1992. Occupational and environmental causes of parkinsonism. *Occup Med* **7**:503–513.

Tanner CM, Ottman R, Goldman SM et al. 1999. Parkinson disease in twins: an etiologic study. *J Am Med Assoc* **281**:341–346.

Tilley BC, Palesch YY, Kieburtz K et al. 2006. Optimizing the ongoing search for new treatments for Parkinson disease: using futility designs. *Neurology* **66**:628–633.

Valente EM, Abou-Sleiman PM, Caputo V et al. 2004. Hereditary early-onset Parkinson's disease caused by mutations in PINK1. *Science* **304**:1158–1160.

Volkmann J, Allert N, Voges J et al. 2001. Safety and efficacy of pallidal or subthalamic nucleus stimulation in advanced PD. *Neurology* **56**:548–551.

Volkmann J, Sturm V, Weiss P et al. 1998. Bilateral high-frequency stimulation of the internal globus pallidus in advanced Parkinson's disease. *Ann Neurol* **44**:953–961.

Waldmeier P, Bozyczko-Coyne D, Williams M, Vaught JL. 2006. Recent clinical failures in Parkinson's disease with apoptosis inhibitors underline the need for a paradigm shift in drug discovery for neurodegenerative diseases. *Biochem Pharmacol* **72**:1197–1206.

Ward CD, Duvoisin RC, Ince SE et al. 1983. Parkinson's disease in 65 pairs of twins and in a set of quadruplets. *Neurology* **33**:815–824.

Watts R, Pahwa R, Lyons K, Boroojerdi B, Wallen L. 2006. Long-term safety and efficacy of the rotigotine transdermal patch in early-stage Parkinson's disease. *Poster presented at the American Academy of Neurology meeting*, San Diego, CA, April 2–8.

West AB, Moore DJ, Biskup S et al. 2005. Parkinson's disease-associated mutations in leucine-rich repeat kinase 2 augment kinase activity. *Proc Natl Acad Sci USA* **102**:16842–16847.

West AB, Moore DJ, Choi C *et al.* 2007. Parkinson's disease-associated mutations in LRRK2 link enhanced GTP-binding and kinase activities to neuronal toxicity. *Hum Mol Genet* **16**:223–232.

Wu DC, Jackson-Lewis V, Vila M *et al.* 2002. Blockade of microglial activation is neuroprotective in the 1-methyl-4-phenyl-1,2,3,6-tetrahydropyridine mouse model of Parkinson disease. *J Neurosci* **22**:1763–1771.

Wu SS, Frucht SJ. 2005. Treatment of Parkinson's disease: what's on the horizon? *CNS Drugs* **19**:723–743.

Xu K, Xu YH, Chen JF, Schwarzschild MA. 2002. Caffeine's neuroprotection against 1-methyl-4-phenyl-1,2,3,6-tetrahydropyridine toxicity shows no tolerance to chronic caffeine administration in mice. *Neurosci Lett* **322**:13–16.

Yang Y, Gehrke S, Haque ME *et al.* 2005. Inactivation of *Drosophila* DJ-1 leads to impairments of oxidative stress response and phosphatidylinositol 3-kinase/Akt signaling. *Proc Natl Acad Sci USA* **102**:13670–13675.

Youdim MB, Geldenhuys WJ, Van der Schyf CJ. 2007. Why should we use multifunctional neuroprotective and neurorestorative drugs for Parkinson's disease? *Parkinsonism Relat Disord* **13**(Suppl. 3): S281–S291.

Zimprich A, Biskup S, Leitner P *et al* 2004. Mutations in LRRK2 cause autosomal-dominant parkinsonism with pleomorphic pathology. *Neuron* **44**:601–607.

Chapter 12
Amyotrophic lateral sclerosis

Nicholas J. Maragakis

The challenges of translational medicine

Heterogeneity of sporadic amyotrophic lateral sclerosis

Amyotrophic lateral sclerosis (ALS) is the most common form of adult motor neuron disease. It is an uncommon but not particularly rare disease with an incidence of 1/100,000 to 3/100,000 individuals (Yoshida et al. 1986) and a male:female ratio of 1.4:2.5 (Mitsumoto et al. 1998). The prognosis of patients with ALS remains poor, with the mean duration of disease from onset to death approximately 2–5 years. Most patients with ALS die from complications of respiratory failure as a result of diaphragmatic paralysis. Factors suggested as predictors of survival include age at onset, gender, clinical presentation (bulbar vs. spinal), and rate of disease progression. Age at onset appears to be a powerful predictor of disease duration, with younger patients surviving longer. Patients with bulbar onset ALS progress to death more quickly (Eisen et al. 1993a; Haverkamp et al. 1995). In another subset of patients with ALS, a significant percentage (19–39%) survive 5 years and a smaller percentage (8–22%) survive 10 years without ventilator use for respiratory failure.

The majority (over 90%) of patients have "sporadic" ALS, that is, ALS without a defined family history of disease. Although it is thought of historically as a neuromuscular disease, current theories based on pathophysiology and natural history suggest that ALS is a neurodegenerative disease. This designation is more appropriate and places ALS in the category of other neurodegenerative diseases including Parkinson's disease, Alzheimer's disease, and Huntington's disease. Whereas each of these disorders has a unique clinical presentation and pathological characteristics, one sees significant overlap in pathophysiological and clinical features.

Although the majority of cases are sporadic, 5–10% are familial ALS, with 20% of those familial cases linked to autosomal dominant mutations in the Cu/Zn superoxide dismutase 1 (SOD1) gene (Mitsumoto et al. 1998). Transgenic mice (Bruijn et al. 1998; Gurney 1994; Wong et al. 1995) and rats (Howland et al. 2002) carrying mutant human SOD1 genes recapitulate many, although not all, features of the human disease and have been used in an attempt to translate medical therapeutics to the human ALS population.

The diagnosis of ALS is sometimes delayed because of the heterogeneous presentation of the disease with either prominent dysfunction or death of spinal cord motor neurons (lower motor neuron signs and symptoms) or, conversely, primarily death or dysfunction of motor neurons in the primary motor cortex (upper motor neuron signs and symptoms). Indeed, in two motor neuron disease variants, clinical features are limited largely to either lower motor neurons (progressive muscular atrophy) or upper motor neurons (primary lateral sclerosis). Many consider these motor neuron diseases to be distinct clinical entities. In general, patients with these diseases have a better prognosis than patients diagnosed with ALS. However, the purely upper motor neuron or lower motor neuron disorders often progress to more typical ALS over time and thus may also be considered to be at either end of the ALS spectrum of disease.

ALS is also often categorized anatomically as either spinal or bulbar onset. The spinal form of the disease may present with lower motor neuron symptoms including weakness and muscle atrophy. These symptoms may have an insidious onset and are

---

Translational Neuroscience, ed. James E. Barrett, Joseph T. Coyle and Michael Williams. Published by Cambridge University Press. © Cambridge University Press 2012.

progressive over time. The spinal form may affect one limb asymmetrically with subsequent spread to adjacent limbs and eventually affect muscles of respiration. Upper motor neuron signs and symptoms in the spinal form include hyperreflexia, extensor plantar responses, and limb spasticity. Bulbar ALS initially and prominently affects muscles of speech (tongue and facial weakness), swallowing (tongue and pharyngeal muscles), and respiration (diaphragm). Dyspnea can be an early symptom with shortness of breath after exertion or when lying supine.

Historically, ALS patients were told that cognition was largely spared in the disease. However, emerging data suggest that the coexistence of dementia is higher than previously thought. A particular association has been made between ALS and frontotemporal lobar dementia (Lomen-Hoerth *et al.* 2002, 2003).

These findings highlight the heterogeneity of ALS and reinforce its classification as a neurodegenerative disease rather than only a neuromuscular disease and suggest that perhaps a single therapeutic agent for all types of ALS is unlikely. However, an increased understanding of the heterogeneity of this disease may translate into more specific targets for therapeutic interventions.

Mouse models: shortcomings

It now appears that SOD1 mutations account for about 15–20% of all familial cases of ALS. Several SOD1 mutations have been used to generate transgenic mutant (Tg m) SOD1 mouse models; G93A, G37R, and G85R all produce reliable motor neuron degeneration in transgenic mice overexpressing the mutant protein (Bruijn *et al.* 1998; Gurney 1994; Wong *et al.* 1995). Today, these are the most reliable and accurate animal models of the disease; they recapitulate the relative selective loss of motor neurons. Nevertheless, they are not perfect. As with the human disease, motor neurons are largely but not entirely selectively affected in the model; small interneurons degenerate in the mouse models – a feature also observed in humans. The mouse has been used extensively to determine the exact pathogenic cascade by which the presence of mutant SOD1 leads to cell death. Therefore, no single insult can explain all cases of ALS because only about 1% of all ALS patients carry SOD1 mutations. Instead, multiple mechanisms and cellular pathways are likely to be responsible for motor neuron degeneration in ALS.

Indeed, several pharmacological compounds that have had effects in Tg mSOD1 mice studies have not been efficacious in human ALS trials (Benatar 2007). Several factors could account for this finding, including the well-known appreciation that the Tg mSOD1 mice carry a familial form of the disease and may not recapitulate either the etiology or course of sporadic ALS. However, other factors may also be in play.

For example, one therapeutic attempt to lessen glutamate excitotoxicity involved administration of the compound nordihydroguaiaretic acid. This compound increased glutamate transport in wild-type mice, but on examination of tissues from Tg mSOD1 mice, P-glycoprotein (also known as multidrug resistance 1) increased as the disease progressed, resulting in an absence of concomitant increases in glutamate transport in Tg mSOD1 mice (Boston-Howes *et al.* 2008). This protein is known as a drug-efflux transporter that is particularly abundant in neuroinflammatory disorders. Although drug-efflux transporters have not been thoroughly studied either in human ALS neural tissues or in animal models of the disease such as the Tg mSOD1 mouse, poor drug responses in other disorders have been studied more extensively (Loscher and Potschka 2005). Therefore, it is possible that, although effective translational therapeutic agents for ALS have already been tested, the negative results for therapeutic efficacy may not be due to lack of efficacy or appropriate target but rather to the inadequate delivery of the drug to the target tissues because of efflux transporters.

In summary, the transgenic mutant SOD1 mouse model represents only a small proportion of the biological processes responsible for ALS but does recapitulate many factors of human ALS including, at the most basic level, a motor neuron disease with progressive limb paresis, respiratory failure, and a reduced lifespan. Although at this time it is the most reliable model of a motor neuron disease available to the research community, the development of other animal models of ALS will allow comparison of therapeutic compounds across more than one model and possibly result in more accurate predictions of clinical efficacy.

Absence of biomarkers for diagnosis or determining therapeutic efficacy

One of the hurdles in ALS is making an early diagnosis that could make neuroprotective strategies more efficacious. ALS remains largely a clinical diagnosis based on the presence of upper and lower motor neuron signs that can be observed on physical examination and bolstered by electrophysiological study. Because many of these findings are subjective and dependent on the clinical acumen of the examiner, objective markers for early diagnosis are being sought so that one can initiate potential treatments early in the disease. Biomarkers obtained from tissue or fluids may allow us to fill in that gap in time to diagnosis. Another potentially useful role for biomarkers is to establish early in the course of disease whether progression will be slow or more rapid. Separation of ALS subtypes is also important because, as a general rule, patients with spinal onset ALS have a better prognosis than those with bulbar ALS. An earlier assessment of ALS subtypes could allow ALS clinicians to appropriately and in a timely fashion anticipate the needs of their patients. For example, those with bulbar ALS presenting with dysphagia are more likely to require a feeding tube or noninvasive positive pressure ventilation earlier in the course of ALS than a patient who has limb weakness and is categorized as having spinal onset ALS. Biomarkers could also be used to monitor response to drug therapy. Oncologists routinely rely on tumor size to gauge the efficacy of a particular chemotherapeutic agent. Yet, although pharmacokinetic monitoring of a specific drug target has been undertaken in ALS, no universal marker for drug efficacy has been established for the disease. Finally, differentiating between ALS and other neurodegenerative disorders is also a consideration, particularly if dementia is a prominent part of the clinical presentation.

Biomarkers can be measured in the blood; several reports identify either increases or decreases in particular compounds in the blood of ALS patients. The cerebrospinal fluid (CSF) also would appear to have the potential for biomarker assessment. One shortcoming of CSF assessment is that a lumbar puncture is required, making it more time consuming and in theory a greater risk than blood analysis (Turner *et al.* 2009). Biomarkers do not have to be biological samples. The use of more sophisticated magnetic resonance imaging (MRI) techniques including diffusion tensor imaging, magnetic resonance spectroscopy, functional MRI, and other methods may fulfill many of the biomarker criteria outlined previously.

Other electrophysiological measures such as motor unit number estimate and electrical impedance myography can also be used to monitor a variety of ALS-relevant assessments. The specific biomarkers studied in ALS are beyond the scope of this chapter but have been reviewed by Turner and colleagues (2009).

Advances in identifying relevant therapeutic targets
Genetic advances

As noted in the opening paragraphs, sporadic ALS probably accounts for 90% of all cases of ALS. However, the other 10% that inherit the disease are an important subset of ALS patients. Identification of the genes that encode for these familial forms of ALS can offer powerful clues into the broad mechanisms of cell death in sporadic disease. Identification of these genes also offers the opportunity to generate new animal models of ALS either through transgenic models that overexpress the mutant forms or as knockout mouse models that can relay an increased understanding of loss of function in the disease. Finally, understanding the part these newly identified genes play in specific pathways can translate into new therapeutic compounds targeting these gene products. A brief overview of some of the more important genes identified in familial ALS follows.

Superoxide dismutase 1 (ALS1)

Superoxide dismutase 1 is a highly abundant free radical scavenging enzyme that forms a major component of the intracellular defense mechanisms used by most cells to guard against free radical species produced during cellular metabolism. Mutations in SOD1 were identified in 1993 as associated with the autosomal dominant form of ALS (Rosen *et al.* 1993). Despite the identification of this mutation over 15 years ago, the exact mechanism by which mutant SOD1 causes disease is yet to be determined. Nevertheless, given that this is the most common gene mutation in human ALS and because animal models of this mutation are the most widely used, this gene mutation may be the most likely to provide clues to ALS pathogenesis and treatment in the near future.

Alsin (ALS2)

The *ALS2* gene is expressed ubiquitously and encodes the protein alsin, a guanine nucleotide exchange factor known to activate small guanosine triphosphatase belonging to the Ras superfamily. Deletion mutations in this gene have been associated with ALS2 – a juvenile onset form of ALS primarily associated with upper motor neuron findings and inherited in an autosomal recessive pattern (Hadano *et al.* 2001; Yang *et al.* 2001). The mechanism behind the ability of alsin to cause disease has not yet been identified.

Senataxin (ALS4)

Mutations in the senataxin gene are responsible for a juvenile form of ALS inherited in an autosomal dominant form. It is characterized by distal muscle weakness and atrophy, normal sensation, and pyramidal signs. Individuals affected with ALS4 usually have an onset of symptoms before the age of 25, a slow rate of progression, and a normal lifespan. Missense mutations in senataxin (a DNA/RNA helicase) were found in this gene, implicating a potential part for dysfunction in DNA helicase activity or RNA processing in the development of this disorder (Chen *et al.* 2004).

FUS/TLS (ALS6)

An additional approximately 4% of familial ALS cases were also recently attributed to the *FUS* (fused in sarcoma) gene, also known as the *TLS* (translocation in liposarcoma) gene, identified in a family with an autosomal dominant missense mutation (Vance *et al.* 2009) and a family who inherited the gene in an autosomal recessive pattern (Kwiatkowski *et al.* 2009). Cytoplasmic inclusions have been found in the cytoplasm of neurons in those families. These inclusions are not seen in patients with ALS with SOD1 mutations or in those with sporadic ALS. Like TDP-43, early evidence suggests that the *FUS/TLS* gene may play a role in RNA processing.

VAPB (ALS8)

Missense mutations in the vesicle-associated protein (*VAPB*) gene have been associated with an autosomal dominant form of ALS (Nishimura *et al.* 2004). These mutations are associated with a motor neuron disease that has features of an atypical slowly progressing case of ALS with features of an essential tremor, typical ALS, or late-onset spinal muscular atrophy. The *VAPB* gene appears to act during endoplasmic reticulum (ER)-Golgi transport, and it has been proposed that the mutant VAP protein accumulates in the ER and becomes ubiquitinated and that normal proteins become trapped in the inclusions. These protein inclusions result in reduced cell viability and in a decrease in the secretion of a protein domain (MSP – a ligand for the ephrin receptor). Therefore, toxicity may be related to a combination of reduced paracrine signaling and protein accumulation within the cell (Tsuda *et al.* 2008).

Angiogenin (ALS9)

Angiogenin induces new blood vessel formation. Angiogenin is induced by hypoxia to elicit angiogenesis and, although it is expressed in motor neurons, its role in these cells has not been definitively established. Missense mutations in the angiogenin gene were identified in Scottish and Irish populations, suggesting that angiogenin may be a susceptibility gene for the development of ALS (Greenway *et al.* 2006).

TDP-43 (ALS10)

Identification of the TARDNA-binding protein (TDP-43) in ubiquitinated protein aggregates found in many patients with sporadic ALS (but not in those with familial SOD1-mediated ALS), or with the most common form of frontotemporal dementia called frontotemporal lobar degeneration with ubiquitinated inclusions, has been an important recent advance in ALS not only with respect to genetic implications but also in the implication of this protein as either a byproduct or initiator of sporadic ALS (Arai *et al.* 2006; Neumann *et al.* 2006). However, dominant mutations of TDP-43 have now been found and may account for up to 3% of cases of familial ALS. Although the exact mechanisms behind why TDP-43 mutations cause motor neuron loss in ALS have yet to be elucidated, TDP-43 is believed to be involved in RNA processing. Spinal muscular atrophy, another motor neuron disorder, is associated with the SMN (survival of motor neuron) protein also associated with RNA processing. This association may offer a therapeutic target because the *SMN* gene has already been the target of translational therapeutics. Whether these RNA processing pathways are relevant and can be manipulated in ALS remains to be determined.

Cell-specific targets for drug intervention and discovery

Because motor neuron loss accounts for the progressive muscle weakness and atrophy observed in the disease, attention has been focused on cellular pathways inherent in motor neuron biology. Over the last two decades, however, emerging data suggest that motor neuron death in ALS is non-cell autonomous. Whereas motor neuron death is still the end point of disease, other nonneuronal cell types like microglia and astrocytes appear to be key drivers of disease progression. Studies with chimeric mice showed that increasing the proportion of healthy, wild-type non-neuronal cells in proximity to mutant human SOD1-expressing motor neurons reduces the mortality of those motor neurons and extends survival in these animals (Clement *et al.* 2003). More recently, researchers found that a reduction in mutant human SOD1 selectively from microglia or astrocytes using a CRE-lox system in mice prolongs disease progression but has no effect on disease onset (Boillee *et al.* 2006; Yamanaka *et al.* 2008).

The role of other cell types in disease manifestations may not be limited to neural cells alone. In a set of studies, Beers and colleagues sought to identify the potential role of $CD4^+$ T cells in motor neuron injury by performing bone marrow transplants on mutant Tg mSOD1 mice crossed with several mouse lines deficient in their capacity for immune modulation. The results established that the lack of T-cell recruitment accelerated disease progression and death. However, the reconstitution of the T-cell population through bone marrow transplantation resulted in neuroprotection in the Tg mSOD1 models, possibly through elaboration of trophic factors and reduction of cytotoxic factors (Beers *et al.* 2008). Other cell types implicated in the development or progression of ALS (at least in animal models) include endothelial cells (Zhong *et al.* 2008) and Schwann cells (Lobsiger *et al.* 2009). The identification of these cell types as potential contributors to disease offers not only a new set of potential pathways but also a new set of cellular targets for translational medicine.

Role of translational medicine

To date, riluzole is the only drug that has demonstrated efficacy in patients with ALS. This efficacy was established in two clinical trials. In the first trial, a robust effect on survival was seen in patients with bulbar-onset disease. In the riluzole-treated group, 74% of patients were alive at 12 months compared with 58% in the placebo-treated group (Bensimon *et al.* 1994). In a second and larger human clinical trial, in which ALS patients were treated for 18 months, the survival rates were 50.4% for placebo and 56.8% for riluzole (100 mg/day). Adjustment for baseline prognostic factors showed a 35% decreased risk of death with the 100-mg dose compared with placebo (Lacomblez *et al.* 1996). Because of these findings, riluzole is considered standard of care in the pharmacological treatment of ALS.

This single success has, however, been overshadowed by numerous failures of traditional therapeutic agents used for ALS. Targeted pathways have included apoptotic cascades (sodium phenylbutyrate); growth factor regulation/dysregulation (insulin-like growth factor-1) (Borasio *et al.* 1998; Lai *et al.* 1997); glial cell-derived neurotrophic factor (GDNF), brain-derived neurotrophic factor (BDNF), and ciliary neurotrophic factor (CNTF) (BDNF Study Group 1999; Miller *et al.* 1996a); mitochondrial dysfunction (creatine); neuroinflammation (minocycline, thalidomide, celecoxib); and immunomodulatory therapies (total lymphoid irradiation; Drachman *et al.* 1994), cyclophosphamide (Smith *et al.* 1994), and cyclosporine (Appel *et al.* 1988). The relative efficacy of riluzole also spawned the study of other antiglutamatergic agents including topiramate, lamotrigine (Eisen *et al.* 1993b), dextromethorphan (Gredal *et al.* 1997), and gabapentin (Miller *et al.* 2001), none of which has proven beneficial in human clinical trials. Table 12.1 summarizes past key therapeutic clinical trials.

The reason these compounds have not achieved efficacy is probably multifactorial. As noted in the opening section, the heterogeneity of ALS may preclude a single efficacious treatment for all types of ALS. The unique challenges in ALS clinical trial design have a learning curve; identification of the potential mechanisms and the means for overcoming these challenges are discussed in the section "Clinical trial design."

Potential opportunities for translational medicine
Clinical trial design

One of the most challenging aspects in translating candidate therapeutic agents for ALS to clinical use is the appropriate clinical trial design. Many factors, such as adequately powered statistical analysis of the number of patients required to see an effect, selection of the appropriate dosage and route of delivery, and a pharmacodynamic marker for assessing whether the

Chapter 12: Amyotrophic lateral sclerosis

Table 12.1. Summary of past key therapeutic clinical trials for amyotrophic lateral sclerosis.

Drug	Mechanism of action/indication
Riluzole (Bensimon et al. 1994; Lacomblez et al. 1996)	Modulates glutamate excitotoxicity through inhibition of glutamate release, blockade of amino acid receptors, and inhibition of voltage-dependent sodium channels on dendrites and cell bodies
Topiramate (Cudkowicz et al. 2003)	Inhibits glutamate release from neurons, AMPA glutamate receptor antagonist
Lamotrigine (Eisen et al. 1993b)	Inhibits glutamate release from neurons
Dextromethorphan (Gredal et al. 1997)	Acts as NMDA-glutamate receptor antagonist
Gabapentin (Miller et al. 2001)	Exhibits antiexcitotoxic activity through a number of mechanisms
Celecoxib (Cudkowicz et al. 2006)	Inhibits cyclooxygenase-2, which may result in reduced glutamate release and reduced free radical formation
Minocycline	Antibiotic that inhibits microglial activation
Insulin-like growth factor 1 (IGF-1) (Borasio et al. 1998; Lai et al. 1997; Sorenson et al. 2008)	Trophic factor
Ciliary neurotrophic factor (CNTF) (Miller et al. 1996a)	Trophic factor
Brain-derived neurotrophic factor (BDNF) (BDNF Study Group 1999)	Trophic factor
Xaliproden (Meininger et al. 2004)	Neurotrophism
Omigapil (TCH 346) (Miller et al. 2007)	Antiapoptotic – prevents degeneration of neurons from programmed cell death
CoEnzyme Q_{10} (Ferrante et al. 2005)	Energy metabolism, antioxidant
Creatine monohydrate (Groeneveld et al. 2003; Shefner et al. 2004)	Modulates mitochondrial dysfunction, swelling, apoptotic cascades, and energy metabolism
Sodium phenylbutyrate (Cudkowicz et al. 2009)	Regulates DNA transcription and is effective in models of neurodegeneration
Verapamil (Miller et al. 1996c)	Calcium channel blocker
Nimodipine (Miller et al. 1996b)	Calcium channel blocker
Pentoxifylline (Meininger et al. 2006)	Inflammatory mediator, antiapoptotic
Vitamin E (Desnuelle 2001)	Antioxidant
Glutathione (Chio et al. 1998)	Antioxidant
N-acetyl-L-cysteine (Louwerse et al. 1995)	Antioxidant
Total lymphoid irradiation (Drachman et al. 1994)	Immune modulation
Cyclophosphamide (Smith et al. 1994)	Immune modulation
Cyclosporine (Appel et al. 1988)	Immune modulation

therapeutic agent is having some effect on its drug target, by necessity need to be addressed before initiation of a clinical trial. Many of the past "failures" in developing drugs to treat ALS may have been due to trials whose designs failed to address one or more of these factors. Part of this process has been an evolution in understanding ALS-specific challenges. One scenario demonstrating this learning process was an

ALS study using the drug celecoxib. This drug inhibits cyclooxygenase 2. The rationale for studying the compound celecoxib in ALS was partially based on the observation that a small sample of ALS patients had elevated levels of prostaglandin E2 in their CSF (Almer *et al.* 2002; Ilzecka 2003). Therefore, it was hypothesized that reducing the levels of prostaglandins would have a beneficial effect. However, during the study, repeat CSF analyses did not show similar elevations (Cudkowicz *et al.* 2006) in subjects participating in the trial; thus, the pharmacological target reductions were not realized.

As outlined by Aggarwal and Cudkowicz (2008), one of the greatest challenges, even after a target therapeutic has been identified, is designing an appropriate trial. Given the fact that patients with ALS have a poor prognosis, one might assume that enrollment in clinical trials would be high. This is, however, not the case. Only 8% of patients with ALS are enrolled in clinical trials. Possible reasons for the low enrollment rates include overly rigorous inclusion criteria based on the El Escorial criteria of the World Federation of Neurology (the criteria used for ALS diagnosis), stringent requirements for excellent respiratory function, frequent off-label uses of medications that make people trial-ineligible, and lack of information among community physicians, participants, their families, and possibly investigators. Study retention and the use of off-label study medications confound recruitment and the interpretation of any findings.

In a phase III clinical trial in which a measure of efficacy is sought, one of the current challenges is how to define a primary end point. Whereas a statistically significant improvement in survival rates would be considered a "home run," the use of survival rates requires long trial periods. Other measures have been used, including the ALS functional rating scale (ALSFRS) and measurement of pulmonary forced vital capacity (FVC). Recent analyses have supported their use as primary outcome measures. Another consideration that needs to be explained clearly to ALS patients is the need for placebo groups. Patients often say "If there is no cure for the disease, why doesn't everyone receive the experimental drug?" Critical to the doctor/patient relationship is an explanation of the power of the placebo effect. It is also an appropriate time to discuss safety issues and provides an opportunity to explain that some drugs may in fact speed the course of the disease. This situation occurred with a clinical trial of minocycline in which the functional measures of ALS patients who took minocycline declined more rapidly than those of people who took the placebo (Aggarwal and Cudkowicz 2008).

Traditional drug targets and deliveries

"Traditional" drug targets and deliveries refer primarily to well-identified methods for administering therapeutic agents including oral, intravenous, and subcutaneous routes and represent the bulk of translational medicine for ALS in the last two decades. This section focuses on those methods whereas the sections "Gene therapy," "Stem-cell therapies for transplantation and drug discovery," and "RNAi and antisense oligonucleotides" focus on emerging technologies. Although these emerging technologies may garner attention from the lay press, it is equally, if not more likely, that efficacious therapies for ALS lie in traditional therapeutic agents targeting ALS-relevant pathways.

Although the cause of the relatively selective death of motor neurons in ALS has remained elusive, several mechanisms that probably contribute to disease pathogenesis have been proposed. These include oxidative damage, glutamate excitotoxicity, mitochondrial dysfunction, cytoskeletal abnormalities, impaired neurotrophic support, mutant SOD1 and neurofilament protein aggregation, axonal transport defects, activation of apoptotic pathways, altered microglial function and, more recently, impairment of the blood–brain/spinal cord barrier (Bruijn *et al.* 2004; Zhong *et al.* 2008).

Therapeutic agents for each of these pathways have been studied in preclinical ALS models like the Tg mSOD1 mouse resulting in the translation of several study compounds to human ALS clinical trials.

The overall summary of the efforts using traditional therapeutic agents for a variety of targets is disappointing. However, it is worth noting that the failure of therapeutic agents targeting the pathways noted in Table 12.1 does not mean that these compounds are either not efficacious or that the pathways are not relevant. More likely, in retrospect, issues related to challenges of ALS clinical trial design may underlie the lack of efficacy. Furthermore, identification of other genetic forms of the disease will reveal new pathways, and novel therapeutics will undergo preclinical study. Current clinical trials in ALS and their targets are detailed in Table 12.2.

Chapter 12: Amyotrophic lateral sclerosis

Table 12.2. Current clinical trials for amyotrophic lateral sclerosis and their targets.

Drug	Mechanism of action/indication
Ceftriaxone	Antibiotic, promotes glutamate transporter protein synthesis and modulates glutamate excitotoxicity
ONO-2506	Glutamate antagonist, reduces astrocytosis
CoQ$_{10}$	Energy metabolism, antioxidant
Memantine	NMDA (glutamate receptor) antagonist
Talampanel	AMPA (glutamate receptor) antagonist
(R)-pramipexole	Antioxidant
Pioglitazone (Schutz et al. 2005)	Anti-inflammatory [peroxisome proliferator-activated receptor gamma (PPAR-γ) agonist]
Tauroursodeoxycholic acid	Inhibits apoptosis and is an antioxidant

AMPA, α-amino-3-hydroxyl-5-methyl-4-isoxazole-propionate; NMDA, N-methyl-D-aspartic acid.

What is the state of current ALS clinical trial thinking? Given the failure of a number of compounds targeting a variety of molecular mechanisms to have any real efficacy in the disease thus far, the focus is primarily on *slowing* disease progression through neuroprotection. Targeting the processes involved in motor neuron *regeneration* and *functional improvement* in ALS, although the subject of numerous preclinical efforts, has not translated into any formal phase III human clinical trials.

Gene therapies

Identification of potential pathways contributing to ALS-related biological processes also lends itself to creative approaches in translating these processes to human ALS clinical trials. Perhaps the best examples are related to the use of gene therapy to deliver growth factors of interest to ALS tissues.

Vascular endothelial cell growth factor (VEGF) is a critical factor that controls the growth and permeability of blood vessels. Studies in a transgenic mouse model in which the VEGF gene had the specific hypoxia-response element deleted indicated that, whereas mice maintained normal baseline levels of VEGF expression, they exhibited a severe reduction in the ability to induce VEGF during bouts of hypoxia. This finding resulted in a mouse model with motor deficits and many of the hallmark pathological features of ALS. In addition, when a VEGF mutant mouse was crossed with a Tg mSOD1 mouse, the course of the disease was accelerated, thus suggesting a potential neuroprotective role for VEGF. VEGF was found potentially to be a modifier of ALS: patients who were homozygous for some VEGF haplotypes showed an increased risk of developing the disease (Lambrechts et al. 2003), although these findings do not appear to be consistent among all groups (Van Vught et al. 2005). VEGF levels were also found to be decreased in the CSF of ALS patients (Devos et al. 2004), and lack of VEGF upregulation in hypoxemic ALS patients suggests VEGF dysregulation (Moreau et al. 2006). In light of VEGF as an ALS-relevant factor, preclinical gene therapies were designed to deliver VEGF to ALS animal models. Azzouz and colleagues demonstrated that a single injection of a VEGF-expressing lentiviral vector into multiple muscles delayed onset and slowed progression in Tg mSOD1 mice. Perhaps more impressive was the fact that the effect was seen even after injection at the onset of paralysis rather than at a presymptomatic stage (Azzouz et al. 2004).

The delivery of other factors by intramuscular, intraspinal, or ex vivo cellular gene therapy approaches included gene transfer of neurotrophin-3 (NT-3) in the mouse mutant progressive motor neuronopathy model (Haase et al. 1997), and CNTF (Aebischer et al. 1996), insulin-like growth factor-1 (Kaspar et al. 2003; Lepore et al. 2007), GDNF (Acsadi et al. 2002; Wang et al. 2002), and Bcl-2 in Tg mSOD1 models (Azzouz et al. 2000; Bordet et al. 2001). A human clinical trial of SB-509 (clinicaltrials.gov identifier: NCT00748501; www.clinicaltrials.gov), a gene encoding a zinc finger DNA-binding protein transcription factor that can induce VEGF

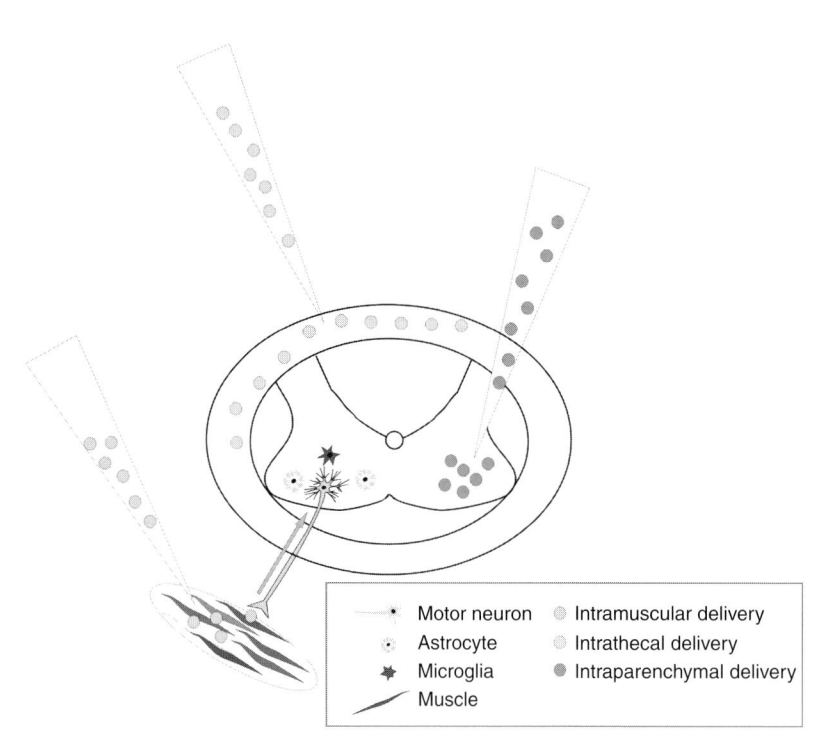

Figure 12.1. Gene therapy applications. Previous studies in animal models and humans with ALS included intraparenchymal spinal cord delivery of viral vectors with genes encoding for growth factors and antiapoptotics (orange circles). Intramuscular injection of viral vectors or transcription factors activating endogenous growth factors (blue circles) result in retrograde transport to the host motor neurons and spinal cord (blue arrow). Ex vivo polymer capsules containing hamster kidney cells expressing CNTF were injected into the CSF space (yellow circles). This figure is reproduced in color in the color plate section.

transcription, is currently underway in patients with ALS. Previous animal and human studies of ALS demonstrating potential gene therapy approaches to the spinal cord are shown in Fig. 12.1.

Stem-cell therapies for transplantation and drug discovery

The observation that multiple nonneuronal cell subtypes contribute to varying aspects of the ALS (at least in Tg mSOD1 animal models) has opened the door for translating these observations into therapies designed to replace cells using cell-transplantation biology. To date, stem-cell replacement strategies for ALS are not ready for "prime time," needing to overcome numerous regulatory hurdles including, first and foremost, rigorous safety testing. One of the greatest concerns with cell transplantation is uncontrolled cell growth or migration to other regions and subsequent tumor formation. Optimal cell dose, source, route of delivery, and an ideal immunosuppressive regimen must be carefully considered.

Several ALS rodent studies using stem-cell transplantation strategies have highlighted the potential for replacing cell types involved in the disease. Given that astrocytes may play a role in ALS disease progression, Lepore and colleagues transplanted rodent glial restricted precursor (GRP) cells derived from developing embryonic spinal cord into the spinal cords of Tg mSOD1 rats. Multiple, targeted injections were aimed at specific motor neuron pools of the cervical spinal cord involved in respiratory function – because respiratory failure is the main cause of death in patients with ALS (Lepore et al. 2008). Transplantation of GRPs led to extensive differentiation of transplanted cells into mature astrocytes that prevented host motor neuron loss and reduced microgliosis. Transplanted GRPs extended survival and disease duration and slowed declines in forelimb motor and respiratory physiological functions. These effects may be related to the ability of these transplanted cells to maintain normal levels of the glutamate transporter protein GLT-1. These results demonstrate that stem-cell transplantation-based astrocyte replacement is a potentially viable option for ALS therapy.

Microglial replacement from hematopoietic stem cells (HSC) via bone marrow transplantation has been used in a clinical trial of patients with ALS. Although no significant clinical benefit was found following treatment with HSC, transplanted HSCs infiltrated areas of motor neuron injury and neuroinflammation

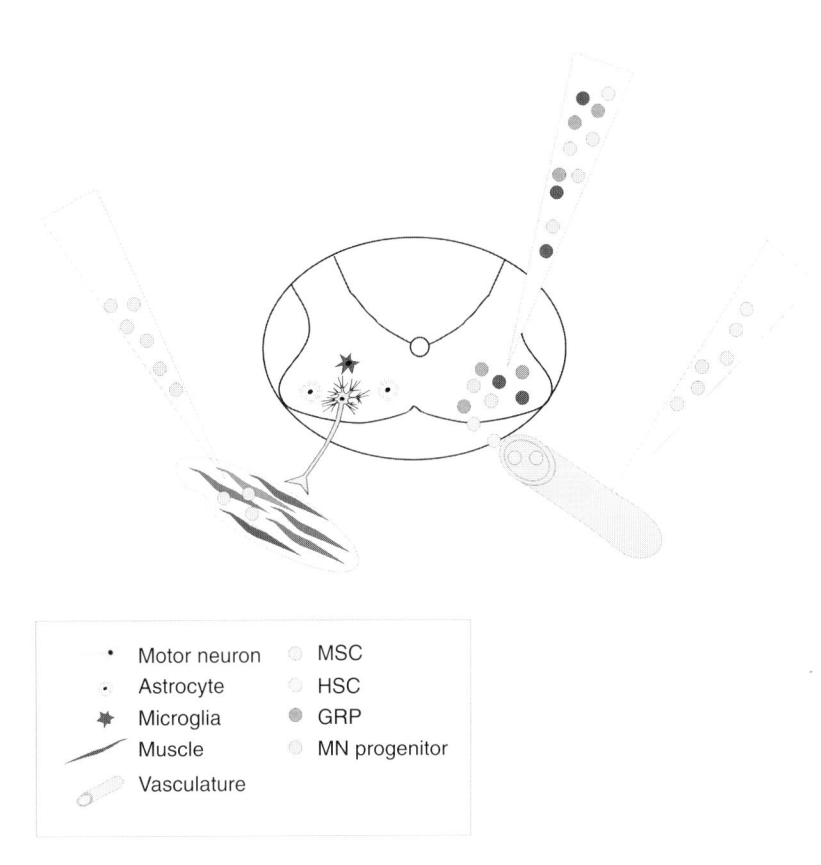

Figure 12.2. Cell transplantation approaches. Potential strategies for cell replacement include direct intraparenchymal delivery of motor neuron, astrocyte, or microglial progenitor cells (red, orange, green circles). Intraparenchymal or muscle delivery of mesenchymal stem cells could provide trophic support to host motor neurons (blue circles). Hematopoietic stem-cell delivery via bone marrow transplantation and delivery of cells into the vasculature offer benefits of lower surgical risk and widespread distribution (yellow circles). MSC, mesenchymal stem cells; HSC, hematopoietic stem cells; GRP, glial restricted precursors; MN, motor neuron progenitors. This figure is reproduced in color in the color plate section.

and engrafted as immunomodulatory cells (Appel et al. 2008). This approach is appealing in that the delivery of HSCs through bone marrow transplantation has been performed innumerable times for the treatment of other disorders and therefore has a well-identified safety profile. Whether such a strategy will be efficacious in patients with ALS is not yet known.

If motor neuron loss is a prominent feature of ALS, it would seem that motor neuron replacement would be a reasonable translational opportunity for stem-cell transplantation. However, for a neurodegenerative disorder in which motor axon outgrowth into target muscle must outpace ALS patient death from diaphragmatic paralysis and respiratory failure, the biological underpinnings for adequate regenerative capacities do not currently exist. At this time, the most appropriate translational targets for cell transplantation are probably cells that will support motor neuron function and prevent motor neuron cell death. Potential strategies and cell types for targeted cell replacement are detailed in Fig. 12.2.

Interfering RNA and antisense oligonucleotides

The ability to silence specific genes has been used in animal models to study the role of gene products in the development of a variety of disorders. Yet the use of gene silencing strategies may have therapeutic applications as well. Although the majority of cases of ALS appear to be sporadic ALS, identification of a subset of ALS patients with familial ALS-related mutations in the superoxide dismutase gene may allow for a unique approach to ALS treatment.

Previous studies have shown that therapeutic benefits can be achieved via adenovirus-, lentivirus-, herpes simplex virus-, and adeno-associated virus-based delivery of genes targeting SOD1. Investigators using a lentiviral vector to deliver interfering RNA (RNAi) to spinal motor neurons of the Tg mSOD1 mouse by injection into the muscle showed that the RNAi was transported retrogradely into the spinal cord, resulting in the downregulation of SOD1 and an impressive prolongation of motor strength and survival (Ralph *et al.* 2005). Similar results were obtained using adeno-associated virus delivery of small RNAi to muscle (Miller *et al.* 2005). The direct intraspinal injection of RNAi using a lentivirus also demonstrated an improvement in survival in Tg mSOD1 mice (Raoul *et al.* 2005).

Because these RNAi methods target a specific protein (SOD1), this selective method does not have a broad therapeutic potential for sporadic ALS, but it may serve those patients with SOD1 mutations and, as a result, provide an important understanding about the potential for reversing clinical symptoms resulting from motor neurons that carry mutations and are dysfunctional but not dead.

Antisense methods targeting SOD1 are also being used. The intraventricular administration of antisense oligonucleotides into the CSF of the Tg mSOD1 rat model slowed disease progression and reduced SOD1 protein and mRNA levels in the CNS (Smith *et al.* 2006). The demonstration that antisense oligonucleotides have biological and behavioral effects in rodent models of SOD1 has resulted in the translation of this strategy to patients with ALS. Preclinical studies are underway to evaluate the safety of antisense oligonucleotides targeting SOD1 with the intention of translating this method to a subset of familial ALS patients carrying SOD1 mutations.

Conclusions

Translational approaches to drug development may be more relevant than ever for ALS. Our increased understanding of relevant ALS pathological pathways and the identification of several new genes presenting novel targets are the first steps toward translational medicine. However, several key elements for effectively assessing these translational approaches require further development. No consistent reliable biomarker from the blood or the CSF has been identified, leaving more crude measures of drug efficacy, including functional outcomes such as the ALSFRS, pulmonary FVC, and quantitative strength measurements, as the most widely accepted methods for assessment. However, the use of viral vectors for gene delivery of a variety of different ALS-relevant compounds has recently increased, and the potential for RNAi and antisense technologies to target a specific but well-characterized (mutant SOD1) protein responsible for many cases of familial ALS may offer proof of the principle that ALS can be effectively treated if the upstream causative etiologies are identified. Finally, recent advances in stem cell research, including the development of induced pluripotent stem cells, offer the potential for autologous cell transplantation as well as drug discovery.

References

Acsadi G, Anguelov RA, Yang H *et al.* 2002. Increased survival and function of SOD1 mice after glial cell-derived neurotrophic factor gene therapy. *Hum Gene Ther* **13**:1047–1059.

Aebischer P, Schluep M, Déglon N *et al.* 1996. Intrathecal delivery of CNTF using encapsulated genetically modified xenogeneic cells in amyotrophic lateral sclerosis patients. *Nature Med* **2**:696–699.

Aggarwal S, Cudkowicz M. 2008. ALS drug development: reflections from the past and a way forward. *Neurotherapeutics* **5**:516–527.

Almer G, Teismann P, Stevic Z *et al.* 2002. Increased levels of the pro-inflammatory prostaglandin PGE2 in CSF from ALS patients. *Neurology* **58**:1277–1279.

Appel SH, Engelhardt JI, Henkel JS *et al.* 2008. Hematopoietic stem cell transplantation in patients with sporadic amyotrophic lateral sclerosis. *Neurology* **71**:1326–1334.

Appel SH, Stewart SS, Appel V *et al.* 1988. A double-blind study of the effectiveness of cyclosporine in amyotrophic lateral sclerosis. *Arch Neurol* **45**:381–386.

Arai T, Hasegawa M, Akiyama H *et al.* 2006. TDP-43 is a component of ubiquitin-positive tau-negative inclusions in frontotemporal lobar degeneration and amyotrophic lateral sclerosis. *Biochem Biophys Res Commun* **351**:602–611.

Azzouz M, Hottinger A, Paterna JC *et al.* 2000. Increased motoneuron survival and improved neuromuscular function in transgenic ALS mice after intraspinal injection of an adeno-associated virus encoding Bcl-2. *Hum Mol Genet* **9**:803–811.

Azzouz M, Ralph GS, Storkebaum E *et al.* 2004. VEGF delivery with retrogradely transported lentivector prolongs survival in a mouse ALS model. *Nature* **429**:413–417.

BDNF Study Group 1999. A controlled trial of recombinant methionyl human BDNF in ALS (Phase III). *Neurology* **52**:1427–1433.

Beers DR, Henkel JS, Zhao W, Wang J, Appel SH. 2008. CD4+ T cells support glial, slow disease progression, and modify glial morphology in an animal model of inherited ALS. *Proc Natl Acad Sci USA* **105**:15558–15563.

Benatar M. 2007. Lost in translation: treatment trials in the SOD1 mouse and in human ALS. *Neurobiol Dis* **26**:1–13.

Bensimon G, Lacomblez L, Meininger V. The ALS/Riluzole Study Group. 1994. A controlled trial of riluzole in amyotrophic lateral sclerosis. *N Engl J Med* **330**:585–591.

Boillee S, Yamanaka K, Lobsiger CS et al. 2006. Onset and progression in inherited ALS determined by motor neurons and microglia. *Science* **312**:1389–1392.

Borasio GD, Robberecht W, Leigh PN et al. 1998. A placebo-controlled trial of insulin-like growth factor-I in amyotrophic lateral sclerosis. European ALS/IGF-I Study Group. *Neurology* **51**:583–586.

Bordet T, Lesbordes JC, Rouhani S et al. 2001. Protective effects of cardiotrophin-1 adenoviral gene transfer on neuromuscular degeneration in transgenic ALS mice. *Hum Mol Genet* **10**:1925–1933.

Boston-Howes W, Williams EO, Bogush A et al. 2008. Nordihydroguaiaretic acid increases glutamate uptake in vitro and in vivo: therapeutic implications for amyotrophic lateral sclerosis. *Exp Neurol* **213**:229–237.

Bruijn LI, Houseweart MK, Kato S et al. 1998. Aggregation and motor neuron toxicity of an ALS-linked SOD1 mutant independent from wild-type SOD1. *Science* **281**:1851–1854.

Bruijn LI, Miller TM, Cleveland DW. 2004. Unraveling the mechanisms involved in motor neuron degeneration in ALS. *Annu Rev Neurosci* **27**:723–749.

Chen YZ, Bennett CL, Huynh HM et al. 2004. DNA/RNA helicase gene mutations in a form of juvenile amyotrophic lateral sclerosis (ALS4). *Am J Hum Genet* **74**:1128–1135.

Chio A, Cucatto A, Terreni AA, Schiffer D. 1998. Reduced glutathione in amyotrophic lateral sclerosis: an open, crossover, randomized trial. *Ital J Neurol Sci* **19**:363–366.

Clement AM, Nguyen MD, Roberts EA et al. 2003. Wild-type nonneuronal cells extend survival of SOD1 mutant motor neurons in ALS mice. *Science* **302**:113–117.

Cudkowicz ME, Andres PL, Macdonald SA et al. 2009. Phase 2 study of sodium phenylbutyrate in ALS. *Amyotroph Lateral Scler* **10**:99–106.

Cudkowicz ME, Shefner JM, Schoenfeld DA et al. 2003. A randomized, placebo-controlled trial of topiramate in amyotrophic lateral sclerosis. *Neurology* **61**:456–464.

Cudkowicz ME, Shefner JM, Schoenfeld DA et al. 2006. Trial of celecoxib in amyotrophic lateral sclerosis. *Ann Neurol* **60**:22–31.

Desnuelle C, Dib M, Garrel C, Favier A. 2001. A double-blind, placebo-controlled randomized clinical trial of alpha-tocopherol (vitamin E) in the treatment of amyotrophic lateral sclerosis. ALS riluzole-tocopherol Study Group. *Amyotroph Lateral Scler Other Motor Neuron Disord* **2**:9–18.

Devos D, Moreau C, Lassalle P et al. 2004. Low levels of the vascular endothelial growth factor in CSF from early ALS patients. *Neurology* **62**:2127–2129.

Drachman DB, Chaudhry V, Cornblath D et al. 1994. Trial of immunosuppression in amyotrophic lateral sclerosis using total lymphoid irradiation. *Ann Neurol* **35**:142–150.

Eisen A, Schulzer M, MacNeil M, Pant B, Mak E. 1993a. Duration of amyotrophic lateral sclerosis is age dependent. *Muscle Nerve* **16**:27–32.

Eisen A, Stewart H, Schulzer M, Cameron D. 1993b. Anti-glutamate therapy in amyotrophic lateral sclerosis: a trial using lamotrigine. *Can J Neurol Sci* **20**:297–301.

Ferrante KL, Shefner J, Zhang H et al. 2005. Tolerance of high-dose (3,000 mg/day) coenzyme Q10 in ALS. *Neurology* **65**:1834–1836.

Gredal O, Werdelin L, Bak S et al. 1997. A clinical trial of dextromethorphan in amyotrophic lateral sclerosis. *Acta Neurol Scand* **96**:8–13.

Greenway MJ, Andersen PM, Russ C et al. 2006. ANG mutations segregate with familial and 'sporadic' amyotrophic lateral sclerosis. *Nat Genet* **38**:411–413.

Groeneveld GJ, Veldink JH, van der Tweel I et al. 2003. A randomized sequential trial of creatine in amyotrophic lateral sclerosis. *Ann Neurol* **53**:437–445.

Gurney ME. 1994. Mutant mice, Cu, Zn superoxide dismutase, and motor neuron degeneration. *Science* **266**:1587.

Haase G, Kennel P, Pettmann B et al. 1997. Gene therapy of murine motor neuron disease using adenoviral vectors for neurotrophic factors. *Nature Med* **3**:429–436.

Hadano S, Hand CK, Osuga H et al. 2001. A gene encoding a putative GTPase regulator is mutated in familial amyotrophic lateral sclerosis 2. *Nat Genet* **29**:166–173.

Haverkamp LJ, Appel V, Appel SH. 1995. Natural history of amyotrophic lateral sclerosis in a database population. Validation of a scoring system and a model for survival prediction. *Brain* **118**:707–719.

Howland DS, Liu J, She Y et al. 2002. Focal loss of the glutamate transporter EAAT2 in a transgenic rat model of SOD1 mutant-mediated amyotrophic lateral sclerosis (ALS). *Proc Natl Acad Sci USA* **99**:1604–1609.

Ilzecka J. 2003. Prostaglandin E2 is increased in amyotrophic lateral sclerosis patients. *Acta Neurol Scand* **108**:125–129.

Kaspar BK, Llado J, Sherkat N, Rothstein JD, Gage FH. 2003. Retrograde viral delivery of IGF-1 prolongs survival in a mouse ALS model. *Science* **301**:839–842.

Kwiatkowski TJ Jr, Bosco DA, Leclerc AL et al. 2009. Mutations in the

FUS/TLS gene on chromosome 16 cause familial amyotrophic lateral sclerosis. *Science* **323**:1205–1208.

Lacomblez L, Bensimon G, Leigh PN et al. 1996. A confirmatory dose-ranging study of riluzole in ALS. ALS/Riluzole Study Group-II. *Neurology* **47**:S242–S250.

Lai EC, Felice KJ, Festoff BW et al. 1997. Effect of recombinant human insulin-like growth factor-I on progression of ALS. A placebo-controlled study. The North America ALS/IGF-I Study Group. *Neurology* **49**:1621–1630.

Lambrechts D, Storkebaum E, Morimoto M et al. 2003. VEGF is a modifier of amyotrophic lateral sclerosis in mice and humans and protects motoneurons against ischemic death. *Nat Genet* **34**:383–394.

Lepore AC, Haenggeli C, Gasmi M et al. 2007. Intraparenchymal spinal cord delivery of adeno-associated virus IGF-1 is protective in the SOD1G93A model of ALS. *Brain Res* **1185**:256–265.

Lepore AC, Rauck B, Dejea C et al. 2008. Focal transplantation-based astrocyte replacement is neuroprotective in a model of motor neuron disease. *Nat Neurosci* **11**:1294–1301.

Lobsiger CS, Boillee S, McAlonis-Downes M et al. 2009. Schwann cells expressing dismutase active mutant SOD1 unexpectedly slow disease progression in ALS mice. *Proc Natl Acad Sci USA* **106**:4465–4470.

Lomen-Hoerth C, Anderson T, Miller B. 2002. The overlap of amyotrophic lateral sclerosis and frontotemporal dementia. *Neurology* **59**:1077–1079.

Lomen-Hoerth C, Murphy J, Langmore S et al. 2003. Are amyotrophic lateral sclerosis patients cognitively normal? *Neurology* **60**:1094–1097.

Loscher W, Potschka H. 2005. Drug resistance in brain diseases and the role of drug efflux transporters. *Nat Rev Neurosci* **6**:591–602.

Louwerse ES, Weverling GJ, Bossuyt PM, Meyjes FE, de Jong JM. 1995. Randomized, double-blind, controlled trial of acetylcysteine in amyotrophic lateral sclerosis. *Arch Neurol* **52**:559–564.

Meininger V, Asselain B, Guillet P et al. 2006. Pentoxifylline in ALS: a double-blind, randomized, multicenter, placebo-controlled trial. *Neurology* **66**:88–92.

Meininger V, Bensimon G, Bradley WR et al. 2004. Efficacy and safety of xaliproden in amyotrophic lateral sclerosis: results of two phase III trials. *Amyotroph Lateral Scler Other Motor Neuron Disord* **5**:107–117.

Miller R, Bradley W, Cudkowicz M et al. 2007. Phase II/III randomized trial of TCH346 in patients with ALS. *Neurology* **69**:776–784.

Miller RG, Moore DH 2nd, Gelinas DF et al. 2001. Phase III randomized trial of gabapentin in patients with amyotrophic lateral sclerosis. *Neurology* **56**:843–848.

Miller RG, Petajan JH, Bryan WW et al. 1996a. A placebo-controlled trial of recombinant human ciliary neurotrophic (rhCNTF) factor in amyotrophic lateral sclerosis. rhCNTF ALS Study Group. *Ann Neurol* **39**:256–260.

Miller RG, Shepherd R, Dao H et al. 1996b. Controlled trial of nimodipine in amyotrophic lateral sclerosis. *Neuromuscul Disord* **6**:101–104.

Miller RG, Smith SA, Murphy JR et al. 1996c. A clinical trial of verapamil in amyotrophic lateral sclerosis. *Muscle Nerve* **19**:511–515.

Miller TM, Kaspar BK, Kops GJ et al. 2005. Virus-delivered small RNA silencing sustains strength in amyotrophic lateral sclerosis. *Ann Neurol* **57**:773–776.

Mitsumoto H, Chad DA, Pioro EP. 1998. *Amyotrophic Lateral Sclerosis*. Philadelphia, PA: F.A. Davis, pp. 19–21.

Moreau C, Devos D, Brunaud-Danel V et al. 2006. Paradoxical response of VEGF expression to hypoxia in CSF of patients with ALS. *J Neurol Neurosurg Psychiatry* **77**:255–257.

Neumann M, Sampathu DM, Kwong LK et al. 2006. Ubiquitinated TDP-43 in frontotemporal lobar degeneration and amyotrophic lateral sclerosis. *Science* **314**:130–133.

Nishimura AL, Mitne-Neto M, Silva HC et al. 2004. A mutation in the vesicle-trafficking protein VAPB causes late-onset spinal muscular atrophy and amyotrophic lateral sclerosis. *Am J Hum Genet* **75**:822–831.

Ralph GS, Radcliffe PA, Day DM et al. 2005. Silencing mutant SOD1 using RNAi protects against neurodegeneration and extends survival in an ALS model. *Nat Med* **11**:429–433.

Raoul C, Abbas-Terki T, Bensadoun JC et al. 2005. Lentiviral-mediated silencing of SOD1 through RNA interference retards disease onset and progression in a mouse model of ALS. *Nat Med* **11**:423–428.

Rosen DR, Siddique T, Patterson D et al. 1993. Mutations in Cu/Zn superoxide dismutase gene are associated with familial amyotrophic lateral sclerosis. *Nature* **362**:59–62.

Schutz B, Reimann J, Dumitrescu-Ozimek L et al. 2005. The oral antidiabetic pioglitazone protects from neurodegeneration and amyotrophic lateral sclerosis-like symptoms in superoxide dismutase-G93A transgenic mice. *J Neurosci* **25**:7805–7812.

Shefner JM, Cudkowicz ME, Schoenfeld D et al. 2004. A clinical trial of creatine in ALS. *Neurology* **63**:1656–1661.

Smith RA, Miller TM, Yamanaka K et al. 2006. Antisense oligonucleotide therapy for neurodegenerative disease. *J Clin Invest* **116**:2290–2296.

Smith SA, Miller RG, Murphy JR, Ringel SP. 1994. Treatment of ALS with high dose pulse cyclophosphamide. *J Neurol Sci* **124** (Suppl.):84–87.

Sorenson EJ, Windbank AJ, Mandrekar JN et al. 2008. Subcutaneous IGF-1 is not beneficial in 2-year ALS trial. *Neurology* **71**:1770–1775.

Tsuda H, Han SM, Yang Y et al. 2008. The amyotrophic lateral sclerosis 8 protein VAPB is cleaved, secreted, and acts as a ligand for Eph receptors. *Cell* **133**:963–977.

Turner MR, Kiernan MC, Leigh PN, Talbot K. 2009. Biomarkers in amyotrophic lateral sclerosis. *Lancet Neurol* **8**:94–109.

Van Vught PW, Sutedja NA, Veldink JH et al. 2005. Lack of association between VEGF polymorphisms and ALS in a Dutch population. *Neurology* **65**:1643–1645.

Vance C, Rogelj B, Hortobágyi T et al. 2009. Mutations in FUS, an RNA processing protein, cause familial amyotrophic lateral sclerosis type 6. *Science* **323**:1208–1211.

Wang LJ, Lu YY, Muramatsu S et al. 2002. Neuroprotective effects of glial cell line-derived neurotrophic factor mediated by an adeno-associated virus vector in a transgenic animal model of amyotrophic lateral sclerosis. *J Neurosci* **22**:6920–6928.

Wong PC, Pardo CA, Borchelt DR et al. 1995. An adverse property of a familial ALS-linked SOD1 mutation causes motor neuron disease characterized by vacuolar degeneration of mitochondria. *Neuron* **14**:1105–1116.

Yamanaka K, Chun SJ, Boillee S et al. 2008. Astrocytes as determinants of disease progression in inherited amyotrophic lateral sclerosis. *Nat Neurosci* **11**:251–253.

Yang Y, Hentati A, Deng HX et al. 2001. The gene encoding alsin, a protein with three guanine-nucleotide exchange factor domains, is mutated in a form of recessive amyotrophic lateral sclerosis. *Nat Genet* **29**:160–165.

Yoshida S, Mulder DW, Kurland LT, Chu CP, Okazaki H. 1986. Follow-up study on amyotrophic lateral sclerosis in Rochester, Minn., 1925 through 1984. *Neuroepidemiology* **5**:61–70.

Zhong Z, Deane R, Ali Z, Parisi M et al. 2008. ALS-causing SOD1 mutants generate vascular changes prior to motor neuron degeneration. *Nat Neurosci* **11**:420–422.

Chapter 13
Epilepsy

Maciej Gasior and Frank Wiegand

Epilepsy is one of the most common of the serious brain disorders and can occur at all ages, with incidence rates peaking in early childhood and in the elderly population. The disease is characterized by an enduring predisposition to generate epileptic seizures and by the neurobiological, cognitive, psychological, and social consequences of this condition. Epilepsy can be diagnosed if a patient has two or more unprovoked seizures. An epileptic seizure is a transient occurrence of signs and/or symptoms related to abnormal excessive or synchronous neuronal activity in the brain (Fisher *et al.* 2005).

Worldwide the yearly incidence rate of epilepsy is estimated to be 48 per 1,000,000 population (Hirtz *et al.* 2007) and the prevalence is between 0.4% and 1.0% of the population (Forsgren *et al.* 2005; Sander 2003). The World Health Organization estimates that more than 50 million people have epilepsy worldwide (Reynolds 2005). People with epilepsy have an increased risk of premature death (Lhatoo *et al.* 2001) and symptomatic epilepsy can reduce life expectancy by up to 18 years (Gaitatzis *et al.* 2004). Sudden death, trauma, suicide, pneumonia, and status epilepticus are more common in people who have epilepsy than in those without the disorder (Gaitatzis and Sander 2004). In addition to the morbidity and mortality associated with seizures, patients with epilepsy may suffer a significant emotional, social, and economic burden.

The pathophysiology of epilepsy has been described in a crude oversimplification as a disruption of the normal balance between excitation and inhibition in the brain. An accurate description involves the understanding that brain function is highly dependent on the oscillatory cooperation of disparate neuronal networks. The occurrence of epileptic activity within neuronal networks is thought to be caused by greater spread and neuronal recruitment secondary to a combination of enhanced connectivity, enhanced excitatory transmission, a failure of inhibitory mechanisms, and changes in intrinsic neuronal properties (Duncan *et al.* 2006).

Conditions that among others cause seizures or epilepsy in humans include the following (Schachter 2002):

Genetic predisposition.
Head injury.
Stroke or other conditions that affect the vascular system in the brain.
Brain tumors.
Brain infection, such as meningitis or encephalitis.
Alzheimer's disease.
Alcohol or drug abuse or withdrawal.

Epilepsies can be divided into three major etiological categories: idiopathic, symptomatic, and presumed symptomatic (previously called "cryptogenic") (Engel Jr. 2001). Idiopathic epilepsies are thought to be caused mainly by genetic factors. Classic examples are hereditary channelopathies, which can have a major causative role in the development of seizures. Symptomatic epilepsies can be diagnosed by identifying the localized lesion in the brain that triggers seizures. The lesion can be a genetically programmed cellular alteration such as neuronal migration disorder in the cortex (e.g., tuberous sclerosis; see "Future Directions") or an acquired lesion such as traumatic brain injury (TBI) or stroke (Pitkanen *et al.* 2007). Presumed symptomatic epilepsies are most likely caused by a localization-related lesion but currently available diagnostic tools do not allow for a final proof (Engel Jr. 2001).

Symptomatic epilepsies typically develop in three phases: (1) The occurrence of an initial brain-

Translational Neuroscience, ed. James E. Barrett, Joseph T. Coyle and Michael Williams. Published by Cambridge University Press. © Cambridge University Press 2012.

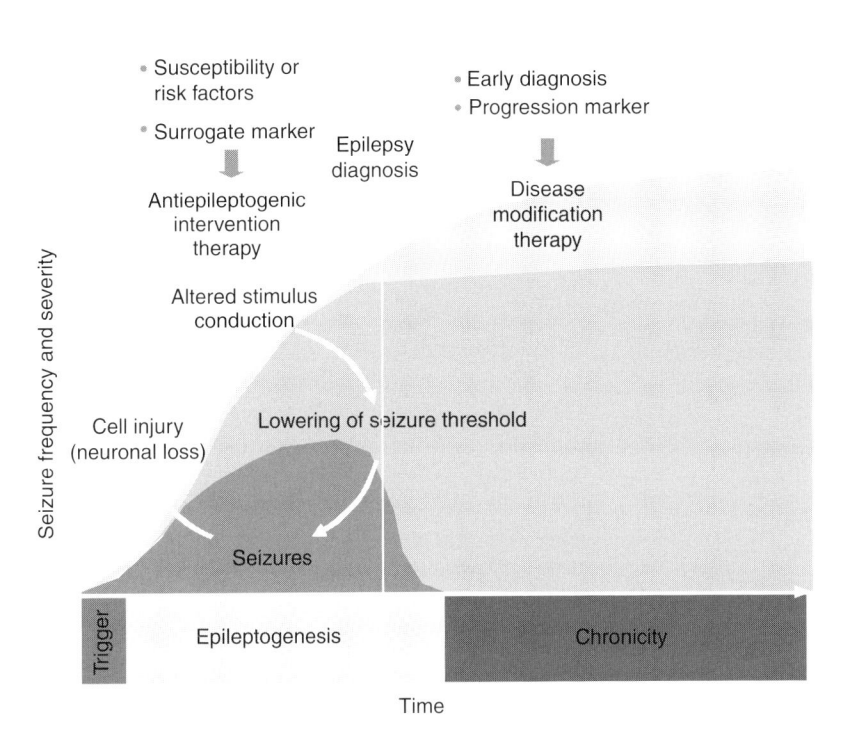

Figure 13.1. In epileptogenesis, increasingly severe and frequent electrical seizure activity occurs during the latency period after an initial insult, which triggers the kindling process. Antiepileptogenic treatment strategies may be developed to prevent epilepsy from occurring initially, and disease-modifying approaches could potentially limit disease progression once the diagnosis is established.

damaging insult (e.g., TBI, stroke); (2) epileptogenesis, also called the latency period, during which neuronal circuits undergo a large number of pathological changes but no overt seizure activity can be detected. Cellular changes described in animal models during this phase include cell death, gliosis, neurogenesis, axonal and dendritic plasticity, rearrangement of the extracellular matrix, and angiogenesis (Jutila *et al.* 2002); (3) the recurrent seizure phase, which characterizes epilepsy.

The epileptogenic process is not well understood. The general concept is that "seizures beget seizures." The initial neuronal injury is believed to trigger a first seizure event or subclinical seizure activity that in turn leads to additional neuronal injury and the subsequent sprouting of excitatory interneurons, which facilitates further excitatory neuronal firing, leading to more seizures. "Kindling" is probably only one of the many parallel and sequential changes taking place while epilepsy develops. Due to the degenerative nature of these events, epilepsy is often coupled with various functional impairments, including sensorimotor, memory, and emotional decline. The epileptogenic period is variable in length and can continue for months and years. Figure 13.1 depicts the epileptogenic period and elaborates on the two primary possibilities for pharmacological intervention, antiepileptogenesis and disease modification. Early intervention during the epileptogenic period requires knowledge of the susceptibility and risk factors involved in the seizure development. Ideally, we will identify general surrogate markers related to ongoing epileptogenic activity and susceptibility or risk factors for individual patients so that targeted antiepileptogenic treatment interventions can be deployed, with the ultimate goal of preventing the disease. After epilepsy has manifested, disease modification would promise to limit further worsening and progression into pharmacological resistance. Depending on the approach, it might be sufficient to target one or a subset of the different molecular mechanisms of cellular alterations that have been described (Pitkanen and Lukasiuk 2009):

Neuroprotection to limit neuronal injury.
  Multiple preclinical models of temporal lobe epilepsy have shown neuronal damage occurring in the hilus and the CA1 pyramidal cell layer and interneurons, with milder damage in the CA3 and CA2 pyramidal cell layer and granule cells of the brain.
Neurogenesis may offer the potential for improved cellular regeneration, although the extent to which neurotrophic mechanisms can potentially worsen seizures is unclear.

- Gliosis: Astrocytes are involved in regulation of the extracellular neuronal milieu; microglia play a crucial role in inflammatory cell responses and can potentially be targeted.
- Axonal sprouting: The role of axonal sprouting in epileptogenesis and ictogenesis is controversial, but the kindling hypothesis is partly founded on this concept.
- Axonal injury: Although axonal injury has been described in several trauma models, whether it directly affects epileptogenesis or increased seizure spread is still controversial.
- Dendritic plasticity: Loss of dendritic spines, changes in spine morphology, and reduced dendritic branching have been described.
- Angiogenesis: Disruption of the blood–brain barrier and angiogenesis have been described during seizure development.
- Changes to the extracellular matrix: A large number of enzymes contributing to extracellular matrix changes have been identified.
- Acquired channelopathies: Brain injury, particularly after status epilepticus, can result in altered function of ligand- and receptor-gated ion channels.

During the epileptogenic process the circuitry reorganization leads to permanent hyperexcitability and the occurrence of recurrent spontaneous seizures. Depending on the localization of pathological networks within the brain, epilepsy can be classified in focal (localization-related) and generalized forms. Focal epilepsies are divided into simple partial seizures (e.g., simple partial motor seizures) and complex partial seizures, located mainly in the temporal lobe of the brain. Focal seizures have the ability to secondarily generalize, which can lead to tonic-clonic seizures, the hallmark of primarily generalized epilepsies. Based on the seizure semiology, the patient's age at onset, the causes of seizures, provoking factors, the seizure frequency and pattern, electroencephalographic (EEG) findings, additional disorders, and other criteria, a multitude of distinct seizure syndromes can be classified and diagnosed (Engel Jr. 2001).

The mainstay of therapy is the use of antiepileptic drugs (AEDs). AEDs increase inhibition, decrease excitation, or prevent aberrant burst-firing of neurons. The aim of antiepileptic treatment is to control seizures as quickly as possible without adverse effects (Sander 2004). AEDs are effective in 60–70% of patients. Unfortunately, 30–40% of patients develop intractable forms of the disease that are refractory to the effects of currently available AEDs (Kwan and Brodie 2000).

Over the past 100 years, several AEDs have been developed. Table 13.1 shows the array of compounds that have been approved for the treatment of epilepsy, the year of their introduction into the US market, as well as the regulatory requirements for approval. Epileptologists define the "older" compounds prior to the development of felbamate as first-generation AEDs. These agents are efficacious but are frequently associated with treatment-limiting side effects or safety issues as well as unfavorable pharmacokinetic properties. "Newer" AEDs, the so-called second-generation AEDs, were developed to overcome some of these issues and are usually better tolerated while maintaining a good efficacy across a broad variety of different seizure types. Most of the compounds were initially discovered serendipitously before predictive translational animal models and screening assays were developed that led to novel molecular entities. One of the consequences of the "untargeted" discovery approach is that in most cases the mechanisms of action of AEDs are not fully understood. Many AEDs have multiple proposed actions. The current understanding of known (classic) drug targets involves molecular effects on sodium channels, potassium channels, glutamate receptors, the γ-aminobutyric acid (GABA)ergic system, synaptic vesical protein 2A (SV2A), intracellular calcium signaling, and carbonic anhydrase inhibition. Figures 13.2 and 13.3 show the proposed mechanisms of action of commonly used drugs on excitatory as well as inhibitory neurons.

Drug development in the twentieth century has focused mainly on the prevention or suppression of recurrent seizures. Given the high unmet medical need associated with this disease, and the improved understanding of its pathophysiology, the twenty-first century provides the opportunity to tackle three important issues: the development of pharmacoresistance leading to intractable forms of epilepsy (seen in 30% of patients); the potential to prevent disease through novel antiepileptogenic compounds (not necessarily AEDs in the classic sense); and the potential to prevent seizure worsening through disease modification. An understanding of the molecular and cellular mechanisms that are common to different etiological types of seizures will likely provide

Chapter 13: Epilepsy

Table 13.1. Antiepileptic drugs in the USA: Year of introduction and regulatory requirements.

Year	Compound	Company	FDA Requirements
1912	Phenobarbital	Winthrop	No requirement for toxicity or efficacy data until 1938 (toxicity) and 1962 (efficacy)
1935	Mephobarbital	Winthrop	
1938	Phenytoin	Parke-Davis	Toxicity but no requirement of efficacy data until 1962, without requirement for double-blind, randomized controlled trials
1947	Mephenytoin	Sandoz	
1954	Primidone	Ayerst	
1957	Methsuximide	Parke-Davis	
1957	Ethotoin	Abbott	
1960	Ethosuximide	Parke-Davis	
1968	Diazepam	Roche	Risk–benefit with toxicity and substantial evidence of efficacy (double-blind, randomized controlled trials)
1974	Carbamazepine	Ciba-Geigy	
1975	Clonazepam	Roche	
1978	Valproate	Abbott	
1981	Clorazepate	Abbott	
1992	Felbamate	Carter-Wallace	Era of double-blind, randomized controlled trials with superiority design to show significant treatment effect, i.e., statistically significant difference between treatment arms
1993	Gabapentin	Parke-Davis	
1994	Lamotrigine	Glaxo-Wellcome	
1997	Topiramate	Ortho-McNeil	
1998	Tiagabine	Abbott	
2000	Zonisamide	Élan to Eisai	
2000	Levetiracetam	UCB Pharma	
2000	Oxcarbazepine	Novartis	
2004	Pregabalin	Pfizer	
2008	Rufinamide	Eisai	
2008	Lacosamide	UCB Pharma	

FDA, Food and Drug Administration.

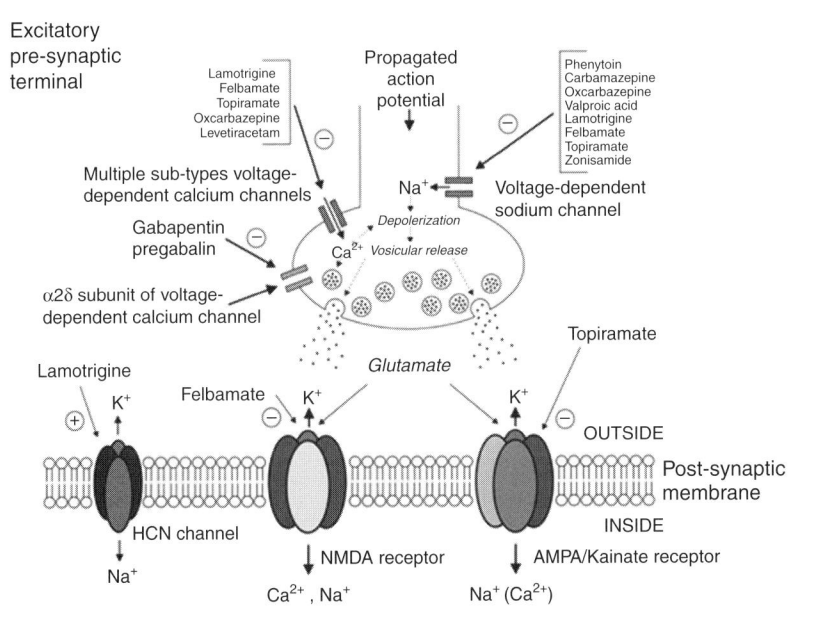

Figure 13.2. The proposed pre- and postsynaptic mechanism of antiepileptic drugs (AEDs) related to excitatory interneurons. AMPA, α-amino-3-hydroxy-5-methyl-4-isoxazole-propionate; HCN, hyperpolarization-activated cation; NMDA, N-methyl-D-aspartate. Courtesy of Dr. Raman Sankar.

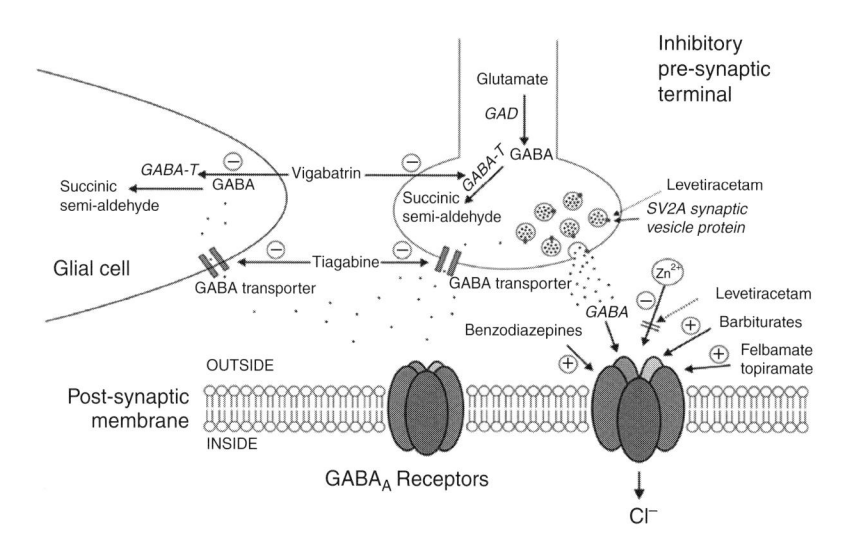

Figure 13.3. Proposed pre- and postsynaptic mechanism of antiepileptic drugs related to inhibitory interneurons. GABA, γ-aminobutyric acid; GABA-T, GABA transaminase; GAD, glutamic acid decarboxylase. Courtesy of Dr. Raman Sankar.

molecular targets that can be used to modify neurobiological changes underlying epileptogenesis using pharmacological or other tools. Table 13.2 summarizes putative targets for future drug development based on a report from Meldrum and Rogawski (2007).

This chapter first describes translational models that have led to the development of classic AEDs and then addresses novel translational approaches to advance our understanding of areas of high unmet medical need. We describe approaches to identifying and validating targets that may be promising in the following areas: antiepileptogenesis, disease modification, pharmacoresistance, genetically determined idiopathic epilepsies, drug utility and drug effectiveness (ability to positively influence a variety of common comorbidities, including psychiatric disorders, cognitive impairment, migraine, and neuropathic pain), and "drugability," or the pharmacokinetic and pharmacodynamic aspects of candidate selection including drug–drug interactions and formulations and delivery options.

We believe that increased focus in these areas and advances in translational models will ultimately lead to third-generation AEDs that will provide superior treatment outcomes for millions of epilepsy patients. Additional clinical challenges not discussed in detail here include the identification of patients at risk for epilepsy after an epileptogenic brain insult through the use of surrogate markers (e.g., proteomics, electrophysiology, imaging); pharmacogenetic approaches to cure genetic forms of epilepsy; predictive endophenotype identification, which would help with drug choice and with individualizing therapy to maximize treatment success and effectiveness and to avoid side effects of treatment; and a better understanding of whether individual patients can be treated with monotherapy or polytherapy and whether the various treatments should be administered in a serial or parallel manner or tailored specifically for each etiological form of disease. After addressing the preclinical translational efforts we address the clinical aspects of translational research related to seizure disorders.

Currently available preclinical screening models

Preclinical research has played a fundamental role in advancing our knowledge of human epilepsy and discovery of novel therapeutic approaches (Kupferberg 2001; Smith *et al.* 2007). The preclinical research in epilepsy relies on both in vivo and in vitro assays (Fisher 1989).

Seizure test vs. epilepsy model

For both in vivo and in vitro models, the terms *seizure test* and *epilepsy model* are often used interchangeably although there are distinct and important differences. If epilepsy research is done in treatment-naïve, non-epileptic animals or tissues harvested from such animals, the term *seizure test* should be used. *Epilepsy model* should be used when epileptic animals (i.e., animals exhibiting spontaneous seizures) are used for in vivo testing or are a source of tissues for

Table 13.2. Novel molecular targets for development of antiepileptic drugs.

Voltage-gated ion channels
Voltage-gated sodium channels
Voltage-gated calcium channels
Voltage-gated potassium channels
HCN channels
Voltage-gated chloride channels

Ligand-gated ion channels
Cys-loop ligand-gated channels
GABA$_A$ receptors
Nicotinic cholinergic receptors
Glycine receptors
Ionotropic glutamate receptors
Structure of ionotropic glutamate receptors
NMDA receptors
AMPA receptors

Acid-sensing ion channels

G protein-coupled receptors
Metabotropic glutamate receptors
GABA$_B$ receptors

Neurotransmitter transporters
Plasma membrane GABA transporters
Plasma membrane glutamate transporters
Vesicular glutamate transporters

Presynaptic proteins influencing synaptic function
Synaptic vesicle proteins
Synaptic anchoring proteins

Enzymes
GABA transaminase
Carbonic anhydrase
Protein kinases and phosphatases

Gap junctions (connexins)

AMPA, α-amino-3-hydroxyl-5-methyl-4-isoxazole-propionate; GABA, γ-aminobutyric acid; HCN, hyperpolarization-activated cation; NMDA, N-methyl-D-aspartate.
Data in this table taken from Meldrum and Rogawski (2007).

in vitro testing. A third group of assays within this category can be classified as neither a seizure test nor an epilepsy model. This group includes assays in animals, or their tissues, that do not exhibit spontaneous seizure activity (thus are not epileptic) but exhibit a higher propensity to seizures due to, for instance, genetic factors or pharmacological manipulations. For clarity, the term *seizure assays* will be used throughout this chapter and *seizure tests* and *epilepsy models* will be distinguished where appropriate.

Characteristics of an ideal seizure assay

The heterogeneity of seizure disorders and the complexity of seizure phenotypes together explain why there is no "ideal" or "ultimate" assay that would answer all relevant questions. In vivo assays have an established function in testing for efficacy of candidate AEDs whereas in vitro assays may be better suited for basic research relevant to fundamental pathophysiological processes causing or resulting from epilepsy (Fisher 1989; Kupferberg 2001).

An ideal assay should exhibit the following characteristics:

Sensitivity: The stimulus produces a response that is quantifiable and monotonically related to stimulus intensity. This response should also be sensitive to manipulations, especially pharmacological ones.

Reliability: The response produced by a stimulus should be consistent when applied under identical or similar conditions.

Reproducibility: The results should be reproducible within the same and across different laboratories.

Validity: Three principal measures of an assay's validity include predictive validity (ability to predict that the effect in the assay will be similar to the condition in humans being modeled); face validity (phenomenological similarity between the assay and the human abnormality being modeled); and construct validity (similar theoretical rationale behind the abnormality in the assay and the abnormality in humans).

Although sensitivity, reliability, and reproducibility relate more to the technical aspects of the assay, validity is the most important criterion for the translational value of a given assay. A good assay should have high predictive, face, and construct validity. Compared with many of the other CNS disorders described in this book, epilepsy models have fortunately demonstrated this high "translational value" in recent decades.

Predictive validity

Due to the similarities of the pathways that govern neuronal excitation and inhibition between primate and nonprimate species, seizure disorders have been in a relatively advantageous position compared with many other neuropsychiatric disorders. Firstly, there are many clinically effective AEDs with unique as well as overlapping mechanisms of action and several newer AEDs are in clinical development (Bialer *et al.* 2009; Meldrum and Rogawski 2007; Rogawski and Löscher 2004*a*). Multiple pharmacological mechanisms have been identified that, when targeted, are likely to produce anticonvulsant effects in humans. These major mechanisms include blockade of sodium or calcium channels, potentiation of GABAergic transmission, and blockade of excitatory neurotransmission through N-methyl-D-aspartate (NMDA), α-amino-3-hydroxyl-5-methyl-4-isoxazole-propionate (AMPA), or kainate receptors (Meldrum and Rogawski 2007). Secondly, many seizure tests and epilepsy models have a good predictive validity for specific types of epilepsy (Kupferberg 2001; Smith *et al.* 2007). All AEDs in clinical use today have been identified as anticonvulsants in a battery of in vivo assays, and no single AED is effective in humans but not effective in several of the commonly used animal assays (Rogawski and Porter 1990). Translation of preclinical findings into the clinical situation is thus facilitated (Smith *et al.* 2007). The reverse – translation from humans into exploratory in vivo models – is also possible. The ketogenic diet, a highly effective intervention in drug-resistant epilepsy in humans, for example, is now being extensively studied preclinically for its pharmacological and other (e.g., metabolic) mechanisms responsible for clinically distinct efficacy (Gasior *et al.* 2006; Hartman *et al.* 2007). In addition, the available assays can be used to validate novel drug targets and predict clinical efficacy of new chemical entities (NCEs) (Meldrum and Rogawski 2007; Rogawski 2006).

Face validity

The basic phenomenology involved in seizure activity and its behavioral manifestation is similar in humans and animals and can be easily quantified through observation or video monitoring (Durand 1993; Engel Jr. 1995; Hughes 1989). Some in vitro assays, however, may fall short of fully capturing and modeling all complexities of neuronal and interneuronal processes involved in seizure initiation and spread, and they clearly lack their behavioral aspect (convulsions). These assays, however, can be successfully used for early target validation (Bernard 2006; Dichter and Pollard 2006; Heinemann *et al.* 2006; Thompson *et al.* 2006).

Construct validity

The difference between seizure test and epilepsy model should be mentioned again with regard to construct validity. In seizure tests, seizure activity is artificially produced in most cases by either electrical or chemical stimulation in a naïve, nonepileptic animal or its tissue. In contrast, in the human condition seizures are spontaneous and develop usually after a prolonged latent period during which specific changes take place at all organizational levels of the brain. Clearly, seizure tests have been instrumental in identifying clinically effective AEDs. However, epilepsy models with pathophysiologies similar to human epilepsy may be better suited for finding novel treatments. Thus, one critique of fully relying on acute classic seizure tests is that they can only identify "me too" drugs that would not be effective in refractory epilepsy, which represents the highest unmet medical need in epilepsy treatment (Löscher 2002*a*; Rogawski 2006).

The preclinical discovery of antiepileptic drugs

The preclinical discovery of NCEs for treating epilepsy relies heavily on in vivo assays. Several in vivo assays are available and this number is still growing (Sarkisian 2001). However, the early preclinical discovery process is limited to several standard assays for primary screening of NCEs for their anticonvulsant efficacy (Kupferberg 2001; Smith *et al.* 2007). These standard assays have been well characterized with a number of clinically used AEDs. They show a good predictive validity for specific types of epilepsy and are amenable to high-throughput screening.

In addition to showing efficacy in seizure assays, a given NCE must also display a couple of crucial biochemical properties in order to qualify as a useful AED. As with other translational models, in vivo studies reasonably predict the ability of NCEs to cross the blood–brain barrier, a key requirement for all

Table 13.3. Correlation between anticonvulsant efficacy in preclinical tests and clinical indications of classic and second-generation antiepileptic drugs.

Preclinical test	Tonic-clonic generalized seizures	Myoclonic/ generalized absence seizures	Generalized absence seizures	Partial seizures
MES[a]	CBZ, PB, PHT, VPA, *FBM, GBP, LTG, TPM, ZNS*			
Subcutaneous PTZ[a]		BZD, ESM, PB[b], VPA, *FBM, GBP, TGB*[b], *VGB*[b]		
Spike-wave discharges[c]			BZD, *ETS*, VPA, *LTG, LVT, TPM*	
Electrical kindling[d]				BZD, CBZ, PB, PHT, VPA, *FBM, GBP, LTG, LVT, TGB, TPM, VGB, ZNS*
6-Hz(44 mA)[e]				VPA, *LVT*

Preclinical tests: MES, maximal electroshock; PTZ, pentylenetetrazole; 6-Hz (44 mA), 6-Hz seizure test performed at 44 mA current intensity.
Classic antiepileptic drugs: BZD, benzodiazepines; CBZ, carbamazepine; PB, phenobarbital; PHT, phenytoin; VPA, valproate.
Second-generation antiepileptic drugs (in italic): ETS, ethosuximide; FBM, felbamate; GBP, gabapentin; LTG, lamotrigine; LVT, levetiracetam; TGB, tiagabine; TPM, topiramate; VGB, vigabatrin; ZNS, zonisamide.
[a] Data from White (2003).
[b] PB, TGB, and VGB block seizures induced by subcutaneous PTZ but are ineffective in generalized absence seizures and may exacerbate spike-wave discharges.
[c] Data summarized from the γ-butyrolactone seizure test, the genetic absence epileptic rat of Strasbourg, and the lethargic (lh/lh) mouse test in Hosford *et al.* (1992), Hosford and Wang (1997), Marescaux and Vergnes (1995), Snead III (1992).
[d] Data from Löscher (2002b).
[e] Data from Barton *et al.* (2001).
With kind permission from Springer Science+Business Media: *Neurotherapeutics, Discovery of Antiepileptic Drugs*, Vol. 4, 2007, pp. 12–17, Smith M, Wilcox KS, White HS, Table 1, © The American Society for Experimental NeuroTherapeutics, Inc.

CNS-active compounds. The careful assessment of a therapeutic range, or therapeutic window, is another crucial element in identifying suitable and efficacious novel compounds. In contrast to some of the other CNS disorders, epilepsy treatment specifically requires compounds with a long half-life and with a pharmacokinetic profile that ideally generates a completely flat plasma-level profile in humans to avoid steep peak and trough-level fluctuations. Fluctuations of the plasma levels, especially rapid clearance of AEDs, are known to trigger so-called withdrawal or breakthrough seizures and should be avoided. The ideal profile of a novel AED would encompass once-daily dosing, linear pharmacokinetics, good bioavailability, and limited or no drug–drug interaction propensity. Interactions are of particular concern because about one-third of patients with epilepsy are on a combination of two or more AEDs. This chapter focuses not on these essential prerequisites of new compounds but on the efficacy assays at our disposal.

The assays currently used in the primary screening include the maximal electroshock (MES), the subcutaneous pentylenetetrazol (PTZ) test, spike-wave discharges, electrical kindling, and the 6-Hz seizure test. Basic parameters of these assays are relatively standard across various laboratories, making them very reliable, reproducible, and easy to set up and validate. As Table 13.3 shows, these primary screening assays predict clinical utility of first- as well as second-generation AEDs.

The maximal electroshock and subcutaneous pentylenetetrazol tests

The MES and subcutaneous PTZ tests are both seizure tests and have been the two most frequently used in vivo assays since the early years of screening programs for AEDs. In 1937, Putnam and Merritt demonstrated the efficacy of phenytoin in the cat MES test. Later, demonstration of phenytoin's efficacy in human generalized tonic-clonic seizures provided the necessary clinical validation of the MES assay as predictive for clinical efficacy against human generalized tonic-clonic seizures. Likewise, the utility of the subcutaneous PTZ assay was established by demonstrating first the ability of trimethadione, but not phenytoin, to block PTZ-induced convulsions and then later clinical efficacy of trimethadione, but not phenytoin, in human myoclonic and generalized absence seizures. Thanks to those early preclinical and clinical studies, the MES and subcutaneous PTZ tests were established as reasonably predictive for clinical efficacy in, at least, generalized tonic-clonic seizures (MES) and in myoclonic and generalized absence seizures (subcutaneous PTZ) (Smith et al. 2007).

Despite the early enthusiasm, the predictive validity of these assays turned out to be imperfect and can now be challenged by several exceptions. The profile of lamotrigine can serve as an example of false-negative results the subcutaneous PTZ test can yield. Specifically, lamotrigine is inactive in the subcutaneous PTZ test and, therefore, would be predicted to be ineffective against human generalized absence seizures; but in fact, lamotrigine is effective in treating these seizures clinically. There are also several AEDs (e.g., phenobarbital, gabapentin, tiagabine) that are effective in the subcutaneous PTZ test but not in human generalized absence seizures. Thus, false positives can be yielded by the PTZ test as well.

Spike-wave discharges

The false-negative and false-positive results of these seizure models underscore the need for additional in vivo assays that are true epilepsy models in order to improve predictive validity of the preclinical screening process for new AEDs effective in human generalized absence seizures. Assays with better predictive validity in this regard are now customarily included in the search for new AEDs against generalized absence seizures. Such assays include the γ-butyrolactone seizure test and the genetic absence epileptic rat of Strasbourg (GAERS) as well as the WAG/Rij rats and the lethargic (lh/lh) mouse (Coenen and Van Luijtelaar 2003; Hosford and Wang 1997; Marescaux and Vergnes 1995; Snead III 1992). Unlike the MES and subcutaneous PTZ tests, some of these assays (e.g., GAERS and WAG/Rij rats) are true epilepsy models with seizures occurring spontaneously and with construct validity similar, in at least some aspects, to human epilepsy.

Electrical kindling

The term *kindling* has been used almost exclusively in the epilepsy field. Kindling shares many similarities with behavioral sensitization resulting from repeated exposure to psychostimulant drugs (Pierce and Kalivas 1997; Post and Weiss 1989). Kindling occurs when repeated exposures to initially subconvulsive stimuli result in progressively increasing seizure response with accompanying durable neuronal changes (Löscher 2002a). Of all possible types of stimulations (e.g., chemical or electrical) and sites (e.g., amygdala, cornea, hippocampus, or olfactory bulb), electrical stimulations of the hippocampus or amygdala have been most frequently employed in research and compound testing. Such local stimulations are associated with a progressive increase in seizure sensitivity, severity, and duration. At the end of the kindling procedure, animals' spontaneous seizures can also occur, even in the absence of the triggering stimulus. Adding to its construct validity, kindling can result in neuronal degeneration in limbic brain regions similar to those in human temporal lobe epilepsy. From the predictive validity perspective, the rat kindling models predicted clinical utility of levetiracetam, which was ineffective in the MES and subcutaneous PTZ tests. The kindling model described here is used to convert healthy animals into epileptic ones and is thus a true epilepsy model. Due to the time it takes before the seizure susceptibility is maximal (usually about 10–14 days), it is also possible to interfere with the ongoing kindling process before it is complete. Any treatment that might slow the development of epilepsy or even prevent kindling from being successful could indicate disease-modifying or antiepileptogenic properties of NCEs.

Epileptogenesis

Kindling models provide a unique opportunity to study processes involved in the development of epilepsy and spontaneous seizures (epileptogenesis) as well as to identify potential antiepileptogenic treatments (Dichter 2006; Löscher and Schmidt 2004), an area of high unmet medical need (see Table 13.4). The concept is to prevent or slow the deleterious effects of the ongoing kindling procedure. Usually kindling

Table 13.4. Translational animal models used to investigate epileptogenesis and antiepileptogenic properties of new molecular entities.

Model	Neuronal degeneration	Mossy fiber sprouting	Chronic hyperexcitability	Latent period	Spontaneous seizures
Kindling					
Classical kindling	Present	Present	Yes	No[a]	No
Rapid kindling	Absent	Absent	Yes	Compressed	No
Status epilepticus (i.e., kainic acid, pilocarpine, Li-pilocarpine, PPS, SAS)	Marked	Marked	Yes	Days – weeks	Yes
Traumatic brain injury					
Cortical undercut	Yes	?	Yes	Yes	Yes
FeCl$_2$	Yes	?	Yes	Yes	Yes
Fluid percussion	Yes	Yes	Yes	No	No
Neonatal hypoxia	No	Minimal	Yes	No	No
Neonatal hyperthermia	No	No	Yes	No	No

[a] Spontaneous seizures do develop with prolonged kindling stimulation.
PPS, perforant path stimulation; SAS, sustained amygdala stimulation.
Reprinted from *Neurology*, Vol. **59**, 9 Suppl. 5, White HS, Animal models of epileptogenesis, pp. S7–S14, with permission from Wolters Kluwer Health. © 2002 by AAN Enterprises, Inc.

occurs in animals in the presence of a presumably protective compound, which if effective should prevent stage 5 seizures (generalized tonic-clonic seizures) from occurring. To prove the causality of the treatment, researchers stop giving the test compound after a short break in the kindling stimulation to see whether the continuation of kindling will eventually also render the partly protected animals epileptic or whether the temporary protection was able to completely stop the progression of seizure worsening. Most of the compounds tested so far were able to slow the seizure acquisition but did not completely prevent kindling. One of the open questions using the kindling model to investigate compounds with disease-modifying properties is the interaction that can occur between the antiseizure activity of a compound and its antiepileptogenic properties. Very efficacious antiseizure drugs could in theory alleviate the amount of damage that is induced during each kindling procedure and thus mimic the effect of a disease modifier. Because of this criticism as well as concerns that spontaneous seizures, the hallmark of true epilepsy, are rarely seen in kindled animal models, additional models for epileptogenesis have been developed. The most prominent is the status epilepticus model (Curia et al. 2008; Grabenstatter et al. 2005; Leite et al. 2002; Morimoto et al. 2004; Münller et al. 2009). This model takes advantage of the fact that status epilepticus of sufficient duration can induce the pathological changes that after a latent period lead to the development of spontaneous seizures, a model with presumably high face and construct validity. Status epilepticus models allow early pharmacological intervention, which can be applied during the latent period between the epilepsy-causing insult and fully developed epilepsy with spontaneous seizures and permanent neuronal changes.

Efforts are also ongoing to develop and further refine kindling models. Examples of such models include spontaneous seizures induced by pilocarpine or kainic acid, rapid kindling, TBI, neonatal hyperthermic seizures, and hypoxia (Sharma et al. 2007; Stables et al. 2002; White 2003). Some of these models are not associated with spontaneous seizures; nevertheless they can provide insight into various mechanisms involved in epileptogenesis. Until a drug with proven antiepileptogenic properties in humans is available, however, predictive validity of all such models awaits verification.

Genetic models of human epilepsy

In recent years, several mouse genetic models of human epilepsy have been developed (Bialer and White 2010; Catterall *et al.* 2008; Frankel 2009). These mouse models carry mutations of the genes that cause specific epilepsy syndromes in humans. Such mouse models recapitulate many characteristics of the corresponding epilepsy syndromes in humans and thus should have a better construct validity. Specific gene mutations encoding different subunits of voltage-gated sodium, potassium, or calcium channels are involved in various epilepsy syndromes with corresponding mouse models (Bialer and White 2010). For example, severe myoclonic epilepsy of infancy is associated with a mutation of the *SCN1A* gene that encodes voltage-gated sodium channel $Na_v1.1$. (also known as SCN1A) and a mouse model carrying the same mutation and exhibiting many features of this syndrome is available (Mullen and Scheffer 2009). Likewise, there are known polymorphisms of ligand-gated channels of the $GABA_A$ or neuronal nicotinic acetylcholine receptors that produce specific types of epilepsies in humans and mice. For example, adult nocturnal frontal lobe epilepsy is associated with mutations of *CHRNA4* or *CHRNB2* genes encoding α or β subunits, respectively, of the nicotinic acetylcholine receptor; the same mutations in mice result in epileptic phenotypes (Fonck *et al.* 2005; Manfredi *et al.* 2009; Marini and Guerrini 2007; Raggenbass and Bertrand 2002). Such models can provide a wealth of information relevant to the pathophysiology of epilepsy syndromes and can be used to identify novel targets. However, those models are not typically used in screening programs and their predictive validity in identifying novel, not "me too," NCEs needs to be established.

Drug resistance

Approximately 30% of patients with epilepsy are estimated to have drug-resistant epilepsy. Drug resistance is defined as a failure to respond to at least two AEDs at tolerable doses. Even the approval of many second-generation AEDs since 1993, marked by the approval of felbamate in the USA (Table 13.1), failed to substantially improve the prognosis for drug-resistant epilepsy, making drug resistance another area of high unmet medical need in epilepsy (Stables *et al.* 2003).

A handful of in vivo assays model drug resistance (Löscher 2002*a*). Notwithstanding, kindling models have played a critical role in the development of several models of drug resistance. These models include phenytoin-resistant kindled rats and lamotrigine-resistant kindled rats. Other, nonkindling models are the 6-Hz seizure model of psychomotor seizure (see below), post-status epilepticus models of temporal epilepsy, and the methylazoxymethanol acetate in utero model of nodular heterotopias (Barton *et al.* 2001; Brandt *et al.* 2004; Glien *et al.* 2002; Löscher *et al.* 1993; Postma *et al.* 2000; Rundfeldt and Löscher 1993; Smyth *et al.* 2002).

One of the better characterized models that originated from traditional kindling procedures is that of kindled seizures resistant to phenytoin, a method developed by Löscher, Rundfeldt, and colleagues nearly 20 years ago (Rundfeldt *et al.* 1990). They first observed that kindled rats were less responsive to anticonvulsant treatment than were animals undergoing the traditional MES test. The second pivotal observation was that amygdala kindled rats could be differentiated on the basis of their response to phenytoin challenge into responders and nonresponders. The rats that did not respond to phenytoin and other drugs (e.g., carbamazepine) fulfilled the criterion of drug resistance. This development allowed the use of nonresponding rats (drug-resistant rats) for comparative testing of NCEs.

Another interesting model of drug resistance is the lamotrigine-resistant kindled rat model (Postma *et al.* 2000). Unlike the models of phenytoin resistance, resistance to lamotrigine is not inherited but is induced by repeated exposure to low doses of lamotrigine during kindling development. Exposure to lamotrigine during the process of epileptogenesis results in a diminished response to higher doses of lamotrigine in fully kindled rats. These resistant animals also show cross-resistance to carbamazepine, topiramate, and phenytoin (Srivastava *et al.* 2003, 2004).

The 6-Hz seizure test of psychomotor seizures has been used increasingly in drug screening programs. The 6-Hz test differs from the MES test only in regard to specific electrical parameters such as frequency (6 vs. 50 Hz), stimulus duration (3 vs. 0.2 seconds), and shape of the electric wave (square vs. sine) (Giardina and Gasior 2009). Compared with MES-type stimulation, this low-frequency and long-duration stimulation results in qualitatively different convulsions and, more importantly, in different sensitivity to treatments (Barton *et al.* 2001, 2003). Levetiracetam was effective in the 6-Hz test, whereas other AEDs were not, when high currents (44 mA) of electrical stimulation were applied (Barton *et al.* 2001). This finding, together with the fact that levetiracetam was not effective in traditional MES and subcutaneous PTZ tests, led to the conclusion that the 6-Hz seizure may be sensitive to pharmacological interventions that would have failed efficacy tests in traditional models such as the MES or subcutaneous PTZ tests. In support of this argument is the finding that the 6-Hz test in mice is very sensitive in demonstrating anticonvulsant properties of the ketogenic diet (Hartman *et al.* 2008), which is used very effectively in human drug-resistant epilepsy (Kossoff 2004).

Combination therapy

Additional work is also needed to fully understand the pharmacokinetic and pharmacodynamic interaction of combination therapies. In clinical practice most patients with refractory epilepsy are treated with more than one AED. Some epileptologists suggest a "rational polypharmacy" approach combining AEDs based on their presumed mode of action (Czuczwar and Borowicz 2002; Deckers *et al.* 2000; Kwan and Brodie 2006; Patsalos *et al.* 2002; Schmidt 1996). The assumption is that synergies occur when several pathophysiological elements of neuronal hyperexcitability are addressed at once, for example, by combining a sodium channel antagonist with a GABAergic drug. An additional clinical advantage of this approach could be the fact that lower dosages of each individual compound might be used, which potentially avoids treatment-limiting side effects. Translational models to investigate advantageous combinations are using isobolographic analysis but are in general labor intensive and do not necessarily lead to the discovery of novel molecular targets (Czuczwar *et al.* 2009).

All these models serve as tools for studying molecular mechanisms involved in drug resistance as well as for testing drugs. In addition, most models can be used to identify relevant biomarkers that could be used clinically for measuring efficacy of drug treatment. As with models of epileptogenesis, models of drug resistance will remain clinically not fully validated until clinically effective drugs are available to provide backvalidation of these models. This significant limitation should not, however, stop the use and further development of these models. Contrarily, they should be used increasingly in order to better understand the phenomenon of drug resistance and to facilitate bidirectional translation between preclinical and clinical findings. Even without the validation of the models available today, their use for preclinical testing of NCEs can provide important information differentiating some NCEs from others. This kind of information can then be used to backvalidate these models once relevant clinical data are available.

Side effects of antiepileptic drugs

All AEDs have CNS-related side effects, most prominently somnolence, dizziness, nausea, vertigo, ataxia, and diplopia in addition to cognitive adverse events. Intolerable side effects limit the use of AEDs considerably, and in their quest to enhance the quality of life of patients with epilepsy, neurologists are weighing the extent of seizure reduction that particular AEDs provide against the side effect burden introduced by the treatments. Often the dose of an AED is limited by adverse events and treatment-associated side effects are a major contributor to reduced quality of life. Epilepsy is also frequently associated with neuropsychiatric comorbidities such as mood disorders, anxiety, and depression, making drug choice even more complicated. AEDs may have a positive as well as a negative influence on some of these comorbidities (Lagae 2006; Schmitz 2006). AEDs such as lamotrigine can have a positive influence on depressive and bipolar symptoms; others such as topiramate might have a positive influence on migraine headaches, which have a higher incidence in patients with epilepsy compared with the general public (Rogawski and Löscher 2004*b*).

During preclinical testing, a differentiation between untoward and anticonvulsant effects is always evaluated to predict the therapeutic index of drug candidates. This distinction is customarily made by evaluating a drug's effect on simple motor functions, typically in the open field or roto-rod tests (Löscher and Nolting 1991; Wlaz and Löscher 1998). The therapeutic index is then calculated by dividing the dose that produces behavioral impairment by an effective or median anticonvulsant dose in the seizure test. Although this approach provides an easy way to comparatively evaluate NCEs for their safety margins, it may have limited clinical value. The behavioral effects measured in the open field or roto-rod tests may be more relevant to gross behavioral side effects in humans (e.g., inability to walk, impairment of motor coordination, muscle weakness, somnolence). These measures do not reproduce subtle behavioral effects of concern in epileptic patients. For example, testing for the effects of AEDs on cognitive functions and comorbid neuropsychiatric disorders is labor intensive and is not routinely done. Rare examples of such studies can be found in the literature (Higgins *et al.* 2010; Hudzik and Palmer 1995; Picker *et al.* 1985; Renfrey *et al.* 1989; Shannon and Love 2004, 2005, 2007). Sophisticated behavioral assays need to be introduced into the screening programs to characterize NCEs more comprehensively, rather than focusing on simple motor function impairment. It would be very beneficial to extend testing of NCEs for their potentially bidirectional effects on cognition, depression, and anxiety, as well as others.

Strategies for discovery of new antiepileptic drugs

Three major approaches are used to identify new AEDs: (1) random screening of NCEs, (2) structural derivatives of approved AEDs, and (3) rational, target-based drug discovery and optimization. Success stories are associated with each of the three approaches. Random screening has been employed successfully to discover most of the classic and several second-generation AEDs. Phenytoin represents the first AED approved in humans based on its efficacy in preclinical testing. Phenytoin emerged from the search for nonsedating barbiturates and demonstrated efficacy in the MES test and then in human generalized tonic-clonic seizures. Carbamazepine was discovered about 20 years later. Another classic AED, valproate, was discovered based on its efficacy in the subcutaneous PTZ test. As discussed earlier, the MES and subcutaneous PTZ tests have been instrumental in discovering many AEDs; however, this approach carries many limitations as exemplified by the experience with levetiracetam.

Developing derivatives of the existing AEDs has been successful in the search for safer and more efficacious AEDs (Bialer *et al.* 2009). This approach yielded drugs such as trimethadione, ethosuximide, and fosphenytoin (structural analogs of phenytoin) and oxcarbamazepine and eslicarbazepine (structural analogs of carbamazepine). Structural analogs of several second-generation AEDs also yielded new and promising AEDs. For example, JZP-4 and brivaracetam are structural analogs of lamotrigine and levetiracetam, respectively. In many cases, these structural analogs not only offer improved side-effect and efficacy profiles but also display different mechanisms of action (Bialer *et al.* 2009; Landmark and Johannessen 2008). Conversely, however, this approach might also be misleading because focusing on only one target mechanism of action and identifying follow-up compounds with higher binding affinity to this receptor does not take into account the multifaceted nature of the disease itself and our limited understanding of which of the many modes of action of an individual AED contributes most to its clinical efficacy.

A better understanding of the pharmacological mechanisms that are involved in ictal activity and that are responsible for the anticonvulsant properties of AEDs resulted in an effort to optimize NCEs for their activities at selected pharmacological targets. Most activity in this regard was focused on either enhancing GABAergic inhibitory neurotransmission or decreasing excitatory neurotransmission. Rational, target-based drug discovery and optimization has not been as successful as the other two approaches, perhaps with the exception of vigabatrin, which was specifically developed to increase brain levels of GABA. The compound is a selective, irreversible inhibitor of the GABA transaminase that by inhibiting the enzyme that breaks down GABA in the synaptic cleft can effectively make this inhibitory neurotransmitter more available to its receptor site.

The targeted discovery approach has proved less useful because epilepsy encompasses a vastly divergent group of symptoms with episodic abnormal electrical activity often being the only common feature. Thus, we should expect that not one but many different mechanisms of action can be simultaneously involved in seizure activity and different pharmacological mechanisms can be differently affected in different types of epilepsy. It is not surprising therefore that all clinically available AEDs display multiple mechanisms of action. Likewise, polytherapy is routinely used in order to improve the outcome of epilepsy treatment. Perhaps the only exception to this rule is the newly developed analog of levetiracetam, brivaracetam, which was optimized for its activity at a high-affinity ligand for the synaptic vesicle protein, SV2A (Matagne *et al.* 2008; Rogawski 2008). Because the role of SV2A in epilepsy and seizure activity is still not well understood, other mechanisms of action (e.g., sodium channels blockade) may be involved in the net anticonvulsant effects of brivaracetam. Mixed negative and positive results from phase III studies of this compound have recently been published, calling target discovery and its predictive validity further into question (Briton *et al.* 2010).

Another example of a targeted discovery effort is related to inherited epileptic syndromes. The ability to use novel and more cost-effective sequencing approaches has led to the discovery of several genes that predispose for heritable forms of epilepsies and other CNS disorders. The most prominent examples are probably the mutations of genes coding for the CNS-specific voltage-gated sodium channel alpha1 subunit gene (SCN1A), which lead not only to seizure syndromes but also to familial hemiplegic migraine. Gain-of-function missense mutations in the brain type I sodium channel $Na_V1.1$ are a primary cause of generalized epilepsy with febrile seizures plus (GEFS+). Loss-of-function mutations in $Na_V1.1$ channels cause severe myoclonic epilepsy of infancy, an intractable childhood epilepsy (Catterall *et al.* 2008). Recently developed animal models of *SCN1A* mutants have demonstrated that the downstream effects are cell type-dependent and that some mutations can lead to a reduction in interneuron excitability, which, if located on inhibitory interneurons, might contribute to overexcitation and may therefore explain the pathophysiological correlate of the condition (Tang *et al.* 2009). For future drug development we will need to completely understand the pathways that lead from the genotype to the phenotype of the disease, before reasonable targets amenable to pharmacological interventions can be identified. The example cited above signifies again the complexity of epilepsy itself and the issue of how to target a specific neuronal population without interfering with other networks.

Preclinical assessment of seizure liability

Many psychoactive drugs can affect an individual's sensitivity to seizures and carry black box warnings for their seizure liability (e.g., the antipsychotic clozapine). These proconvulsant properties of drugs are particularly important for patients with epilepsy and individuals at a high risk of seizures due to predisposing factors (e.g., neurodevelopmental abnormalities, severe head trauma, cerebrovascular diseases, cerebral tumors, substance abuse, or family history of epilepsy). Seizure tests can be used to identify proconvulsant properties of NCEs or the existing approved medications (Easter *et al.* 2009; Giardina and Gasior 2009; Löscher 2009). The preclinical seizure risk assessment is typically done by employing modified versions of the traditional MES and subcutaneous PTZ tests, which allows for the detection of both pro- and anticonvulsant properties. It is not rare that certain psychoactive drugs (e.g., some antipsychotic agents) display anticonvulsant effects at lower doses and proconvulsant effects at higher doses (Löscher 2009).

Proconvulsant effects are also relevant for drugs considered as AEDs. For example, phenobarbital, tiagabine, or vigabatrin can block seizures in the subcutaneous PTZ test but exacerbate seizures in generalized absence models (White 2003).

Beyond small molecules for epilepsy treatment

Treatment of epilepsy has been dominated by small-molecule AEDs since the discovery of the anticonvulsant properties of bromide, and 25 such drugs are now approved. However, other nonpharmacological approaches are gaining attention. Several approaches may offer therapeutic benefit when small molecule-based therapies are ineffective (Rogawski and Holmes 2009). Such approaches include, for example, brain stimulation and cooling, cell and gene therapies, novel methods to deliver therapeutics either peripherally (e.g., rapid intranasal delivery for emergency treatments) or directly into the epileptic zone (e.g., convection delivery method), and hormonal therapies for specific types of epilepsy (e.g., progesterone and its metabolites, neuroactive steroids for catamenial epilepsy associated with menstrual exacerbation of seizures), and dietary therapies (ketogenic diet for refractory epilepsy). Stimulation of the vagal nerve has also proven to be efficacious in some patients. Many of these approaches are still at early stages of preclinical development (e.g., cell and gene therapies) whereas others have already been successfully used in patients with epilepsy (e.g., vagal nerve stimulation or ketogenic diet). These methods are likely to offer therapeutic benefit when pharmacological treatments fail. The ketogenic diet not only is effective in drug-resistant epilepsy but may also offer long-term neuroprotective and disease-modifying benefits after it is discontinued (Gasior *et al.* 2006; Kossoff and Rho 2009). From a translational point of view, ketogenic diet research is extremely promising. Building on the clinical proof of concept for the efficacy of the ketogenic diet in drug-resistant epilepsy and its potential disease-modifying long-term effects in humans, an extensive effort has been directed into preclinical study of the effects of the ketogenic diet at in vitro and in vivo levels. Such an effort can aid the discovery of novel targets for anticonvulsant or antiepileptogenic drugs. Ketogenic diet-initiated research has already identified novel therapeutic approaches for treating epilepsy that interfere with the body's glucose and ketone metabolism (Lian *et al.* 2007; Stafstrom *et al.* 2009), mechanisms not typically targeted by the known AEDs.

Researchers are also seeking better understanding of inflammatory processes and how they contribute to epileptogenesis (Vezzani and Granata 2005). Recently developed epilepsy models use procedures that induce massive CNS inflammation (e.g., a newly developed model for infantile spasms; Scantlebury *et al.* 2009), and in models of status epilepticus pilocarpine has been shown to compromise the blood–brain barrier and stimulate the adhesion of white blood cells that contribute to seizure aggravation (Fabene *et al.* 2008). Progress will depend on understanding the immunomodulatory effects of novel targets and the involvement of these pathways.

Antiepileptic drugs for the treatment of nonepileptic conditions

Many AEDs are commonly prescribed for a variety of nonepileptic indications (Rogawski and Löscher 2004*b*). Clinical efficacy has been demonstrated for many AEDs for managing neuropathic pain and trigeminal neuralgia, migraine prophylaxis, neuromuscular disorders (essential tremor, myotonia, myokymia, restless leg syndrome, or dystonia), and psychiatric disorders (insomnia, anxiety, bipolar disorders, or substance abuse) (Rogawski and Löscher 2004*b*). In these medical conditions, as in epilepsy, the AEDs interfere with the impaired balance between excitatory and inhibitory neurotransmission, affect targets that are pathologically changed, or interfere with mechanisms involved in neuronal plasticity. Because many overlapping molecular mechanisms are involved in these conditions and epilepsy, we can reasonably predict that any new AED might also be effective in one or several nonepileptic conditions. Therefore, almost all new candidate AEDs are now additionally evaluated in preclinical models predictive of efficacy in pain, neuromuscular, or psychiatric disorders, as the other chapters of this book describe.

Translating into humans: proof-of-concept studies, regulatory pathways, and future directions

Proof-of-concept studies

Once preclinical models have identified suitable NCEs, the next hurdle and translational challenge is the clinical development of new drug candidates. After the preclinical toxicology program has been passed, initial single and multiple ascending dose studies have demonstrated adequate tolerability, and no apparent safety issues have arisen, a drug candidate may advance further into the clinic. Initially a proof-of-concept (POC) or a phase IIa trial may be performed to evaluate efficacy under clinical conditions.

The following criteria should routinely be used in the design of adequate POC studies in general and in epilepsy specifically.

Positive predictive value

Positive predictive value is the ability of a clinical trial to predict efficacy of the phase III studies and ultimately to predict regulatory approval. Because the regulatory pathway for new drug applications requires the demonstration of efficacy as adjunctive treatment of partial-onset seizures (see "Regulatory pathways and requirements"), POC models that are relevant surrogates of the standard seizure rate reduction end point should be kept in mind. Over the past decades, acute efficacy in POCs has usually translated well into long-term effects of AEDs. POCs with a low positive predictive value can be very misleading, as they might lead to further investment in an NCE that is useless. The ability to predict efficacy accurately is arguably the most important criterion by which to judge a POC design. The initial POC does not necessarily reflect the target population, nor does it necessarily have the same end point or trial conditions of a regulatory trial.

Negative predictive value

Negative predictive value is the ability of a POC to adequately and with high certainty predict that a potential NCE does not work in the condition tested.

The second most important attribute of a good POC is its ability to rule out the possibility that a compound will ever be a successful epilepsy drug if the POC results are negative. POCs with a low negative predictive value might exclude compounds from being developed that fail the POC although in reality they might be very efficacious.

Low cost
Keeping the initial cost for a POC study low will allow for a more streamlined development and may facilitate the simultaneous evaluation of an NCE in several POCs for different disease areas, which ultimately leads to a more cost-efficient research and development process. Because study costs are related to the number of subjects, visits, and trial-related procedures, expensive diagnostics and examinations (e.g., imaging, long-term EEGs, hospitalizations) should be avoided if possible.

Adequate timelines
The shorter the exposure of patients to a potentially useless or even harmful new compound the better. Timing also relates to the ease and speed of recruitment into the clinical trial. High prevalence rates of the subpopulation of epilepsy patients recruited are beneficial and will facilitate study enrollment. Unrestrictive inclusion and exclusion criteria as well as a high unmet medical need for novel compounds due to limited treatment alternatives can be incentives for patients to participate in a trial.

Ability to predict the final dose
Dose-ranging studies are usually phase II studies, but the necessity to slowly titrate most AEDs in order to alleviate CNS side effects may provide a welcome opportunity to investigate the differential effects of different dosages on the primary end point already during the POC study. Subjects with a high seizure frequency might show a dose-related decrease that can potentially be evaluated during the slow uptitration. Information regarding adequate target dosages will ultimately facilitate the design of the phase II program.

Ability to learn about potential efficacy in other indications
Antiepileptic drugs are usually efficacious in multiple CNS diseases. Patients with epilepsy also have a high rate of comorbid conditions. Through intelligent trial design and careful patient selection, combined with detailed assessment of potential positive effects on some of these conditions, a POC can help generate evidence for efficacy in other disease areas. Benefits may be documented in mood enhancement, headache or migraine frequency, or neuropathic pain or substance abuse (alcohol or nicotine). A qualitative appraisal of these diverse end points can be potentially revealing.

Ability to learn about additional product properties
Drugs sometimes have beneficial effects that are not related to their primary efficacy on seizures but are valuable product attributes that warrant further exploration. A POC trial may provide the first opportunity to learn about these beneficial effects. Patient-reported outcome scales as well as so-called exit interviews have proven useful to identify favorable effects that subjects notice during their exposure to the medication. The weight loss related to topiramate is a good example of a side effect that was perceived as beneficial by some patients. Other favorable effects include the mood-elevating or antianxiety properties of certain AEDs. Ultimately the side effects of an NCE as well as its positive attributes are important differentiators in the marketplace, especially if the primary end point of regulatory trials is as rigid as seizure frequency reduction and leaves little room for further differentiation.

Availability of comparative data (either active or historical)
In a highly competitive marketplace such as epilepsy drugs, the effect size of a novel AED should be classified early in development to avoid investment in "me too" compounds. Ideally a POC study should include an active comparator with known efficacy and performance, or the trial design should be standardized in a way that allows comparison with historical control data to make early inferences regarding the magnitude of effect.

Designing POCs that optimally fulfill all the criteria described here is difficult if not impossible. Recently several companies have used a rare form of seizure disorders, photosensitive epilepsy, as a preferred POC model (Trenite *et al.* 2007). Patients with photoparoxysmal responses to flicker-light or intermittent photic stimulation (IPS) are being evaluated in a nonrandomized, single-blind, placebo-controlled fashion through exposure to single ascending dosages of new AEDs. The study subjects are characterized by a predictable response to standardized IPS and a positive efficacy signal constitutes a suppression in their photosensitivity leading to a complete abolition of the typical EEG synchronization over the occipital brain regions. Typically the suppression is seen at or around the time of peak plasma drug levels and can be long-lasting, with clinically significant reductions in photosensitivity observed as long as 24 hours after exposure. This POC also has the benefit of providing clear evidence for blood–brain barrier penetration and usually uses low patient numbers (approximately 20–30 subjects). How predictive this model is for efficacy against nongeneralized seizure types is unclear.

Several other POC designs have been used and suggested over the past decade. The structured dose escalation trial evaluates the seizure frequency in patients with refractory epilepsy who have a very high and predictable seizure rate during uptitration of the test drug to the maximum tolerated dose (usually weekly increments). This model has several disadvantages, mainly the atypical patient population, a potential regression to the mean, the natural fluctuation of seizure activity, and the short titration and limited exposure to the compound, in addition to the small sample sizes.

Presurgical POC studies rely on hospitalized patients who are rapidly withdrawn from their baseline AEDs in order to facilitate evaluation for surgical removal or isolation of the epileptic focus. These subjects can be randomly allocated to receive a test compound or placebo and fixed criteria related to the seizure or EEG improvement can be used as outcome parameters. Other end points can relate to the percent of patients staying or becoming seizure-free. This POC is hampered mainly by the availability of patients as well as by the diverse nature of individual patients' situations and seizure propensities. Also, the duration of hospitalization or surgical evaluation might not be sufficiently long to achieve adequate dosages, further limiting the utility of this model.

Patients with frequent interictal EEG activity may be recruited for study using another POC model. Focal or generalized interictal spike-wave discharges can function as a surrogate marker for seizure activity or for efficacy in a crossover fashion vs. placebo or compared with baseline. The primary outcome would be the number of spike counts obtained during a standard observation interval. Downsides of this model include the heterogeneity of the study population and the high and rapid intraindividual and diurnal variability in combination with unproven clinical validity.

Transcranial magnetic stimulation (TMS) has also been suggested as a tool to measure the state of neuronal hyperexcitability of cortical interneurons. The minimal threshold for motor responses, the amplitude, the silence period, and the intracortical inhibition can potentially be used in healthy volunteers as surrogate markers for brain excitability after single or paired pulses are applied over the motor cortex. The pattern of TMS evoked responses is unfortunately highly variable and the relevance of findings in healthy volunteers may have limited predictive value in epilepsy.

The time to nth seizure design is a dose-ranging study with a different end point that facilitates a faster efficacy evaluation of individual patients, but it is not necessarily a true POC. The trial design resembles a standard placebo-controlled fixed dose-ranging study with a different end point. Instead of seizure reduction, the time to the occurrence of the nth seizure (usually the fourth to sixth seizure event) has been suggested as a primary end point (Dichter 2007). The study design takes advantage of the fact that AEDs usually work rapidly and that initial signs of efficacy can potentially be detected early during titration through a shift in the interval between adjacent seizure events. Instead of recording a prospective baseline seizure rate and comparing it with the double-blind phase of the treatment period, the time to nth seizure design does not require a baseline period and the study population is less restricted, thereby facilitating enrollment. Reanalysis of prior study data with this new end point suggests that the sample size necessary to provide enough power to detect significant efficacy must be slightly larger than in standard phase II designs, while the trial duration is appreciably shorter due to the lack of a 4- to 8-week baseline period and a shorter double-blind phase of about 6 instead of 12 weeks. The downside of this approach is the slightly greater sample size, the lack of historical control data, and the unfamiliarity with the end point, which make it more difficult to interpret the results. Also, compounds that have a slower onset of efficacy or that must be titrated to effect will be unduly disadvantaged with this design.

Regulatory pathways and requirements

After the initial POC, drug development in epilepsy follows strict regulatory guidelines and a sequenced approach of standard trials. Both the US Food and Drug Administration (FDA) and the European authorities require clear evidence of efficacy and a positive risk–benefit evaluation including replication and evidence of incremental dose response demonstrated in epilepsy patients with refractory partial-onset seizures (temporal lobe epilepsy, simple partial motor seizures with and without secondary generalization). Study subjects must remain on their baseline AED regimen, which is presumably optimal but still insufficient to control seizures, and the novel AED must include a substantial additional seizure reduction compared with placebo over the treatment duration of 3–4 months. Subjects currently enrolling in these standard trials are usually about 30–40 years of age, with their epilepsy diagnosed approximately 15–20 years previously; an average of 5–9 prior AEDs have failed in their treatment and they are on 1–3 baseline AEDs. Their mean baseline seizure frequency is about 8–10 seizures per month, with a slightly lower median number of baseline seizures. A meaningful improvement required for FDA approval is defined as a substantial seizure reduction, compared with the prospective baseline (usually 2 months in duration) over placebo. European authorities require a substantial elevation of the responder rate compared with placebo treatment. Responders are defined as patients who experience at least a 50% reduction in their mean or median monthly seizure counts compared with baseline. The exposure of the study subjects to placebo for an extended duration (5–6 months) can be justified only by the fact that patients have presumably already exhausted all other potential treatment options and "tested" a fair number of available drugs, before being eligible for experimental drugs. Only after initial proof of efficacy in this difficult-to-treat patient population are regulatory agencies willing to allow the exploration of NCEs in generalized forms of epilepsy (e.g., tonic-clonic seizures) or the development of a monotherapy indication through additional large studies.

Special requirements also apply to studies in children and infants. Monotherapy studies follow three different design pathways depending on the regulatory body governing the development. The FDA does require placebo-controlled designs, which imposes the ethical dilemma of exposing a patient with newly diagnosed epilepsy to placebo and leaving him or her unprotected. Because of this restriction, researchers have used low, presumably minimally effective, dosages of the compound under investigation, so-called pseudo-placebo. The efficacy of this low dose will then be compared with the standard dose and the time to the first seizure will be used as an end point using a Kaplan–Meier survival analysis approach. Recently the FDA has agreed to also accept "placebo-less" trial designs as long as they use a patient population and a trial design that allow a comparison with historical controls. Regulatory bodies in Europe prohibit the use of placebo and demand active controls in monotherapy studies. For this reason a novel compound in Europe is compared in a noninferiority design against a standard monotherapy drug, usually carbamazepine or valproate, using the time-to-first-seizure end point. In addition, complex pediatric investigational plans must be negotiated and agreed upon prior to the filing of a new drug application in Europe.

Because of these regulations and requirements, proof of efficacy in the adjunctive treatment of partial-onset seizures has become a bottleneck in the costly development of new AEDs. Furthermore, due to the restrictive inclusion and exclusion criteria and the number of drugs currently in development, the pool of potential subjects for regulatory trials can be quite limited. Because of the tight timelines, companies have started to recruit subjects in a multitude of different countries and cultures. Accordingly the variability of the data has increased and the study population is less homogeneous than 20 years ago. As a consequence of increased confidence intervals, the sample size grew in order to preserve adequate power and the number of investigators per trial doubled or tripled, making it more important to select adequate study sites with well-trained personnel. Another phenomenon observed in recent AED trials is the "refractoriness creep" within the patient population available for drug trials. Over the past decade, patients with epilepsy have benefitted from the introduction of multiple new compounds with diverse modes of action. Presumably twenty-first century patients in whom six AEDs have failed are only partially comparable to similar subjects 20 to 30 years ago, when limited treatment choice affected the quality of care. Because of this and other factors, the average net-over-placebo gain in seizure reduction has decreased steadily over the past decade, making it increasingly difficult and expensive to develop novel compounds for patients with epilepsy. Because of the limited patient pool and the low drug share a compound can summon over its life cycle, pharmaceutical companies have unfortunately started to shift focus from epilepsy to other more "attractive" indications that AEDs can serve, such as neuropathic pain or psychiatric indications. This trend needs to be reversed.

Future directions

Novel approaches are needed to identify target treatment options that lead to improved effectiveness compared with our currently available treatment options. Science must guide the way from symptomatic treatments that suppress seizures toward approaches that affect the underlying condition. Future challenges are related to advances in antiepileptogenesis, disease modification, pharmacoresistance, and targeted treatment approaches addressing certain subpopulations determined, for example, by the genetic underpinning of their epilepsy (e.g., genetically determined idiopathic epilepsies).

Novel clinical trial designs should dovetail with the preclinical research but such designs are often difficult to establish. The following trial methodology questions must be answered to design adequate studies of disease-modifying or antiepileptogenic properties in the clinical setting in the future:

Which population should be studied?
How homogeneous can the study population be?
What are the right inclusion and exclusion criteria?
What is the appropriate sample size?
Which dose is sufficient?
When should prophylactic treatment start?
What is the therapeutic window of opportunity?
What is the length of the treatment and the observation period?
Which end points can be used that are meaningful and will ultimately be accepted as evidence for disease modification by regulatory agencies?
How can functional recovery be evaluated systematically?
Is there enough equipoise for a certain trial design?
Will the study be ethically sound?
How can logistical hurdles that might hamper trial execution be overcome?
Is an active comparator or placebo as control acceptable and/or necessary?
Which markers clearly define a study population at risk for the development of epilepsy or its progression?
Which EEG and imaging technologies can be used as potential surrogate markers?
Should a POC or definitive trial be conducted?

Multiple attempts have been made to evaluate whether early treatment with AEDs has protective effects against the development of epilepsy in several human models of epileptogenesis. The most prominent model that has been used is TBI. Based on preclinical evidence, researchers hypothesized not only that early posttraumatic treatment with AEDs could prevent acute trauma-induced seizures but also that prolonged exposure could prevent the development of posttraumatic epilepsy itself.

Advantages of the TBI model

Relatively well-defined risk.
Large numbers of patients.
Possible in single center.
2-year follow-up seems sufficient.
Precedents in literature.
Mostly younger population.
Animal models exist.

Disadvantages of the TBI model

Multiple traumas can cause complications.
Informed consent may be difficult if treatment is immediate.
Use of additional drug and procedures.
Requires interactions with multiple departments.
Follow-up can be problematic.
Multiple procedures early can interfere with monitoring.
Cognitive/behavioral issues need close monitoring.

Clinical studies have evaluated the efficacy of phenytoin, phenobarbital, valproic acid, and carbamazepine in the prevention of late posttraumatic seizures or epilepsy (Temkin 2009). Many of the studies initiated treatment within 24 hours of injury, and the duration of treatment ranged from 1 week to 2 years. Follow-up continued for 6 months to 3 years after the injury. The majority of studies included patients considered at high risk for posttraumatic seizures (i.e., patients with penetrating injuries, depressed skull fractures, subdural hematomas, or seizures within the first week after injury). The bulk of evidence shows that although these AEDs reduce the incidence of early seizures relative to placebo, none reduces the incidence of late posttraumatic seizures, and therefore the routine use of prophylactic AEDs beyond the first week after injury is not supported by the current evidence.

Other models of antiepileptogenesis that have been investigated to a lesser extent with, unfortunately, also mainly negative outcome include brain tumors, craniotomy, hypoxic-ischemic brain injury (perinatal hypoxia, hypoxic-ischemic encephalopathy), and febrile seizures. More work needs to be done to adequately translate preclinical findings into the right human models, and AEDs may ultimately not be the right compounds to interfere with the underlying pathophysiological pathways of the epileptogenic process.

Ideal characteristics for a POC study in disease modification/antiepileptogenesis are a relatively common event that facilitates the accessibility of patients, the homogeneity of the disease group, a predictable and high risk for worsening, surrogate markers or risk factors that reliably predict or indicate disease progression or worsening, the ability to interfere with underlying pathology, a short latency, absence of secondary issues (no recovery from other processes; no concurrent illness; no progressive condition underlying epilepsy), and an adult patient population to be studied.

The use of novel biomarkers may in the future help to design adequate and successful clinical trials. A nonexhaustive list of potential biomarkers that could be used not only to measure the risk for progression or epileptogenesis but also as primary or secondary outcome parameters includes the following:

Electrophysiology

- Early spikes.
- Subclinical seizures.
- Interictal spikes.
- High-frequency oscillations.
- Excitability marker.

Imaging

- Hippocampal sclerosis.
- Changes in fiber tract trajectories.
- Magnetoencephalography.

Biochemical

- Proteomics.
- Inflammatory markers.
- Markers for acute vs. continuing neuronal damage.

An encouraging development in recent years points toward our ability to potentially translate appropriately "from bedside to bench to bedside." Tuberous sclerosis is an autosomal dominant inherited disease that predisposes, among other symptoms, to the development of subependymal giant-cell astrocytomas. This disease has become a good example of how advances in our understanding of the underlying pathophysiology can lead to the development of adequate animal models and how the exploration of pathways and the identification of potential drug candidates might successfully be translated into disease-modifying treatments (Wong 2010). Patients with tuberous sclerosis have a loss of *TSC1* and *TSC2* gene function and their corresponding proteins TSC1 (hamartin) and TSC2 (tuberin), a loss that in knock-out animals is directly related to enhanced cell size, altered cell proliferation, and abnormal organogenesis. The loss of TSC1 or TSC2 protein function leads to constitutive activation of the mammalian target of rapamycin (mTOR) cascade, which governs the regulation of cell growth. Activated mTOR serves as a kinase and phosphorylates several downstream proteins. Proteins in this cascade exert control over cell size, via regulation of gene transcription and protein translation, and are responsible for the pathogenesis of the tuberous sclerosis complex. In mouse models of tuberous sclerosis complex, mTOR inhibitors prevent the development of epilepsy and underlying brain abnormalities associated with epileptogenesis. The macrolide antibiotic rapamycin, a powerful inhibitor of mTOR, has shown positive effects in several in vitro and in vivo studies of tuberous sclerosis complex. In addition there is evidence that mTOR-inhibition with rapamycin also suppresses seizure activity in acquired epilepsy models (pilocarpine) in which seizure acquisition had already been established, raising the possibility of an expanded therapeutic window for this disease-modifying treatment approach (Huang *et al.* 2010). Encouraging results with everolimus, a rapamycin derivative approved for the treatment of certain cancers, from a recent single-arm, open-label study in 28 patients with tuberous sclerosis showed a clinically meaningful reduction in volume of primary subependymal giant-cell astrocytomas and an improvement in seizure frequency (Krueger *et al.* 2010). Based on these findings, the FDA granted an orphan drug approval for the use of the mTOR inhibitor everolimus for patients with subependymal giant-cell astrocytomas associated with tuberous sclerosis. This example of successful bedside-to-bench-to-bedside translational research underlines the importance of the integration of translational medicine in our attempt to develop meaningful new therapeutic options for patients with epilepsy.

Conclusions

Epilepsy constitutes a complex and heterogeneous group of diseases with the common symptom of recurrent unprovoked seizures. Animal models have led to a better understanding of the underlying pathology of epilepsy and have been valuable in the identification of AEDs that downregulate pathological excitation or upregulate inhibitory pathways. Seizure tests as well as epilepsy models have a high translational value and good face validity. In the past, most AEDs were identified through screening batteries without concrete knowledge of their mode of action. Recently, several drug targets related to neuronal ion channels and neurotransmitter systems have been identified, furthering the discovery of NCEs with better tolerability and efficacy profiles.

Thus far neuronal targets have been the focus of model development, but other brain cells (glia and microglia) certain to also play important roles in signal transduction and the formation of epileptic circuits must be targeted. Because patients with refractory disease usually need combination therapy, models must be developed that help predict potential synergistic or antagonistic pharmacodynamic interactions of novel compounds given together with older AEDs. Furthermore, novel models need to be developed and validated to facilitate the discovery of compounds with some of the following characteristics: disease modification and antiepileptogenesis; utility in special epilepsy syndromes and childhood epilepsies; ability to affect comorbid conditions; and exceptional side-effect profiles, especially related to cognitive and behavioral adverse events.

The adequate design of proof-of-concept studies is difficult and multifaceted, and because the clinical development process of AEDs is strictly regulated, historical approaches leave limited room for product differentiation. Future clinical trial designs should be developed that better facilitate the evaluation of potential disease-modifying and antiepileptogenic drugs that fulfill high unmet medical needs. Tuberous sclerosis has been shown to be the first disease leading to epilepsy in which a successful development of a disease-modifying treatment approach has come to fruition. These results follow unsuccessful attempts to achieve the same goal in TBI.

References

Barton ME, Klein BD, Wolf HH, White HS. 2001. Pharmacological characterization of the 6 Hz psychomotor seizure model of partial epilepsy. *Epilepsy Res* 47:217–227.

Barton ME, Peters SC, Shannon HE. 2003. Comparison of the effect of glutamate receptor modulators in the 6 Hz and maximal electroshock seizure models. *Epilepsy Res* 56:17–26.

Bernard C. 2006. Hippocampal slices: designing and interpreting studies in epilepsy research. In *Models of Seizures and Epilepsy*. Pitkanen A, Schwartzkroin PA, Moshe SL, eds. New York: Elsevier Academic Press, pp. 59–72.

Bialer M, Johannessen SI, Levy RH *et al.* 2009. Progress report on new antiepileptic drugs: a summary of the Ninth Eilat Conference (EILAT IX). *Epilepsy Res* 83:1–43.

Bialer M, White HS. 2010. Key factors in the discovery and development of new antiepileptic drugs. *Nat Rev Drug Discov* 9:68–82.

Brandt C, Volk HA, Löscher W. 2004. Striking differences in individual anticonvulsant response to phenobarbital in rats with spontaneous seizures after status epilepticus. *Epilepsia* 45:1488–1497.

Briton V, Werhahn K, Johnson M *et al.* 2010. Brivaracetam as adjunctive treatment of refractory partial-onset seizures in adults: results from two randomized, double-blind, placebo-controlled trials [abstract]. *Epilepsia* 50S11 (106): abstract 1.216.

Catterall WA, Dib-Hajj S, Meisler MH, Pietrobon D. 2008. Inherited neuronal ion channelopathies: new windows on complex neurological diseases. *J Neurosci* 28:11768–11777.

Coenen AM, Van Luijtelaar EL. 2003. Genetic animal models for absence epilepsy: a review of the WAG/Rij strain of rats. *Behav Genet* 33:635–655.

Curia G, Longo D, Biagini G, Jones RSG, Avoli M. 2008. The pilocarpine model of temporal lobe epilepsy. *J Neurosci Methods* 172:143–157.

Czuczwar SJ, Borowicz KK. 2002. Polytherapy in epilepsy: the experimental evidence. *Epilepsy Res* **52**:15–23.

Czuczwar SJ, Kaplanski J, Swiderska-Dziewit G et al. 2009. Pharmacodynamic interactions between antiepileptic drugs: preclinical data based on isobolography. *Expert Opin Drug Metab Toxicol* **5**:131–136.

Deckers CL, Czuczwar SJ, Hekster YA et al. 2000. Selection of antiepileptic drug polytherapy based on mechanisms of action: the evidence reviewed. *Epilepsia* **41**:1364–1374.

Dichter MA. 2006. Models of epileptogenesis in adult animals available for antiepileptogenesis drug screening. *Epilepsy Res* **68**:31–35.

Dichter MA. 2007. Innovative clinical trial designs for future antiepileptic drugs. *Epilepsia* **48** (Suppl. 1):26–30.

Dichter MA, Pollard J. 2006. Cell culture models for studying epilepsy. In *Models of Seizures and Epilepsy*. Pitkanen A, Schwartzkroin PA, Moshe SL, eds. New York: Elsevier Academic Press, pp. 23–34.

Duncan JS, Sander JW, Sisodiya SM, Walker MC. 2006. Adult epilepsy. *Lancet* **367**:1087–1100.

Durand D. 1993. Ictal patterns in experimental models of epilepsy. *J Clin Neurophysiol* **10**:281–297.

Easter A, Bell ME, Damewood J et al. 2009. Approaches to seizure risk assessment in preclinical drug discovery. *Drug Discov Today* **14**:876–884.

Engel J Jr. 1995. Critical evaluation of animal models for localization-related epilepsies. *Ital J Neurol Sci* **16**:9–16.

Engel J Jr. 2001. A proposed diagnostic scheme for people with epileptic seizures and with epilepsy: report of the ILAE Task Force on Classification and Terminology. *Epilepsia* **42**:796–803.

Fabene PF, Mora GN, Martinello M et al. 2008. A role for leukocyte-endothelial adhesion mechanisms in epilepsy. *Nat Med* **14**:1377–1383.

Fisher RS. 1989. Animal models of the epilepsies. *Brain Res Brain Res Rev* **14**:245–278.

Fisher RS, van Emde BW, Blume W et al. 2005. Epileptic seizures and epilepsy: definitions proposed by the International League Against Epilepsy (ILAE) and the International Bureau for Epilepsy (IBE). *Epilepsia* **46**:470–472.

Fonck C, Cohen BN, Nashmi R et al. 2005. Novel seizure phenotype and sleep disruptions in knock-in mice with hypersensitive alpha 4* nicotinic receptors. *J Neurosci* **25**:11396–11411.

Forsgren L, Beghi E, Oun A, Sillanpaa M. 2005. The epidemiology of epilepsy in Europe: a systematic review. *Eur J Neurol* **12**:245–253.

Frankel WN. 2009. Genetics of complex neurological disease: challenges and opportunities for modeling epilepsy in mice and rats. *Trends Genet* **25**:361–367.

Gaitatzis A, Johnson AL, Chadwick DW, Shorvon SD, Sander JW. 2004. Life expectancy in people with newly diagnosed epilepsy. *Brain* **127**:2427–2432.

Gaitatzis A, Sander JW. 2004. The mortality of epilepsy revisited. *Epileptic Disord* **6**:3–13.

Gasior M, Rogawski MA, Hartman AL. 2006. Neuroprotective and disease-modifying effects of the ketogenic diet. *Behav Pharmacol* **17**:431–439.

Giardina WJ, Gasior M. 2009. Acute seizure tests in epilepsy research: electroshock- and chemical-induced convulsions in the mouse. *Curr Protoc Pharmacol* **45**:5.22.1–5.22.37.

Glien M, Brandt C, Potschka H, Löscher W. 2002. Effects of the novel antiepileptic drug levetiracetam on spontaneous recurrent seizures in the rat pilocarpine model of temporal lobe epilepsy. *Epilepsia* **43**:350–357.

Grabenstatter HL, Ferraro DJ, Williams PA, Chapman PL, Dudek FE. 2005. Use of chronic epilepsy models in antiepileptic drug discovery: the effect of topiramate on spontaneous motor seizures in rats with kainate-induced epilepsy. *Epilepsia* **46**:8–14.

Hartman AL, Gasior M, Vining EP, Rogawski MA. 2007. The neuropharmacology of the ketogenic diet. *Pediatr Neurol* **36**:281–292.

Hartman AL, Lyle M, Rogawski MA, Gasior M. 2008. Efficacy of the ketogenic diet in the 6-Hz seizure test. *Epilepsia* **49**:334–339.

Heinemann U, Kann O, Schuchmann S. 2006. An overview of in vitro seizure models in acute and organotypic slices. In *Models of Seizures and Epilepsy*. Pitkanen A, Schwartzkroin PA, Moshe SL, eds. New York: Elsevier Academic Press, pp. 35–44.

Higgins G, Breysse N, Undzys E et al. 2010. Comparative study of five antiepileptic drugs on a translational cognitive measure in the rat: relationship to antiepileptic property. *Psychopharmacology (Berl)* **207**:513–527.

Hirtz D, Thurman DJ, Gwinn-Hardy K et al. 2007. How common are the "common" neurologic disorders? *Neurology* **68**:326–337.

Hosford DA, Clark S, Cao Z et al. 1992. The role of $GABA_B$ receptor activation in absence seizures of lethargic (lh/lh) mice. *Science* **257**:398–401.

Hosford DA, Wang Y. 1997. Utility of the lethargic (lh/lh) mouse model of absence seizures in predicting the effects of lamotrigine, vigabatrin, tiagabine, gabapentin, and topiramate against human absence seizures. *Epilepsia* **38**:408–414.

Huang X, Zhang H, Yang J et al. 2010. Pharmacological inhibition of the mammalian target of rapamycin pathway suppresses acquired epilepsy. *Neurobiol Dis* **40**:193–199.

Hudzik TJ, Palmer GC. 1995. Effects of anticonvulsants in a novel operant learning paradigm in rats: comparison of remacemide hydrochloride and FPL 15896AR to other anticonvulsant agents. *Epilepsy Res* **21**:183–193.

Hughes JR. 1989. The significance of the interictal spike discharge: a review. *J Clin Neurophysiol* **6**:207–226.

Jutila L, Immonen A, Partanen K *et al.* 2002. Neurobiology of epileptogenesis in the temporal lobe. *Adv Tech Stand Neurosurg* **27**:5–22.

Kossoff EH. 2004. More fat and fewer seizures: dietary therapies for epilepsy. *Lancet Neurol* **3**:415–420.

Kossoff EH, Rho JM. 2009. Ketogenic diets: evidence for short- and long-term efficacy. *Neurotherapeutics* **6**:406–414.

Krueger DA, Care MM, Holland K *et al.* 2010. Everolimus for subependymal giant-cell astrocytomas in tuberous sclerosis. *N Engl J Med* **363**:1801–1811.

Kupferberg H. 2001. Animal models used in the screening of antiepileptic drugs. *Epilepsia* **42** (Suppl. 4):7–12.

Kwan P, Brodie MJ. 2000. Early identification of refractory epilepsy. *N Engl J Med* **342**:314–319.

Kwan P, Brodie MJ. 2006. Combination therapy in epilepsy: when and what to use. *Drugs* **66**:1817–1829.

Lagae L. 2006. Cognitive side effects of anti-epileptic drugs. The relevance in childhood epilepsy. *Seizure* **15**:235–241.

Landmark CJ, Johannessen SI. 2008. Modifications of antiepileptic drugs for improved tolerability and efficacy. *Perspect Medicin Chem* **2**:21–39.

Leite JP, Garcia-Cairasco N, Cavalheiro EA. 2002. New insights from the use of pilocarpine and kainate models. *Epilepsy Res* **50**:93–103.

Lhatoo SD, Johnson AL, Goodridge DM *et al.* 2001. Mortality in epilepsy in the first 11 to 14 years after diagnosis: multivariate analysis of a long-term, prospective, population-based cohort. *Ann Neurol* **49**:336–344.

Lian XY, Khan FA, Stringer JL. 2007. Fructose-1,6-bisphosphate has anticonvulsant activity in models of acute seizures in adult rats. *J Neurosci* **27**:12007–12011.

Löscher W. 2002a. Animal models of drug-resistant epilepsy. *Novartis Found Symp* **243**: 149–159.

Löscher W. 2002b. Animal models of epilepsy for the development of antiepileptogenic and disease-modifying drugs. A comparison of the pharmacology of kindling and post-status epilepticus models of temporal lobe epilepsy. *Epilepsy Res* **50**:105–123.

Löscher W. 2009. Preclinical assessment of proconvulsant drug activity and its relevance for predicting adverse events in humans. *Eur J Pharmacol* **610**:1–11.

Löscher W, Nolting B. 1991. The role of technical, biological and pharmacological factors in the laboratory evaluation of anticonvulsant drugs. IV. Protective indices. *Epilepsy Res* **9**:1–10.

Löscher W, Rundfeldt C, Honack D. 1993. Pharmacological characterization of phenytoin-resistant amygdala-kindled rats, a new model of drug-resistant partial epilepsy. *Epilepsy Res* **15**:207–219.

Löscher W, Schmidt D. 2004. New horizons in the development of antiepileptic drugs: the search for new targets. *Epilepsy Res* **60**:77–159.

Manfredi I, Zani AD, Rampoldi L *et al.* 2009. Expression of mutant beta2 nicotinic receptors during development is crucial for epileptogenesis. *Hum Mol Genet* **18**:1075–1088.

Marescaux C, Vergnes M. 1995. Genetic Absence Epilepsy in Rats from Strasbourg (GAERS). *Ital J Neurol Sci* **16**:113–118.

Marini C, Guerrini R. 2007. The role of the nicotinic acetylcholine receptors in sleep-related epilepsy. *Biochem Pharmacol* **74**:1308–1314.

Matagne A, Margineanu DG, Kenda B, Michel P, Klitgaard H. 2008. Anti-convulsive and anti-epileptic properties of brivaracetam (ucb 34714), a high-affinity ligand for the synaptic vesicle protein, SV2A. *Br J Pharmacol* **154**:1662–1671.

Meldrum BS, Rogawski MA. 2007. Molecular targets for antiepileptic drug development. *Neurotherapeutics* **4**:18–61.

Morimoto K, Fahnestock M, Racine RJ. 2004. Kindling and status epilepticus models of epilepsy: rewiring the brain. *Prog Neurobiol* **73**:1–60.

Mullen SA, Scheffer IE. 2009. Translational research in epilepsy genetics: sodium channels in man to interneuronopathy in mouse. *Arch Neurol* **66**:21–26.

Münller CJ, Bankstahl M, Gröticke I, Löscher W. 2009. Pilocarpine vs. lithium-pilocarpine for induction of status epilepticus in mice: development of spontaneous seizures, behavioral alterations and neuronal damage. *Eur J Pharmacol* **619**:15–24.

Patsalos PN, Froscher W, Pisani F, van Rijn CM. 2002. The importance of drug interactions in epilepsy therapy. *Epilepsia* **43**:365–385.

Picker M, Thomas J, Koch C, Poling A. 1985. Effects of phenytoin, phenobarbital, and valproic acid, alone and in selected combinations, on schedule-controlled behavior of rats. *Pharmacol Biochem Behav* **22**:389–393.

Pierce RC, Kalivas PW. 1997. A circuitry model of the expression of behavioral sensitization to amphetamine-like psychostimulants. *Brain Res Brain Res Rev* **25**:192–216.

Pitkanen A, Kharatishvili I, Karhunen H *et al*. 2007. Epileptogenesis in experimental models. *Epilepsia* **48** (Suppl. 2):13–20.

Pitkanen A, Lukasiuk K. 2009. Molecular and cellular basis of epileptogenesis in symptomatic epilepsy. *Epilepsy Behav* **14** (Suppl. 1):16–25.

Post RM, Weiss SR. 1989. Sensitization, kindling, and anticonvulsants in mania. *J Clin Psychiatry* **50** (Suppl.):23–30.

Postma T, Krupp E, Li XL, Post RM, Weiss SR. 2000. Lamotrigine treatment during amygdala-kindled seizure development fails to inhibit seizures and diminishes subsequent anticonvulsant efficacy. *Epilepsia* **41**:1514–1521.

Putnam TJ, Merritt HH. 1937. Experimental determination of the anticonvulsant properties of some phenyl derivatives. *Science* **85**:525–526.

Raggenbass M, Bertrand D. 2002. Nicotinic receptors in circuit excitability and epilepsy. *J Neurobiol* **53**:580–589.

Renfrey G, Schlinger H, Jakubow J, Poling A. 1989. Effects of phenytoin and phenobarbital on schedule-controlled responding and seizure activity in the amygdala-kindled rat. *J Pharmacol Exp Ther* **248**:967–973.

Reynolds EH. 2005. *Atlas: Epilepsy Care in the World*, p. 20 and http://www.who.int/mental_health/neurology/epilepsy/en/index.html, World Health Organization [accessed July 5, 2011].

Rogawski MA. 2006. Molecular targets versus models for new antiepileptic drug discovery. *Epilepsy Res* **68**:22–28.

Rogawski MA. 2008. Brivaracetam: a rational drug discovery success story. *Br J Pharmacol* **154**:1555–1557.

Rogawski MA, Holmes GL. 2009. Nontraditional epilepsy treatment approaches. *Neurotherapeutics* **6**:213–217.

Rogawski MA, Löscher W. 2004a. The neurobiology of antiepileptic drugs. *Nat Rev Neurosci* **5**:553–564.

Rogawski MA, Löscher W. 2004b. The neurobiology of antiepileptic drugs for the treatment of nonepileptic conditions. *Nat Med* **10**:685–692.

Rogawski MA, Porter RJ. 1990. Antiepileptic drugs: pharmacological mechanisms and clinical efficacy with consideration of promising developmental stage compounds. *Pharmacol Rev* **42**:223–286.

Rundfeldt C, Honack D, Löscher W. 1990. Phenytoin potently increases the threshold for focal seizures in amygdala-kindled rats. *Neuropharmacology* **29**:845–851.

Rundfeldt C, Löscher W. 1993. Anticonvulsant efficacy and adverse effects of phenytoin during chronic treatment in amygdala-kindled rats. *J Pharmacol Exp Ther* **266**:216–223.

Sander JW. 2003. The epidemiology of epilepsy revisited. *Curr Opin Neurol* **16**:165–170.

Sander JW. 2004. The use of antiepileptic drugs: principles and practice. *Epilepsia* **45** (Suppl. 6):28–34.

Sarkisian MR. 2001. Overview of the current animal models for human seizure and epileptic disorders. *Epilepsy Behav* **2**:201–216.

Scantlebury MH, Galanopoulou AS, Chudomelova L *et al*. 2009. A model of symptomatic infantile spasms syndrome. *Neurobiol Dis* [epub ahead of print].

Schachter SC. 2002. Epilepsy: Etiology and manifestations. In *Manual of Neurologic Practice*. Evans RW, ed. Philadelphia, PA: WB Saunders, pp. 244–265.

Schmidt D. 1996. Modern management of epilepsy: rational polytherapy. *Baillieres Clin Neurol* **5**:757–763.

Schmitz B. 2006. Effects of antiepileptic drugs on mood and behavior. *Epilepsia* **47** (Suppl. 2):28–33.

Shannon HE, Love PL. 2004. Effects of antiepileptic drugs on working memory as assessed by spatial alternation performance in rats. *Epilepsy Behav* **5**:857–865.

Shannon HE, Love PL. 2005. Effects of antiepileptic drugs on attention as assessed by a five-choice serial reaction time task in rats. *Epilepsy Behav* **7**:620–628.

Shannon HE, Love PL. 2007. Effects of antiepileptic drugs on learning as assessed by a repeated acquisition of response sequences task in rats. *Epilepsy Behav* **10**:16–25.

Sharma AK, Reams RY, Jordan WH *et al*. 2007. Mesial temporal lobe epilepsy: pathogenesis, induced rodent models and lesions. *Toxicol Pathol* **35**:984–999.

Smith M, Wilcox KS, White HS. 2007. Discovery of antiepileptic drugs. *Neurotherapeutics* **4**:12–17.

Smyth MD, Barbaro NM, Baraban SC. 2002. Effects of antiepileptic drugs on induced epileptiform activity in a rat model of dysplasia. *Epilepsy Res* **50**:251–264.

Snead OC III. 1992. Pharmacological models of generalized absence seizures in rodents. *J Neural Transm Suppl* **35**:7–19.

Srivastava D, Franklin MR, Palmer BS, White HS. 2004. Carbamazepine, but not valproate, displays pharmaco-resistance in lamotrigine-resistant kindled rats. *Epilepsia* **45** (Suppl. 7):12.

Srivastava D, Woodhead JH, White HS. 2003. Effects of lamotrigine, carbamazepine and sodium valproate on lamotrigine-resistant kindled rats. *Epilepsia* **44** (Suppl. 9):42.

Stables JP, Bertram E, Dudek FE *et al*. 2003. Therapy discovery for pharmacoresistant epilepsy and for disease-modifying therapeutics: summary of the NIH/NINDS/AES models II workshop. *Epilepsia* **44**:1472–1478.

Stables JP, Bertram EH, White HS *et al*. 2002. Models for epilepsy and epileptogenesis: Report from the NIH Workshop, Bethesda, Maryland. *Epilepsia* **43**:1410–1420.

Stafstrom CE, Ockuly JC, Murphree L *et al*. 2009. Anticonvulsant and antiepileptic actions of 2-deoxy-D-glucose in epilepsy models. *Ann Neurol* **65**:435–447.

Tang B, Dutt K, Papale L *et al*. 2009. A BAC transgenic mouse model reveals neuron subtype-specific effects of a Generalized Epilepsy with Febrile Seizures Plus (GEFS+) mutation. *Neurobiol Dis* **35**:91–102.

Temkin NR. 2009. Preventing and treating posttraumatic seizures: the human experience. *Epilepsia* **50** (Suppl. 2):10–13.

Thompson SM, Cai X, Dinocourt S, Nestor W. 2006. The use of brain slice cultures for the study of epilepsy. In *Models of Seizures and Epilepsy*. Pitkanen A, Schwartzkroin PA, Moshe SL, eds. New York, NY: Elsevier, pp. 45–58.

Trenite DG, French JA, Hirsch E *et al*. 2007. Evaluation of carisbamate, a novel antiepileptic drug, in photosensitive patients: an exploratory, placebo-controlled study. *Epilepsy Res* **74**:193–200.

Vezzani A, Granata T. 2005. Brain inflammation in epilepsy: experimental and clinical evidence. *Epilepsia* **46**:1724–1743.

White HS. 2002. Animal models of epileptogenesis. *Neurology* **59** (9 Suppl. 5):S7–S14.

White HS. 2003. Preclinical development of antiepileptic drugs: past, present, and future directions. *Epilepsia* **44**:2–8.

Wlaz P, Löscher W. 1998. Evaluation of associated behavioral and cognitive deficits in anticonvulsant drug testing. In *Neuropharmacology Methods in Epilepsy Research*. Peterson SL, Albertson TE, eds. Boca Raton, FL: CRC Press, pp. 171–192.

Wong M. 2010. Mammalian target of rapamycin (mTOR) inhibition as a potential antiepileptogenic therapy: from tuberous sclerosis to common acquired epilepsies. *Epilepsia* **51**:27–36.

Chapter 14

Section summary and perspectives: Translational medicine in neurology

James E. Barrett and Joseph T. Coyle

The collective societal burden of the diseases covered in Chapters 8 to 13 is staggering and is worldwide in scope. In 2010, for example, in the USA, approximately 5 million people were afflicted with Alzheimer's disease (AD) at a cost of over $170 billion. The number of individuals with AD is predicted to rise to between 11 and 15 million in the USA by 2050 in the absence of any further therapeutic breakthroughs (Alzheimer's Association 2009, 2010). This potential increase has been designated as the "challenge of the second century," having been first described a little more than 100 years ago (Holtzman et al. 2011). Worldwide, approximately 34 million people have AD with the prevalence expected to triple over the next 40 years (Barnes and Yaffe 2011). Although the patient numbers and societal costs are smaller, increases in all of the other neurological and neurodegenerative disease categories are also predicted to occur in the absence of any therapeutic interventions that either stop disease progression or prevent onset. As Finkbeiner (2010) has pointed out, there are currently no disease-modifying therapies for the majority of neurodegenerative or neurological diseases discussed in the preceding chapters nor are there drugs for other diseases not specifically discussed in this volume such as Huntington's disease and stroke. Collectively, these disorders are among the most challenging to address from the perspectives of understanding the underlying pathophysiology and of providing either disease-modifying or symptomatic treatment. Although tremendous gains have been made in elucidating the genetics of these disorders and in increasing information on potential targets for new therapeutics, a growing gap remains between the number of individuals afflicted with these disorders and effective treatment opportunities.

Despite the wide range and diversity of neurological disorders covered in the preceding six chapters, a number of recurring themes emerge that appear to provide common threads for creating the framework for further developments in translational neurology research. Each of these areas is seeking validated *biomarkers* that permit reliable identification of the disease and its course, ideally ones that predict significant risk or that occur early enough to comfortably initiate appropriate intervention. This goal appears to be particularly the case for AD and Parkinson's disease (PD) as well as for amyotrophic lateral sclerosis (ALS), in which intervention with effective agents must be initiated before too much irreversible neuronal damage has occurred. Additionally, all of the areas covered in this section address the need for and reliance on *preclinical animal models* of the various disorders. Despite the tremendous advances in the development of transgenic animal models and in the identification of the genetics underlying these conditions, none of the current animal models fully recapitulate the complexity of the human pathological condition or its time course. There remains a pressing need to better understand the pathophysiology and the disease mechanisms of these conditions to be able to more effectively guide the development of appropriate model systems and to identify relevant drug targets. Without a more adequate understanding of the mechanisms that initiate and then lead to the neurodegenerative cascades, the development of translational approaches to these neurological disorders falls far short of the ultimate aim of using that mechanistic information to design new drugs against those targets and to use that information to guide the further development of animal models.

Another thread running through these chapters is the need for improvements in *clinical trial design* that

---

Translational Neuroscience, ed. James E. Barrett, Joseph T. Coyle and Michael Williams. Published by Cambridge University Press. © Cambridge University Press 2012.

reduce cost, minimize exposure to noneffective compounds, and expedite development and decision making without compromising patient safety. Although there have been advances in this area and receptivity on the part of the regulatory bodies, there is a clear need for further progress in this area.

Finally, there is a recognition in each of the disorders covered in this section that *combination therapies* are likely essential to fully address the diverse symptoms associated with their complex manifestations. This need has multiple dimensions that include not only an understanding of the disease but also the need to appreciate drug–drug interactions, regulatory approaches to combination therapies and, at the medicinal chemistry level, how to design drugs that interact with multiple targets. Each of these themes is discussed in more detail in the sections that follow.

Biomarkers

The Biomarkers Definitions Working Group (2001) arrived at a consensus definition of a biomarker as "a characteristic that is objectively measured and evaluated as an indicator of normal biological processes, pathogenic processes, or pharmacologic responses to a therapeutic intervention." This definition has been elaborated over the past decade and has now been incorporated into several phases of the drug discovery and development process. The development and use of biomarkers are anticipated to add needed objective rationale to decision making, provide insights into a drug's mechanism of action, and allow for the assessment of target engagement. This last step is critical in that, if positive results are obtained for target engagement and clinical outcome, these findings provide a strong validation of the target. Alternatively, if negative results are obtained for both target engagement and clinical outcome, the target may still be valid but the compound may not be appropriate. The ability to dissect these different aspects early in the developmental stages of a compound's life is critical to being able to make decisions that can save both time and expense.

Biomarkers are also expected to provide enhanced diagnostic tools and to have utility as safety markers in the early stages of drug development. Finally, the availability of well-qualified, disease-related biomarkers has the potential to tie together preclinical and clinical data, which can aid in the validation of animal models and can facilitate early proof of concept together with the added ability to select appropriate dose regimens. Together, these attributes of biomarkers will increase the efficiency of early clinical development and enhance the ability to make appropriate decisions (Wagner 2008). If available and then incorporated into the drug development process, biomarkers will also assist in stratifying patients for clinical trials and can more definitively assess responders and nonresponders.

Despite the many advantages that biomarkers bring to the discovery and development process, there is a recognized paucity of predictive biomarkers for most of the neurological disorders described in the preceding chapters. Treatments for many of these disorders are largely inadequate, particularly treatments that prevent onset or stem further disease progression, which raises the question of the utility of a biomarker in the absence of a beneficial therapeutic. This situation is particularly true for AD, for which there have been considerable advances in imaging technologies and methods to label Aβ plaques (Frank and Hargreaves 2003). Yet, at the present time, no drug is available to prevent further decline or to reverse the disease process. The failure of many of the agents that have been evaluated in AD clinical trials thus far, as suggested in the chapters by Williams and Coyle (Chapter 7) and Price (Chapter 8), may be due to any number of factors, including the possibility that the target (e.g., γ-secretase, Aβ plaque removal) may not be the key mechanism in the etiology or treatment of this disease. It may also be the case that AD is a disorder with many underlying pathologies, a view that is supported by the recent finding that AD has distinct clinicopathological subtypes that need to be considered in the design and interpretation of biomarker studies (Murray *et al.* 2011). Moreover, it is estimated that AD pathology likely begins 10–20 years before the onset of clinical symptoms and that by the time most treatments are initiated the disease process is well established. It is critical, therefore, to develop biomarkers that can detect the early pathological steps in the cascade leading eventually to dementia (Jack *et al.* 2010; Morris and Price 2001; Perrin *et al.* 2009). Although the disease process starts early, when therapeutic intervention is likely to be more effective, current diagnostic criteria identify patients at more advanced stages of the disease with significant neuropathology. At that late stage, significant neuronal loss, disruption of synaptic connections, transmitter deficits, and marked protein aggregation are likely, all of which interact in complex ways while also providing opportunities for therapeutic strategies as these cascades unfold. Thus, developing a better understanding of the pathological cascade and coupling these steps to the identification of valid biomarkers are essential for identifying intervention strategies and for discovering preventive therapeutics. Hampel *et al.* (2010) have called for a collaborative effort between industry, academia, and regulatory organizations to establish standards by which appropriate biomarkers can be identified to aid in the identification of patients likely to respond to therapies for AD, to aid in patient stratification, and to quantify treatment benefits.

The approaches and principles summarized in the preceding discussion on the relevance of biomarkers to translational medicine are underscored with regard to multiple sclerosis (MS) by Sandrock and Rudick in Chapter 10. The authors describe five factors that improve the efficiency of translational research in MS: (1) the identification of drug targets within well-validated, disease-relevant biological pathways; (2) the use of pharmacodynamic markers, especially in early proof-of-concept and dose-ranging clinical trials; (3) the appropriate use of animal models of disease; (4) the availability of surrogate imaging biomarkers of disease activity in proof-of-concept clinical trials; and (5) the use of validated clinical outcome measures that confirm clinically meaningful treatment effects. These areas would gain widespread regulatory approval and adoption by treating neurologists. Indeed, these approaches could also be applied to AD, PD, pain, and ALS.

Perhaps in no other area of neurology has the progress been as substantial as it has been in MS. Despite the complexity of this disease, disease-modifying agents are available, and the animal models of EAE have been reasonably predictive of clinical outcome. In addition to imaging techniques, other approaches to biomarker development for MS are underway and include optic neuritis, as assessed by optical coherence tomography, along with pupillometry, both of which permit the assessment of demyelinating and neurodegenerative events affecting the optic nerve. These techniques can also be assessed in rodents, thereby providing some potential early-stage translational biomarkers (Stüve *et al.* 2010).

With regard to ALS, the point is made by Maragakis (Chapter 12) that biomarkers identified early in the course of disease may permit the determination of whether progression will be slow or more rapid and may also allow for the separation of ALS subtypes, as it is often the case that patients with spinal-onset ALS have a better prognosis than those with bulbar ALS. Thus, an early assessment of ALS subtypes could allow appropriate intervention and perhaps the timely identification and anticipation of patients' needs. Maragakis also makes the point that biomarkers could be used to monitor response to drug therapy in ALS and may permit the differentiation of ALS from other neurodegenerative disorders, particularly when dementia is a prominent component of the clinical presentation.

Preclinical animal models

A great deal has been written in this book and elsewhere about the shortcomings of animal models in neurological and psychiatric disorders. This theme recurs throughout many of the chapters in this section. Hackham (2007) concluded that only one-third of highly cited animal research translates at the level of success in clinical trials. Despite their widespread use, animal models of various neurological disorders frequently do not fully recapitulate the clinical features typically occurring in the disease. For instance, α-synuclein transgenic mice show progressive age-dependent neuropathology along with cognitive deficits and motor dysfunction but the relationship between these symptoms and the α–synuclein lesions is unclear (Dawson *et al.* 2010). Even in mouse models with α-synuclein expression confined to the substantia nigra, dopamine neuron loss in the nigrostriatal system that resembles one of the hallmarks of PD, is not apparent (Kahle 2008; Obeso *et al.* 2010; Jucker 2010). A key issue in PD and in many of the other progressive neurodegenerative diseases is that of distinguishing between changes that are causal and those that are correlated with the disease. Different mutant models, termed "incomplete models" of the disease (Jucker 2010), may provide mechanistic insight and clarity with regard to these questions by selectively focusing on the various components of the disease and then by combining various mutant models.

Criticism of animal models has been extensive, and a number of suggestions have been provided as to how they might be improved. Of interest is the point that the models should more closely parallel clinical study protocols and procedures. For example, in a systematic review of animal studies on PD, MS, and ALS, 2–25% of the studies used randomization and 11–25% included clinical outcome assessments (van der Worp *et al.* 2010). Jucker (2010) also noted that the inconsistencies between the effects obtained using mouse models and clinical outcomes may be a consequence of inadequate preclinical studies and misinterpretation of the results obtained with those models, a point also emphasized by van der Worp *et al.* (2010). These issues include failure to randomize assignments to treatment groups, insufficient reporting or inclusion of gender in published studies, and failure to report whether the experimenter was blinded to treatment and outcome evaluation. The fidelity of animal models and the challenges of translational research for analgesics continue to draw concern with regard to the many deficiencies that exist, with Quessy (2010) proposing a number of specific recommendations.

Atkinson (2011) elaborated further on such disconnects in translating preclinical animal models to clinical outcome in the area of type 1 diabetes. These points are applicable to animal models in general when the latter are used to guide therapeutic decisions for clinical trials. The discovery of the nonobese diabetic mouse (NOD), a spontaneous animal model for type 1 diabetes in the 1980s, led to a large number of studies with this mouse that predicted positive therapeutic outcomes. Despite the widespread use of this model system, with over 125 reports of successful therapeutic outcomes using NOD mice, there has not been a single successful therapeutic to prevent the disease (Couzin-Frankel 2011). Atkinson (2011) has suggested a careful, critical evaluation of this model and proposes the adoption of experimental standards when this model is used to assess efficacy. These standards include a specific definition of onset, duration of disease reversal when efficacy is demonstrated, specification of sample sizes, observation of the frequency of type 1 diabetes in the animal colony in the absence of any intervention, and other standards including the number of control animals and controls for diurnal variation. In general, the proposal is to adopt meaningful efficacy standards both for mouse model studies and for human trials. The suggestion is that preclinical studies that parallel much more closely the methodological features in the conduct of clinical trials will lead to greater predictive and translational value for the animal models, but this idea has not yet been experimentally validated.

Alternatively, focusing on the clinical side of the inconsistency, van der Worp *et al.* (2010) described a number of possible reasons for the translational disparity between preclinical data and clinical outcome. One suggestion for the disparity may be related to the shortcomings of the clinical trial, which may have been insufficiently powered to detect a clinical benefit. Alternatively, the clinical trial may not have acknowledged known limitations or constraints obtained in the animal studies, including, for example, the time when treatment was initiated. The animal studies may have been flawed, extrapolations made without adequate data, and the number of subjects, although sufficient to produce a statistically significant effect, might not have been replicated in a different cohort. In addition, although not specifically mentioned, it may also be the case that there is a tacit perspective that animal models are not a reliable indicator of clinical outcome but are inserted into the drug development evaluation scheme to demonstrate a positive outcome or to complete a developmental step. Once that step has been achieved, the compound is viewed as having passed a key hurdle and can progress to the next phase.

The general question surrounding the validity or utility of animal models arises repeatedly, and with increasing frequency, during the screening stage of compounds and is intimately related to the concepts of target identification and validation. In recent years, considerable effort has been focused on the identification of the target and validation of that target's involvement in the mechanism of action of the drug. As mentioned previously, proof of target engagement is one of the hallmarks of biomarker development and of establishing proof of concept. Several new techniques have been developed to establish the validity of a target that include molecular approaches such as RNA interference, genetically modified animals, chemical probes, and other means of evaluating and characterizing a specific target in an effort to assure its involvement in the disease. Early drug discovery did not have available many of the resources currently used for characterizing the engagement of a compound with its target and often proceeded without knowledge of the mechanism of action of a drug. Prior to the introduction of these technologies, compounds were often evaluated by phenotypic screening using whole animal assays. Indeed, some have pointed to the "target-centric" approach that evolved, with the advances in molecular biology and genomics being one factor in the decline in productivity associated with the pharmaceutical industry (Enna and Williams 2009). Swinney and Anthony (2011) analyzed the number of new medical entities for the 10-year period between 1999 and 2008 during which the Food and Drug Administration approved 183 small-molecule drugs and 56 new biologics. Phenotypic screening, which refers to the effect of a compound on the whole organism or on cells, was the most successful approach for first-in-class drugs, with 37% (28) of the new medical entities being discovered by phenotypic screens compared with 23% (17) for target-based screening. For follow-on drugs, this relationship was reversed, with 51% (83) of the follow-on drugs being discovered using target-based screening and only 18% (30) of the follow-on drugs coming from phenotypic screens. With regard to central nervous system drugs that were included in the analysis for this time period, seven were based on phenotypic screens, and only one compound (ramelteon [Rozerem], a melatonin receptor agonist) came from a target-based approach. This outcome might not seem terribly surprising, considering the evolution of psychopharmacology, the reliance on phenotypic assays, and the poor understanding of the pathophysiological mechanisms associated with disorders of the central nervous system (see Williams and Barrett, Chapter 1).

Finally, there is the issue of publication bias in stroke models (Sena *et al.* 2010) where the focus is on publishing only positive experimental outcomes, creating a distorted perception of the validity of a model and of the compound(s) under evaluation that has resulted in numerous clinical failures (O'Collins *et al.* 2006). Although a comparable analysis has not been performed for those indications covered in the series of articles in this section, it would seem to have generality across other therapeutic preclinical animal models.

Clinical trial design

One of the most challenging aspects in translating candidate therapeutic agents from preclinical models to clinical use is the selection of an appropriate clinical trial design. Many factors, such as adequately powered statistical analysis of the number of patients required to observe an effect, selection of the appropriate dosage and route of delivery, and a pharmacodynamic marker for assessing whether the therapeutic agent is having some effect on its target, by necessity, need to be addressed before a clinical trial is initiated. Many of the past "failures" in developing drugs to treat neurological disorders may have been due to trials whose designs failed to address one or more of these factors.

Standard clinical trial protocols are typically executed without modification of the initial detailed protocol, which includes the timing of dose administration, the number of doses and subjects, and inclusion/exclusion criteria. These factors are all described prospectively, and the trial then proceeds without modification. Adaptive trials, however, use incoming information, e.g., are data-driven, to evaluate outcome measures and to change parameters such as discontinuing a dose or adding more subjects. The design of such trials calls for meticulous planning, sophisticated statistical techniques, including modeling, and a clear delineation of the assessments that are to be made as well as of decision points that are data driven. Orloff *et al.* (2009) argued that clinical development can be improved considerably by adopting a more integrated approach that increases flexibility and maximizes the use of accumulated knowledge gained as the trial progresses. Adaptive trial designs, as is the case with traditional trial designs, use preplanned protocols but build in flexibility that, because of the proscribed criteria and independent monitoring, does not reduce the validity or the integrity of the data.

One of the first large-scale demonstrations of the successful use of an adaptive trial design was the ASTIN stroke study: The study was terminated 4 months early, yielding a cost savings and a reduction of patient exposure to an ineffective drug (Grieve and Krams 2005). The increased use and acceptance of adaptive clinical trials is likely as they continue to demonstrate the attributes of cost savings, efficiency, and minimization of patient exposure to noneffective compounds. In some cases, for example in MS and ALS, where patient populations are smaller, it is even more essential to incorporate trial designs that maximize information and minimize the number of patients required to demonstrate efficacy. The challenge lies in areas in which the clinical end point is disease modification, which may require more lengthy trials to establish effectiveness.

Pathophysiology and combination therapies

Many of the preceding chapters have focused on the complexity and heterogeneous nature of the neurological and neurodegenerative disorders. All of the disorders covered in these chapters involve multiple pathways, impact multiple systems, and have many different dimensions. Pain and epilepsy, for example, as pointed out in the chapters by Bannon (Chapter 9) and by Gasior and Wiegand (Chapter 13), respectively, are not homogeneous in their etiology or in their individual pathophysiological mechanisms. Cancer pain, for example, differs significantly from neuropathic pain in terms of its expression, persistence, and responsivity to pharmacological treatment. It has become increasingly apparent that many of these disorders, as well as others covered elsewhere in this book, are not best treated by a drug acting on a single receptor or enzyme target; in many cases, the more effective drugs will be "broad-spectrum" agents (e.g., clozapine for the treatment of schizophrenia). An enhanced understanding of the heterogeneity of the neurological disorders, as is the case with neuropsychiatric disorders, suggests strongly that to be truly effective a multitarget approach or combination therapy may be necessary to treat the composite disease, which may include cognitive deficits, motor dysfunction, progressive neuronal loss, and other features. The enthusiasm for combination therapies has been offset by concerns about enhanced toxicity when two or more agents are combined; but, there are arguments and experimental data, including computational modeling approaches based on systems and network pharmacology, to suggest that toxicity actually can be decreased and selectivity increased (Hopkins 2008; Lehar *et al.* 2009a, 2009b). Woodcock *et al.* (2011) have suggested that the use of combination drugs may have certain advantages over single compounds but that the development of combination therapies will require a revision of the typical paradigm for developing and evaluating drugs that focus on a single therapeutic target with a single agent and will require careful regulatory guidelines for evaluating combination therapies. Others (Podolsky and Greene 2011), however, have added a cautionary note to an approach based on the use of combination therapies and provide a historical perspective to the development and use of drug combinations where the latter were actually less effective than either of the individual agents. Clear regulatory guidelines are now in place for the development and evaluation of combination products that should preclude the introduction of drug combinations that do not meet the criterion of showing efficacy that is greater than that of the individual drugs and where the contributions of the individual drugs to the effect can be ascertained.

The approach of using drug combinations in which two or more drugs are given together, either as a single tablet or by the administration of two or more individual drugs to achieve an enhanced or broader therapeutic effect, differs from the approach of using a single molecule acting at multiple targets or pathways. There is a growing recognition and movement away from the notion that a drug acting at a single target minimizes off-target effects, therefore reducing side effects due to their selectivity (Zimmermann *et al.* 2007). This view is supported by the heightened acknowledgment that complex disorders involving multiple pathways and different systems, such as those neurological disorders covered in the preceding chapters, can be appropriately addressed only by drugs with multimechanisms of action (Geldenhuys *et al.* 2011). Complex pathologies such as those involving neurodegenerative and neurological disorders require drugs that engage multiple targets. The recognition that the development of "promiscuous" drugs necessitates new approaches to drug discovery will require a more sophisticated understanding of chemical and systems biology, drug design, and screening approaches for drug activity and a dramatic revision of the drug discovery paradigm, perhaps reverting to the pharmacologically driven research approach that provided the serendipity for the golden age of psychopharmacology of the mid twentieth century (Klein 2008). Suggestions and approaches are already in place for the implementation of systems biology approaches to screening end points with the use of diverse cell types that capture the different pathways and networks that are related to various disease states (Butcher 2005). In addition, a number of efforts are underway to incorporate computational models into the drug discovery and development processes. These models incorporate data from neuropharmacology, medicinal chemistry, neuroanatomy, and pathways, and, when available, data from clinical trials to generate algorithms to guide drug design and evaluation (Ferrante *et al.* 2008; Geerts 2011). Ultimately, these approaches may be beneficial in integrating vast amounts of information and using that information beneficially in drug design and evaluation to better optimize outcome and the prediction of a successful translation from preclinical to clinical stages of development.

Summary and conclusions

Many factors have thwarted our progress toward an understanding of neurological and neurodegenerative disorders. The current poor understanding of the pathophysiology of the different disorders greatly impedes our ability to develop drugs to address the pressing need for disease-modifying and preventive agents. Progress in the discovery of drugs to treat these disorders has been slow and frustrating because of repeated drug failures, which are costly and which occur after extensive research and effort has been applied. Although there has been noteworthy progress and new introductions in treatment options for MS and epilepsy, these advances are not paralleled for other disorders that include AD, PD, pain, and ALS. New approaches are being developed that take into account the complexity of these diseases and that may contribute significantly to the eventual unraveling of these disorders and to the identification of safe and therapeutically effective compounds. The integration of chemical biology and systems biology with computational neuroscience network analysis is capturing considerable attention and may ultimately be successfully incorporated into the drug discovery and development scheme, but it is too early to determine the true value of these initiatives. It is clear, however, that innovative approaches are needed both in understanding the pathophysiology of these complex disorders and in successfully translating that information into more successful clinical outcomes. Unfortunately, the promise of these newer approaches comes against a backdrop of several other novel approaches that have included the use of combinatorial libraries, high-throughput screening, and the successful sequencing of the genome that have not yet yielded many of the advances that were anticipated at the time of their implementation. However, as in many cases in the past, these developments help to set the iterative stages for potential advances where they can be integrated into the more recent evolution of approaches based on chemical biology and systems biology. Using information from the human genome for drug repositioning, that is, evaluating existing drugs for potential use in other indications, is underway (Lussier and Chen 2011) as are efforts to use systems pharmacology and genomic information to identify pathways for pharmaceutical intervention (Wist *et al.* 2009). Although it is not specifically addressed in this section, recognition is growing of the importance of epigenetic regulation in neurodegenerative disorders, a topic covered in the chapter by Gupta *et al.* (Chapter 18) and in the summary by Barrett and Coyle (Chapter 19) that follows that section. Although these approaches are in the early stages and are yet to be firmly established either as academic disciplines or as key initiatives in the drug discovery process, they offer promise and may well herald a new era in the application of new technologies and approaches to established disciplines, all of which will eventually find their way into the introduction of safe and effective drugs to treat these serious disorders.

References

Alzheimer's Association 2009. 2009 Alzheimer's disease facts and figures. *Alzheimer's Dement* 5:234–270.

Alzheimer's Association 2010. 2010 Alzheimer's disease facts and figures. *Alzheimer's Dement* 6:158–194.

Atkinson MA. 2011. Evaluating preclinical efficacy. *Sci Trans Med* 3:96cm22.

Barnes DE, Yaffe K. 2011. The projected effect of risk factor reduction on Alzheimer's disease prevalence. *Lancet Neurol* 10:819–828.

Biomarkers Definitions Working Group. 2001. Biomarkers and surrogate endpoints: preferred definitions and conceptual framework. *Clin Pharmacol Ther* 69:89–95.

Butcher EC. 2005. Can cell systems biology rescue drug discovery? *Nat Rev Drug Discov* 4:461–467.

Couzin-Frankel JA. 2011. Clinical studies. Trying to reset the clock on type I diabetes. *Science* 333:819–821.

Dawson TM, Ko HS, Dawson VL. 2010. Genetic animal models of Parkinson's disease. *Neuron* 66:646–661.

Enna SJ, Williams M. 2009. Challenges in the search for drugs to treat central nervous system disorders. *J Pharmacol Exp Ther* 329:404–411.

Ferrante M, Blackwell KT, Migliore M, Ascoli GA. 2008. Computational models of neuronal biophysics and the characterization of potential neuropharmacological targets. *Curr Med Chem* 15:2456–2471.

Finkbeiner S. 2010. Bridging the valley of death of therapeutics for neurodegeneration. *Nat Med* 16:1227–1232.

Frank R, Hargreaves R. 2003. Clinical biomarkers in drug discovery and development. *Nat Rev Drug Discov* **2**:566–580.

Geerts H. 2011. Mechanistic disease modeling as a useful tool for improving CNS drug research and development. *Drug Dev Res* **72**:66–73.

Geldenhuys WJ, Youdim MBH, Carrol RT, Van der Schyf CJ. 2011. The emergence of designed multiple ligands for neurodegenerative disorders. *Prog Neurobiol* **94**:347–359.

Grieve AP, Krams M. 2005. ASTIN: a Bayesian adaptive dose-response trial in acute stroke. *Clin Trials* **2**:340–351.

Hackham DG. 2007. Translating animal research into clinical benefit. *Br Med J* **334**:163–164.

Hampel H, Frank R, Broich K et al. 2010. Biomarkers for Alzheimer's disease: academic, industry and regulatory perspectives. *Nat Rev Drug Discov* **9**:560–574.

Holtzman DN, Morris JC, Goate AM. 2011. Alzheimer's disease: the challenge of the second century. *Sci Transl Med* **3**:1–17.

Hopkins AL. 2008. Network pharmacology: the next paradigm in drug discovery. *Nat Chem Biol* **4**:682–690.

Jack CR, Knopman DS, Jagust WJ et al. 2010. Hypothetical model of dynamic biomarkers of the Alzheimer's pathological cascade. *Lancet Neurol* **9**:119–128.

Jucker M. 2010. The benefits and limitations of animal models for translational research in neurodegenerative diseases. *Nat Med* **16**:1210–1214.

Kahle PJ. 2008. alpha-Synucleinopathy models and human neuropathology: similarities and differences. *Acta Neuropathol* **115**:87–95.

Klein DF. 2008. The loss of serendipity in psychopharmacology. *J Am Med Assoc* **299**:1063–1065.

Lehar J, Krueger AS, Zimmermann GR, Borisy AA. 2009a. Therapeutic selectivity and the multi-node drug target. *Discov Med* **8**:185–190.

Lehar J, Krueger AS, Avery W, et al. 2009b. Synergistic drug combinations tend to improve therapeutically relevant selectivity. *Nat Biotechnol* **27**:659–666.

Lussier YA, Chen JL. 2011. The emergence of genome-based drug repositioning. *Sci Transl Med* **3**:96ps35.

Morris JL, Price JL. 2001. Pathologic correlates of nondemented aging, mild cognitive impairment and early-stage Alzheimer's disease. *Nature* **461**:916–922.

Murray ME, Graff-Radford NR, Ross OA et al. 2011. Neuropathologically defined subtypes of Alzheimer's disease with distinct clinical characteristics: a retrospective study. *Lancet Neurol* **10**:785–796.

Obeso JA, Rodriguez-Oroz MC, Goetz CG et al. 2010. Missing pieces in the Parkinson's disease puzzle. *Nat Med* **16**:653–661.

O'Collins VE, Macleod MR, Donnan GA et al. 2006. 1,026 experimental treatments in acute stroke. *Ann Neurol* **59**:467–477.

Orloff J, Douglas F, Pinheiro J et al. 2009. The future of drug development: advancing clinical trial design. *Nat Rev Drug Discov* **8**:949–957.

Perrin RJ, Fagan AM, Holtzman DM. 2009. Multi-modal techniques for diagnosis and prognosis of Alzheimer's disease. *Nature* **461**:916–922.

Podolsky SH, Greene JA. 2011. Combination drugs – hype, hope and harm. *N Engl J Med* **365**:488–491.

Quessy SN. 2010. The challenges of translational research for analgesics: the state of knowledge needs upgrading and some uncomfortable deficiencies remain to be urgently addressed. *J Pain* **11**:698–700.

Sena ES, Van der Worp HB, Bath PMW, Howells DW, Macleod MR. 2010. Publication bias in reports of animal stroke studies leads to overstatement of efficacy. *PLoS Biol* **8**:e1000344.

Stüve O, Kieseier BC, Hemmer B et al. 2010. Translational research in neurology and neuroscience 2010. *Arch Neurol* **67**:1307–1315.

Swinney DC, Anthony J. 2011. How were new medicines discovered? *Nat Rev Drug Discov* **10**:507–519.

Van der Worp HB, Howells DW, Sena ES et al. 2010. Can animal models of disease reliably inform human studies? *PLoS Med* **7**:1–8.

Wagner JA. 2008. Strategic approach to fit-for-purpose biomarkers in drug development. *Ann Rev Pharmacol Toxicol* **48**:631–651.

Wist AD, Berger SI, Iyengar R. 2009. Systems pharmacology and genome medicine: a future perspective. *Genome Med* **1**:11.

Woodcock J, Griffin JP, Behrman RE. 2011. Development of novel combination therapies. *N Engl J Med* **364**:985–987.

Zimmermann GR, Lehar J, Keith CT. 2007. Multi-target therapeutics: when the whole is greater than the sum of the parts. *Drug Discov Today* **12**:34–42.

Chapter 15

Historical perspectives on the use of therapeutic agents to treat neurodevelopmental disorders

Kimberly A. Stigler, Craig A. Erickson, David J. Posey, and Christopher J. McDougle

We provide a historical overview of the evolution of drug therapy in autistic disorder (autism), fragile X syndrome (FXS), and attention deficit hyperactivity disorder (ADHD). Often, the discovery of a pharmacological treatment is serendipitous, particularly for ADHD. In contrast, neurobiological findings, in part, have led the way to a consideration of certain therapeutic agents for autism and FXS. The intriguing early history behind our understanding of the pharmacotherapy of these disorders is described, with an emphasis on landmark studies in their respective fields.

Neurobiology and pharmacotherapy of autistic disorder

Autism is a severe neuropsychiatric disorder characterized by impairments in social skills and communication as well as repetitive interests and activities. Individuals with autism often suffer from interfering associated symptoms that range from aggression and self-injurious behavior to a profound need for sameness and repetition that can negatively impact meaningful participation in activities of everyday life. In an effort to better understand the neurobiological basis of autism, investigators looked to research methods that would elucidate the neurochemistry of this lifelong disorder.

Historical perspectives

Research into the neurobiology of autism initially focused on the monoamine neurotransmitter serotonin (5-hydroxytryptamine [5-HT]), largely due to its known prominent role in mammalian brain development. The 5-HT system is one of the first neuronal systems to develop and is extensively distributed throughout the brain. In the immature mammalian brain, 5-HT functions as a growth factor to guide brain proliferation and maturation (Whitaker-Azmitia 1993). Given the importance of the 5-HT system in human brain development, investigators hypothesized that 5-HT dysregulation may contribute to the emergence of autism early in life.

Hyperserotonemia

In 1961, Schain and Freedman published their landmark paper describing hyperserotonemia in a subset of children with autism. In this study, 23 children (mean age, 10.8 years; age range, 6–18 years) with "infantile autism" underwent testing to determine levels of 5-HT in blood (whole blood serotonin [WBS]) and levels of 5-hydroxyindoleacetic acid (5-HIAA; primary metabolite of 5-HT) in urine. The study included other children who were matched for age and sex. Altogether, they had three groups of participants: group A ("mildly retarded children"; IQ = 60–80); group B (children diagnosed with "infantile autism who functioned on a severely retarded level"); and group C ("severely retarded children without a diagnosis of autism"; IQ < 20).

Several blood samples were obtained from each child to ascertain levels of WBS. Within the blood, approximately 95% of the 5-HT is carried in platelets (Campbell and Todrick 1973). In group A ("mildly retarded children") (n = 12), WBS levels averaged 0.072 gamma/cc, similar to the normal values obtained in their laboratory (0.02–0.15 gamma/cc). Group B (children with "infantile autism") (n = 23) participants had a mean level of WBS of 0.141 gamma/cc. Six children (26%) in this group exhibited mean WBS levels over 0.200 gamma/cc, a value

Translational Neuroscience, ed. James E. Barrett, Joseph T. Coyle and Michael Williams. Published by Cambridge University Press. © Cambridge University Press 2012.

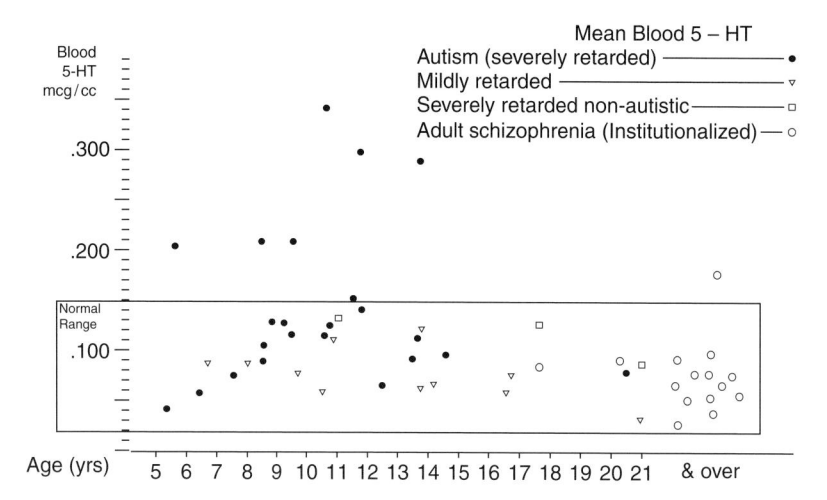

Figure 15.1. Mean blood serotonin levels for subjects of each group. Reprinted from *Journal of Pediatrics*, Vol. **58**, Schain RJ, Freedman DX, Studies on 5-hydroxyindole metabolism in autistic and other mentally retarded children, pp. 315–320, copyright 1961, with permission from Elsevier.

considered significantly above the normal range (Fig. 15.1). Finally, group C ("severely retarded children without a diagnosis of autism") (n = 7) children had a mean level of WBS of 0.128 gamma/cc, which was not significantly different from that of group B participants.

In addition, four of the children diagnosed with "infantile autism" received tryptophan loads (1 g of L-tryptophan/day) for 3 days. Tryptophan is an essential amino acid necessary for central nervous system production of 5-HT. The authors reported no consistent change in WBS levels in response to administration of tryptophan.

In addition to obtaining WBS levels, Schain and Freedman (1961) also tested urine samples for levels of 5-HIAA. They reported that 5-HIAA levels were higher in the group with "infantile autism" (group B) (5.9 gamma/mg of creatinine) (n = 12) than in the "mildly retarded children" (group A) (1.6 gamma/mg of creatinine) (n = 6). In both groups, the absolute amount of 5-HIAA/ml of urine was similar. However, creatinine values were much lower in the children with autism, signifying greater dilution of urine. Urine 5-HIAA levels were not reported for group C. None of the urine 5-HIAA results was considered to be significantly abnormal.

Schain and Freedman's paper was the first to identify hyperserotonemia in whole-blood samples of a subset of children with autism, namely those described as "more severely defective." Whereas the mean level of WBS in the "severely retarded" group did not significantly differ from that of the autistic group, consistent elevations of WBS were recorded only in the children with autism. When the presenting symptoms of six autistic children with the highest WBS levels were compared with those who had normal levels, no differences were found. However, the researchers noted an absence of seizure disorders.

In light of Schain and Freedman's intriguing results, additional research was conducted on WBS in autism. In 1970, Ritvo and colleagues measured levels of WBS in 24 children with autism (age range, 33–91 months) and 82 child and adult controls (age range, 23–360+ months). An inverse relationship between age and levels of both WBS and platelet values was identified in the control group. When WBS levels were compared between the 24 children with autism and 36 matched controls, the authors found that the children with autism exhibited significantly higher mean values of WBS (0.263 ± 0.063 μg/ml vs. 0.216 ± 0.061 μg/ml). No significant difference was found in mean 5-HT platelet values between participants with autism and age-matched controls.

In 1987, investigators from Yale University published findings from their laboratory as well as a summary of research that had been conducted to date on WBS in autism (Anderson et al. 1987). Levels of WBS and tryptophan were determined for 40 participants with autism and 87 typical controls. The sample consisted of children and young adults, with a similar age distribution between groups. Significantly higher mean WBS concentrations were found in the drug-free participants (n = 21) with autism compared with controls (n = 87) (205 ± 16 ng/ml and 136 ± 5.4 ng/ml, respectively). The authors then defined hyperserotonemia as the 95th percentile of the control group (WBS > 220 ng/ml). They reported that, when this definition was applied, 38% of the participants with autism were considered hyperserotonemic. An age effect was recorded, but only in the typical control group, with young boys exhibiting higher WBS levels than adult men. They found no significant difference in mean tryptophan levels or platelet counts between the group with autism and the control group. The authors hypothesized that differences in platelet function in the participants with autism could account for the hyperserotonemia. They also acknowledged that additional research was necessary to understand the link between central and peripheral regulation of 5-HT metabolism before any meaningful conclusions could be drawn from their findings.

A study by Leboyer and colleagues (1999) also pointed to possible developmental differences in 5-HT levels between individuals with autism and typical controls. Levels of WBS were measured in 60 participants with autism aged 3–23 years (mean age, 9.2 years), 91 typical controls aged 2–16 years, and 118 typical controls greater than 16 years of age. Participants were determined to be hyperserotonemic if they had WBS values above 0.90 µmol/L. On the basis of this definition, the authors found that 29 (48%) of the 60 participants with autism were hyperserotonemic, exhibiting significantly higher mean WBS levels than those of typical controls older than 16 years of age (1.02 ± 0.77 µmol/L vs. 0.42 ± 0.14 µmol/L, respectively).

The investigators then compared participants with autism younger than 16 years of age with typical controls matched for age and gender. The autism group had higher mean levels of WBS than the controls (0.97 ± 0.70 µmol/L vs. 0.86 ± 0.30 µmol/L), but the difference was not statistically significant. Of interest, however, was the finding that the distribution of WBS levels between age-matched participants with autism and controls differed (Fig. 15.2). Whereas WBS concentrations decreased with age in the control group, they were age-independent in the patients with autism.

In general, early research suggested that 5-HT dysregulation may play a role in the pathophysiology of autism. WBS levels were higher in younger participants with autism and appeared to remain elevated across the age range compared with typical controls. Furthermore, typical controls exhibited an inverse relationship between age and WBS level, with decreasing WBS values documented with increasing age. These findings were hypothesized to be the result of aberrant 5-HT system maturation in individuals with autism (Anderson et al. 1987; Leboyer et al. 1999).

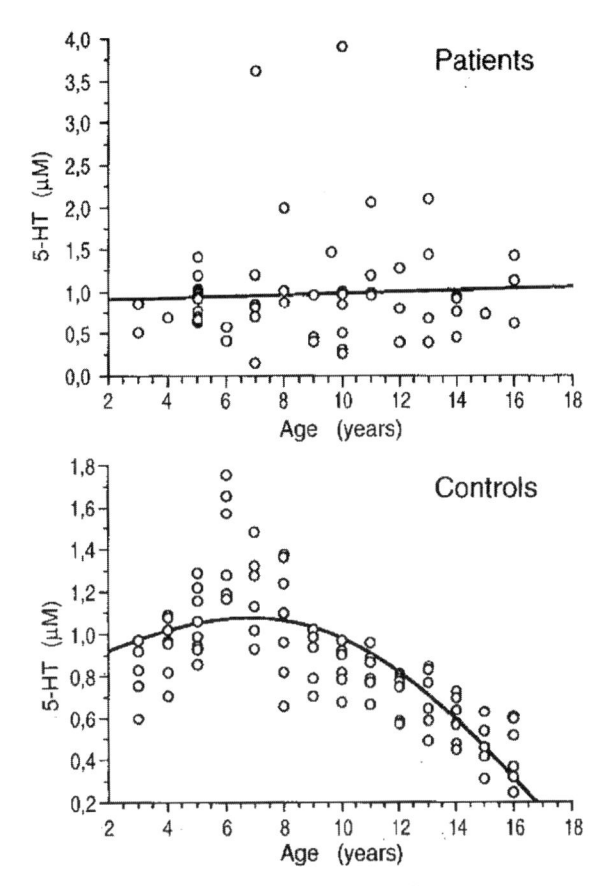

Figure 15.2. Whole blood serotonin levels of patients with autism (< 16 years) and controls according to age. Reprinted from *Biological Psychiatry*, Vol. **45**, Leboyer M, Philippe A, Bouvard M et al., Whole blood serotonin and plasma beta-endorphin in autistic probands and their first-degree relatives, pp. 158–163, copyright 1999, with permission from Elsevier.

Tryptophan depletion

To better understand central 5-HT function in autism, McDougle and colleagues (1996a) conducted an acute tryptophan-depletion study in 17 drug-free adult participants with autism. Participants received tryptophan-free amino acid mixtures via a protocol that has been shown to deplete plasma tryptophan levels and cerebrospinal fluid (CSF) levels of tryptophan and 5-HIAA within 5 hours (Carpenter et al. 1998).

Administration of the tryptophan-free amino acid mixture resulted in a significant reduction in plasma free and total tryptophan levels, whereas administration of a mixture containing tryptophan (sham depletion) resulted in a significant increase in these levels. Potential behavioral effects of tryptophan depletion were captured in a double-blind fashion using standardized, validated rating scales. A significant increase in sensory motor symptoms (e.g., hand flapping, pacing, body rocking, hitting self, spinning, toe walking) following tryptophan depletion was recorded in 11 (65%) of 17 participants, whereas none of the 17 participants exhibited a clinical change after sham depletion (Fig. 15.2). These findings observed after experimental manipulation of central nervous system 5-HT levels pointed investigators toward a model of reduced central 5-HT function in adult patients with autism.

Selective serotonin reuptake inhibitors

The advent of selective serotonin reuptake inhibitors (SSRIs) provided researchers with a pharmacological probe to investigate the 5-HT system in autism. Similar to the results with WBS presented above, developmental differences in the efficacy and tolerability of SSRIs have become apparent in individuals with autism. In the first double-blind, placebo-controlled study of a SSRI in patients with autism, McDougle and colleagues (1996b) found fluvoxamine (mean dose, 277 mg/day) significantly more effective than placebo for treating repetitive thoughts and behavior, disruptive behavior, and aggression in 30 adults with autism. After 12 weeks of treatment, 8 (53%) of 15 participants in the fluvoxamine group responded, compared with 0 of 15 participants in the placebo group. Adverse effects were mild and included sedation and nausea. In light of these encouraging results, McDougle et al. (2000) conducted a 12-week, double-blind, placebo-controlled trial of fluvoxamine (mean dose, 107 mg/day) in 34 children and adolescents (mean age, 9.5 years; age range, 5–18 years) with autism and related disorders. In comparison to the favorable findings in adults, the drug was poorly tolerated and of minimal to no efficacy in the children and adolescents. Only one (6%) of 18 participants in the fluvoxamine group and 0 of 16 participants in the placebo group were considered responders. Adverse effects were reported frequently and included agitation, impulsivity, hyperactivity, aggression, and insomnia. These discrepant findings between youth and adult participants suggested that brain 5-HT system development may be a critical factor in drug response and tolerability with respect to fluvoxamine and other SSRIs. Indeed, results of recent large-scale, double-blind, placebo-controlled trials of two other SSRIs, fluoxetine and citalopram, indicate that they are ineffective and poorly tolerated in children with autism (Autism Speaks 2009; King et al. 2009). These observations may not be unexpected in light of the developmental differences that have been uncovered regarding WBS in autism.

Summary

Over the past 50 years, studies of 5-HT function in patients with autism have led to additional research that has advanced our understanding of 5-HT dysregulation in autism. Measures of WBS levels demonstrated hyperserotonemia in a subset of individuals with autism. In addition, the impact of development on both 5-HT levels and drug response in autism became apparent via well-designed controlled research. Despite these findings, much remains unknown and further investigation into the role of 5-HT function in autism is warranted.

The pharmacology of fragile X syndrome

Fragile X syndrome (FXS) is the most common inherited form of mental retardation. The disorder is a form of X-linked mental retardation and is the result of the silencing of a single gene on the X chromosome known as the fragile X mental retardation 1 gene (*FMR1*) (Cornish et al. 2008). This silencing occurs as a result of a cysteine-guanine-guanine (CGG) trinucleotide repeat expansion (> 200 repeats) within the *FMR1* gene, which is located near the long arm of the X chromosome. Translation of the *FMR1* gene leads to the synthesis of fragile X mental retardation protein (FMRP) in healthy individuals, whereas mutations in *FMR1* lead to a lack of FMRP, resulting in FXS (Loesch et al. 2004; Pieretti et al. 1991; Tassone et al. 1999). Physical features of FXS include macroorchidism, large or prominent ears, enlarged head circumference, and an elongated face, among others. In addition to mental retardation, FXS is often associated with behavioral symptoms that include anxiety (shyness, social phobia, obsessive compulsive/perseverative behaviors), emotional lability, attention-deficit/hyperactivity disorder (ADHD), and aggression/self-injurious behaviors (Berry-Kravis and Potanos 2004). Importantly, FXS represents the most common known cause of autism and related disorders (Rogers et al. 2001).

Chapter 15: Historical perspectives on the use of therapeutic agents to treat neurodevelopmental disorders

Historical perspectives

Exploration into the history of the discovery of FXS leads us back to early observations of mental retardation in males made in the late 1800s (Sherman 2002). In 1897, Johnson reviewed US census figures and noted a 24% excess of mentally retarded males in comparison with females. This observation was also made by Penrose in 1938, on examination of the gender ratio in the Colchester survey of institutionalized persons. Penrose believed that the high ratio of male to female patients with mental retardation was likely due to ascertainment bias (Sherman 2002). This bias was explained, in part, by differences between male and female members of society at the time; namely, that expectations were higher for males than for females and that males were more likely to exhibit disruptive behavior that would lead to institutionalization.

Although it would be many years before investigators would hypothesize a genetic cause for the observed gender imbalance of mental retardation, reports of X-linked forms of mental retardation began to surface in 1943. In the first report, Martin and Bell (1943) documented sex-linked inheritance in connection with severe mental retardation in a group of 11 males over two generations. Later, other investigators published reports of X-linked mental retardation pedigrees (Dunn *et al.* 1963; Losowsky 1961; Renpenning *et al.* 1962; Snyder and Robinson 1969). These findings, in part, led Lehrke (1974) to first propose a genetic cause for the preponderance of males with mental retardation, stating that X-linked genes may be a key factor resulting in the gender imbalance of mental retardation.

The fragile X site

In 1969, Lubs published the first report identifying a cytogenetic marker on the X chromosome after studying a family that included four males with mental retardation over three generations. This marker, the fragile X site, was initially believed to be an isolated finding because it was not documented again for several years in the USA (Sherman 2002). This delay was likely due to the fact that a specialized tissue culture medium was required for its detection.

In 1977, Sutherland published a landmark paper that demonstrated that the type of culture medium used to prepare chromosomes was a key factor in determining whether fragile sites were discovered in a sample. In this report, Sutherland found that when cells with known fragility were recultured on enriched medium, the fragility was no longer apparent. However, when they were subsequently recultured on the original deficient medium (medium 199), fragility was again shown. The fragile X site is known as such because of its appearance as a site of constriction on the long arm of the X chromosome, a site that is prone to breakage when cultured in deficient medium.

Sutherland next set out to determine what factors in medium 199 were responsible for these intriguing findings. In contrast to the enriched medium, medium 199 is deficient in folic acid. Early research had found that folic acid inhibited, and methotrexate (folic acid antagonist) induced, the expression of some sites. Furthermore, researchers determined that when thymidine, glycine, and hypoxanthine were available, some mutant cell lines grew in the presence of folic acid inhibitors (Sutherland and Basilico 1966). After careful testing, only thymidine was found to affect expression of fragile sites. Further research clarified that folic acid and thymidine needed to be restricted in tissue culture medium for the fragile X site to manifest itself (Sutherland 1979*a*, 1979*b*, 2003).

The concept of an X-linked syndrome grew with reports describing the physical characteristics of certain male patients with X-linked mental retardation, in particular the association of the fragile X chromosome with macroorchidism (Sutherland and Ashforth 1979; Turner *et al.* 1978). In the 1980s, a number of reports supported and elaborated on these observations, suggesting that up to 50% of cases of X-linked mental retardation are associated with the fragile X chromosome and distinct phenotypic features, the constellation of which became known as FXS (Herbst and Miller 1980; Jacobs *et al.* 1980; Richards *et al.* 1981; Turner *et al.* 1980; Venter *et al.* 1981).

Folic acid

After the discovery of FXS, investigators began to search for potential pharmacological treatments in an attempt to remediate the adverse developmental and behavioral effects of the disorder. Given the known research demonstrating that folate-deficient medium was needed to reveal the fragile X site, many wondered whether individuals with FXS suffered from a folic acid deficiency or were unable to adequately use folic acid. The possibility that folic acid supplementation might alleviate symptoms of this condition led to the first therapeutic trials in patients with FXS.

In 1981, Lejeune reported on the use of high-dose folic acid in the treatment of patients with FXS. The author found that folic acid dramatically reduced the percent fragility of the X chromosome when administered to patients in an open-label fashion. More importantly, Lejeune observed positive clinical effects with folic acid, finding "psychosis-like" symptoms to be significantly improved after only a few weeks of treatment (Lejeune 1982). In this report, eight of 16 patients demonstrated severe behaviors, described as ranging from "psychotic complication of mental retardation" to "autistic status noted from infancy." Given their symptoms, Lejeune administered an intramuscular form of folic acid, 5-formyltetrahydrofolate (0.5 mg/kg/day), to the eight symptomatic patients. Overall, seven (88%) of eight patients were found to exhibit significant behavioral improvement. Three (38%) of the eight patients were considered "close to a total recovery." In light of these encouraging preliminary findings, the author suggested that a study be conducted to test for any long-term benefits from folic acid, such as improvement in mental retardation. This suggestion was followed by Harpey's report of improvement in learning ability and behavior in three patients with FXS after oral or intramuscular doses of folic acid (Harpey 1982). Lejeune and colleagues (1984), in a larger open-label study of 42 participants with FXS, again reported behavioral improvement with folic acid treatment.

Although these reports appeared promising, none had been carried out in a double-blind, placebo-controlled fashion. Investigators quickly identified the need to further explore the potential role of folic acid in FXS via controlled trials. At the same time, studies of folic acid metabolism found no evidence for folate deficiency or aberrant folate pathways in patients with FXS (Brondum-Nielsen et al. 1983; Popovich et al. 1983; Wang and Erbe 1984). To date, at least 10 published controlled trials of folic acid in patients with FXS, in general, have found no statistically significant improvements in symptoms (Hagerman 2002).

Two of the largest controlled studies of folic acid in FXS were conducted by Hagerman and colleagues (1986) and Strom et al. (1992). In the study by Hagerman et al. (1986), the investigators conducted a 12-month, double-blind, placebo-controlled crossover study of folic acid in 25 males (mean age, 16 years; age range, 1–31 years) with FXS. Participants were maintained on their previously prescribed psychotropic medications throughout the study, whereas all vitamin supplements were discontinued prior to baseline. The participants were randomized to 6-month blocks of treatment with folic acid (10 mg/day) or matched placebo. As a whole, standardized tests of intelligence, behavior, and language revealed no statistically significant differences between those taking folic acid and those taking a placebo. The report noted that when prepubertal males were analyzed separately, a statistically significant improvement in intellectual performance was found. In addition, parent reports reflected some improvement in behavioral symptoms. Overall, folic acid was well tolerated.

Strom and colleagues (1992) completed a 24-week, double-blind, placebo-controlled crossover study of folinic acid for the treatment of FXS. In their study, 21 males (mean age, 8.3 years; age range, 2–22 years) with FXS received 15 mg/day of folinic acid or placebo. Because folinic acid bypasses the steps of folic acid metabolism, they hypothesized that it would lead to greater effects in comparison with folic acid. However, they observed no improvements from a clinical, cognitive, or social standpoint. Indeed, standardized tests of cognitive functioning, as well as behavioral rating scales, showed no statistically significant differences between folic acid treatment and placebo. No significant adverse effects were recorded.

Summary

The history of the discovery of FXS spans more than 100 years, from general observations of an increased ratio of male to female patients with mental retardation, to the identification of the fragile site on the long arm of the X chromosome in folate-deficient medium. As a whole, controlled trials have not revealed significant improvements in outcomes with folic acid treatment compared with placebo in patients with FXS. Although folic acid is not currently considered an effective treatment for FXS, it was the first medication to be used in the FXS population. Over time, an increased understanding of the molecular biology of FXS has begun to inform the development of novel treatments. One such example involves the discovery of excessive metabotropic glutamate receptor 5 (mGluR5) activation in FXS and the ensuing theory that treatment with mGluR5 antagonists will reverse aspects of the FXS phenotype (Bear 2005; Bear et al. 2004; Cornish et al. 2008; McBride et al. 2005; Yan et al. 2005).

Emergence of drug therapy in attention-deficit/hyperactivity disorder

Attention-deficit/hyperactivity disorder (ADHD) is a heterogeneous condition characterized by interfering symptoms of hyperactivity, impulsivity, and inattention. The disorder is one of the most commonly diagnosed childhood neuropsychiatric disorders, persisting into adolescence in a majority of children (Barkley et al. 1990; Biederman et al. 1996; Claude and Firestone 1995; Kessler et al. 2005). ADHD often negatively impacts functioning in children across multiple aspects of life, leading to difficulties at home and school as well as with peers. In light of the significant impairments associated with ADHD, investigators have been drawn to research the disorder for over a century. Similar to many important discoveries, serendipity led to the first effective pharmacological agent for ADHD and to the drug class that would become the "gold standard" treatment.

Historical perspectives

George Still (1902) and Alfred Tredgold (1908) were the first individuals to seriously consider the clinical entity known today as ADHD. Still and Tredgold presaged current treatment perspectives when they wrote that although behavior may be temporarily improved through environmental modifications or pharmacological approaches, the underlying disorder would remain relatively unchanged.

The pharmacotherapy of ADHD was set in motion by a series of reports published from 1937 to 1941 (Bradley 1937; Bradley and Bowen 1940; Molitch and Eccles 1937). In 1937, Bradley described the first clinical use of psychostimulant medication (stimulants) for disruptive behavior in children and adolescents at the Emma Pendleton Bradley Home for Children in Rhode Island. Thirty children (21 boys, 9 girls; ages 5–14 years) with brain injuries whose "behavior disorders were severe enough to have warranted hospitalization" received pneumoencephalograms as a part of their diagnostic evaluation, a procedure often associated with severe headaches. Looking to successfully treat the headaches, Bradley decided to administer the racemic form of amphetamine "benzedrine" (D,L-amphetamine) to his patients. Fourteen of the children responded "in a spectacular fashion," displaying rapid improvements in disruptive behavior, academic performance, impulsivity, and inattention. This landmark paper incited numerous additional publications that have described the effectiveness of stimulants for ADHD symptoms (Connor 2006).

The first double-blind, placebo-controlled trials of stimulants took place in the 1960s. These studies of dextroamphetamine and methylphenidate supported the findings by Bradley and others. Since then, hundreds of controlled trials have been conducted that have overwhelmingly continued to demonstrate the efficacy and tolerability of stimulants in patients with ADHD (Connor 2006; Connor and Steingard 2004; Spencer et al. 1996).

Biochemical studies

The marked effects observed with stimulant treatment led researchers to consider its mechanism of action in an attempt to understand the neurobiology of ADHD. In 1970, Kornetsky was the first to describe the catecholamine hypothesis of ADHD. The author suggested that because stimulants have marked effects on brain catecholamine levels, the examination of the levels of catecholamine in urine may help guide future research directions. Then, in 1979, Brozoski and colleagues published a landmark study that provided evidence of the important role of catecholamines in the functioning of the prefrontal cortex (PFC). In this study, regional biochemical depletion of dopamine in the PFC of rhesus monkeys significantly impaired working memory function to a degree similar to that produced by surgical ablation. This deficit in working memory was reversed after administration of dopamine agonists. The author suggested that these findings provided clear evidence of the importance of dopamine in PFC function. Even though Brozoski's paper placed an emphasis primarily on dopamine, the potential importance of both dopamine and norepinephrine in PFC function has come to be appreciated over time.

Dopamine

Investigations into the role of dopamine in the pathophysiology of ADHD have involved peripheral and central measures of dopamine and its main metabolite, homovanillic acid (HVA). Studies have shown that peripheral measures of plasma and urine levels exhibit a limited relationship to central dopamine system activity and that stimulants have little effect on the levels of HVA in urine (Pliszka 2005; Pliszka et al. 1996). As a result, research has focused on central measures of dopamine, namely CSF levels of HVA.

In 1977, Shaywitz and colleagues used the probenecid loading technique to ascertain CSF levels of HVA in six children with minimal brain dysfunction versus 26 controls. Probenecid prevents the passage of HVA from the CSF. Concentration of HVA (ng/ml) per unit of probenecid (mcg/ml) was found to be significantly lower in children with minimal brain dysfunction (9.8 ± 1.5) compared with controls (16.5 ± 1.5), suggesting reduced turnover of brain dopamine in the group with minimal brain dysfunction. However, levels of probenecid varied between study groups. In a small study of ten hyperactive children, levels of CSF HVA were measured before and after treatment with dextroamphetamine (Shetty and Case 1976). A significant decline in the levels of HVA in CSF was recorded after treatment, and the extent of this decline correlated with the amount of clinical improvement. Castellanos and colleagues (1996) conducted a 9-week, double-blind, placebo-controlled, crossover trial of dextroamphetamine and methylphenidate in 45 boys with ADHD. A subset of 16 participants also took part in a subsequent 4-week, open-label trial of pemoline. During the study, levels of HVA in the CSF were measured at baseline and after treatment. A positive correlation was found between the concentration of HVA in the CSF at baseline and the degree of behavioral improvement after treatment with a stimulant, as measured by parent and teacher hyperactivity ratings. The authors suggested that central dopaminergic activity plays a mediating role in the efficacy of treatment with a stimulant in children with ADHD.

Given the potential role of dopamine in ADHD, dopamine agonists that stimulate postsynaptic dopamine receptors, such as piribidel, amantadine, and L-dopa were studied. A small pilot trial of piribidel in eight children with ADHD found the drug ineffective at both low and high dosages (Pliszka 2005). In another small trial (n = 9), no significant improvement in ADHD symptoms was recorded with treatment with amantadine (Pliszka 2005). Langer and colleagues (1982) conducted a 3-week, double-blind, crossover trial of carbidopa/levodopa in 8 boys with ADHD. Although modest improvement in hyperactivity with drug treatment was recorded via teacher ratings, no improvement in motor activity was captured by actometry. Carbidopa/levodopa was also ineffective for symptoms of inattention. At the time, these studies were considered important in that they suggested that ADHD was due not only to a dysregulation in the central dopamine system. Indeed, another monoaminergic system would begin to capture the attention of investigators in their efforts to more fully understand the neurobiology of ADHD.

Norepinephrine

Kornetsky (1970) was the first to suggest a possible noradrenergic hypothesis of ADHD. In this work, the effects of amphetamine on behavior in the laboratory setting were highlighted, specifically its ability to cause norepinephrine release and lead to increased hyperactivity. This observation was extended to ADHD, with the author hypothesizing that an increase in norepinephrine leads to the core symptom of hyperactivity in this disorder. Preclinical research demonstrated that the stimulants dextroamphetamine, methylphenidate, and pemoline increased release and reuptake inhibition of both dopamine and norepinephrine (Fuller et al. 1978; Kuczenski 1983). After these insightful findings, investigators began to pursue clinical research that involved obtaining peripheral measures, most often urinary levels of norepinephrine and its metabolites. However, these early studies involving 24-hour measures of urinary norepinephrine produced inconsistent results (Zametkin and Rapoport 1987).

In 1981, Mikkelsen and colleagues further investigated this line of research by examining the acute effects of stimulant treatment on plasma catecholamines in children with ADHD. The authors found that plasma norepinephrine levels increased after a single dose of dextroamphetamine. Instead of measuring plasma levels, however, many subsequent investigators focused on urinary levels of norepinephrine and its metabolites (normetanephrine [NM], 3-methoxy, 5-hydroxyphenylglycol [MHPG], vanillylmandelic acid [VMA]) (Pliszka et al. 1996). For example, in a double-blind, placebo-controlled crossover study of 14 boys with ADHD, 24-hour urinary norepinephrine and its metabolites were measured after 4 weeks of treatment with the stimulant dextroamphetamine or the monoamine oxidase inhibitor tranylcypromine (Zametkin et al. 1985). Both drugs were found to consistently generate striking changes in levels of norepinephrine and its metabolite MHPG. Over time, additional preclinical and clinical research has supported a role for the noradrenergic effects of stimulants in targeting cognitive impairment in ADHD (Solanto 1998).

In addition to stimulants, other medications emerged as potential therapeutic treatments for ADHD. Since the early 1970s, tricyclic antidepressants (TCAs) have been considered an alternative to stimulants. Like stimulants, TCAs, in part, block the reuptake of norepinephrine, but they do not block the reuptake of dopamine (Pliszka 2005). Although TCAs (clomipramine, imipramine, desipramine) were found to effectively target ADHD symptoms, the stimulants demonstrated greater efficacy in comparative studies (Pliszka 1987). Biederman and colleagues (1989) conducted the largest controlled study of a TCA to date involving 62 children with ADHD. During this 6-week trial, 68% of participants in the desipramine group (mean dose, 4.6 mg/kg/day) were considered significantly improved versus only 10% of placebo-treated patients.

These early findings led the TCAs to become recognized as viable treatment alternatives for ADHD, particularly the more noradrenergic compounds, desipramine and nortriptyline (Spencer 2006). This recognition, in turn, led to research into other agents targeting norepinephrine in ADHD. These agents have included such drugs as the alpha-2 adrenergic agonists clonidine and guanfacine, and the atypical mixed noradrenergic-dopaminergic antidepressant bupropion. More recently, the norepinephrine reuptake inhibitor atomoxetine became the first nonstimulant approved by the FDA for the treatment of ADHD. Although investigations into novel compounds targeting the symptoms of ADHD are ongoing, thus far the stimulants remain the "gold standard" treatment for children and adolescents with ADHD.

Summary

Research into the pharmacotherapy of ADHD began in earnest after Bradley's serendipitous finding in 1937. His discovery propelled researchers to thoroughly investigate stimulant compounds to develop an appreciation of their mechanism of action in an attempt to gain some insights into the neurobiology of ADHD. Preclinical and clinical research, some of which included studies measuring central and peripheral levels of monoamines, suggested a role for dopamine and norepinephrine in this disorder. In addition to the stimulants, several other medications have been studied in an attempt to broaden treatment alternatives and further elucidate the pathophysiology of ADHD.

Conclusions

We provide unique historical insights into the evolution of drug therapy in three disorders of childhood onset: autism, FXS, and ADHD. In autism and FXS, the identification of a potentially effective therapeutic agent was, in part, driven by knowledge of the disorder's underlying neurobiology. This pathway to drug discovery, from bench to bedside, is known today as translational research. Through such research, investigators from multiple disciplines actively collaborate to create advances in pharmacological treatment. Whereas translational research methods hold great promise, to date, serendipity has been the primary pathway to drug discovery in neuropsychiatry, as was the case with ADHD. Although multiple paths may lead to the identification of a novel pharmacotherapy, with each new discovery comes the opportunity to meaningfully impact the lives of individuals suffering from these neurodevelopmental disorders.

Acknowledgments

This work was supported in part by a Research Grant (RO1 MH072964) from the National Institute of Mental Health (NIMH) (Dr. McDougle), a Career Development Award (K23), and a Daniel X. and Mary Freedman Foundation in Academic Psychiatry Fellowship Award (Dr. Stigler).

References

Anderson GM, Freedman DX, Cohen DJ et al. 1987. Whole blood serotonin in autistic and normal subjects. *J Child Psychol Psychiatry* 28:885–900.

Autism Speaks Press Release 2009. Autism Speaks announces results reported for the Study of Fluoxetine in Autism (SOFIA). www.autismspeaks.org/press/as_announces_sofia_results.php. [Accessed July 18, 2011].

Barkley RA, Fischer M, Edelbrock CS, Smallish L. 1990. The adolescent outcome of hyperactive children diagnosed by research criteria: I. An

Chapter 15: Historical perspectives on the use of therapeutic agents to treat neurodevelopmental disorders

8-year prospective follow-up study. *J Am Acad Child Adolesc Psychiatry* **29**:546–557.

Bear MF. 2005. Therapeutic implications of the mGluR theory of fragile X mental retardation. *Genes Brain Behav* **4**:393–398.

Bear MF, Huber KM, Warren ST. 2004. The mGluR theory of fragile X mental retardation. *Trends Neurosci* **27**:370–377.

Berry-Kravis E, Potanos K. 2004. Psychopharmacology in fragile X syndrome – present and future. *Ment Retard Dev Disabil Res Rev* **10**:42–48.

Biederman J, Baldessarini RJ, Wright V, Knee D, Harmatz JS. 1989. A double-blind placebo controlled study of desipramine in the treatment of ADD: I. Efficacy. *J Am Acad Child Adolesc Psychiatry* **28**:777–784.

Biederman J, Faraone S, Milberger S et al. 1996. A prospective 4-year follow-up study of attention-deficit hyperactivity and related disorders. *Arch Gen Psychiatry* **53**:437–446.

Bradley C. 1937. The behavior of children receiving Benzedrine. *Am J Psychiatry* **94**:577–585.

Bradley W, Bowen C. 1940. School performance of children receiving amphetamine (Benzedrine) sulfate. *Am J Orthopsychiatry* **10**:782–788.

Brondum-Nielsen K, Tommerup N, Friis B, Hjelt K, Hippe E. 1983. Folic acid metabolism in a patient with fragile X. *Clin Genet* **30**:45–47.

Brozoski T, Brown RM, Rosvold HE, Goldman PS. 1979. Cognitive deficit caused by regional depletion of dopamine in prefrontal cortex of rhesus monkey. *Science* **205**:929–931.

Campbell IC, Todrick A. 1973. On the pharmacology and biochemistry of the amine-uptake mechanism in human blood platelets. *Br J Pharmacol* **49**:279–287.

Carpenter LL, Anderson GM, Pelton GH et al. 1998. Tryptophan depletion during continuous CSF sampling in healthy human subjects. *Neuropsychopharmacology* **19**:26–35.

Castellanos FX, Elia J, Kruesi MJP et al. 1996. Cerebrospinal homovanillic acid predicts behavioral response to stimulants in 45 boys with attention-deficit hyperactivity disorder. *Neuropsychopharmacology* **14**:125–137.

Claude D, Firestone P. 1995. The development of ADHD boys: a 12 year follow-up. *Can J Behav Sci* **27**:226–249.

Connor DF. 2006. Stimulants. In *Attention-Deficit Hyperactivity Disorder*. Barkley RA, ed. New York, NY: Guilford Press, pp. 608–647.

Connor DF, Steingard RJ. 2004. New formulations of stimulants for attention-deficit hyperactivity disorder: therapeutic potential. *CNS Drugs* **18**:1011–1030.

Cornish K, Turk J, Hagerman R. 2008. The fragile X continuum: new advances and perspectives. *J Intellect Disabil Res* **52**:469–482.

Dunn HG, Renpenning H, Gerrard JW et al. 1963. Mental retardation as a sex-linked defect. *Am J Ment Defic* **67**:827–848.

Fuller RW, Perry KW, Bymaster FP, Wong DT. 1978. Comparative effects of pemoline, amfoelic acid, and amphetamine on dopamine uptake and release in vitro on brain 3,4-dihydroxyphenylacetic acid concentration on spiperone-treated rats. *J Pharm Pharmacol* **30**:197–198.

Hagerman RJ. 2002. Medical follow-up and pharmacotherapy. In *Fragile X Syndrome: Diagnosis, Treatment, and Research*, 3rd edn. Hagerman RJ, Hagerman PJ, eds. Baltimore, MD: The Johns Hopkins University Press, pp. 136–168.

Hagerman RJ, Jackson AW, Levitas A et al. 1986. Oral folic acid versus placebo in the treatment of males with the fragile X syndrome. *Am J Med Genet* **23**:241–262.

Harpey JP. 1982. Treatment of fragile X. *Pediatrics* **69**:670.

Herbst D, Miller J. 1980. Nonspecific X-linked mental retardation. II. The frequency in British Columbia. *Am J Med Genet* **7**:461–469.

Jacobs P, Glover T, Mayer M. 1980. X-linked mental retardation: a study of seven families. *Am J Med Genet* **7**:471–489.

Johnson GE. 1897. Contribution to the psychology and pedagogy of feeble-minded children. *J Psycho-asthenics* **2**:26–32.

Kessler RC, Chin WT, Demler O, Walters EE. 2005. Prevalence, severity, and comorbidity of 12-month DSM-IV disorders in the National Comorbidity Survey Replication. *Arch Gen Psychiatry* **62**:617–627.

King BH, Hollander E, Sikich L et al. 2009. Lack of efficacy of citalopram in children with autism spectrum disorders and high levels of repetitive behavior: citalopram ineffective in children with autism. *Arch Gen Psychiatry* **66**:583–590.

Kornetsky C. 1970. Psychoactive drugs in the immature organism. *Psychopharmacologia* **17**:105–136.

Kuczenski R. 1983. Biochemical actions of amphetamines and other stimulants. In *Stimulants: Neurochemical, Behavior, and Clinical Perspectives*. Crease I, ed. New York, NY: Raven Press, pp. 31–63.

Langer DH, Rapoport JL, Brown GL, Ebert MH, Bunney WE Jr. 1982. Behavioral effects of carbidopa/levodopa in hyperactive boys. *J Am Acad Child Psychiatry* **21**:10–18.

Leboyer M, Philippe A, Bouvard M et al. 1999. Whole blood serotonin and plasma beta-endorphin in autistic probands and their first-degree relatives. *Biol Psychiatry* **45**:158–163.

Lehrke RG. 1974. X-linked mental retardation and verbal disability. In *Birth Defects: Original Article Series*.

Chapter 15: Historical perspectives on the use of therapeutic agents to treat neurodevelopmental disorders

Bergsma D, ed. New York, NY: National Foundation, pp. 1–100.

Lejeune J. 1981. Metabolisme des monocarbones et syndrome de l'X fragile. *Bull Acad Natl Med (Paris)* **165**:1197–1206.

Lejeune J. 1982. Is the fragile X syndrome amenable to treatment? *Lancet* **1**:273–274.

Lejeune J, Rethore MO, de Blois MC, Ravel A. Trial of folic acid treatment in fragile X syndrome. 1984. *Ann Genet* **27**:230–232.

Loesch DZ, Huggins RM, Hagerman RJ. 2004. Phenotypic variation and FMRP levels in fragile X. *Ment Retard Dev Disabil Res Rev* **10**:31–41.

Losowsky MS. 1961. Hereditary mental defect showing the pattern of sex influence. *J Ment Defic Res* **5**:60–62.

Lubs HA. 1969. A marker X chromosome. *Am J Hum Genet* **21**:231–244.

Martin JP, Bell J. 1943. A pedigree of mental defect showing sex linkage. *J Neurol Psychiatry* **6**:154–157.

McBride SM, Choi CH, Wang Y et al. 2005. Pharmacological rescue of synaptic plasticity, courtship behavior, and mushroom body defects in a *Drosophila* model of fragile X syndrome. *Neuron* **45**:753–764.

McDougle CJ, Kresch L, Posey DJ. 2000. Repetitive thoughts and behavior in pervasive developmental disorders: treatment with serotonin reuptake inhibitors. *J Autism Dev Disord* **30**:427–435.

McDougle CJ, Naylor ST, Cohen DJ et al. 1996. Effects of tryptophan depletion in drug-free adults with autistic disorder. *Arch Gen Psychiatry* **53**:993–1000.

McDougle CJ, Naylor ST, Cohen DJ et al. 1996. A double-blind, placebo-controlled study of fluvoxamine in adults with autistic disorder. *Arch Gen Psychiatry* **53**:1001–1008.

Mikkelsen E, Lake RC, Brown GL, Ziegler MG, Ebert MH. 1981. The hyperactive child syndrome: peripheral sympathetic nervous system function and the effect of d-amphetamine. *Psychiatry Res* **4**:157–169.

Molitch M, Eccles AK. 1937. Effect of benzedrine sulphate on intelligence scores of children. *Am J Psychiatry* **94**:587–590.

Penrose LS. 1938. A clinical and genetic study of 1,280 cases of mental defect. *Ment Res Council Special Report*; Ser. 229.

Pieretti M, Zhang FP, Fu YH et al. 1991. Absence of expression of the FMR1 gene in fragile X syndrome. *Cell* **66**:817–822.

Pliszka SR. 1987. Tricyclic antidepressants in the treatment of children with attention deficit disorder. *J Am Acad Child Adolesc Psychiatry* **26**:127–132.

Pliszka SR. 2005. The neuropsychopharmacology of attention-deficit/hyperactivity disorder. *Biol Psychiatry* **57**:1385–1390.

Pliszka SR, McCracken JT, Maas JW. 1996. Catecholamines in attention deficit hyperactivity disorder: current perspectives. *J Am Acad Child Adolesc Psychiatry* **35**:264–272.

Popovich BW, Rosenblatt DS, Cooper BA, Vekemans M. 1983. Intracellular folate distribution in cultured fibroblasts from patients with fragile X syndrome. *Am J Hum Genet* **35**:869–878.

Renpenning H, Gerrard JW, Zaleski A, Tabata T. 1962. Familial sex-linked mental retardation. *Can Med Assoc J* **87**:954–956.

Richards BW, Sylvester PE, Brooker C. 1981. Fragile X-linked mental retardation: the Martin-Bell syndrome. *J Ment Defic Res* **25**:253–256.

Ritvo ER, Yuwiler A, Geller E et al. 1970. Increased blood serotonin and platelets in early infantile autism. *Arch Gen Psychiatry* **23**:566–572.

Rogers SJ, Wehner DE, Hagerman R. 2001. The behavioral phenotype in fragile X: symptoms of autism in very young children with fragile X syndrome, idiopathic autism, and other developmental disorders. *J Dev Behav Pediatr* **22**:409–417.

Schain RJ, Freedman DX. 1961. Studies on 5-hydroxyindole metabolism in autistic and other mentally retarded children. *J Pediatr* **58**:315–320.

Shaywitz SE, Cohen DJ, Bowers MB Jr. 1977. CSF monoamine metabolites in children with minimal brain dysfunction: evidence for alteration of brain dopamine. *J Pediatr* **90**:67–71.

Sherman S. 2002. Epidemiology. In *Fragile X Syndrome: Diagnosis, Treatment, and Research*, 3rd edn. Hagerman RJ, Hagerman PJ, eds. Baltimore, MD: The Johns Hopkins University Press, pp. 136–168.

Shetty T, Chase TN. 1976. Central monoamines and hyperactivity of childhood. *Neurology* **26**:1000.

Snyder RD, Robinson A. 1969. Recessive sex-linked mental retardation in the absence of other recognizable abnormalities. *Clin Pediatr* **8**:669–674.

Solanto MV. 1998. Neuropsychopharmacological mechanisms of stimulant drug action in attention-deficit hyperactivity disorder: a review and integration. *Behav Brain Res* **94**:127–152.

Spencer TJ. 2006. Antidepressant and specific norepinephrine reuptake inhibitor treatments. In *Attention-Deficit Hyperactivity Disorder*. Barkley RA, ed. New York, NY: Guilford Press, pp. 648–657.

Spencer T, Biederman J, Wilens T et al. 1996. Pharmacotherapy of attention-deficit hyperactivity disorder across the life cycle. *J Am Acad Child Adolesc Psychiatry* **35**:409–432.

Still GF. 1902. Some abnormal psychical conditions in children.

Lancet i:1008–1012, 1077–1082, 1163–1168.

Strom CM, Brusca RM, Pizzi WJ. 1992. Double-blind, placebo-controlled crossover study of folinic acid (Leucovorin) for the treatment of fragile X syndrome. *Am J Med Genet* **44**:676–682.

Sutherland GR. 1977. Fragile sites on human chromosomes: demonstration of their dependence on the type of tissue culture medium. *Science* **197**:265–266.

Sutherland GR. 1979*a*. Heritable fragile sites on human chromosomes. I. Effect of composition of culture media on expression. *Am J Hum Genet* **31**:125–135.

Sutherland GR. 1979*b*. Heritable fragile sites on human chromosomes. II. Distribution, phenotypic effects and cytogenetics. *Am J Hum Genet* **31**:136–148.

Sutherland GR. 2003. Rare fragile sites. *Cytogenet Genome Res* **100**:77–84.

Sutherland GR, Ashforth PL. 1979. X-linked mental retardation with macro-orchidism and the fragile site at Xq27 or 28. *Hum Genet* **48**:117–120.

Sutherland GR, Basilico C. 1966. Infection of thymidine kinase-deficient BHK cells with polyoma virus. *Nature* **211**:250–252.

Tassone F, Hagerman RJ, Ikle DN et al. 1999. FMRP expression as a potential prognostic indicator in fragile X syndrome. *Am J Med Genet* **84**:250–261.

Tredgold AF. 1908. *Mental Deficiency (Amentia)*. New York, NY: William Wood.

Turner G, Daniel A, Frost M. 1980. X-linked mental retardation, macroorchidism and the Xq27 fragile site. *J Pediatr* **96**:836–841.

Turner G, Till R, Daniel A. 1978. Marker X chromosomes, mental retardation and macroorchidism. *N Engl J Med* **299**:1472.

Venter PA, Gericke GS, Dawson B, Op't Hof J. 1981. A marker X chromosome associated with nonspecific male mental retardation. *S Afr Med J* **21**:807–811.

Wang JCC, Erbe RW. 1984. Folate metabolism in cells from fragile X syndrome patients and carriers. *Am J Med Genet* **17**:303–310.

Whitaker-Azmitia PM. 1993. The role of serotonin and serotonin receptors in development of the mammalian nervous system. In *Receptors in the Developing Nervous System, Vol. 2, Neurotransmitters*. Zagon IS, McLaughlin PJ, eds. London: Chapman & Hall, pp. 43–53.

Yan QJ, Rammal M, Tranfaglia M, Bauchwitz RP. 2005. Suppression of two major fragile X syndrome mouse model phenotypes by the mGluR5 antagonist MPEP. *Neuropharmacology* **49**:1053–1066.

Zametkin AJ, Rapoport JL. 1987. Neurobiology of attention deficit disorder with hyperactivity: where have we come in 50 years? *J Am Acad Child Adolesc Psychiatry* **26**:676–686.

Zametkin AJ, Rapoport JL, Murphy DL et al. 1985. Treatment of hyperactive children with monoamine oxidase inhibitors. II. Plasma and urinary monoamine findings after treatment. *Arch Gen Psychiatry* **42**:969–973.

Chapter 16
Autism spectrum disorders

Timothy P.L. Roberts, Michael Gandal, Steven J. Siegel, Paulo Vianney-Rodrigues, and John P. Welsh

Autism spectrum disorders (ASD) comprise a devastating array of developmental disorders, characterized by hallmark impairments in three broad domains: social reciprocity, language and communication, and stereotypic and repetitive behaviors. Additionally, nonspecific conditions are often comorbid, including anxiety, irritability, and aggression. The core phenotypes represent a broad array of degrees of severity, leading some to suggest that the heterogeneous disorder should be known as the *autisms*. Diagnosis of autism is rarely made before a child reaches 2–3 years of age, with the median age of diagnosis in the USA being 4.5 years. At the point of diagnosis, intensive behavioral therapy is the most widely accepted but, sadly, only partially successful, therapeutic approach. Pharmaceutical approaches targeting the core phenotypes are not available. Diagnosis is made by an experienced clinician, typically on the basis of extensive direct observation and parent reports, using instruments such as the Autism Diagnostic Observation Schedule (Lord *et al.* 2000) and the Autism Diagnostic Interview, Revised (Lord *et al.* 1994), which may be supplemented by neuropsychological and clinical assessment tools. No clear-cut, quantitative, objective indices of autism exist: there is no simple "test" for autism.

Nevertheless, autism spectrum disorders are widely considered to be associated with brain dysfunction, secondary to structural and microstructural developmental anomalies. The leading emerging theories implicate abnormal local and distant brain connectivity, abnormal sensory processing, or abnormal brain electrical oscillatory activity. Such hypotheses lend themselves to evaluation with advanced neuroimaging and electrophysiological techniques, in particular, magnetic resonance imaging (MRI) and electroencephalography (EEG) and magnetoencephalography (MEG).

In general, the pursuit of objective, quantitative, noninvasive indices of "brain-level" features of autism that may be considered "signatures," "endophenotypes," or even "biomarkers" yields many potential benefits spanning both the clinical and basic research realms: diagnostic utility (including the potential for early detection), prognostic (symptom severity) prediction, neurobiological insight, targets for treatment, and indices of response. An additional role that such indices can play is to validate the relevance of experimental (rodent) models developed to study the neurobiology of autism and as a platform to identify, develop, and evaluate therapeutic approaches. Given the widespread appreciation that the biological basis is in large part genetic but that the genetic contribution is complex, with many genes implicated and interactions with environmental factors (such as in utero exposure to toxins) also significant, a tremendous array of mouse and rat models have been proposed. A fundamental question applied to all such models is how to validate their relevance to autism. Although "parallel" behavioral traits are used with elaborate mechanisms to quantify social interactions, the interspecies gulf places a limit on interpretability of findings and extrapolation to the clinical setting. The central tenet of this chapter is the fact that advanced imaging techniques, in particular, electrophysiological methods of characterizing ASD, may identify a set of "brain traits" that might serve to tie more closely the experimental models to the clinical population, thereby enabling or facilitating translational research and interpretation. Reflecting the bedside–bench–bedside nature of translational research, candidate "signatures" may be identified in a clinical population, replicated in an experimental model (thereby offering electrophysiological validation of the model's relevance), and evaluated in the

---

Translational Neuroscience, ed. James E. Barrett, Joseph T. Coyle and Michael Williams. Published by Cambridge University Press. © Cambridge University Press 2012.

controlled setting of the experimental laboratory before selecting lead approaches (e.g., drug candidates) perhaps with concomitant measures of efficacy for implementation in the clinic.

The chapter begins with an introduction to candidate neuroimaging and electrophysiological measures drawn from large-scale studies of children with ASD conducted with high-field MRI and MEG (Roberts *et al.* 2010). We then illustrate the components of translational electrophysiological research in ASD with studies in rats and in a specific mouse model incorporating environmental exposure to toxins. The general philosophy, rationale, and approach can be extrapolated to any of the plethora of experimental models under development.

Electrophysiological signatures and imaging biomarkers of autism

Given the hypotheses relating brain dysfunction in ASD to issues of neural connectivity, response timing, oscillatory activity, and networks, in the absence of gross structural abnormalities, we focus on the following approaches, individually and, more powerfully, when integrated into a multimodal characterization.

Magnetoencephalographic studies of auditory processing – M100, magnetic mismatch field

Magnetoencephalography, often considered the magnetic counterpart of EEG, detects the tiny magnetic fields ($\sim 10^{-15}$ T) emerging from the brain secondary to neuronal intracellular electrical currents. Demanding synchrony and spatial superposition of current sources in order to achieve adequate signal, it is likely that the fields detected by MEG are associated with excitatory and inhibitory postsynaptic potentials (relatively slower, and therefore more synchronous) rather than with action potentials. Nonetheless, with arrays of several hundred magnetic field detectors [typical biomagnetometers use a helmet design (Fig. 16.1) with over 200 detectors], MEG offers a spatial as well as a temporal depiction of brain activity in real time (with submillisecond temporal resolution). Source modeling techniques such as dipole modeling, minimum norm estimation, and beamforming (beyond the scope of this chapter, but see Hamalainen 1992 and Hillebrand

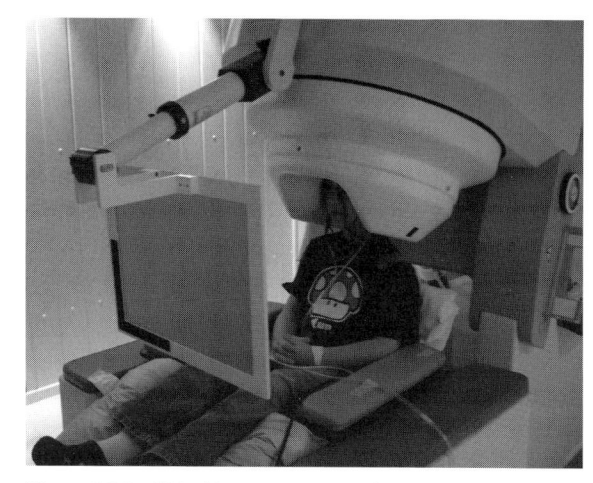

Figure 16.1. Clinical biomagnetometer for recording magnetoencephalographic data.

et al. 2005 for reviews) allow sensor-detected signals to be interpreted in terms of activity of specific brain regions, in many cases, down to a "voxel" resolution of a few millimeters.

In particular, MEG studies of auditory processing are most promising; they focus on the ~100-ms component of the auditory evoked response elicited by simple tones, complex tones, or vowel stimuli. The latency of this component (often referred to as N100M or M100) is known to reflect acoustic and perceptual features of the stimulus (see, e.g., Roberts *et al.* 2000) that mature (shorten) with developmental age (Roberts *et al.* 2009) but also, of particular importance, are prolonged in children with ASD compared with age-matched, typically developing peers (Roberts *et al.* 2010) (Fig. 16.2). Other studies probe rapid temporal processing (that is, the response to two closely spaced stimuli), revealing diminished evoked responses in children with ASD (Oram Cardy *et al.* 2005a). Incrementally more complex paradigms include the use of "oddball" designs, such as the presentation of an infrequent "deviant" stimulus in a stream of "standard" stimuli, to elicit a response known as the magnetic mismatch field, the magnetic counterpart of mismatch negativity (Naatanen *et al.* 1987), thought to be a neural indicator of change detection and thus a marker of successful recognition of phoneme or syllable change (critical for spoken speech comprehension). The latency of the magnetic mismatch field induced by either tonal or vowel contrasts has been shown to be significantly delayed in children with autism, with concomitant clinical

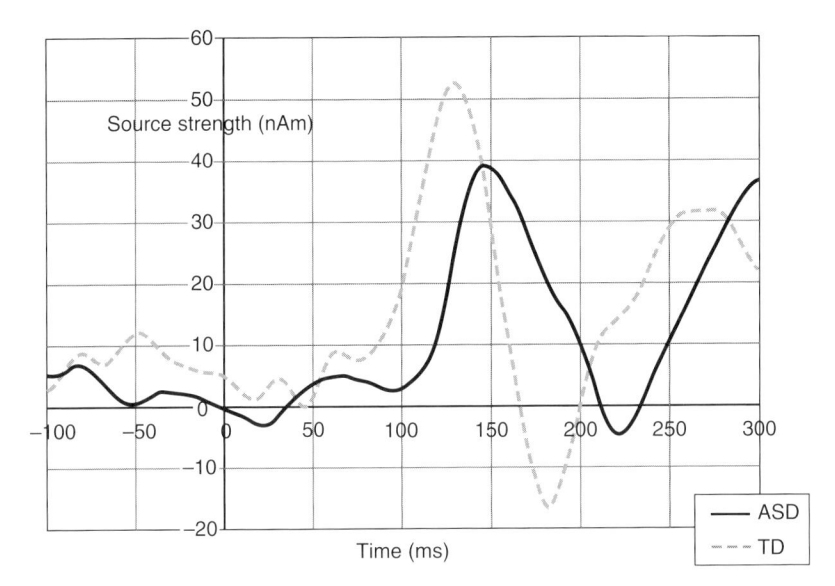

Figure 16.2. Latency prolongation of the M100 auditory evoked response component (shown as the time activity of the modeled auditory cortex neuronal response to a brief 500 Hz sinusoidal tone) in a child with autism spectrum disorder (unbroken line), compared to an age-matched typically developing peer (dotted line). ASD, autism spectrum disorder; TD, typically developing.

language impairment (Oram Cardy et al. 2005b). This finding supports the contention that these measures can be considered neural correlates of behavior that have some relevance not merely for diagnosis but also for predicting symptom severity on a specific dimensional axis (e.g., language impairment). The ability of the auditory system to adequately process auditory input, even nonspeech, appears to correlate with language impairment (Oram Cardy et al. 2005b, 2008), offering the tantalizing possibility of studying *in rodents* a feature of direct relevance to *human* language ability.

Resting state magnetoencephalography

Electrophysiological studies of brain activity are not restricted to studies of activity evoked by a stimulus. Rather, spontaneous activity can also be probed, analogous to the resting EEG. In this case, spectral analysis can offer insight into the spatial patterns of activity across various frequency bands, e.g., delta (1–4 Hz), theta (5–8 Hz), alpha (8–12 Hz), beta (12–30 Hz), and gamma (>30 Hz). Whole-brain maps of oscillatory power within a single frequency band can be generated and interrogated to establish patterns of coherence (synchronized oscillations) across distinct regions, with interpretation in terms of functional connectivity. Although this field is emerging, it appears that the brains of children with ASD may be associated with abnormally high levels of "resting state" oscillatory power across frequency bands, with posterior alpha and frontal delta/theta being particularly pronounced.

Diffusion tensor imaging

Functional connectivity and indeed all interaction between functional centers at different brain locations are predicated on effective white matter connection. The techniques of diffusion tensor MRI (often termed diffusion tensor imaging) exploit the nonuniform diffusion properties of water in the spatially ordered environment of white matter fibers to extract a voxel-wise measure of amplitude properties of diffusion, such as the mean diffusivity, relative, or fractional, anisotropy of diffusion, but also, in the setting of significant anisotropy, the direction of preferred diffusion. This finding can be interpreted locally as the orientation of white matter fiber bundles, and connectivity can be inferred from step-wise propagation from a starting voxel in the direction of preferred diffusion. These observations have given birth to the field of MR-based white matter tractography, which allows interrogation of the interconnectivity between nodes of networks and circuits. Furthermore, by examining the magnitude of diffusion parameters (such as mean diffusivity or fractional anisotropy) computed along the direction of a tract representation, some inference about the quality, integrity, or development of that white matter structure can be drawn. Given the prevailing discussion of ASD as a disorder with hypo- or hyperconnectivity within the brain, diffusion-based techniques are achieving prominence in this field (Lange et al. 2010). Consideration of the developmental trajectory of diffusion changes, as reported by Roberts et al. (2009), offers an interpretation of concomitant electrophysiological changes (e.g., M100 latency maturation), providing a biophysically relevant integration of modalities.

Magnetic resonance spectroscopy of γ-aminobutyric acid

Animal (Roopun et al. 2006; Yamawaki et al. 2008) and noninvasive human studies (Hall et al. 2005; Jensen et al. 2005) have demonstrated a strong relationship between cortical electrical oscillations and the inhibitory neurotransmitter γ-aminobutyric acid (GABA); observations have recently shown that visual cortex gamma activity (~40 Hz) is associated with magnetic resonance spectroscopy-derived visual cortex GABA concentrations in adults (Muthukumaraswamy et al. 2009). To estimate GABA levels in vivo, a special form of magnetic resonance spectroscopy is emerging as a viable technique. Using the same magnet that is used for clinical MRI (typically a 3T), a modified magnetic resonance spectroscopic experiment known as spectral editing, usually based on the MEGAPRESS approach (Mescher et al. 1998), exploits the chemical environment (and scalar J-coupling) of the protons on the GABA molecule, such that under precise circumstances (echo time TE = 68 ms), two appropriately acquired spectra can be subtracted to reveal a resonance associated with GABA (a 14.6-Hz doublet at a spectral location of 3.0 ppm) after elimination of the dominant obscuring resonance associated with creatine (which does not exhibit a similar J-coupling, and therefore is removed by subtraction) (Fig. 16.3). Quantification of the GABA resonance may then be relative (to the subtracted NAA resonance, for example) or absolute, by reference to a simultaneously scanned phantom of known concentration. Although tantalizing as a bridge between electrophysiological oscillations and cellular biochemistry, present implementations limit resolution of GABA determination to sublobar (~20 cc) volumes. Nonetheless, the way ahead is paved for multimodal integration of structure, function, and neurochemistry.

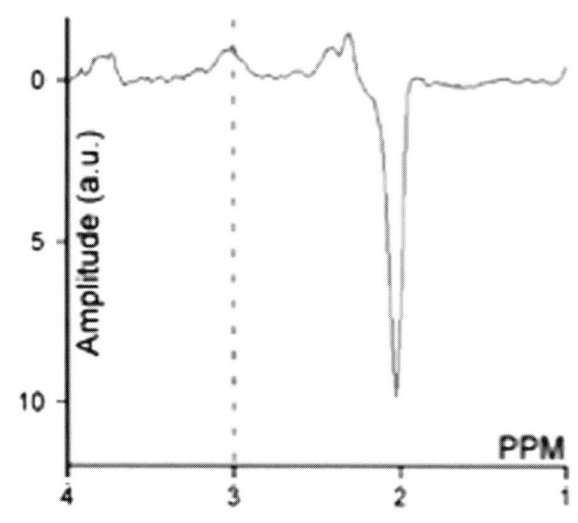

Figure 16.3. A γ-aminobutyric acid (GABA) spectrum obtained using the MEGAPRESS spectral editing approach from the motor cortex of a healthy volunteer. The GABA resonance is marked with a dashed line at 3.0 ppm. Also visible is the inverted (subtracted) resonance of N-acetyl aspartate, a neuronal marker.

Heterogeneity and strategies for translational research in autism

One of the challenges for translational research in autism is in implementing a nonhuman animal model system that allows meaningful translation. The utility of a whole-animal model for translational research is enhanced when it can overcome the "heterogeneity problem" so that it can address general mechanisms of brain dysfunction that may exist throughout the ASD spectrum and that may be targets for therapy. Children with ASD exhibit phenotypic heterogeneity, and the factors that cause ASD (causal heterogeneity) are heterogeneous. Causal heterogeneity is represented by heterogeneity in genetic risk factors that affect synaptic functions, intracellular signaling pathways, and neurodevelopment and that can enhance sensitivity to environmental risks. The range of environmental risks linked to ASD is large (i.e., mutagens, teratogens, infections, maternal antibodies, birth complications). Their heterogeneity also suggests that effects on most neurotransmitter receptors, ion channels, and major developmental processes contribute to ASD (Kinney et al. 2010; Pessah et al. 2008). Moreover, exposures to environmental risk factors have been implicated at every stage of development (gestational, perinatal, and preconceptual), suggesting more or less global influences on the developing nervous system depending on the time of exposure (Currenti 2010). Thus, the heterogeneity problem is embodied in multiple gene × environment × exposure time interactions that can bias a developing nervous system toward ASD through multiple biological pathways. A second major source of heterogeneity that is not often appreciated is "compensatory heterogeneity," which refers to the behavioral adaptations that individual children acquire in response to their ASD. Compensatory heterogeneity reflects each child's unique learning ability and learning history, which shapes his behavioral response to his unique ASD disease state. The combination of causative and compensatory heterogeneity results in the extremely diverse phenotypic profile that defines the ASD spectrum and complicates the development of animal models for translational research to a far greater extent than for other neurological disorders.

Two approaches to translational research in ASD attempt to reduce the heterogeneity in order to elucidate fundamental mechanisms of brain dysfunction. The first approach reduces heterogeneity by engineering rodents that express candidate ASD gene mutations, by exposing them to candidate environmental risk factors, or both, and then working forward to establish brain dysfunction. This approach has the advantage of producing a highly defined animal model in the hope that any brain dysfunction might generalize to a large fraction of the human ASD spectrum. The approach usually involves searching for a behavioral phenotype in a rodent that models one or more of the core symptoms of human ASD that are used to validate the model and prove causal effects of the risk factors. One challenge of this approach is that there are as many potential ASD models as there are different genetic and environmental causes of ASD. Thus, animals generated with this approach may only model a small fraction of the ASD population, and their utility as a general model becomes an empirical question. Another challenge of this approach is that there is not always a straightforward relation between behavioral phenotypes of rodents and core symptoms of children with ASD. This finding is due to the fact that the behavioral repertoires of rodents and humans differ and have evolved under different evolutionary pressures. The identification of relevant behavioral variables in rodents that map onto higher language and social function in humans can be difficult and susceptible to anthropomorphic bias. Ultimately, the goal of this approach is to generate animal models of ASD that allow discovery of neurophysiological endophenotypes that may be considered candidate dysfunctions for ASD.

A second approach reduces heterogeneity by establishing electrophysiological signatures of brain dysfunction using MEG or EEG in children with ASD and working backward into an animal model to understand neurophysiological mechanisms. This approach addresses the problem of ASD pathophysiology as an inverse problem and differs from the first because it does not rely on knowing the genetic or environmental causes of ASD. A key to this approach is to determine an electrophysiological endophenotype of ASD that is broadly represented across the ASD spectrum that is used to inform animal experiments. By focusing primarily on pathophysiological issues, the approach overcomes the challenge of relating complex social and language behavior across species by removing them from the analysis. The electrophysiological endophenotype generates a "common currency" that can be related between children and an animal model. An advantage of this approach is that there may be fewer electrophysiological signatures of ASD than permutations of genetic and environmental risk factors that induce ASD. From a translational perspective, the approach works best when the electrophysiological endophenotype of ASD is measured in children using highly defined sensory paradigms that are devoid of language and social content. Removing social and language content from clinical tests allows the identical paradigm to be implemented in nonhuman animals during high-density microelectrode array recordings. Intracranial microelectrode array recordings in rodents experiencing the same tests performed in the clinic increase spatial resolution by at least 20-fold over MEG and can record identified neuron types whose dendritic orientation does not contribute to the MEG signal. High-resolution microelectrode array recordings can then be used to elucidate microcircuit functions that are required for sensory or motor tasks in which ASD children are impaired. Once established, the electrophysiological signatures of normal function may serve as a preclinical screening tool for candidate therapeutics that can be selected for their ability to enhance the electrophysiological signature that is lost in ASD. Candidate therapeutics found to enhance electrophysiological function in the animal model can be tested in children with ASD using whole-head MEG monitoring to ascertain benefit. Real-time feedback using MEG is an essential component of this approach because it can verify the effect of a candidate therapeutic agent on the electrophysiological phenotype that may precede behavioral improvement or be necessary for behavioral therapy to become effective.

We recently began to apply the second approach to understanding ASD pathophysiology *in vivo* (Gandal *et al.* 2010; Vianney-Rodrigues *et al.* 2011; Welsh *et al.* 2010). MEG recordings from the superior temporal sulcus in children were related to microelectrode array recordings directly from primary auditory cortex (A1) of rats as both passively listened to a tone. Children with ASD showed electrophysiological signatures of dysfunction as a delayed evoked response to the tone (Roberts *et al.* 2010) (Fig. 16.2) and reduced phase locking of gamma oscillation (Gandal *et al.* 2010). Under the identical paradigm, awake rats passively listened to the tone while 16 microelectrodes were individually inserted into 1 mm^2 of the A1 (Vianney-Rodrigues *et al.* 2011). Each microelectrode placed into the rat A1 recorded both action potentials and local field potentials (LFPs). The LFP of the rat primary auditory cortex (i.e., depth EEG) was directly comparable to the superior temporal sulcus magnetic response in the children measured with MEG. It has been estimated that extracellular microelectrodes record single neuron action potentials within a radius of 140 microns (Henze *et al.* 2000) and that the LFP is composed of synaptic activity over approximately twice that distance (Berens *et al.* 2008; Katzner *et al.* 2009). LFPs showed a short-latency negativity at 30 ms followed by a longer-latency component at 100 ms, almost identical to the magnetic response in the children (Fig. 16.4A). After filtering in the gamma band (30–140 Hz), the LFP showed an evoked gamma response and multiple induced gamma responses with variable latencies up to 350 ms after tone onset (Fig. 16.4B). At short latency, the dominant contributor to the LFP is synaptic input from the auditory thalamus, whereas longer latency components largely reflect intracortical processing. The LFP findings confirmed the MEG findings in typically developed children by showing that passive listening is associated with robust gamma activity in A1 and also showed that gamma oscillations were represented in the action potentials of A1 neurons (Fig. 16.4C).

Coherence analysis of simultaneously recorded LFP sites and individual neurons demonstrated a fine spatial structure to gamma oscillations within A1 whose temporal disruption may contribute to ASD pathophysiology (Vianney-Rodrigues *et al.* 2011). In rats, intracortical coherence in the gamma band during listening was generated locally and restricted to areas no wider than 300 μm (Fig. 16.4D). The finding suggested that multiple domains of gamma oscillation are involved in passive listening and that they can operate independently. The impairment in gamma phase locking observed using MEG in children with ASD is therefore consistent with an inability of thalamic input to coherently recruit multiple gamma domains across the A1 field in a stereotypic manner. This finding suggests that the pathophysiology of ASD involves dysfunction in the ability of intracortical circuitry to synchronize the gamma activity of spatially separated domains. Electrotonic coupling of GABAergic neurons is known to be essential for the production of coherent gamma oscillation (Buhl *et al.* 2003) and is therefore suggested as a candidate therapeutic target for ASD.

Translational models of autism

Given the high degree of heritability of ASD, ASD models in preclinical settings that introduce the orthologous genetic perturbations identified in the clinical population show great promise for uncovering the pathophysiology of the disease and new targets for therapeutic intervention. However, one encounters a number of significant challenges when trying to model a complex, human behavioral disorder in rodents. First, the genetics of ASD have been difficult to decipher, making it a challenge to develop a valid, generalizable preclinical model of autism. Second, autism is diagnosed purely by behavioral criteria, without the aid of an accepted, validated biological marker. As such, primary outcome measures in preclinical studies are generally behavioral phenotypes, despite the lack of clear analogy between some complex murine and human behaviors, such as language. Third, autism often shows great clinical heterogeneity as well as frequent medical and neuropsychiatric comorbidities. Special care must be taken to assess phenotypic specificity as well as potential confounders for observed behavioral deficits. Finally, given its neurodevelopmental origin, it is unclear whether targeted therapeutic interventions will be successful in fully reversing behavioral deficits after disease presentation, although recent successes have been reported in preclinical studies.

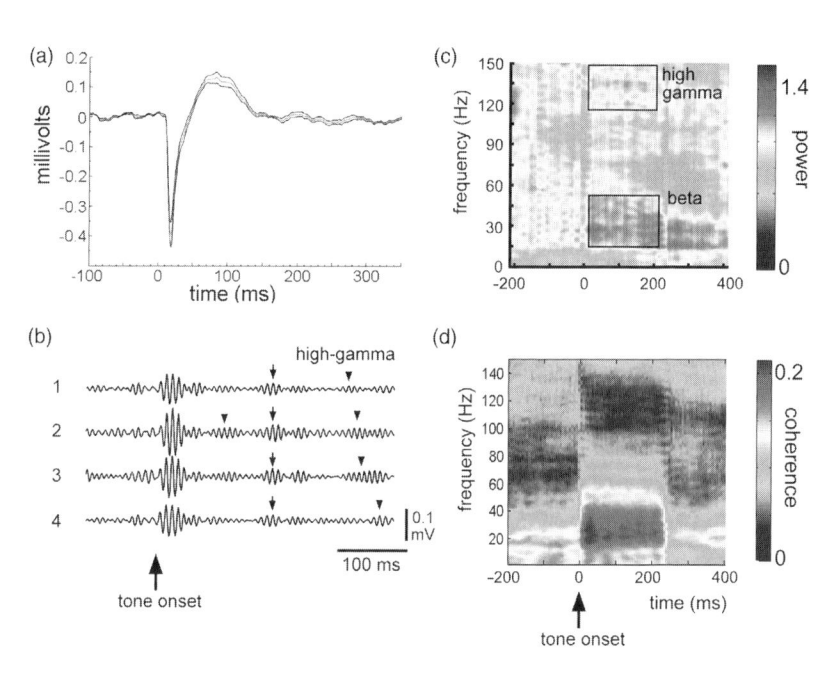

Figure 16.4. Gamma (30–140 Hz) oscillation and coherence within primary auditory cortex (A1) during listening in the awake rat. (A) Wideband local field potential. (B) Gamma oscillations in four simultaneously recorded sites triggered by tone onset. (C) Peristimulus time spectrogram of a characteristic multispike unit recorded from A1 during passive listening. (D) Mean peristimulus time coherogram of single neuron spiking with simultaneously recorded local field potentials during passive listening. Modified from *European Journal of Neuroscience*, Vol. 33, Vianney-Rodrigues P, Iancu OD, Welsh JP. Gamma oscillations in the auditory cortex of awake rats, pp. 119–129, copyright 2011, with permission from John Wiley and Sons. This figure is reproduced in color in the color plate section.

This section reviews preclinical approaches to autism, highlighting the role of translational disease endophenotypes as a currently underutilized means to provide insight into disease pathophysiology and identify new targets for therapeutic development (Fig. 16.5). Neural endophenotypes (i.e., biomarkers) are quantitative, heritable metrics that are considered to be more closely associated with, and predictive of, the neural abnormalities of a gene-based neuropsychiatric illness than the behavioral phenotype alone (Braff et al. 2007; Gottesman and Shields 1973). Endophenotypes help elucidate gene–brain–behavior relationships in complex genetic disorders by quantifying prebehavioral traits, bypassing broad and often heterogeneous diagnostic categories. Importantly, such quantitative, laboratory-based measures can often be directly assessed in preclinical models, overcoming a number of the inherent challenges of extrapolating rodent behaviors to a complex human behavioral disorder.

Criteria for validating preclinical models of autism

When investigating rodent models of autism, it is important to establish the validity of the model before extrapolating observed findings to the clinical population (Chadman et al. 2009; Crawley 2008). "Construct validity" indicates that the preclinical model incorporates an analogous biological perturbation (e.g., genetic mutation, environmental insult) that is associated with the human disease. This stipulation is relatively straightforward, given the number of such insults that have been linked to ASD. For genetic mutations, it is important that the orthologous genetic change is introduced into the mouse instead of just knocking out the gene, because human disease-causing mutations can be gain-of-function mutations (Tabuchi et al. 2007). "Face validity" indicates that the preclinical model shows phenotypes (and endophenotypes) analogous to those seen in the human disorder. Importantly, this criterion should also incorporate specificity: that is, a valid animal model should not show neural abnormalities that are not observed in the clinical syndrome. Finally, "predictive validity" indicates that therapeutics that are effective in a preclinical setting translate successfully to the clinical population (and vice versa). Because antipsychotics like risperidone are the only drugs approved by the US Food and Drug Administration to treat the core symptoms of autism, this criterion is likely the least important. However, specificity is important as well – a drug that has failed to improve core symptoms in children with autism

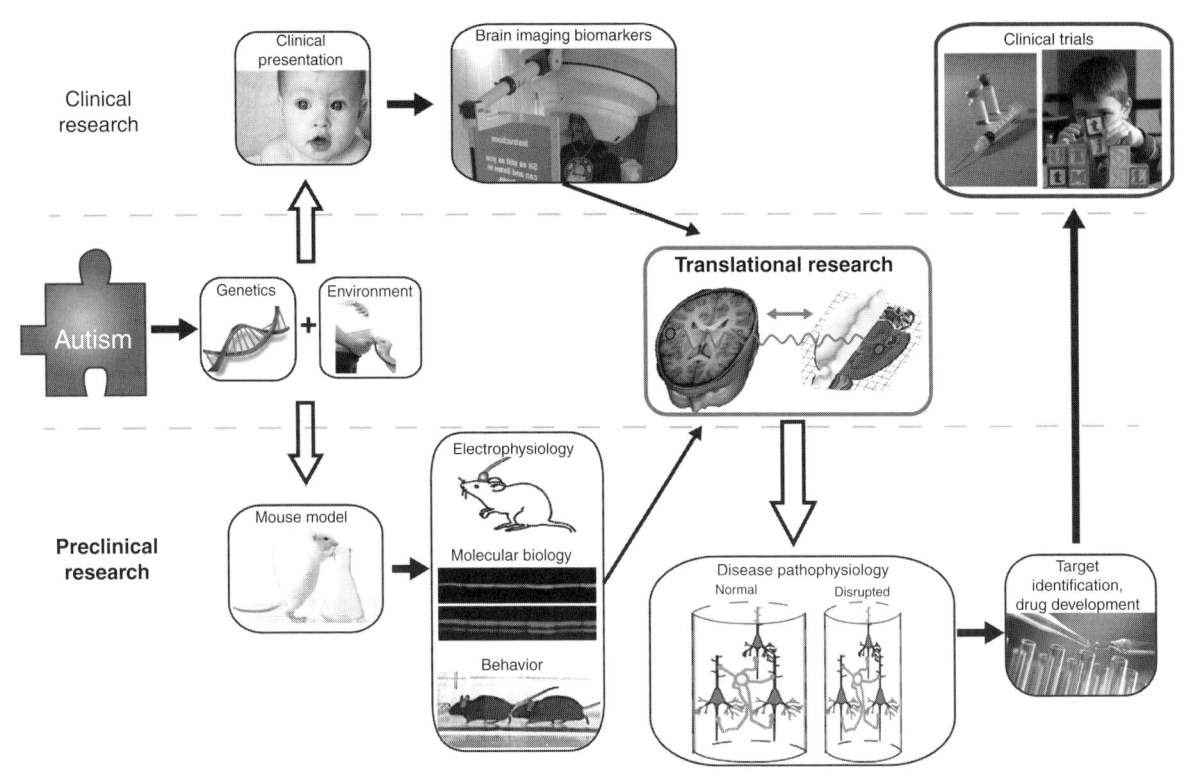

Figure 16.5. Approach to translational research in autism spectrum disorders. Clinical epidemiological studies have identified several autism candidate genes and environmental risk factors. Preclinical mouse models are being developed to recreate these genetic perturbations or environmental exposures. Such rodent models can then be investigated for alterations in molecular and cellular biology, behavior, and electrophysiology. Clinical studies, in particular those involving brain imaging and electrophysiology, are being done to identify autism endophenotypes. These heritable, quantitative metrics are more closely related to the abnormal brain dynamics of autism spectrum disorders than are the behavioral criteria and can help dissect gene–brain–behavior relationships in a complex genetic disorder. Endophenotypes can often be measured directly in preclinical models to help provide insight into the pathophysiology of disease and to provide new targets for preclinical therapeutic development. This figure is reproduced in color in the color plate section.

(e.g., selective serotonin reuptake inhibitors or secretin) should not be effective in valid animal models (Williams *et al.* 2005, 2010).

Developing animal models

Over the past decade, there has been a strong effort to develop mouse and rat models of autism, driven in large part by advances in genetic screening technologies that have helped to identify numerous autism risk genes. As discussed in detail below, modeling autism-like phenotypes in preclinical settings relies on three strategies: (1) introduction to orthologous genetic perturbations; (2) exposure to associated environmental risk factors, or (3) use of mouse screens.

Genetic mutations

The genetics of autism are extremely complex, but the discovery of autism risk genes has been aided by multiple parallel, complementary approaches. The first insights into the genetics of autism came from the identification of several "syndromic" forms of autism, a group of rare monogenetic disorders (i.e., tuberous sclerosis; Rett syndrome [RTT]; fragile X syndrome [FXS]) that share a high degree of overlap with ASD. In addition, chromosomal abnormalities consisting of *de novo* and inherited copy number variations (e.g., 16p11 deletion, 22q11 duplication/deletion, and 15q11–13 duplication syndromes) have been associated with autism. Together, these syndromes are thought to explain 10–25% of cases of autism. Recent work estimates that there are more than 100 such genetic disorders associated with autism (Abrahams and Geschwind 2008; Betancur 2011; Betancur *et al.* 2009). None of these syndromes, however, is fully penetrant for ASD, and they are often characterized by additional features not seen in "idiopathic autism." More recently, several rare, nonsyndromic autism risk genes have been identified (*NLGN3*, *NLGN4X*, *NRXN1*, *SHANK3*) through family linkage studies followed by resequencing (Durand *et al.* 2007; Jamain *et al.* 2003). These mutations are highly penetrant but extremely rare, accounting for less than 1–2% of total cases of autism and are often associated with additional neuropsychiatric disorders (Bozdagi *et al.* 2010). The search for common variants associated with autism has been much more difficult, probably due to the considerable heterogeneity of the disease and the small effect sizes. Several genome-wide linkage studies have reported significant loci, but only a few (17q11–22) have been replicated across studies (Cantor *et al.* 2005). Likewise, genome-wide association studies have begun to identify novel autism risk loci, including common variants (such as polymorphisms between cadherins 9 and 10), but these studies tend not to replicate each other's findings (Anney *et al.* 2010; Morrow *et al.* 2008; Szatmari *et al.* 2007; Wang *et al.* 2009; Weiss *et al.* 2009). Pathway analyses have shown that many of these variants share functionally interrelated cellular mechanisms, such as synaptic cell adhesion (Betancur *et al.* 2009), ERK and PI3K signaling (Levitt and Campbell 2009), transcriptional regulation and chromatin remodeling (Persico and Bourgeron 2006), neurotransmitter receptors and transporters (Lam *et al.* 2006), excitatory–inhibitory balance (Rubenstein and Merzenich 2003), calcium signaling (Krey and Dolmetsch 2007), synaptic plasticity (Bourgeron 2009), and neurotrophic factor regulation (Nickl-Jockschat and Michel 2011), among others.

Given the complexities outlined above, the search for a valid model of idiopathic autism has been difficult. Preclinical models are available for many of the syndromic forms of autism. FXS, which accounts for ~3% of total cases of autism, is caused by a loss of function of the X-linked transcription factor *FMR1* (Lugenbeel *et al.* 1995). Knockout of *Fmr1* orthologs in mice (Kooy 2003) and *Drosophila* (Dockendorff *et al.* 2002; Morales *et al.* 2002) causes behavioral and molecular deficits similar to those seen in the clinical syndrome, including social and cognitive impairments, seizures, and neurostructural abnormalities. Tuberous sclerosis accounts for ~2% of all cases of autism and is caused by loss of function mutations in *TSC1* or *TSC2*, which negatively regulate the mammalian target of rapamycin (mTOR) activity (European Chromosome 16 Tuberous Sclerosis Consortium 1993; Orlova and Crino 2010). *TSC1* and *TSC2* knockout mice have been characterized extensively, demonstrating cognitive and social impairments, altered vocalizations, epilepsy, reduced lifespan, and significant other neuronal abnormalities (Goorden *et al.* 2007; Young *et al.* 2010; Zeng *et al.* 2008). RTT is a neurodevelopmental disorder caused by missense and nonsense mutations in the X-linked transcription factor *MeCP2* (Amir *et al.* 1999). RTT is clinically characterized by autistic behaviors, epilepsy, cognitive deficits, developmental regression, and respiratory dysfunction. Mice harboring null mutations in *MeCP2* show neurological phenotypes similar to those seen in the clinical syndrome (Chen *et al.* 2001; Guy *et al.* 2001). Finally, transgenic mice have been developed to model the genetic changes seen in 22q11.2 deletion and duplication syndromes (Hiroi *et al.* 2005; Sigurdsson *et al.* 2010) and show significant behavioral abnormalities. Despite the strong face and construct validity of these preclinical models, there are questions about how generalizable findings are to ASD, given that these disorders are not fully penetrant for ASD and often show additional behavioral and neurological phenotypes not seen in "idiopathic autism."

Several mouse models recapitulating genetic changes from rare, highly penetrant nonsyndromic forms of autism have also been developed, including the mutations in genes *NLGN1*, *NLGN3*, *NLGN4*, *NRXN1*, *PTEN*, *EN2*, *GABRB3*, *OXT*, *SLAC6A4*, and *SHANK3* (Blundell *et al.* 2010; Bozdagi *et al.* 2010; Cheh *et al.* 2006; DeLorey *et al.* 2008; Etherton *et al.* 2009; Ferguson *et al.* 2000; Jamain *et al.* 2008; Kwon *et al.* 2006; Page *et al.* 2009; Tabuchi *et al.* 2007). Nearly all of these transgenic mice demonstrate ASD-relevant behavioral abnormalities (Moy and Nadler 2008; Silverman *et al.* 2010b) as well as alterations in excitatory or inhibitory signaling, although not all findings have been replicated (Chadman *et al.* 2008). However, the generalizability of these models is also unclear, given that most of these mutations are observed in only a small number of families with ASD. Likewise, several of these genes (e.g., *NRXN1*) have been associated with elevated risk for other neuropsychiatric disorders like schizophrenia (Rujescu *et al.* 2009). Investigating many of these rare, genetic causes of autism in parallel may help uncover an overlapping, final common pathway that contributes to disease pathogenesis.

Environmental insults

Although environmental contributions to the pathogenesis of autism are likely multifactorial, a few specific insults have been reproducibly identified as significant disease risk factors (Herbert 2010; Landrigan 2010). These include prenatal exposure to several drugs, including thalidomide (Miller *et al.* 2005; Stromland *et al.* 1994), valproic acid (VPA) (Bromley *et al.* 2008; Rasalam *et al.* 2005), and misoprostol (Miller *et al.* 2005). For example, *in utero* exposure to the anticonvulsant VPA has been associated with adverse neurodevelopmental outcomes, including lower IQ, poor language functioning, and a tenfold increase in the relative risk for ASD (Bromley *et al.* 2008, 2009; Meador *et al.* 2009; Rasalam *et al.* 2005). More recent evidence has implicated prenatal exposure to beta-2 adrenergic agonists (Witter *et al.* 2009) and the organophosphate insecticide chlorpyrifos (Rauh *et al.* 2006) with elevated risk for ASD, although the clinical evidence is less well established. Maternal infection during pregnancy has been associated with modestly increased risk for ASD (Wilkerson *et al.* 2002), most notably for congenital rubella (Chess *et al.* 1978). Finally, recent work has identified maternal autoantibodies targeting neural tissue that are present at elevated levels in autism (Goines and Van de Water 2010). This observation fits with increased rates of immune/autoimmune dysfunction in subjects with autism and their families (Libbey *et al.* 2005). It appears that risk of ASD is most elevated when such prenatal exposures occur during the first trimester of pregnancy (Arndt *et al.* 2005).

The identification of these environmental risk factors has allowed for the development of animal models with strong construct validity for autism. Indeed, significant behavioral deficits have been identified in a number of such insult-based preclinical models, including prenatal autoantibody exposure (Singer *et al.* 2009), prenatal viral infection (Shi *et al.* 2003), neonatal exposure to the beta-2 adrenergic agonist terbutaline (Zerrate *et al.* 2007), and in utero administration of chlorpyrifos (Levin *et al.* 2001). Whereas thalidomide does not produce the same teratogenic effects in rodents as it does in humans (Schumacher *et al.* 1972), prenatal exposure to VPA has been studied extensively as a model of ASD in rodents (Markram *et al.* 2007). In rats, a single injection of VPA in utero is sufficient to cause well-replicated, lasting behavioral deficits that mimic the human disorder, including reduced social preference, increased repetitive behaviors, and deficits in sensorimotor integration (Gandal *et al.* 2010; Markram *et al.* 2008; Schneider and Przewlocki 2005). Rodents exposed to VPA show cerebellar and brainstem pathological characteristics as well as synaptic and molecular changes consistent with autism, including hyperexcitability, serotonergic dysregulation, and reduced expression of neuroligin-3 (Gogolla *et al.* 2009; Ingram *et al.* 2000; Kolozsi *et al.* 2009; Markram *et al.* 2007, 2008; Rinaldi *et al.* 2007; Rodier *et al.* 1996; Rubenstein and Merzenich 2003). A downside to these insult-based models of autism is the fact that such environmental exposures likely account for only a small percentage of cases of ASD. Likewise, such environmental risk factors lack specificity for autism, because many have been associated with a host of neuropsychiatric disorders. However, as noted above, similar caveats apply to most preclinical genetic models of autism.

Mouse screens

Finally, several groups have used mouse behavioral screening strategies to identify genetic strains, environmental exposures, and brain regions that may be relevant to disease pathophysiology. Screening inbred mice has identified several strains with abnormally low sociability, including the BTBR (Moy *et al.* 2007) and BALB/Cj (Brodkin *et al.* 2004) strains. Further testing has identified several additional ASD-like phenotypic deficits in these mice, bolstering the face validity of such models (Glessner *et al.* 2009; McFarlane *et al.* 2008). However, until causative genetic alterations are identified, questions will remain about their construct validity for the clinical disease. Nevertheless, such models are useful for mapping the neural circuitry involved in regulation of social behaviors in rodents.

Screening environmental toxins with putative relevance to autism has also been frequently used in model organisms. For example, injection of the common food preservative propionic acid has caused social impairments in rats (Shultz *et al.* 2008). Likewise, chronic ingestion of heavy metals by prairie voles also caused reduced social preference (Curtis *et al.* 2010). However, until these compounds are definitively linked to autism in clinical and epidemiological studies, care must be taken when extrapolating such preclinical results to the clinical population. For example, despite overwhelming clinical evidence that the mercury-containing vaccine preservative thimerosal is not associated with increased risk for autism (Dyer 2010; Price et al. 2010; Schechter and Grether 2008; Thompson et al. 2007), preclinical studies reported that the drug causes behavioral abnormalities in mice (Hornig et al. 2004).

Behavioral phenotypes in preclinical models

Assessing the face validity of preclinical models of autism requires the development and validation of appropriate tasks that assess rodent behaviors analogous to the core symptoms of ASD, namely (1) reduced social interactions, (2) language impairments, and (3) repetitive or restricted interests and behaviors. Great progress has been made over the past decade to develop and validate paradigms that evaluate such behavior domains (Brodkin et al. 2004; Crawley 2004, 2007b; Moy et al. 2008; Scattoni et al. 2009; Silverman et al. 2010a). However, difficulty in directly modeling complex, human behaviors in rodents continues to remain a significant obstacle for translational research, especially for language impairment, which is frequently the most disabling core symptom of autism.

Social interactions

Autism is characterized by a lack of social reciprocity, with reduced interest in and ability to maintain social interactions. Fortunately, mice and rats naturally engage in a number of social behaviors, ranging from affiliative social play and communal nesting, to a host of sexual and aggressive interactions. As such, investigation of social behaviors in rodent models of autism has been relatively straightforward and well validated by genetic and pharmacological manipulations. For example, a number of genetic mouse models of autism have shown reduced social interactions (for review, see Silverman et al. 2010a). Likewise, the neuropeptide oxytocin has been shown to enhance affiliative social behaviors in both humans and mice (Insel 1997; Kosfeld et al. 2005).

A number of tests have been developed to assess appropriate social functioning in rodents. Most simply, one can investigate reciprocal social interactions between two rodents by placing them together in a neutral cage for a defined period of time. Videotaped interactions are then scored for various types of physical contact, including sniffing (nose to nose or nose to anogenital), following, mutual grooming, crawling under or over, and others (DeLorey et al. 2008). Mouse pairs should be of the same sex, age, genotype, and treatment. Likewise, mice should be unrelated (to avoid the "litter effect") and unfamiliar. It is often recommended that mice be tested during adolescence (postnatal days 21–45) to avoid potentially confounding sexual and aggressive tendencies that develop in adult animals.

More recently, social choice paradigms have been developed to evaluate approach-and-avoidance behaviors in individual mice (Brodkin et al. 2004; Nadler et al. 2004). This task uses a three-chambered apparatus with two immobile cylinders located in the outer partitions of the cage (Fig. 16.6). In the first phase of the experiment, a test mouse is placed in the center of the apparatus and tracked for 10 minutes by video. In phase 2, an unfamiliar, same-sex, wild-type stimulus mouse is placed inside one of the immobile cylinders. Gonadectomized A/J are often used as stimulus mice to minimize sexual and aggressive tendencies (Brodkin et al. 2004). The cylinders allow for visual, auditory, and olfactory investigation but require the social approach to be initiated by the test mouse while preventing sexual or aggressive acts. Finally, in phase 3 of the experiment, the immobile cylinders are removed to allow free interaction between test and stimulus animals. Dependent measures include time spent sniffing social and nonsocial cylinders, time spent in social and nonsocial chambers, locomotor activity, and aggressive behaviors. A variation of this paradigm can be used to assess social novelty and recognition (Winslow 2003). In this situation, a second unfamiliar stimulus mouse is placed in the nonsocial cylinder while the familiar stimulus remains under the social cylinder. The test mouse should spend more time investigating the novel stimulus mouse.

Finally, many other measures have been developed to investigate social behaviors in rodents. Whisker trimming, also termed barbering, is a commonly observed behavior in many strains of mice that is thought to reflect social dominance (Lijam et al. 1997; Strozik and Festing 1981). Mice with more, longer whiskers when caged in pairs are thought to have reduced social interaction leading to less mutual whisker trimming. Likewise, nest building is a shared social behavior that can easily be quantified (Schneider and Chenoweth 1970). Finally, tests of social dominance have been created and shown to correlate

283

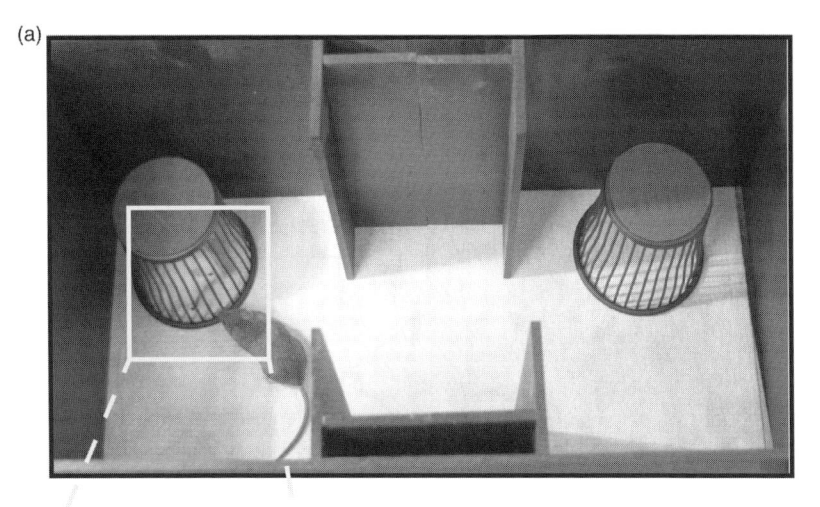

Figure 16.6. Social choice testing in rodents measures affiliative approach-and-avoidance behaviors. (A) A three-chambered social approach/avoidance apparatus is shown with an immobile (white) stimulus mouse and a freely moving (brown) test mouse. A video camera above (not shown) tracks the movements and the sniffing behavior of the test mouse. (Inset) The test mouse can engage in olfactory, auditory, and visual investigation of the stimulus mouse. (B) A heat map indicates where the test mouse is located during a 10-minute session. As shown, the test mouse spends significantly more time investigating the social cylinder than the nonsocial cylinder. This figure is reproduced in color in the color plate section.

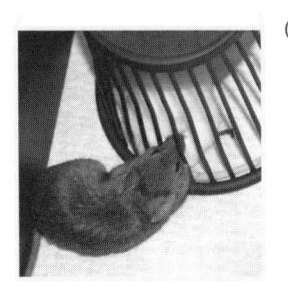

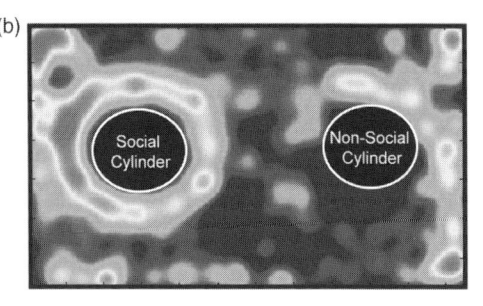

with other social behaviors, like whisker-trimming behavior (Lijam *et al.* 1997; Lindzey *et al.* 1961; Messeri *et al.* 1975). In the social dominance paradigm, two same-sex mice of different experimental manipulations are placed at the opposite ends of a narrow tube and allowed to interact. Dominance is attributed to the remaining mouse when the other mouse backs out of the tube.

Communicative function

The second core symptom domain of autism is characterized by deficits in language function, including delay in verbal language, impairments in pragmatic language use, and stereotyped or repetitive communication. Differences in prosody and tonality, which are frequently instantly recognizable features of the disorder, are often present in individuals with ASD (Page *et al.* 2009). Although symptom severity is heterogeneous, 20–40% of autistic individuals never acquire fully developed speech beyond a few words (Hollander *et al.* 2011; Young *et al.* 2010). Despite this observation, few treatments target communication problems, and an understanding of how genetic and environmental factors contribute to the development of this core deficit remains poor.

Investigating language functioning in rodent models of autism has been a significant obstacle for preclinical studies. Mice communicate using olfactory and acoustic signals. Rodent ultrasonic vocalizations (USVs) have been investigated as a communicative behavior analogous to that of human language, despite the fact that mice only emit such calls in a limited number of contexts. The current standard for assessing vocal communication in mice is to record ultrasonic distress calls emitted from pups temporarily separated from their litter. Pups make 30 to 90 kHz distress USVs between postnatal days 2 to 12 when temporally isolated from the litter (Hofer *et al.* 2002) (Fig. 16.7). Such calls have been shown to have communicative significance in mice, because they induce approach behaviors by the dam to retrieve the isolated pup (Ehret 1987). Interestingly, reduced USV distress calls were observed in mice expressing a mutant form of the transcription factor *FoxP2*, which causes severe speech and language disorders in humans (Shu *et al.* 2005). Likewise, introduction of the humanized

Chapter 16: Autism spectrum disorders

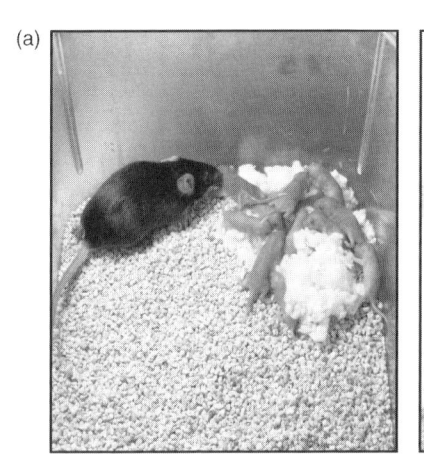

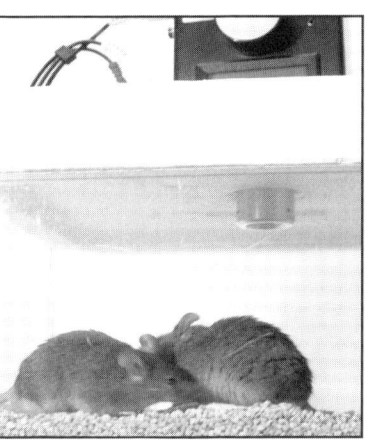

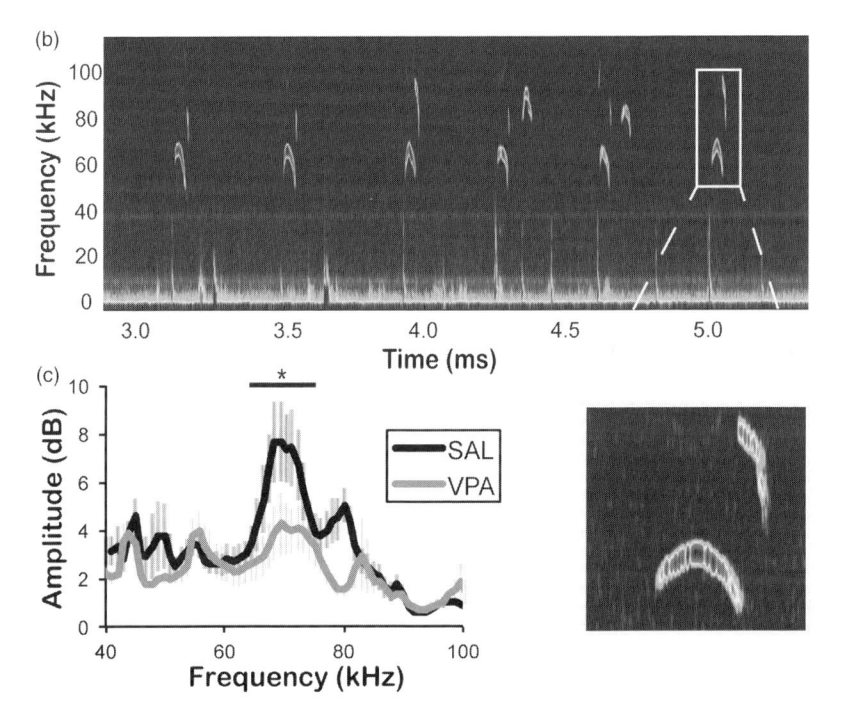

Figure 16.7. Rodent ultrasonic vocalizations are used as a measure of communicative function in preclinical models of autism. (A) In mice, ultrasonic vocalizations are generally investigated in two types of paradigms (Messeri et al. 1975). Neonatal "distress" vocalizations are elicited by temporarily removing a single mouse pup from the litter. Ultrasonic calls emitted by the isolated infant serve as a signal for the dam to come retrieve the pup (Szatmari et al. 2007). Adult same-sex mice will emit ultrasonic vocalizations when paired together after several days of social isolation. In addition, male mice will emit characteristic 70-kHz premating vocalizations and 40-kHz mating vocalizations when paired with a receptive female. (B) Sonogram demonstrating the time and frequency characteristics of mouse vocalizations. Calls can be characterized by density, duration, frequency, intensity, and spectral shape (e.g., prosody). (C) A spectrogram of adult male premating vocalizations recorded from male mice exposed to prenatal valproic acid (VPA) or saline (SAL) when paired with a wild-type receptive female mouse. SAL-exposed mice demonstrate a characteristic peak at 70 kHz that is notably absent in the group exposed to VPA. Modified from *Biological Psychiatry*, Vol. 68, Gandal MJ, Edgar JC, Ehrlichman RS, Mehta M, Roberts TP, Siegel SJ. Validating gamma oscillations and delayed auditory responses as translational biomarkers of autism, pp. 1100–1106, copyright 2010, with permission from Elsevier. This figure is reproduced in color in the color plate section.

version of *FoxP2* (two amino acid substitutions) into mice, which is thought to reflect the evolutionary development of human language, induces alterations in the types (but not absolute numbers) of neonatal USVs (Enard et al. 2009; White et al. 2006). Given these findings, preclinical studies of autism have increasingly investigated such neonatal distress calls as a measure of "protolanguage" function in mice (Scattoni et al. 2009), many of which have found significant differences (Gandal et al. 2010; Scattoni et al. 2008). Dependent measures typically involve measuring the number, intensity, latency, and spectral content with little understanding of the meaning of such calls (Liu et al. 2003). In addition, as is true in relation to an infant's crying, how much these calls directly reflect language is unclear. Finally, several potential confounders have been shown to affect such neonatal distress vocalizations, including state anxiety, body temperature, and deficits in motor coordination (e.g., orofacial and verbal dyspraxia) (Hofer et al. 2002; Scattoni et al. 2011; Shu et al. 2005).

Researchers have begun recently to investigate vocalizations emitted by adult mice, which may have more direct relevance to human language, although again such a connection will be difficult to directly establish (Lahvis *et al.* 2011). Vocalizations emitted in male–female mating pairings have been studied the most. In such a paradigm, males elicit characteristic 70-kHz "premating" vocalizations prior to mount, followed by 40-kHz "mating" calls during copulation (Nyby 1983; White *et al.* 1998). Such vocalizations, which can be elicited simply by exposure to female urine during estrus, are emitted exclusively by males and have been shown to be disrupted in multiple mouse models of autism (Gandal *et al.* 2010; Holy and Guo 2005). Vocalizations emitted by same-sex dyads have been less well characterized. Following social isolation, adolescent and adult male–male and female–female pairs have been shown to emit USVs during social investigation (Lahvis *et al.* 2011; Panksepp *et al.* 2007). Indeed, multiple studies have shown a correlation between number of emitted vocalizations and time of social exploration, suggesting that USVs may be an index of social communication (Moles *et al.* 2007; Nyby 1983; Panksepp *et al.* 2007; Scattoni *et al.* 2011). Although USVs emitted during female–female pairings appear to reflect affiliative behavior and social recognition (Ricceri *et al.* 2007), some controversy exists about the underlying behavioral intention of calls produced by male–male dyads. Some groups have found that such calls are associated with affiliative interactions (Panksepp *et al.* 2007; Scattoni *et al.* 2011). Other groups have shown them to be predictive of aggressive encounters (Gourbal *et al.* 2004; Lahvis *et al.* 2011), and some groups failed to detect any vocalizations from male–male pairings (Ferguson *et al.* 2000). Such divergent results may reflect strain effects, differences in experiment parameters (bedding, length of isolation, age, lighting, handling), or potential state confounders such as anxiety. That fact that adult vocalizations are so sensitive to experimental conditions makes comparisons across groups difficult. Likewise, the fact that adult USV emissions tend to occur only after social isolation and last only for the first few minutes following mouse pairing (unlike other social behaviors) is potentially problematic given that human communication does not follow a similar pattern.

Repetitive restricted interests and behaviors

The third core domain of symptomatic deficits in autism consists of stereotyped, repetitive behaviors

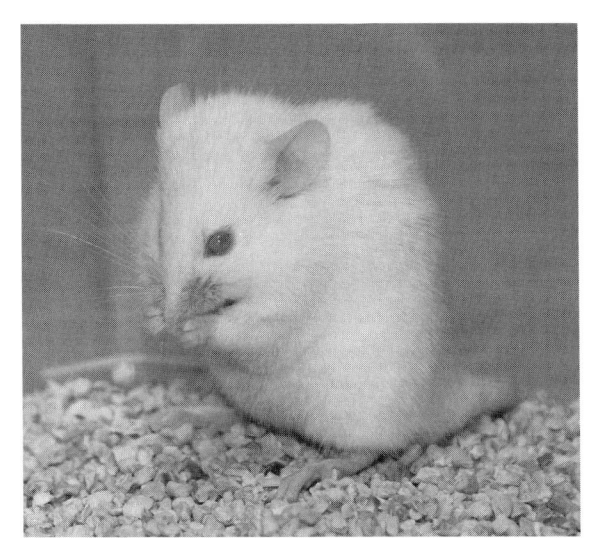

Figure 16.8. Spontaneous self-grooming is often assessed as a stereotypic, repetitive behavior in mice analogous to the third core symptom domain in autism.

and mannerisms as well as restricted, rigid interests and behaviors. Several preclinical assays have been developed to assess analogous behaviors in mice (Crawley 2008; Moy *et al.* 2008). Mice engage in a host of repetitive behaviors (i.e., stereotypies), including self-grooming, circling, forelimb clasping, and spontaneous marble burying (Lewis *et al.* 2007; Thomas *et al.* 2009). Repetitive self-grooming behavior is easy to quantify and has been shown to be elevated in several mouse models of autism, sometimes to the point of self-injury (Chao *et al.* 2010; Etherton *et al.* 2009; Gandal *et al.* 2010; Glessner *et al.* 2009) (Fig. 16.8). Reversal learning in mice, such as with T-maze or water maze paradigms, has been proposed as a means to assess behavioral rigidity seen in autism. Finally, limited exploration in a hole-board paradigm has been proposed as a measure of restricted interests (Moy *et al.* 2008).

Associated phenotypes

Autism is associated with increased incidence of a host of neurological and psychiatric comorbidities, including epilepsy (5–49%), intellectual disability (40–80%), anxiety (43–84%), attention deficit hyperactivity disorder (ADHD, 59%), sensory hypersensitivity (tactile: 80–90%; auditory: 5–47%), and sleep disruption (52–73%), among others (Levy *et al.* 2009). Although these comorbid disorders are nondiagnostic, assessing analogous preclinical phenotypes is informative for the pathophysiology of autism and its overlap with other diseases. Well-validated behavioral paradigms exist to assess each of these phenotypes, including seizures (electroencephalography to record spontaneous, audiogenic, or drug-induced seizures), spatial learning and memory function (Morris water navigation task, Barnes maze, novel object recognition), emotional learning and memory (cued and contextual fear conditioning), anxiety-related behaviors (open-field assay, elevated plus maze, light/dark box), ADHD-related behaviors (spontaneous or amphetamine-induced locomotor activity, 5-choice serial reaction time task), sensory hypersensitivity (tactile and auditory startle), and sleep disruption (EEG, home cage activity monitoring) (Crawley 2004, 2007; Silverman *et al.* 2010*b*).

Assessing model specificity

When assessing the behavioral effects of genetic or environmental perturbations relevant to autism in rodents, it is important to assess the specificity of such deficits. Autism is not caused by comprehensive neurological impairment. Global brain dysfunction in a mouse could, however, manifest itself with autism-like phenotypes. Therefore, it is important to rule out nonspecific developmental, sensory, and motor deficits. Comprehensive characterization of developmental milestones in infant rodents includes assessment of physical landmarks (weight, eye opening, fur development), developmental reflexes (righting reflex, rooting reflex), and locomotor activity (Heyser 2004; Morrow *et al.* 2008). Measures of sensory function in rodents include auditory brain-stem responses and acoustic startle paradigms, olfactory preference tasks, and visual discrimination paradigms (Prusky *et al.* 2000; Witt *et al.* 2009). Motor coordination and motor learning can be tested using an accelerating rotorod protocol. Such comprehensive phenotypic characterization helps rule out potential behavioral confounders that could contribute to false positive results. For example, reduced social activity could be caused by deficits in olfactory function or reduced locomotor activity.

Translational approaches to preclinical investigation

The importance of developing new therapeutic strategies to target symptoms of autism highlights the need to identify neural biomarkers (e.g., endophenotypes) that are associated with these deficits. Because the autism phenotype is heterogeneous and complex, it unlikely that reliable direct relationships will be observed between the complex disease phenotype and brain, symptom, cognitive, and genetic measures. Individual endophenotypes are presumably determined by fewer genes than the more complex behavioral phenotype and would therefore reduce the complexity of genetic analysis (Gottesman and Gould 2003; Viding and Blakemore 2007). These measures are heritable, quantitative, disease-associated, prebehavioral traits that are thought to be in the intermediate pathway between genetic etiology and clinical syndrome. Endophenotypes can also be used to track treatment progress over time, provide insight into, and more closely reflect neurophysiological disease mechanisms than behavioral symptoms alone (Braff *et al.* 2007). Indeed, support for this approach is strengthened by recent findings that unaffected relatives of autistic children often show autism-like phenotypes to a lesser degree (Constantino *et al.* 2006). Unlike behavioral phenotypes, endophenotypes can often be measured in preclinical settings using directly analogous methods.

Cognitive endophenotypes

Several cognitive measures have been proposed as endophenotypes of autism, including "mindblindness" (i.e., mentalizing impairments), "weak central coherence," and deficits in emotional face processing (Viding and Blakemore 2007; Wallace *et al.* 2010). The measure "age of first word" has been successfully used in a genome-wide scan across several hundred affected families to identify potential genetic contributions to language-related deficits (Alarcon *et al.* 2005). Although these endophenotypes are generally heritable and well-replicated in autism, they are not amenable to translational investigation in model organisms. However, emerging evidence suggests that delayed language acquisition in autism may stem from underlying attentional deficits (Charman *et al.* 2003; Page *et al.* 2009), which have recently been identified in first-degree unaffected relatives (Mosconi *et al.* 2010). In preclinical settings, several attentional measures have been developed, including latent inhibition testing and the 5-choice serial reaction time task (Higgins and Breysse 2008; Yamada 2010). Using similar paradigms, attentional deficits have been identified in a mouse model relevant to autism (Moon *et al.* 2006).

Neuroanatomical endophenotypes

One of the most consistently reported neuroanatomical abnormalities in autism is early, enlarged head circumference (Muscarella *et al.* 2007). Such findings have been reported in unaffected relatives, associated with specific genetic polymorphisms, linked to immune system and serotonergic dysfunction, and correlated with symptom domains (Conciatori *et al.* 2004; Fidler *et al.* 2000; Muscarella *et al.* 2007; Wassink *et al.* 2007). Likewise, macrocephaly has been demonstrated in both genetic and environmental insult-based mouse models of autism (Fatemi *et al.* 2002; Kwon *et al.* 2006). However, head size, which is a static measure, seems less useful as a translational biomarker because it provides little insight into the abnormal neural dynamics underlying phenotypic deficits in autism.

Molecular endophenotypes

Complex immune system dysfunction has been proposed as a molecular endophenotype of autism. Individuals with ASD and their healthy siblings show altered profiles of immune cells and increased serum levels of inflammatory cytokines (Saresella *et al.* 2009; Schwarz *et al.* 2010). These data fit with evidence of an association between autism and specific human leukocyte antigen subtypes (Lee *et al.* 2006) and autoimmune disease (Enstrom *et al.* 2009). Whereas hosts of studies have identified immunological abnormalities in autism, there has been a lack of consistent and unifying data with associations to clinical symptoms and established connections to disease pathogenesis (Zimmerman 2005).

Serotonergic (5-HT) abnormalities have been identified in patients with autism and first-degree relatives, including reduced receptor density in the cortex and elevated blood levels of serotonin (Goldberg *et al.* 2009; Piven *et al.* 1991). These findings have been linked to polymorphisms in serotonin transporter genes (Devlin *et al.* 2005). Brain-imaging studies demonstrated that children with autism lack the appropriate peak of brain serotonin synthesis during development (Chandana *et al.* 2005). Interestingly, a recent study demonstrated that deficits in serotonin transporter binding are significantly associated with impairments in social cognition and elevated repetitive, obsessive behaviors (Nakamura *et al.* 2010). Demonstrating translational ability, serotonergic abnormalities have been demonstrated in several mouse models of autism (Brodkin 2007; Cheh *et al.* 2006; Winter *et al.* 2008). However, it remains to be determined how (or if) serotonergic abnormalities contribute to the pathophysiology of autism. Some have speculated that serotonergic modulation of other neurotransmitter systems (e.g., glutamate) and of neurotrophic factors (e.g, BDNF) may be its role in autism, although this has yet to be proved (Blue 2009). Establishing a mechanistic connection is especially relevant given a recent meta-analysis demonstrating that selective serotonin reuptake inhibitors are not effective for treatment of autism (Williams *et al.* 2010).

Neurophysiological endophenotypes

Prepulse inhibition (PPI) of the auditory startle response is a measure of sensorimotor integration and inhibitory control that has been well characterized in humans and rodents (Swerdlow *et al.* 1999). This paradigm assesses preattentive sensory adaptation and, importantly, can be measured in humans and rodents using highly consistent methods (Geyer *et al.* 2002). Several studies have demonstrated PPI deficits in children and adults with ASD (Frankland *et al.* 2004; McAlonan *et al.* 2002; Perry *et al.* 2007), although this measure has yet to be examined in unaffected relatives (Mosconi *et al.* 2010). PPI deficits have been linked to several ASD risk genes (Frankland *et al.* 2004; Levin *et al.* 2009; Sobin *et al.* 2005) as well as to neurocognitive outcome measures (Frankland *et al.* 2004; Sobin *et al.* 2005). PPI deficits have been reported in several preclinical ASD models (de Vrij *et al.* 2008; DeLorey *et al.* 2011; Gandal *et al.* 2010; Kwon *et al.* 2006; Markram *et al.* 2007; Moy *et al.* 2009; Paylor *et al.* 2006; Shi *et al.* 2003). Interestingly, reversal of PPI deficits with a metabotropic glutamate receptor (mGluR5) antagonist has been demonstrated in both preclinical (de Vrij *et al.* 2008; Gandal *et al.* 2010) and clinical settings (Berry-Kravis *et al.* 2009), suggesting strong predictive validity for these measures. However, it is unclear how disruption of PPI relates to core behavioral symptoms of autism. In addition, such findings are hardly specific to autism, as PPI deficits have been observed in a host of other neuropsychiatric disorders (Swerdlow *et al.* 1999).

Smooth-pursuit and saccadic eye movement impairments have been proposed as an endophenotype of autism, given well-replicated findings in subjects with autism and their relatives (Mosconi *et al.* 2010; Takarae *et al.* 2004) coupled with evidence of heritability (Bell *et al.* 1994). Deficits in these quantitative metrics have implicated cerebellar and frontoparietal dysfunction in autism (Mosconi *et al.* 2010; Takarae *et al.* 2004), in accordance with histopathological evidence of cerebellar abnormalities (Palmen *et al.* 2004). Whereas saccadic dysmetria in autism provides important insight into dysfunctional neural networks in the disorder, it is unclear how these findings relate to core symptomatic deficits. In addition, the difficulty in developing analogous paradigms for rodents reduces the translatability of this biomarker.

Neuroimaging endophenotypes

Using auditory evoked response EEG/MEG paradigms (as discussed in section 1), several studies have demonstrated that early auditory encoding processes are abnormal in autism (Jeste and Nelson 2009; Roberts *et al.* 2008). Using simple pure-tone or click paradigms, recent work has demonstrated delayed profiles of auditory processing in subjects with autism (Bruneau *et al.* 1999; Gage *et al.* 2003; Roberts *et al.* 2010; Sokhadze *et al.* 2009a) as well as in unaffected relatives, to a lesser degree (Maziade *et al.* 2000). In particular, one MEG study found such robust differences in the latency of the M100 auditory evoked response that classification of autism was possible with accuracy of 75% (Roberts *et al.* 2010). At least one study has reported an association between delayed auditory evoked responses and oral language ability (Oram Cardy *et al.* 2008), although a later study did not replicate this finding (Roberts *et al.* 2010). The development of appropriate language is contingent on proper development of the auditory cortex, as delays in such maturation are known to cause deteriorated speech and language processing capabilities (Wang 2004). Deficits in auditory processing (e.g., delayed peak latencies) have also been demonstrated in studies of dyslexic individuals (Alonso-Bua *et al.* 2006; van Herten *et al.* 2008), children with specific language impairment (Benasich and Tallal 2002), and children with language-based learning problems (Diedler *et al.* 2009). These recording paradigms are passive and thus can be assessed in infants or animals.

Similar to human evoked-potential studies, rodents can be examined for endophenotypes of preattentive auditory processing, assessing the ability to discriminate between tones presented at different frequencies or temporal proximity. Since mice

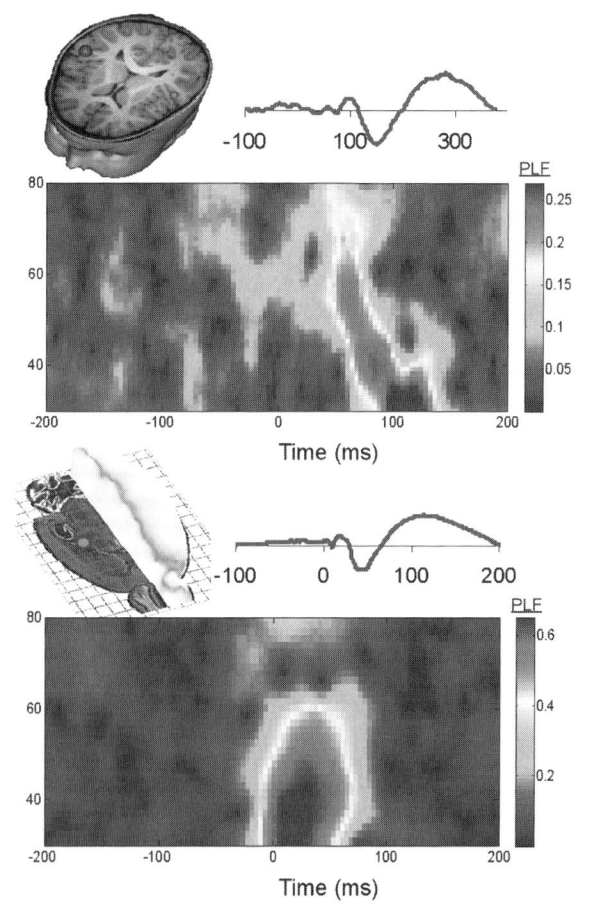

Figure 16.9. Pure-tone auditory evoked responses recorded around the auditory cortex are demonstrated in humans (top) using magnetoencephalography and in mice (bottom) using intracranial electrodes. Top plots show time-domain grand averages of auditory evoked responses, which demonstrate corresponding P1/M50 and N1/M100 peaks. Bottom plots show transient gamma-band phase-locking, with peak responses in both groups occurring at ~40 Hz. Modified from *Biological Psychiatry*, Vol. 68, Gandal MJ, Edgar JC, Ehrlichman RS, Mehta M, Roberts TP, Siegel SJ. Validating gamma oscillations and delayed auditory responses as translational biomarkers of autism, pp. 1100–1106, copyright 2010, with permission from Elsevier. This figure is reproduced in color in the color plate section.

communicate with auditory signals, deficiencies in auditory processing would be detrimental to communicative abilities. Auditory evoked responses have been extensively explored in rats (Simpson and Knight 1993) and mice (Siegel *et al.* 2003; Umbricht *et al.* 2004), with highly analogous waveforms observed across species (Fig. 16.9). Recent work has demonstrated the translational potential of auditory evoked response endophenotypes in autism research (Gandal *et al.* 2010). It was shown that both children with autism and the VPA-insult model of autism demonstrate strikingly similar delays in the mid-latency N1/M100 auditory evoked response, without significant changes in other peak amplitudes or latencies. This endophenotype can then be used as a target for therapeutic intervention and to investigate potential pathophysiological neural mechanisms.

Auditory evoked responses have been assessed in more complex paradigms in autism, eliciting similar results. Using an auditory oddball (i.e., mismatch negativity) paradigm, which characterizes the brain's response to deviant stimuli, multiple studies have shown latency delays in children with autism, suggesting further deficits in auditory cortical function (Kasai et al. 2005; Kujala et al. 2005; Oram Cardy et al. 2005a). During a rapid temporal processing paradigm, ASD subjects failed to show an evoked response to the second stimulus (Oram Cardy et al. 2005a). This paradigm assesses the ability to mount a neural response to the second of two rapidly presented stimuli. Taken together, these studies indicate that autism is characterized by abnormalities in rapid auditory processing. Auditory mismatch negativity recordings have been characterized in mice (Ehrlichman et al. 2008; Umbricht et al. 2005) and rats (Tikhonravov et al. 2008) and been shown to be sensitive to N-methyl-D-aspartic acid (NMDA)-receptor signaling (Ehrlichman et al. 2008; Tikhonravov et al. 2008) as demonstrated in humans (Umbricht et al. 2002). Mismatch negativity has not been investigated as a neurophysiological biomarker in preclinical models of autism, although it has been assessed in mouse models of other neuropsychiatric disorders (Ehrlichman et al. 2009). Rapid temporal processing has yet to be directly investigated in lower order species.

Abnormalities in lateralization of receptive language function have also been reported in ASD, with autistic children demonstrating rightward lateralization as opposed to typical left hemispheric dominance observed in healthy controls (Escalante-Mead et al. 2003; Flagg et al. 2005; Kleinhans et al. 2008). Such findings have been linked to deficits in language function as measured by neuropsychological testing (Bigler et al. 2007). Interestingly, mice also show left hemisphere lateralization when recognizing ultrasonic vocalizations, which can induce approach behaviors (Ehret 1987). To date, this neural phenotype has not been assessed in a mouse model of autism or related neuropsychiatric diseases.

In contrast to traditional EEG/MEG studies, which have generally analyzed neural responses in the time domain, recent work has begun to investigate neural synchrony in autism (Uhlhaas and Singer 2006, 2007; Welsh et al. 2005). Neural oscillatory activity serves to synchronize neural networks within and across brain structures to facilitate coherent cognitive routines. In particular, high-frequency, gamma-band (30–80 Hz) oscillations have been shown to mediate a host of cognitive and sensory functions, including sensory encoding (i.e., perceptual 'feature binding'), selective attention, and memory (Herrmann et al. 2010). In addition, emerging evidence indicates that gamma-band activity mediates certain aspects of social and communicative functioning (Benasich et al. 2008; Braeutigam et al. 2001; Meyer et al. 2005; Williams et al. 2009). Several studies have identified gamma-band abnormalities in autism during visual (Milne et al. 2009; Orekhova et al. 2007; Sokhadze et al. 2009b) and auditory (Braeutigam et al. 2008; Gandal et al. 2010; Rojas et al. 2008; Wilson et al. 2007) paradigms, thought to reflect abnormal cognitive and perceptual functioning in the disorder. Other frequency bands have been investigated in autism, albeit to a lesser degree. Significant abnormalities in the beta rhythm have been observed in autism during motor movement execution or observation, thought to reflect mirror neuron system dysfunction (Honaga et al. 2010; Puzzo et al. 2010). Alterations in lower frequencies (e.g., theta and alpha) have also been reported (Coben et al. 2008; Isler et al. 2010; Murias et al. 2007; Thatcher et al. 2009), although findings are somewhat more mixed and preliminary.

Recent work has begun to investigate neural synchrony as a biomarker in preclinical models. In parallel human and mouse auditory evoked response studies, children with autism and mice exposed in utero to valproic acid demonstrated analogous reductions in the transient auditory-evoked gamma-band response (Gandal et al. 2010), which is thought to reflect perceptual encoding in the auditory cortex (Pantev et al. 1991) (Fig. 16.10). These findings fit with previous work demonstrating that prenatal VPA exposure causes a loss of parvalbumin-expressing interneurons (Gogolla et al. 2009), which are necessary and sufficient generators of the gamma rhythm (Sohal et al. 2009). As such, gamma synchrony is highly sensitive to the ratio of excitation to inhibition in the cortex, which is thought to be

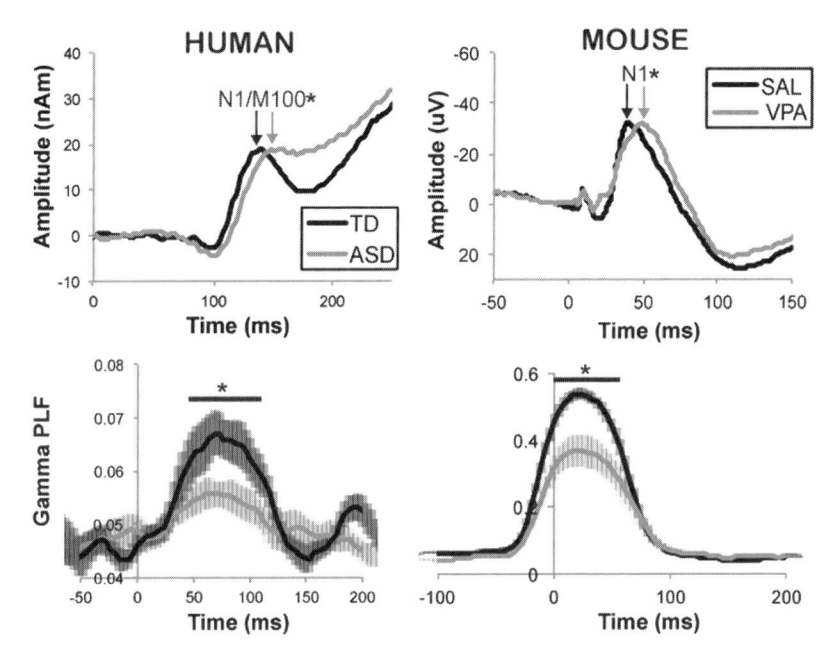

Figure 16.10. The translational potential of auditory evoked-response endophenotypes is demonstrated. (Left column) Pure-tone auditory evoked responses were recorded in children with autism (ASD) and in typically developing (TD) controls. (Right column) Auditory evoked potentials were recorded using analogous methods in the prenatal valproic acid (VPA)-mouse model of autism and in saline (SAL)-treated controls. (Top row) Children with autism and VPA-exposed mice show a significant, ~10% delay in the latency of the N1/M100 auditory evoked response, indicating similar deficits in the temporal precision of auditory stimulus encoding. (Bottom row) Children with autism and VPA-treated mice demonstrate deficits in the transient auditory gamma-band response, suggesting deficient excitatory–inhibitory balance. Modified from *Biological Psychiatry*, Vol. 68, Gandal MJ, Edgar JC, Ehrlichman RS, Mehta M, Roberts TP, Siegel SJ. Validating gamma oscillations and delayed auditory responses as translational biomarkers of autism, pp. 1100–1106, copyright 2010, with permission from Elsevier. This figure is reproduced in color in the color plate section.

disrupted in favor of excitation in autism (Rubenstein and Merzenich 2003). In accordance with this hypothesis, local excitation is elevated in the VPA model (Markram et al. 2007, 2008; Rinaldi et al. 2007). In addition, gamma oscillatory abnormalities following VPA exposure were highly correlated with expression of the autism risk gene *NLGN3*, which regulates excitatory and inhibitory synapse function (Gandal et al. 2010; Varoqueaux et al. 2006). Similar results were observed in vitro, where cultured neurons harboring an autism-related mutation in *NLGN3* showed altered local circuit synchrony and structure as well as a reduction in GABAergic interneurons (Gutierrez et al. 2009). Gamma oscillations are also disrupted in the *Fmr1*-knockout mouse model of fragile X syndrome, which also shows hyperexcitability likely due to loss of inhibition (Gibson et al. 2008). Likewise, *Df*(16)A+/− mice, which model the human 22q11.2 microdeletion associated with autism, have shown significant deficits in neural synchrony during cognitive activation (Sigurdsson et al. 2010). Although gamma (or neural) synchrony has not been explicitly investigated in other preclinical ASD models, several show alterations in excitatory/inhibitory balance and thus would likely demonstrate gamma abnormalities. These models include *NRXN1α* knockout mice (Etherton et al. 2009), *MeCP2*-null mice (Zhang et al. 2008), *TSC1*-deficient mice (Wang et al. 2007), *NLGN1* deletion (Blundell et al. 2010), *NLGN2* deletion (Blundell et al. 2009), and *NLGN4* missense mutation (Zhang et al. 2009), among others.

Therapeutic development

Current treatment options for autism spectrum disorders are limited. Nearly all effective interventions for ASD involve some form of environmental enrichment or applied behavioral therapy, including specialized educational programs, social skills training, speech and language therapy, as well as parent-based interventions (Levy et al. 2009). Medically, antipsychotic drugs such as risperidone are the only effective, FDA-approved treatments for core symptoms (Jesner et al. 2007). Although risperidone is beneficial for irritability and repetitive behaviors in autism, it has no effect on the core social and communicative deficits that are generally most debilitating. Despite evidence for serotonergic dysfunction, a recent meta-analysis of clinical trials for SSRIs in autism concluded that these drugs are not effective for core behavioral deficits, although they may still be useful for comorbid anxiety disorders (Levy et al. 2009; Williams et al. 2010). Methylphenidate is effective for comorbid ADHD or attentional dysfunction (Jahromi et al. 2009; Network RUoPPA 2005), although effect sizes are relatively modest with a higher incidence of adverse effects. Many complementary and alternative medical treatments have been used in children with autism, despite the fact that most of these approaches have little or no evidence to support their use (Levy and Hyman 2008). As such, there is a great need to develop new, biologically based treatment approaches that target core symptoms of autism. Such a goal requires a robust preclinical drug development approach with well-validated therapeutic targets.

Emerging evidence suggests that core pathogenic insults leading to autism occur *in utero* or during early development, despite the fact that the disorder is typically not diagnosed until around 2 years of age. As such, there is the risk that medical intervention after ASD presentation may be too late because the brain has already been incorrectly wired. However, recent developments from preclinical models of syndromic forms of autism indicate that neural rescue is indeed possible, even after full phenotypic presentation. For example, electrophysiological recordings in *Fmr1* knockout mice identified significant alterations in synaptic plasticity due to overactive signaling through mGluR5s (Huber et al. 2002). Blockade of these receptors was able to rescue both behavioral and electrophysiological deficits in *Drosophila* (McBride et al. 2005) and mouse models (Krueger and Bear 2011; Yan et al. 2005) of FXS, even when administered in adults. On the basis of these results, mGluR5 antagonists and similar compounds are now in clinical trials for FXS. Similarly promising results have been reported in preclinical studies of TSC. Several groups have now shown that treatment with mTOR suppressors like rapamycin reverses many of the behavioral and neurological deficits caused by *TSC1* or *TSC2* haploinsufficiency in mice, even when administered in adulthood (Ehninger et al. 2008; Meikle et al. 2008; Zeng et al. 2008). A number of other autism risk genes serve as negative regulators of mTOR activity, including *PTEN*, *NF1*, and *DISC1* (Ehninger and Silva 2011; Hoeffer and Klann 2010). Rapamycin-mediated reversal of phenotypic deficits has likewise been demonstrated in mouse models with mutations in several of these genes (Kim et al. 2009; Zhou et al. 2009). Finally, in mouse models of RTT, recent work has shown that adult reexpression of *MeCP2* in *MeCP2*-null mice can cause robust reversal of neurological deficits (Guy et al. 2007). In addition, it has been shown that one of the main targets of *MeCP2* is BDNF and that a loss of *MeCP2* leads to reduced levels of BDNF. Interestingly, overexpression of BDNF in *MeCP2*-null mice also leads to phenotypic reversal (Chang et al. 2006). This finding is especially important given the recent identification of several neuroactive compounds that stimulate the BDNF receptor, TrkB, and thus may be effective pharmacological therapies in RTT (Jang et al. 2010; Massa et al. 2010). Taken together, results from preclinical studies of these syndromic forms of autism demonstrate that robust reversal of neurological and behavioral deficits is possible, even well after the presentation of such symptoms. This observation has important implications for idiopathic autism, suggesting that targeted therapies may be effective as well.

Less evidence exists for effective therapeutic reversal of neural deficits in nonsyndromic models of autism. As has been demonstrated in the clinical population, early environmental enrichment is one of the most effective interventions. Likewise, in preclinical studies, early environmental enrichment has successfully improved cognitive and behavioral impairments across multiple models, including *Fmr1* knockout mice (Restivo et al. 2005), *MeCP2* null mice (Lonetti et al. 2010), BTBR mice (Yang et al. 2011), and rats exposed to VPA in utero (Schneider et al. 2006). Other studies have shown that restoring the balance of excitation to inhibition with drugs that modulate glutamatergic signaling can improve some deficits in models of autism. For example, *NLGN1* knockout mice demonstrate reduced NMDA-receptor-mediated excitatory signaling as well as increased repetitive behaviors. Administration of the NMDA-receptor partial agonist d-cycloserine rescued the behavioral deficit (Blundell et al. 2010). In mice exposed to prenatal VPA, which have been shown to have excessive excitatory signaling (Rinaldi et al. 2007), administration of the mGluR5 antagonist

2-methyl-6-(phenylethynyl)-pyridine rescued neural deficits (Gandal *et al.* 2010), including increased repetitive behaviors (unpublished observation). Similar positive results were demonstrated with 2-methyl-6-(phenylethynyl)-pyridine on the excessive self-grooming phenotype in BTBR mice (Silverman *et al.* 2010a). Similarly, emerging evidence suggests that restoring inhibition with selective GABA-receptor modulators may also have beneficial behavioral effects. For example, mice with epigenetic disruption of the autism risk gene *RELN* have impairments in GABAergic circuitry as well as social and PPI deficits, which could be reversed by administration of the GABA(A)-alpha-5 receptor agonist imidazenil (Tremolizzo *et al.* 2005). As such, it seems that identifying the appropriate electrophysiological circuit insult (e.g., too much/too little excitation or inhibition) can lead to successful, targeted pharmacological intervention and phenotypic rescue.

Conclusions

Given the heterogeneity and complex behavioral profile of autism, preclinical modeling is highly challenging, and translational approaches to the disorder are in their infancy. The fact that multiple genome-wide association scans have yet to identify replicable common risk loci has made the development of generalizable rodent models of "idiopathic autism" difficult. Likewise, the investigation of complex human behaviors (e.g., language) in mouse or rat models is inherently difficult. However, the identification and validation of neural endophenotypes in autism have begun to help overcome many of the difficulties associated with preclinical, translational investigation. In addition, recent developments demonstrating therapeutic rescue of neural deficits in mouse models of "syndromic" autism even in adulthood show promise for similar outcomes in idiopathic autism.

References

Abrahams BS, Geschwind DH. 2008. Advances in autism genetics: on the threshold of a new neurobiology. *Nat Rev Genet* **9**:341–355.

Alarcon M, Yonan AL, Gilliam TC, Cantor RM, Geschwind DH. 2005. Quantitative genome scan and Ordered-Subsets Analysis of autism endophenotypes support language QTLs. *Mol Psychiatry* **10**:747–757.

Alonso-Bua B, Diaz F, Ferraces MJ. 2006. The contribution of AERPs (MMN and LDN) to studying temporal vs. linguistic processing deficits in children with reading difficulties. *Int J Psychophysiol* **59**:159–167.

Amir RE, Van den Veyver IB, Wan M *et al.* 1999. Rett syndrome is caused by mutations in X-linked MECP2, encoding methyl-CpG-binding protein 2. *Nat Genet* **23**:185–188.

Anney R, Klei L, Pinto D *et al.* 2010. A genome-wide scan for common alleles affecting risk for autism. *Hum Mol Genet* **19**:4072–4082.

Arndt TL, Stodgell CJ, Rodier PM. 2005. The teratology of autism. *Int J Dev Neurosci* **23**:189–199.

Bell BB, Abel LA, Li W, Christian JC, Yee RD. 1994. Concordance of smooth pursuit and saccadic measures in normal monozygotic twin pairs. *Biol Psychiatry* **36**:522–526.

Benasich AA, Gou Z, Choudhury N, Harris KD. 2008. Early cognitive and language skills are linked to resting frontal gamma power across the first 3 years. *Behav Brain Res* **195**:215–222.

Benasich AA, Tallal P. 2002. Infant discrimination of rapid auditory cues predicts later language impairment. *Behav Brain Res* **136**:31–49.

Berens P, Keliris GA, Ecker AS, Logothetis NK, Tolias AS. 2008. Comparing the feature selectivity of the gamma-band of the local field potential and the underlying spiking activity in primate visual cortex. *Front Syst Neurosci* **2**:2.

Berry-Kravis E, Hessl D, Coffey S *et al.* 2009. A pilot open label, single dose trial of fenobam in adults with fragile X syndrome. *J Med Genet* **46**:266–271.

Betancur C. 2011. Etiological heterogeneity in autism spectrum disorders: more than 100 genetic and genomic disorders and still counting. *Brain Res* **1380**:42–77.

Betancur C, Sakurai T, Buxbaum JD. 2009. The emerging role of synaptic cell-adhesion pathways in the pathogenesis of autism spectrum disorders. *Trends Neurosci* **32**:402–412.

Bigler ED, Mortensen S, Neeley ES *et al.* 2007. Superior temporal gyrus, language function, and autism. *Dev Neuropsychol* **31**:217–238.

Blue ME. 2009. Serotonin dysfunction in autism. In: *Autism: Current Theories and Evidence*. Zimmerman AW, ed. Totowa, NJ: Humana Press, pp. 111–132.

Blundell J, Blaiss CA, Etherton MR *et al.* 2010. Neuroligin-1 deletion results in impaired spatial memory and increased repetitive behavior. *J Neurosci* **30**:2115–2129.

Blundell J, Tabuchi K, Bolliger MF *et al.* 2009. Increased anxiety-like behavior in mice lacking the inhibitory synapse cell adhesion molecule neuroligin 2. *Genes Brain Behav* **8**:114–126.

Bourgeron T. 2009. A synaptic trek to autism. *Curr Opin Neurobiol* **19**:231–234.

Bozdagi O, Sakurai T, Papapetrou D et al. 2010. Haploinsufficiency of the autism-associated Shank3 gene leads to deficits in synaptic function, social interaction, and social communication. *Mol Autism* **1**:15.

Braeutigam S, Bailey AJ, Swithenby SJ. 2001. Phase-locked gamma band responses to semantic violation stimuli. *Brain Res Cogn Brain Res* **10**:365–377.

Braeutigam S, Swithenby SJ, Bailey AJ. 2008. Contextual integration the unusual way: a magnetoencephalographic study of responses to semantic violation in individuals with autism spectrum disorders. *Eur J Neurosci* **27**:1026–1036.

Braff DL, Freedman R, Schork NJ, Gottesman, II. 2007. Deconstructing schizophrenia: an overview of the use of endophenotypes in order to understand a complex disorder. *Schizophr Bull* **33**:21–32.

Brodkin ES. 2007. BALB/c mice: low sociability and other phenotypes that may be relevant to autism. *Behav Brain Res* **176**:53–65.

Brodkin ES, Hagemann A, Nemetski SM, Silver LM. 2004. Social approach–avoidance behavior of inbred mouse strains towards DBA/2 mice. *Brain Res* **1002**:151–157.

Bromley RL, Baker GA, Meador KJ. 2009. Cognitive abilities and behaviour of children exposed to antiepileptic drugs in utero. *Curr OpinNeurol* **22**:162–166.

Bromley RL, Mawer G, Clayton-Smith J, Baker GA. 2008. Autism spectrum disorders following in utero exposure to antiepileptic drugs. *Neurology* **71**:1923–1924.

Bruneau N, Roux S, Adrien JL, Barthelemy C. 1999. Auditory associative cortex dysfunction in children with autism: evidence from late auditory evoked potentials (N1 wave-T complex). *Clin Neurophysiol* **110**:1927–1934.

Buhl DL, Harris KD, Hormuzdi SG, Monyer H, Buzsaki G. 2003. Selective impairment of hippocampal gamma oscillations in connexin-36 knock-out mouse in vivo. *J Neurosci* **23**:1013–1018.

Cantor RM, Kono N, Duvall JA et al. 2005. Replication of autism linkage: fine-mapping peak at 17q21. *Am J Hum Genet* **76**:1050–1056.

Chadman KK, Gong S, Scattoni ML et al. 2008. Minimal aberrant behavioral phenotypes of neuroligin-3 R451C knockin mice. *Autism Res* **1**:147–158.

Chadman KK, Yang M, Crawley JN. 2009. Criteria for validating mouse models of psychiatric diseases. *Am J Med Genet B Neuropsychiatr Genet* **150B**:1–11.

Chandana SR, Behen ME, Juhasz C et al. 2005. Significance of abnormalities in developmental trajectory and asymmetry of cortical serotonin synthesis in autism. *Int J Dev Neurosci* **23**:171–182.

Chang Q, Khare G, Dani V, Nelson S, Jaenisch R. 2006. The disease progression of Mecp2 mutant mice is affected by the level of BDNF expression. *Neuron* **49**:341–348.

Chao HT, Chen H, Samaco RC et al. 2010. Dysfunction in GABA signalling mediates autism-like stereotypies and Rett syndrome phenotypes. *Nature* **468**:263–269.

Charman T, Baron-Cohen S, Swettenham J et al. 2003. Predicting language outcome in infants with autism and pervasive developmental disorder. *Int J Lang Commun Disord* **38**:265–285.

Cheh MA, Millonig JH, Roselli LM et al. 2006. En2 knockout mice display neurobehavioral and neurochemical alterations relevant to autism spectrum disorder. *Brain Res* **1116**:166–176.

Chen RZ, Akbarian S, Tudor M, Jaenisch R. 2001. Deficiency of methyl-CpG binding protein-2 in CNS neurons results in a Rett-like phenotype in mice. *Nat Genet* **27**:327–331.

Chess S, Fernandez P, Korn S. 1978. Behavioral consequences of congenital rubella. *J Pediatr* **93**:699–703.

Coben R, Clarke AR, Hudspeth W, Barry RJ. 2008. EEG power and coherence in autistic spectrum disorder. *Clin Neurophysiol* **119**:1002–1009.

Conciatori M, Stodgell CJ, Hyman SL et al. 2004. Association between the HOXA1 A218G polymorphism and increased head circumference in patients with autism. *Biol Psychiatry* **55**:413–419.

Constantino JN, Lajonchere C, Lutz M et al. 2006. Autistic social impairment in the siblings of children with pervasive developmental disorders. *Am J Psychiatry* **163**:294–296.

Crawley JN. 2004. Designing mouse behavioral tasks relevant to autistic-like behaviors. *Ment Retard Dev Disabil Res Rev* **10**:248–258.

Crawley J. 2007a. *What's Wrong With My Mouse: Behavioral Phenotyping of Transgenic and Knockout Mice*, 2nd edn. Hoboken, NJ: Wiley-Liss.

Crawley JN. 2007b. Mouse behavioral assays relevant to the symptoms of autism. *Brain Pathol* **17**:448–459.

Crawley JN. 2008. Behavioral phenotyping strategies for mutant mice. *Neuron* **57**:809–818.

Currenti SA. 2010. Understanding and determining the etiology of autism. *Cell Mol Neurobiol* **30**:161–171.

Curtis JT, Hood AN, Chen Y, Cobb GP, Wallace DR. 2010. Chronic metals ingestion by prairie voles produces sex-specific deficits in social behavior: an animal model of autism. *Behav Brain Res* **213**:42–49.

de Vrij FM, Levenga J, van der Linde HC et al. 2008. Rescue of behavioral phenotype and neuronal protrusion morphology in Fmr1 KO mice. *Neurobiol Dis* **31**:127–132.

DeLorey TM, Sahbaie P, Hashemi E, Homanics GE, Clark JD. 2008. Gabrb3 gene deficient mice exhibit impaired social and exploratory behaviors, deficits in non-selective attention and hypoplasia of cerebellar vermal lobules: a potential model of autism spectrum disorder. *Behav Brain Res* **187**:207–220.

DeLorey TM, Sahbaie P, Hashemi E, Li WW, Salehi A, Clark DJ. 2011. Somatosensory and sensorimotor consequences associated with the heterozygous disruption of the autism candidate gene, Gabrb3. *Behav Brain Res* **216**:36–45.

Devlin B, Cook EH, Jr., Coon H *et al.* 2005. Autism and the serotonin transporter: the long and short of it. *Mol Psychiatry* **10**:1110–1116.

Diedler J, Pietz J, Brunner M *et al.* 2009. Auditory processing in children with language-based learning problems: a magnetoencephalography study. *Neuroreport* **20**:844–848.

Dockendorff TC, Su HS, McBride SM *et al.* 2002. *Drosophila* lacking dfmr1 activity show defects in circadian output and fail to maintain courtship interest. *Neuron* **34**:973–984.

Durand CM, Betancur C, Boeckers TM *et al.* 2007. Mutations in the gene encoding the synaptic scaffolding protein SHANK3 are associated with autism spectrum disorders. *Nat Genet* **39**:25–27.

Dyer C. 2010. Thiomersal does not cause autism, US court finds. *Br Med J* **340**:c1518.

Ehninger D, Han S, Shilyansky C *et al.* 2008. Reversal of learning deficits in a Tsc2+/–mouse model of tuberous sclerosis. *Nat Med* **14**:843–848.

Ehninger D, Silva AJ. 2011. Rapamycin for treating tuberous sclerosis and autism spectrum disorders. *Trends Mol Med* **17**:78–87.

Ehret G. 1987. Left hemisphere advantage in the mouse brain for recognizing ultrasonic communication calls. *Nature* **325**:249–251.

Ehrlichman RS, Luminais SN, White SL *et al.* 2009. Neuregulin 1 transgenic mice display reduced mismatch negativity, contextual fear conditioning and social interactions. *Brain Res* **1294**:116–127.

Ehrlichman RS, Maxwell CR, Majumdar S, Siegel SJ. 2008. Deviance-elicited changes in event-related potentials are attenuated by ketamine in mice. *J Cogn Neurosci* **20**:1403–1414.

Enard W, Gehre S, Hammerschmidt K *et al.* 2009. A humanized version of Foxp2 affects cortico-basal ganglia circuits in mice. *Cell* **137**:961–971.

Enstrom AM, Van de Water JA, Ashwood P. 2009. Autoimmunity in autism. *Curr Opin Investig Drugs* **10**:463–473.

Escalante-Mead PR, Minshew NJ, Sweeney JA. 2003. Abnormal brain lateralization in high-functioning autism. *J Autism Dev Disord* **33**:539–543.

Etherton MR, Blaiss CA, Powell CM, Sudhof TC. 2009. Mouse neurexin-1alpha deletion causes correlated electrophysiological and behavioral changes consistent with cognitive impairments. *Proc Natl Acad Sci USA* **106**:17998–18003.

European Chromosome 16 Tuberous Sclerosis Consortium 1993. Identification and characterization of the tuberous sclerosis gene on chromosome 16. *Cell* **75**:1305–1315.

Fatemi SH, Earle J, Kanodia R *et al.* 2002. Prenatal viral infection leads to pyramidal cell atrophy and macrocephaly in adulthood: implications for genesis of autism and schizophrenia. *Cell Mol Neurobiol* **22**:25–33.

Ferguson JN, Young LJ, Hearn EF *et al.* 2000. Social amnesia in mice lacking the oxytocin gene. *Nat Genet* **25**:284–288.

Fidler DJ, Bailey JN, Smalley SL. 2000. Macrocephaly in autism and other pervasive developmental disorders. *Dev Med Child Neurol* **42**:737–740.

Flagg EJ, Cardy JE, Roberts W, Roberts TP. 2005. Language lateralization development in children with autism: insights from the late field magnetoencephalogram. *Neurosci Lett* **386**:82–87.

Frankland PW, Wang Y, Rosner B *et al.* 2004. Sensorimotor gating abnormalities in young males with fragile X syndrome and Fmr1-knockout mice. *Mol Psychiatry* **9**:417–425.

Gage NM, Siegel B, Callen M, Roberts TP. 2003. Cortical sound processing in children with autism disorder: an MEG investigation. *Neuroreport* **14**:2047–2051.

Gandal MJ, Edgar JC, Ehrlichman RS *et al.* 2010. Validating gamma oscillations and delayed auditory responses as translational biomarkers of autism. *Biol Psychiatry* **68**:1100–1106.

Geyer MA, McIlwain KL, Paylor R. 2002. Mouse genetic models for prepulse inhibition: an early review. *Mol Psychiatry* **7**:1039–1053.

Gibson JR, Bartley AF, Hays SA, Huber KM. 2008. Imbalance of neocortical excitation and inhibition and altered UP states reflect network hyperexcitability in the mouse model of fragile X syndrome. *J Neurophysiol* **100**:2615–2626.

Glessner JT, Wang K, Cai G *et al.* 2009. Autism genome-wide copy number variation reveals ubiquitin and neuronal genes. *Nature* **459**:569–573.

Gogolla N, Leblanc JJ, Quast KB *et al.* 2009. Common circuit defect of excitatory–inhibitory balance in mouse models of autism. *J Neurodev Disord* **1**:172–181.

Goines P, Van de Water J. 2010. The immune system's role in the biology of autism. *Curr Opin Neurol* **23**:111–117.

Goldberg J, Anderson GM, Zwaigenbaum L et al. 2009. Cortical serotonin type-2 receptor density in parents of children with autism spectrum disorders. *J Autism Dev Disord* **39**:97–104.

Goorden SM, van Woerden GM, van der Weerd L, Cheadle JP, Elgersma Y. 2007. Cognitive deficits in Tsc1 +/− mice in the absence of cerebral lesions and seizures. *Ann Neurol* **62**:648–655.

Gottesman, II, Shields J. 1973. Genetic theorizing and schizophrenia. *Br J Psychiatry* **122**:15–30.

Gottesman, II, Gould TD. 2003. The endophenotype concept in psychiatry: etymology and strategic intentions. *Am J Psychiatry* **160**:636–645.

Gourbal BE, Barthelemy M, Petit G, Gabrion C. 2004. Spectrographic analysis of the ultrasonic vocalisations of adult male and female BALB/c mice. *Naturwissenschaften* **91**:381–385.

Gutierrez RC, Hung J, Zhang Y et al. 2009. Altered synchrony and connectivity in neuronal networks expressing an autism-related mutation of neuroligin 3. *Neuroscience* **162**:208–221.

Guy J, Gan J, Selfridge J, Cobb S, Bird A. 2007. Reversal of neurological defects in a mouse model of Rett syndrome. *Science* **315**:1143–1147.

Guy J, Hendrich B, Holmes M, Martin JE, Bird A. 2001. A mouse Mecp2-null mutation causes neurological symptoms that mimic Rett syndrome. *Nat Genet* **27**:322–326.

Hall SD, Holliday IE, Hillebrand A et al. 2005. The missing link: analogous human and primate cortical gamma oscillations. *Neuroimage* **26**:13–17.

Hamalainen MS. 1992. Magnetoencephalography: a tool for functional brain imaging. *Brain Topogr* **5**:95–102.

Henze DA, Borhegyi Z, Csicsvari J et al. 2000. Intracellular features predicted by extracellular recordings in the hippocampus in vivo. *J Neurophysiol* **84**:390–400.

Herbert MR. 2010. Contributions of the environment and environmentally vulnerable physiology to autism spectrum disorders. *Curr Opin Neurol* **23**:103–110.

Herrmann CS, Frund I, Lenz D. 2010. Human gamma-band activity: a review on cognitive and behavioral correlates and network models. *Neurosci Biobehav Rev* **34**:981–992.

Heyser CJ. 2004. Assessment of developmental milestones in rodents. *Curr Protoc Neurosci* Ch. 8: Unit 8.18.

Higgins GA, Breysse N. 2008. Rodent model of attention: the 5-choice serial reaction time task. *Curr Protoc Pharmacol* **41**: 5.49.41–45.49.20.

Hillebrand A, Singh KD, Holliday IE, Furlong PL, Barnes GR. 2005. A new approach to neuroimaging with magnetoencephalography. *Hum Brain Mapp* **25**:199–211.

Hiroi N, Zhu H, Lee M et al. 2005. A 200-kb region of human chromosome 22q11.2 confers antipsychotic-responsive behavioral abnormalities in mice. *Proc Natl Acad Sci USA* **102**:19132–19137.

Hoeffer CA, Klann E. 2010. mTOR signaling: at the crossroads of plasticity, memory and disease. *Trends Neurosci* **33**:67–75.

Hofer MA, Shair HN, Brunelli SA. 2002. Ultrasonic vocalizations in rat and mouse pups. *Curr Protoc Neurosci* Ch. 8: Unit 8.14.

Hollander E, Kolevzon A, Coyle JT, eds. 2011. *Textbook of Autism Spectrum Disorders*. Washington, DC: American Psychiatric Publishing.

Holy TE, Guo Z. 2005. Ultrasonic songs of male mice. *PLoS Biol* **3**: e386.

Honaga E, Ishii R, Kurimoto R et al. 2010. Post-movement beta rebound abnormality as indicator of mirror neuron system dysfunction in autistic spectrum disorder: an MEG study. *Neurosci Lett* **478**:141–145.

Hornig M, Chian D, Lipkin WI. 2004. Neurotoxic effects of postnatal thimerosal are mouse strain dependent. *Mol Psychiatry* **9**:833–845.

Huber KM, Gallagher SM, Warren ST, Bear MF. 2002. Altered synaptic plasticity in a mouse model of fragile X mental retardation. *Proc Natl Acad Sci USA* **99**:7746–7750.

Ingram JL, Peckham SM, Tisdale B, Rodier PM. 2000. Prenatal exposure of rats to valproic acid reproduces the cerebellar anomalies associated with autism. *Neurotoxicol Teratol* **22**:319–324.

Insel TR. 1997. A neurobiological basis of social attachment. *Am J Psychiatry* **154**:726–735.

Isler JR, Martien KM, Grieve PG, Stark RI, Herbert MR. 2010. Reduced functional connectivity in visual evoked potentials in children with autism spectrum disorder. *Clin Neurophysiol* **121**:2035–2043.

Jahromi LB, Kasari CL, McCracken JT et al. 2009. Positive effects of methylphenidate on social communication and self-regulation in children with pervasive developmental disorders and hyperactivity. *J Autism Dev Disord* **39**:395–404.

Jamain S, Radyushkin K, Hammerschmidt K et al. 2008. Reduced social interaction and ultrasonic communication in a mouse model of monogenic heritable autism. *Proc Natl Acad Sci USA* **105**:1710–1715.

Jamain S, Quach H, Betancur C et al. 2003. Mutations of the X-linked genes encoding neuroligins NLGN3 and NLGN4 are associated with autism. *Nat Genet* **34**:27–29.

Jang SW, Liu X, Yepes M et al. 2010. A selective TrkB agonist with potent neurotrophic activities by

7,8-dihydroxyflavone. *Proc Natl Acad Sci USA* **107**: 2687–2692.

Jensen O, Goel P, Kopell N et al. 2005. On the human sensorimotor-cortex beta rhythm: sources and modeling. *Neuroimage* **26**:347–355.

Jesner OS, Aref-Adib M, Coren E. 2007. Risperidone for autism spectrum disorder. *Cochrane Database Syst Rev*: CD005040.

Jeste SS, Nelson CA, 3rd. 2009. Event related potentials in the understanding of autism spectrum disorders: an analytical review. *J Autism Dev Disord* **39**:495–510.

Kasai K, Hashimoto O, Kawakubo Y et al. 2005. Delayed automatic detection of change in speech sounds in adults with autism: a magnetoencephalographic study. *Clin Neurophysiol* **116**:1655–1664.

Katzner S, Nauhaus I, Benucci A et al. 2009. Local origin of field potentials in visual cortex. *Neuron* **61**:35–41.

Kim JY, Duan X, Liu CY et al. 2009. DISC1 regulates new neuron development in the adult brain via modulation of AKT-mTOR signaling through KIAA1212. *Neuron* **63**:761–773.

Kinney DK, Barch DH, Chayka B, Napoleon S, Munir KM. 2010. Environmental risk factors for autism: do they help cause de novo genetic mutations that contribute to the disorder? *Med Hypotheses* **74**:102–106.

Kleinhans NM, Muller RA, Cohen DN, Courchesne E. 2008. Atypical functional lateralization of language in autism spectrum disorders. *Brain Res* **1221**:115–125.

Kolozsi E, Mackenzie RN, Roullet FI, de Catanzaro D, Foster JA. 2009. Prenatal exposure to valproic acid leads to reduced expression of synaptic adhesion molecule neuroligin 3 in mice. *Neuroscience* **163**:1201–1210.

Kooy RF. 2003. Of mice and the fragile X syndrome. *Trends Genet* **19**:148–154.

Kosfeld M, Heinrichs M, Zak PJ, Fischbacher U, Fehr E. 2005. Oxytocin increases trust in humans. *Nature* **435**:673–676.

Krey JF, Dolmetsch RE. 2007. Molecular mechanisms of autism: a possible role for Ca^{2+} signaling. *Curr Opin Neurobiol* **17**:112–119.

Krueger DD, Bear MF. 2011. Toward fulfilling the promise of molecular medicine in fragile X syndrome. *Annu Rev Med* **62**:411–429.

Kujala T, Lepisto T, Nieminen-von Wendt T, Naatanen P, Naatanen R. 2005. Neurophysiological evidence for cortical discrimination impairment of prosody in Asperger syndrome. *Neurosci Lett* **383**:260–265.

Kwon CH, Luikart BW, Powell CM et al. 2006. Pten regulates neuronal arborization and social interaction in mice. *Neuron* **50**:377–388.

Lahvis GP, Alleva E, Scattoni ML. 2011. Translating mouse vocalizations: prosody and frequency modulation (1). *Genes Brain Behav* **10**:4–16.

Lam KS, Aman MG, Arnold LE. 2006. Neurochemical correlates of autistic disorder: a review of the literature. *Res Dev Disabil* **27**:254–289.

Landrigan PJ. 2010. What causes autism? Exploring the environmental contribution. *Curr Opin Pediatr* **22**:219–225.

Lange N, Dubray MB, Lee JE et al. 2010. Atypical diffusion tensor hemispheric asymmetry in autism. *Autism Res* **3**:350–358.

Lee LC, Zachary AA, Leffell MS et al. 2006. HLA-DR4 in families with autism. *Pediatr Neurol* **35**:303–307.

Levin ED, Addy N, Nakajima A et al. 2001. Persistent behavioral consequences of neonatal chlorpyrifos exposure in rats. *Brain Res Dev Brain Res* **130**:83–89.

Levin R, Heresco-Levy U, Bachner-Melman R et al. 2009. Association between arginine vasopressin 1a receptor (AVPR1a) promoter region polymorphisms and prepulse inhibition. *Psychoneuroendocrinology* **34**:901–908.

Levitt P, Campbell DB. 2009. The genetic and neurobiologic compass points toward common signaling dysfunctions in autism spectrum disorders. *J Clin Invest* **119**:747–754.

Levy SE, Hyman SL. 2008. Complementary and alternative medicine treatments for children with autism spectrum disorders. *Child Adolesc Psychiatr Clin N Am* **17**:803–820, ix.

Levy SE, Mandell DS, Schultz RT. 2009. Autism. *Lancet* **374**:1627–1638.

Lewis MH, Tanimura Y, Lee LW, Bodfish JW. 2007. Animal models of restricted repetitive behavior in autism. *Behav Brain Res* **176**:66–74.

Libbey JE, Sweeten TL, McMahon WM, Fujinami RS. 2005. Autistic disorder and viral infections. *J Neurovirol* **11**:1–10.

Lijam N, Paylor R, McDonald MP et al. 1997. Social interaction and sensorimotor gating abnormalities in mice lacking Dvl1. *Cell* **90**:895–905.

Lindzey G, Winston H, Manosevitz M. 1961. Social dominance in inbred mouse strains. *Nature* **191**:474–476.

Liu RC, Miller KD, Merzenich MM, Schreiner CE. 2003. Acoustic variability and distinguishability among mouse ultrasound vocalizations. *J Acoust Soc Am* **114**:3412–3422.

Lonetti G, Angelucci A, Morando L et al. 2010. Early environmental enrichment moderates the behavioral and synaptic phenotype of MeCP2 null mice. *Biol Psychiatry* **67**:657–665.

Lord C, Risi S, Lambrecht L et al. 2000. The autism diagnostic observation schedule-generic: a standard measure of social and communication deficits associated with the spectrum of autism. *J Autism Dev Disord* **30**:205–223.

Lord C, Rutter M, Le Couteur A. 1994. Autism Diagnostic Interview-Revised: a revised version of a diagnostic interview for caregivers of individuals with possible pervasive developmental disorders. *J Autism Dev Disord* **24**:659–685.

Lugenbeel KA, Peier AM, Carson NL, Chudley AE, Nelson DL. 1995. Intragenic loss of function mutations demonstrate the primary role of FMR1 in fragile X syndrome. *Nat Genet* **10**:483–485.

Markram H, Rinaldi T, Markram K. 2007. The intense world syndrome – an alternative hypothesis for autism. *Front Neurosci* **1**:77–96.

Markram K, Rinaldi T, La Mendola D, Sandi C, Markram H. 2008. Abnormal fear conditioning and amygdala processing in an animal model of autism. *Neuropsychopharmacology* **33**:901–912.

Massa SM, Yang T, Xie Y et al. 2010. Small molecule BDNF mimetics activate TrkB signaling and prevent neuronal degeneration in rodents. *J Clin Invest* **120**:1774–1785.

Maziade M, Merette C, Cayer M et al. 2000. Prolongation of brainstem auditory-evoked responses in autistic probands and their unaffected relatives. *Arch Gen Psychiatry* **57**:1077–1083.

McAlonan GM, Daly E, Kumari V et al. 2002. Brain anatomy and sensorimotor gating in Asperger's syndrome. *Brain* **125**:1594–1606.

McBride SM, Choi CH, Wang Y et al. 2005. Pharmacological rescue of synaptic plasticity, courtship behavior, and mushroom body defects in a *Drosophila* model of fragile X syndrome. *Neuron* **45**:753–764.

McFarlane HG, Kusek GK, Yang M et al. 2008. Autism-like behavioral phenotypes in BTBR T+tf/J mice. *Genes Brain Behav* **7**:152–163.

Meador KJ, Baker GA, Browning N et al. 2009. Cognitive function at 3 years of age after fetal exposure to antiepileptic drugs. *N Engl J Med* **360**:1597–1605.

Meikle L, Pollizzi K, Egnor A et al. 2008. Response of a neuronal model of tuberous sclerosis to mammalian target of rapamycin (mTOR) inhibitors: effects on mTORC1 and Akt signaling lead to improved survival and function. *J Neurosci* **28**:5422–5432.

Mescher M, Merkle H, Kirsch J, Garwood M, Gruetter R. 1998. Simultaneous in vivo spectral editing and water suppression. *NMR Biomed* **11**:266–272.

Messeri P, Eleftheriou BE, Oliverio A. 1975. Dominance behavior: a phylogenetic analysis in the mouse. *Physiol Behav* **14**:53–58.

Meyer P, Mecklinger A, Grunwald T et al. 2005. Language processing within the human medial temporal lobe. *Hippocampus* **15**:451–459.

Miller MT, Stromland K, Ventura L et al. 2005. Autism associated with conditions characterized by developmental errors in early embryogenesis: a mini review. *Int J Dev Neurosci* **23**:201–219.

Milne E, Scope A, Pascalis O, Buckley D, Makeig S. 2009. Independent component analysis reveals atypical electroencephalographic activity during visual perception in individuals with autism. *Biol Psychiatry* **65**:22–30.

Moles A, Costantini F, Garbugino L, Zanettini C, D'Amato FR. 2007. Ultrasonic vocalizations emitted during dyadic interactions in female mice: a possible index of sociability? *Behav Brain Res* **182**:223–230.

Moon J, Beaudin AE, Verosky S et al. 2006. Attentional dysfunction, impulsivity, and resistance to change in a mouse model of fragile X syndrome. *Behav Neurosci* **120**:1367–1379.

Morales J, Hiesinger PR, Schroeder AJ et al. 2002. *Drosophila* fragile X protein, DFXR, regulates neuronal morphology and function in the brain. *Neuron* **34**:961–972.

Morrow EM, Yoo SY, Flavell SW et al. 2008. Identifying autism loci and genes by tracing recent shared ancestry. *Science* **321**:218–223.

Mosconi MW, Kay M, D'Cruz AM et al. 2010. Neurobehavioral abnormalities in first-degree relatives of individuals with autism. *Arch Gen Psychiatry* **67**:830–840.

Moy SS, Nadler JJ. 2008. Advances in behavioral genetics: mouse models of autism. *Mol Psychiatry* **13**:4–26.

Moy SS, Nadler JJ, Poe MD et al. 2008. Development of a mouse test for repetitive, restricted behaviors: relevance to autism. *Behav Brain Res* **188**:178–194.

Moy SS, Nadler JJ, Young NB et al. 2007. Mouse behavioral tasks relevant to autism: phenotypes of 10 inbred strains. *Behav Brain Res* **176**:4–20.

Moy SS, Nonneman RJ, Young NB, Demyanenko GP, Maness PF. 2009. Impaired sociability and cognitive function in Nrcam-null mice. *Behav Brain Res* **205**:123–131.

Murias M, Webb SJ, Greenson J, Dawson G. 2007. Resting state cortical connectivity reflected in EEG coherence in individuals with autism. *Biol Psychiatry* **62**:270–273.

Muscarella LA, Guarnieri V, Sacco R et al. 2007. HOXA1 gene variants influence head growth rates in humans. *Am J Med Genet B Neuropsychiatr Genet* **144B**:388–390.

Muthukumaraswamy SD, Edden RA, Jones DK, Swettenham JB, Singh KD. 2009. Resting GABA concentration predicts peak gamma frequency and fMRI amplitude in response to visual stimulation in humans. *Proc Natl Acad Sci USA* **106**:8356–8361.

Naatanen R, Paavilainen P, Alho K, Reinikainen K, Sams M. 1987. The mismatch negativity to intensity changes in an auditory stimulus sequence. *Electroencephalogr Clin Neurophysiol Suppl* **40**:125–131.

Nadler JJ, Moy SS, Dold G et al. 2004. Automated apparatus for quantitation of social approach behaviors in mice. *Genes Brain Behav* **3**:303–314.

Nakamura K, Sekine Y, Ouchi Y et al. 2010. Brain serotonin and dopamine transporter bindings in adults with high-functioning autism. *Arch Gen Psychiatry* **67**:59–68.

Network RUoPPA. 2005. Randomized, controlled, crossover trial of methylphenidate in pervasive developmental disorders with hyperactivity. *Arch Gen Psychiatry* **62**:1266–1274.

Nickl-Jockschat T, Michel TM. 2011. The role of neurotrophic factors in autism. *Mol Psychiatry* **16**:478–490.

Nyby J. 1983. Ultrasonic vocalizations during sex behavior of male house mice (*Mus musculus*): a description. *Behav Neural Biol* **39**:128–134.

Oram Cardy JE, Flagg EJ, Roberts W, Brian J, Roberts TP. 2005a. Magnetoencephalography identifies rapid temporal processing deficit in autism and language impairment. *Neuroreport* **16**:329–332.

Oram Cardy JE, Flagg EJ, Roberts W, Roberts TP. 2005b. Delayed mismatch field for speech and non-speech sounds in children with autism. *Neuroreport* **16**:521–525.

Oram Cardy JE, Flagg EJ, Roberts W, Roberts TP. 2008. Auditory evoked fields predict language ability and impairment in children. *Int J Psychophysiol* **68**:170–175.

Orekhova EV, Stroganova TA, Nygren G et al. 2007. Excess of high frequency electroencephalogram oscillations in boys with autism. *Biol Psychiatry* **62**:1022–1029.

Orlova KA, Crino PB. 2010. The tuberous sclerosis complex. *Ann NY Acad Sci* **1184**:87–105.

Page DT, Kuti OJ, Prestia C, Sur M. 2009. Haploinsufficiency for Pten and Serotonin transporter cooperatively influences brain size and social behavior. *Proc Natl Acad Sci USA* **106**:1989–1994.

Palmen SJ, van Engeland H, Hof PR, Schmitz C. 2004. Neuropathological findings in autism. *Brain* **127**:2572–2583.

Panksepp JB, Jochman KA, Kim JU et al. 2007. Affiliative behavior, ultrasonic communication and social reward are influenced by genetic variation in adolescent mice. *PLoS One* **2**:**e351**.

Pantev C, Makeig S, Hoke M et al. 1991. Human auditory evoked gamma-band magnetic fields. *Proc Natl Acad Sci USA* **88**:8996–9000.

Paylor R, Glaser B, Mupo A et al. 2006. Tbx1 haploinsufficiency is linked to behavioral disorders in mice and humans: implications for 22q11 deletion syndrome. *Proc Natl Acad Sci USA* **103**:7729–7734.

Perry W, Minassian A, Lopez B, Maron L, Lincoln A. 2007. Sensorimotor gating deficits in adults with autism. *Biol Psychiatry* **61**:482–486.

Persico AM, Bourgeron T. 2006. Searching for ways out of the autism maze: genetic, epigenetic and environmental clues. *Trends Neurosci* **29**:349–358.

Pessah IN, Seegal RF, Lein PJ et al. 2008. Immunologic and neurodevelopmental susceptibilities of autism. *Neurotoxicology* **29**:532–545.

Piven J, Tsai GC, Nehme E et al. 1991. Platelet serotonin, a possible marker for familial autism. *J Autism Dev Disord* **21**:51–59.

Price CS, Thompson WW, Goodson B et al. 2010. Prenatal and infant exposure to thimerosal from vaccines and immunoglobulins and risk of autism. *Pediatrics* **126**:656–664.

Prusky GT, West PW, Douglas RM. 2000. Behavioral assessment of visual acuity in mice and rats. *Vision Res* **40**:2201–2209.

Puzzo I, Cooper NR, Vetter P, Russo R. 2010. EEG activation differences in the pre-motor cortex and supplementary motor area between normal individuals with high and low traits of autism. *Brain Res* **1342**:104–110.

Rasalam AD, Hailey H, Williams JH et al. 2005. Characteristics of fetal anticonvulsant syndrome associated autistic disorder. *Dev Med Child Neurol* **47**:551–555.

Rauh VA, Garfinkel R, Perera FP et al. 2006. Impact of prenatal chlorpyrifos exposure on neurodevelopment in the first 3 years of life among inner-city children. *Pediatrics* **118**:e1845–1859.

Restivo L, Ferrari F, Passino E et al. 2005. Enriched environment promotes behavioral and morphological recovery in a mouse model for the fragile X syndrome. *Proc Natl Acad Sci USA* **102**:11557–11562.

Ricceri L, Moles A, Crawley J. 2007. Behavioral phenotyping of mouse models of neurodevelopmental disorders: relevant social behavior patterns across the life span. *Behav Brain Res* **176**:40–52.

Rinaldi T, Kulangara K, Antoniello K, Markram H. 2007. Elevated NMDA receptor levels and enhanced postsynaptic long-term potentiation induced by prenatal exposure to valproic acid. *Proc Natl Acad Sci USA* **104**:13501–13506.

Roberts TP, Ferrari P, Stufflebeam SM, Poeppel D. 2000. Latency of the auditory evoked neuromagnetic field components: stimulus dependence and insights toward perception. *J Clin Neurophysiol* **17**:114–129.

Roberts TP, Khan SY, Blaskey L et al. 2009. Developmental correlation of diffusion anisotropy with auditory-evoked response. *Neuroreport* **20**:1586–1591.

Roberts TP, Khan SY, Rey M et al. 2010. MEG detection of delayed auditory evoked responses in autism spectrum disorders: towards an imaging biomarker for autism. *Autism Res* **3**:8–18.

Roberts TP, Schmidt GL, Egeth M et al. 2008. Electrophysiological signatures: magnetoencephalographic studies of the neural correlates of language impairment in autism spectrum disorders. *Int J Psychophysiol* **68**:149–160.

Rodier PM, Ingram JL, Tisdale B, Nelson S, Romano J. 1996. Embryological origin for autism: developmental anomalies of the cranial nerve motor nuclei. *J Comp Neurol* **370**:247–261.

Rojas DC, Maharajh K, Teale P, Rogers SJ. 2008. Reduced neural synchronization of gamma-band MEG oscillations in first-degree relatives of children with autism. *BMC Psychiatry* **8**:66.

Roopun AK, Middleton SJ, Cunningham MO et al. 2006. A beta2-frequency (20–30 Hz) oscillation in nonsynaptic networks of somatosensory cortex. *Proc Natl Acad Sci USA* **103**:15646–15650.

Rubenstein JL, Merzenich MM. 2003. Model of autism: increased ratio of excitation/inhibition in key neural systems. *Genes Brain Behav* **2**:255–267.

Rujescu D, Ingason A, Cichon S et al. 2009. Disruption of the neurexin 1 gene is associated with schizophrenia. *Hum Mol Genet* **18**:988–996.

Saresella M, Marventano I, Guerini FR et al. 2009. An autistic endophenotype results in complex immune dysfunction in healthy siblings of autistic children. *Biol Psychiatry* **66**:978–984.

Scattoni ML, Crawley J, Ricceri L. 2009. Ultrasonic vocalizations: a tool for behavioural phenotyping of mouse models of neurodevelopmental disorders. *Neurosci Biobehav Rev* **33**:508–515.

Scattoni ML, Gandhy SU, Ricceri L, Crawley JN. 2008. Unusual repertoire of vocalizations in the BTBR T+tf/J mouse model of autism. *PLoS One* **3**: e3067.

Scattoni ML, Ricceri L, Crawley JN. 2011. Unusual repertoire of vocalizations in adult BTBR T+tf/J mice during three types of social encounters. *Genes Brain Behav* **10**:44–56.

Schechter R, Grether JK. 2008. Continuing increases in autism reported to California's developmental services system: mercury in retrograde. *Arch Gen Psychiatry* **65**:19–24.

Schneider CW, Chenoweth MB. 1970. Effects of hallucinogenic and other drugs on the nest-building behaviour of mice. *Nature* **225**:1262–1263.

Schneider T, Przewlocki R. 2005. Behavioral alterations in rats prenatally exposed to valproic acid: animal model of autism. *Neuropsychopharmacology* **30**:80–89.

Schneider T, Turczak J, Przewlocki R. 2006. Environmental enrichment reverses behavioral alterations in rats prenatally exposed to valproic acid: issues for a therapeutic approach in autism. *Neuropsychopharmacology* **31**:36–46.

Schumacher HJ, Terapane J, Jordan RL, Wilson JG. 1972. The teratogenic activity of a thalidomide analogue, EM 12 in rabbits, rats, and monkeys. *Teratology* **5**:233–240.

Schwarz E, Guest PC, Rahmoune H et al. 2010. Sex-specific serum biomarker patterns in adults with Asperger's syndrome. *Mol Psychiatry*. Sep 28. [Epub ahead of print].

Shi L, Fatemi SH, Sidwell RW, Patterson PH. 2003. Maternal influenza infection causes marked behavioral and pharmacological changes in the offspring. *J Neurosci* **23**:297–302.

Shu W, Cho JY, Jiang Y et al. 2005. Altered ultrasonic vocalization in mice with a disruption in the Foxp2 gene. *Proc Natl Acad Sci USA* **102**:9643–9648.

Shultz SR, MacFabe DF, Ossenkopp KP et al. 2008. Intracerebroventricular injection of propionic acid, an enteric bacterial metabolic end-product, impairs social behavior in the rat: implications for an animal model of autism. *Neuropharmacology* **54**:901–911.

Siegel SJ, Connolly P, Liang Y et al. 2003. Effects of strain, novelty, and NMDA blockade on auditory-evoked potentials in mice. *Neuropsychopharmacology* **28**:675–682.

Sigurdsson T, Stark KL, Karayiorgou M, Gogos JA, Gordon JA. 2010. Impaired hippocampal-prefrontal synchrony in a genetic mouse model of schizophrenia. *Nature* **464**:763–767.

Silverman JL, Tolu SS, Barkan CL, Crawley JN. 2010. Repetitive self-grooming behavior in the BTBR mouse model of autism is blocked by the mGluR5 antagonist MPEP. *Neuropsychopharmacology* **35**:976–989.

Silverman JL, Yang M, Lord C, Crawley JN. 2010. Behavioural phenotyping assays for mouse models of autism. *Nat Rev Neurosci* **11**:490–502.

Simpson GV, Knight RT. 1993. Multiple brain systems generating the rat auditory evoked potential. I. Characterization of the auditory cortex response. *Brain Res* **602**:240–250.

Singer HS, Morris C, Gause C et al. 2009. Prenatal exposure to antibodies from mothers of children with autism produces neurobehavioral alterations: a pregnant dam mouse model. *J Neuroimmunol* **211**:39–48.

Sobin C, Kiley-Brabeck K, Karayiorgou M. 2005. Associations between prepulse inhibition and executive visual attention in children with the 22q11 deletion syndrome. *Mol Psychiatry* **10**:553–562.

Sohal VS, Zhang F, Yizhar O, Deisseroth K. 2009. Parvalbumin neurons and gamma rhythms enhance cortical circuit performance. *Nature* **459**:698–702.

Sokhadze E, Baruth J, Tasman A *et al.* 2009. Event-related potential study of novelty processing abnormalities in autism. *Appl Psychophysiol Biofeedback* **34**:37–51.

Sokhadze EM, El-Baz A, Baruth J, Mathai G, Sears L, Casanova MF. 2009. Effects of low frequency repetitive transcranial magnetic stimulation (rTMS) on gamma frequency oscillations and event-related potentials during processing of illusory figures in autism. *J Autism Dev Disord* **39**:619–634.

Stromland K, Nordin V, Miller M, Akerstrom B, Gillberg C. 1994. Autism in thalidomide embryopathy: a population study. *Dev Med Child Neurol* **36**:351–356.

Strozik E, Festing MF. 1981. Whisker trimming in mice. *Lab Anim* **15**:309–312.

Swerdlow NR, Braff DL, Geyer MA. 1999. Cross-species studies of sensorimotor gating of the startle reflex. *Ann NY Acad Sci* **877**:202–216.

Szatmari P, Paterson AD, Zwaigenbaum L *et al.* 2007. Mapping autism risk loci using genetic linkage and chromosomal rearrangements. *Nat Genet* **39**:319–328.

Tabuchi K, Blundell J, Etherton MR *et al.* 2007. A neuroligin-3 mutation implicated in autism increases inhibitory synaptic transmission in mice. *Science* **318**:71–76.

Takarae Y, Minshew NJ, Luna B, Krisky CM, Sweeney JA. 2004. Pursuit eye movement deficits in autism. *Brain* **127**:2584–2594.

Thatcher RW, North DM, Neubrander J *et al.* 2009. Autism and EEG phase reset: deficient GABA mediated inhibition in thalamo-cortical circuits. *Dev Neuropsychol* **34**:780–800.

Thomas A, Burant A, Bui N *et al.* 2009. Marble burying reflects a repetitive and perseverative behavior more than novelty-induced anxiety. *Psychopharmacology (Berl)* **204**:361–373.

Thompson WW, Price C, Goodson B *et al.* 2007. Early thimerosal exposure and neuropsychological outcomes at 7 to 10 years. *N Engl J Med* **357**:1281–1292.

Tikhonravov D, Neuvonen T, Pertovaara A *et al.* 2008. Effects of an NMDA-receptor antagonist MK-801 on an MMN-like response recorded in anesthetized rats. *Brain Res* **1203**:97–102.

Tremolizzo L, Doueiri MS, Dong E *et al.* 2005. Valproate corrects the schizophrenia-like epigenetic behavioral modifications induced by methionine in mice. *Biol Psychiatry* **57**:500–509.

Uhlhaas PJ, Singer W. 2006. Neural synchrony in brain disorders: relevance for cognitive dysfunctions and pathophysiology. *Neuron* **52**:155–168.

Uhlhaas PJ, Singer W. 2007. What do disturbances in neural synchrony tell us about autism? *Biol Psychiatry* **62**:190–191.

Umbricht D, Koller R, Vollenweider FX, Schmid L. 2002. Mismatch negativity predicts psychotic experiences induced by NMDA receptor antagonist in healthy volunteers. *Biol Psychiatry* **51**:400–406.

Umbricht D, Vyssotky D, Latanov A *et al.* 2004. Midlatency auditory event-related potentials in mice: comparison to midlatency auditory ERPs in humans. *Brain Res* **1019**:189–200.

Umbricht D, Vyssotki D, Latanov A, Nitsch R, Lipp HP. 2005. Deviance-related electrophysiological activity in mice: is there mismatch negativity in mice? *Clin Neurophysiol* **116**:353–363.

van Herten M, Pasman J, van Leeuwen TH *et al.* 2008. Differences in AERP responses and atypical hemispheric specialization in 17-month-old children at risk of dyslexia. *Brain Res* **1201**:100–105.

Varoqueaux F, Aramuni G, Rawson RL *et al.* 2006. Neuroligins determine synapse maturation and function. *Neuron* **51**:741–754.

Vianney-Rodrigues P, Iancu OD, Welsh JP. 2011. Gamma oscillations in the auditory cortex of awake rats. *Eur J Neurosci* **33**:119–129.

Viding E, Blakemore SJ. 2007. Endophenotype approach to developmental psychopathology: implications for autism research. *Behav Genet* **37**:51–60.

Wallace S, Sebastian C, Pellicano E, Parr J, Bailey A. 2010. Face processing abilities in relatives of individuals with ASD. *Autism Res* **3**:345–349.

Wang K, Zhang H, Ma D *et al.* 2009. Common genetic variants on 5p14.1 associate with autism spectrum disorders. *Nature* **459**:528–533.

Wang X. 2004. The unexpected consequences of a noisy environment. *Trends Neurosci* **27**:364–366.

Wang Y, Greenwood JS, Calcagnotto ME *et al.* 2007. Neocortical hyperexcitability in a human case of tuberous sclerosis complex and mice lacking neuronal expression of TSC1. *Ann Neurol* **61**:139–152.

Wassink TH, Hazlett HC, Epping EA *et al.* 2007. Cerebral cortical gray matter overgrowth and functional variation of the serotonin transporter gene in autism. *Arch Gen Psychiatry* **64**:709–717.

Weiss LA, Arking DE, Daly MJ, Chakravarti A. 2009. A genome-wide linkage and association scan reveals novel loci for autism. *Nature* **461**:802–808.

Welsh JP, Ahn ES, Placantonakis DG. 2005. Is autism due to brain desynchronization? *Int J Dev Neurosci* **23**:253–263.

Welsh JP, Rodrigues PV, Edgar JC, Roberts TPL. 2010. Gamma band oscillopathy: an electrical signature of language impairment in ASD that impairs active listening. *Intl Meeting for Autism Res (IMFAR), International Society for Autism Research* **109**. [Accessed 25 Apr 2011.] Available at: http://imfar.confex.com/imfar/2010/webprogram/Paper7347.html

White NR, Prasad M, Barfield RJ, Nyby JG. 1998. 40- and 70-kHz vocalizations of mice (*Mus musculus*) during copulation. *Physiol Behav* **63**:467–473.

White SA, Fisher SE, Geschwind DH, Scharff C, Holy TE. 2006. Singing mice, songbirds, and more: models for FOXP2 function and dysfunction in human speech and language. *J Neurosci* **26**:10376–10379.

Wilkerson DS, Volpe AG, Dean RS, Titus JB. 2002. Perinatal complications as predictors of infantile autism. *Int J Neurosci* **112**:1085–1098.

Williams K, Wheeler DM, Silove N, Hazell P. 2010. Selective serotonin reuptake inhibitors (SSRIs) for autism spectrum disorders (ASD). *Cochrane Database Syst Rev*: CD004677.

Williams KW, Wray JJ, Wheeler DM. 2005. Intravenous secretin for autism spectrum disorder. *Cochrane Database Syst Rev*: CD003495.

Williams LM, Whitford TJ, Nagy M et al. 2009. Emotion-elicited gamma synchrony in patients with first-episode schizophrenia: a neural correlate of social cognition outcomes. *J Psychiatry Neurosci* **34**:303–313.

Wilson TW, Rojas DC, Reite ML, Teale PD, Rogers SJ. 2007. Children and adolescents with autism exhibit reduced MEG steady-state gamma responses. *Biol Psychiatry* **62**:192–197.

Winslow JT. 2003. Mouse social recognition and preference. *Curr Protoc Neurosci* Ch. 8: Unit 8.16.

Winter C, Reutiman TJ, Folsom TD et al. 2008. Dopamine and serotonin levels following prenatal viral infection in mouse–implications for psychiatric disorders such as schizophrenia and autism. *Eur Neuropsychopharmacol* **18**:712–716.

Witt RM, Galligan MM, Despinoy JR, Segal R. 2009. Olfactory behavioral testing in the adult mouse. *J Vis Exp* **23**:949.

Witter FR, Zimmerman AW, Reichmann JP, Connors SL. 2009. In utero beta 2 adrenergic agonist exposure and adverse neurophysiologic and behavioral outcomes. *Am J Obstet Gynecol* **201**:553–559.

Yamada K. 2010. Strain differences of selective attention in mice: effect of Kamin blocking on classical fear conditioning. *Behav Brain Res* **213**:126–129.

Yamawaki N, Stanford IM, Hall SD, Woodhall GL. 2008. Pharmacologically induced and stimulus evoked rhythmic neuronal oscillatory activity in the primary motor cortex in vitro. *Neuroscience* **151**:386–395.

Yan QJ, Rammal M, Tranfaglia M, Bauchwitz RP. 2005. Suppression of two major fragile X syndrome mouse model phenotypes by the mGluR5 antagonist MPEP. *Neuropharmacology* **49**:1053–1066.

Yang M, Perry K, Weber MD, Katz AM, Crawley JN. 2011. Social peers rescue autism-relevant sociability deficits in adolescent mice. *Autism Res* **4**:17–27.

Young DM, Schenk AK, Yang SB, Jan YN, Jan LY. 2010. Altered ultrasonic vocalizations in a tuberous sclerosis mouse model of autism. *Proc Natl Acad Sci USA* **107**:11074–11079.

Zeng LH, Xu L, Gutmann DH, Wong M. 2008. Rapamycin prevents epilepsy in a mouse model of tuberous sclerosis complex. *Ann Neurol* **63**:444–453.

Zerrate MC, Pletnikov M, Connors SL et al. 2007. Neuroinflammation and behavioral abnormalities after neonatal terbutaline treatment in rats: implications for autism. *J Pharmacol Exp Ther* **322**:16–22.

Zhang C, Milunsky JM, Newton S et al. 2009. A neuroligin-4 missense mutation associated with autism impairs neuroligin-4 folding and endoplasmic reticulum export. *J Neurosci* **29**:10843–10854.

Zhang L, He J, Jugloff DG, Eubanks JH. 2008. The MeCP2-null mouse hippocampus displays altered basal inhibitory rhythms and is prone to hyperexcitability. *Hippocampus* **18**:294–309.

Zhou J, Blundell J, Ogawa S et al. 2009. Pharmacological inhibition of mTORC1 suppresses anatomical, cellular, and behavioral abnormalities in neural-specific Pten knock-out mice. *J Neurosci* **29**:1773–1783.

Zimmerman AW. 2005. The immune system. In *The Neurobiology of Autism*. Bauman ML, Kemper TL, eds. Baltimore, MD: Johns Hopkins University Press, pp. 371–386.

Chapter 17
Attention deficit hyperactivity disorder

Craig W. Berridge, David M. Devilbiss, Robert C. Spencer, Brooke E. Schmeichel, and Amy F.T. Arnsten

Attention deficit hyperactivity disorder (ADHD), first described by Still in 1902, is a behavioral syndrome associated with attentional deficits, hyperactivity, and impulsivity. Initially viewed as a childhood disorder, ADHD is now known to occur in adults, with a sizeable proportion of adult ADHD reflecting a continuance of the disorder from childhood (Barkley et al. 2002a; Biederman et al. 1993; Mannuzza et al. 1991; Spencer et al. 1994; Weiss et al. 1985). The prevalence rate of ADHD is estimated to be 3–8% (Visser et al. 2007). Importantly, this disorder is associated with increased risk in a number of domains including academic, social, and health related (Barkley 2002; Barkley et al. 2002b; Hechtman et al. 2004; Mannuzza et al. 1997, 1993). Thus, it is important that ADHD patients be identified and treated to mitigate these risks.

Pharmacological treatment of ADHD is remarkably effective. Currently, the psychostimulants (methylphenidate, amphetamine) are the most widely used form of treatment for this disorder, with millions of prescriptions written annually (Greenhill 2001). When explicitly examined, these drugs are generally more effective than behavioral interventions alone (Abikoff et al. 2004; Jensen et al. 2005; Newcorn et al. 2008). Psychostimulants not only reduce symptoms of ADHD but also improve socioacademic outcome measures in several domains (Hechtman et al. 2004; Scheffler et al. 2009; Tannock et al. 1989).

Despite the effectiveness of these drugs, psychostimulants are not without risk, possessing the potential for both toxicity and abuse. Widespread use of psychostimulants is thus of concern, particularly in children, and also limits the use of these drugs for the treatment of cognitive dysfunction outside ADHD (e.g., sleep deprivation, aging, narcolepsy). Moreover, stimulant use is contraindicated in some patients, particularly those with tics or a history of substance abuse. Finally, not all patients in whom ADHD is diagnosed respond well to psychostimulants.

These observations indicate a need for additional treatment options for ADHD. To better identify new pharmacological treatments for ADHD, we must first understand the neural mechanisms responsible for the therapeutic actions of psychostimulants and other drugs used in the treatment of ADHD. Surprisingly, until relatively recently this issue received little attention. This chapter reviews the basic pharmacology of the most commonly used drugs in the treatment of ADHD, including the psychostimulants, tricyclic antidepressants, selective norepinephrine (NE) reuptake inhibitors, and α_2 agonists. Of particular interest, relatively recent findings indicate that these differing pharmacological treatments have in common the ability to enhance catecholamine neurotransmission preferentially within the prefrontal cortex (PFC). These modulatory actions of ADHD-related drugs on PFC catecholamines are consistent with known cognitive and behavioral functions of the PFC and the proposed role for the PFC in the pathophysiology of ADHD. Combined, the available evidence suggests a critical role of PFC catecholamines in the therapeutic actions of drugs used in the treatment of ADHD.

Attention deficit hyperactivity disorder and the prefrontal cortex

Although our understanding of the neurobiology of ADHD is evolving, considerable evidence indicates that ADHD is associated with a dysregulation of the PFC and extended frontostriatal circuitry (for review see Castellanos and Tannock 2002). The PFC regulates a variety of behavioral and higher cognitive

Translational Neuroscience, ed. James E. Barrett, Joseph T. Coyle and Michael Williams. Published by Cambridge University Press. © Cambridge University Press 2012

processes involved in goal-directed behavior, particularly under distracting or ambiguous conditions. These processes include planning, inhibiting interference/distraction from irrelevant information, gating sensory inputs based on internal goals, and facilitating sustained attention (Bunge *et al.* 2001; Chao and Knight 1995; Miller and Cohen 2001; Wilkins *et al.* 1987). Consequently, damage to the PFC results in impulsivity, distractibility, poor concentration, and hyperactivity in animals and humans (Arnsten *et al.* 1996; Clark *et al.* 2007; French 1959). The right hemisphere of the PFC may be particularly important in the regulation of behavioral activity and behavioral inhibition (Aron *et al.* 2004; Clark *et al.* 2007). Combined, these and other actions comprise a proposed "executive function" of the PFC associated with the temporal organization of goal-directed behavior.

The cardinal symptoms of ADHD bear a striking similarity to the effects of PFC lesions. As with PFC lesions, ADHD is associated with deficits in tests of executive function, working memory, regulation of attention, and inhibitory control (Clark *et al.* 2007; Loo *et al.* 2007). Structural and functional imaging studies provide direct evidence for a dysregulation of the PFC in ADHD, demonstrating reductions in the size and activity of the PFC in subjects with ADHD, particularly in the right hemisphere (Bush *et al.* 2005; Rubia *et al.* 1999; Sheridan *et al.* 2007). Moreover, recent studies have reported disorganized white matter tracks emanating from the PFC in ADHD, potentially suggesting weaker prefrontal connectivity (Casey *et al.* 2007; Makris *et al.* 2007). Although the PFC matures more slowly than less evolved brain regions, evidence suggests that the delay in prefrontal development is greater in ADHD (Shaw *et al.* 2007). Nonetheless, ADHD does not appear to reflect simply a delay in PFC development, as reductions in PFC activity and size are observed in adults with ADHD (Makris *et al.* 2007; Seidman *et al.* 2006). Interestingly, recent research indicates that long-term stimulant medication, when taken properly, normalizes PFC gray matter in adolescents with ADHD (Shaw *et al.* 2007).

The PFC represents one node of an extended neural network involved in response selection and response evaluation under ambiguous or distracting conditions (Johnson *et al.* 2007). Evidence suggests this network includes the PFC, hippocampus, striatum, cerebellum, and other cortical and subcortical regions (Johnson *et al.* 2007; Dalley *et al.* 2004; Pratt and Mizumori 2001; Vertes 2006). PFC-striatal interactions may be particularly important in a variety of behavioral processes, including cognitive and affective processes (Dalley *et al.* 2004; Gabbott *et al.* 2005; Johnson *et al.* 2007; Pratt and Mizumori 2001; Vertes 2006; Voorn *et al.* 2004). Thus it is of interest that ADHD is also associated with a reduction in the size of the caudate (as well as the cerebellum; Casey *et al.* 2007; Castellanos and Tannock 2002). In contrast to that seen in the frontal cortices, however, the smaller caudate volume seen in children with ADHD disappears across development (i.e., during adolescence; Castellanos *et al.* 2002).

Catecholamines and prefrontal cortex function

The catecholamines, NE and dopamine (DA), are brainstem-originating neuromodulatory systems that project widely throughout the CNS, including across the entire cortical mantle (Lewis 2001). These systems modulate arousal state and a variety of state-dependent behavioral/physiological processes (e.g., Berridge and Waterhouse 2003). NE acts at α_1, α_2, and β receptors, each comprised of multiple subtypes. α_2 receptors display a higher affinity for NE relative to α_1 and β receptors (Arnsten 2000). The three subtypes of α_2 adrenoceptors α_{2A}, α_{2B}, and α_{2C} (MacDonald *et al.* 1997) are expressed both pre-(α_{2C}) and postsynaptically (α_{2A}). The most prominent DA receptors in the PFC are those comprising the D_1 receptor family, which includes D_1 and D_5 receptors (Paspalas and Goldman-Rakic 2004). D_1 and D_5 receptors are similar pharmacologically, and to date there are no drugs that distinguish between them. The D_2 receptor family includes the D_2, D_3, and D_4 receptors. It should be noted, however, that the D_4 receptor binds both NE and DA and thus acts as a generalized catecholamine receptor (Van Tol *et al.* 1991).

The modulatory actions of NE and DA on PFC function follow an "inverted-U" dose–response relationship, with either too little (e.g., drowsiness) or too much (e.g., stress) associated with an impairment in PFC-dependent behavior (Fig. 17.1; Arnsten 2007). Indeed, NE and DA are such critical modulators of PFC function that their depletion in the PFC is as detrimental to PFC-dependent behavior as are lesions to the PFC itself (Brozoski *et al.* 1979). The modulatory actions of these transmitters on PFC function involve actions of postsynaptic NE α_2- and

Chapter 17: Attention deficit hyperactivity disorder

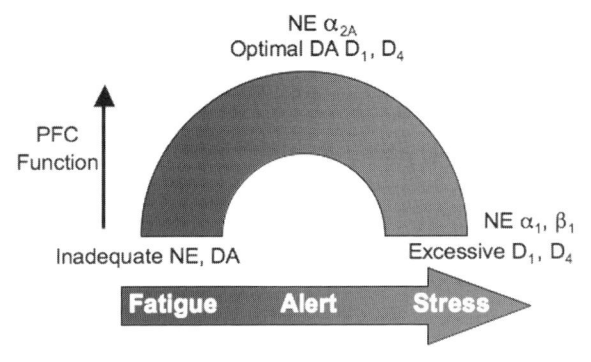

Figure 17.1. Inverted-U shaped modulation of prefrontal cortex (PFC)-dependent function by norepinephrine (NE) and dopamine (DA) receptors. The PFC receives NE inputs from the locus ceruleus in the pons and DA inputs from the substantia nigra/ventral tegmental area complex in the midbrain. Optimal levels of NE and DA, resulting in optimal levels of NE α_{2A} and DA D_1 receptor stimulation, are necessary for optimal PFC-dependent behavior. At low levels of NE and DA release associated with sedation/fatigue, suboptimal levels of α_{2A} and D_1 receptor stimulation occur. High rates of NE and DA release, associated with stress, result in an activation of lower-affinity NE α_1 receptors and excessive D_1 receptor stimulation, leading to an overall suppression in PFC network activity and an impairment in PFC-dependent behavior.

α_1-receptors and DA D_1 receptors within the PFC (Birnbaum et al. 2004; Vijayraghavan et al. 2007; Wang et al. 2007). Early work on α_2 receptors emphasized the presence and actions of presynaptic α_2 receptors, which, acting as autoreceptors, reduce NE cell firing and decrease NE release (Cedarbaum and Aghajanian 1977). Work over the past 30 years, however, indicates that in addition to presynaptic α_{2C} receptors, there exists a high density of postsynaptic α_{2A} receptors (U'Prichard et al. 1979).

Extensive pharmacological studies demonstrate that stimulation of postsynaptic α_{2A} receptors in the PFC promotes PFC-dependent behavior (for review see Arnsten 2007; Arnsten et al. 1996). In contrast, pharmacological stimulation of PFC α_1 receptors produces a stress-like impairment in PFC function while blockade of PFC α_1 receptors prevents stress-related impairment in PFC behavior (Arnsten 2007; Birnbaum et al. 1999, 2004). Based on these and other observations, it is hypothesized that high rates of NE release, associated with stress and impaired PFC function, result in an activation of the lower-affinity α_1 receptors (for review see Arnsten 2007). D_1 receptor stimulation elicits an inverted-U shaped modulation of PFC-dependent processes, with low and high rates of D_1 receptor stimulation associated with impaired PFC function and moderate rates associated with optimal function (Arnsten 2007; Vijayraghavan et al. 2007).

Electron microscopic studies indicate that α_{2A} and D_1 receptors reside on separate dendritic spines on PFC pyramidal cells, near synaptic inputs from other cortical neurons (Smiley et al. 1992; Wang et al. 2007). Electrophysiological evidence suggests that stimulation of these receptors gates synaptic inputs to PFC neurons, with α_{2A} receptor stimulation strengthening behaviorally appropriate inputs and D_1 receptor stimulation weakening inappropriate inputs (Arnsten 2007). For example, one of the most intensively studied aspects of PFC neuronal properties is the sustained discharge displayed by a subset of PFC neurons during the delay portion of delayed-response tasks (working memory tasks; Fuster and Alexander 1971). In the dorsolateral PFC of monkeys, delay-related activity displays spatial tuning, with largest responses observed to stimuli located in a restricted spatial location (Funahashi et al. 1989). Single-unit recordings in monkeys indicate that iontophoretic application of α_{2A} agonists increases delay-related alterations in neuronal activity to stimuli in preferred spatial locations whereas moderate D_1 receptor stimulation decreases neuronal responses to nonpreferred locations (Arnsten 2007; Vijayraghavan et al. 2007). These actions improve the spatial tuning properties of PFC neurons. In contrast, α_1 receptor stimulation or high rates of D_1 receptor stimulation produce a general suppression of PFC neuronal activity, reducing spatial tuning properties (Birnbaum et al. 2004; Wang et al. 2007).

Pharmacology of attention deficit hyperactivity disorder

Pharmacological treatments are currently the most effective form of treatment for ADHD. Several drug classes have been shown to be effective in the treatment of ADHD. These include the psychostimulants (primarily methylphenidate and amphetamine), selective NE reuptake blockers (desipramine, atomoxetine), and α_2 agonists, particularly α_{2A}-preferring, such as guanfacine. Though the neural mechanism involved in the therapeutic actions of these different drug classes has been poorly understood, as reviewed below, recent observations indicate that a common action of these drugs is the enhancement of *both* NE and DA neurotransmission preferentially within the PFC.

305

Psychostimulants

Psychostimulants have been used in the treatment of ADHD since the 1930s. Extensive clinical studies demonstrate that these drugs are effective in treating the attentional and hyperactivity/impulsivity components of ADHD in children, adolescents, and adults (Shenker 1992; Wender et al. 1985). For this reason, stimulants are viewed as the first line of treatment for ADHD. The therapeutic effects of low-dose stimulants are observed acutely and neither pronounced tolerance nor sensitization occurs with repeated treatment over many months (Greenhill 2001; Solanto 1998; Wilens et al. 2004; however, see Swanson and Volkow 2001).

Therapeutic actions of stimulants are not paradoxical

High doses of psychostimulants increase arousal, motor activity, and euphoria, while impairing cognition (Arnsten and Dudley 2005; Berridge and Stalnaker 2002; Rebec and Bashore 1984; McGaughy and Sarter 1995; Segal 1975). The behaviorally activating and cognition-impairing actions of psychostimulants are in distinct contrast to the behavioral and cognitive actions of these drugs seen in the treatment of ADHD. Historically, the behavioral/cognitive actions of low-dose stimulants were viewed as unique to ADHD, the so-called paradoxical effect of these drugs in the treatment of ADHD.

A major advance in our understanding of the pharmacology of ADHD was the discovery that the cognition-enhancing actions of psychostimulants are not confined to ADHD. Low and clinically relevant doses of psychostimulants have been well documented to improve PFC-dependent cognitive function and reduce impulsivity in normal human subjects (Rapoport et al. 1980; Mehta et al. 2000, 2001; Rapoport and Inoff-Germain 2002; Vaidya et al. 1998). Consistent with these findings, low-dose stimulants are commonly used as cognitive enhancers by individuals without ADHD (Maher 2008). These observations demonstrate that the cognition-enhancing and behavior-calming actions of stimulants occur only at low doses, and at these doses, psychostimulants exert similar cognition-enhancing effects in normal subjects and in subjects with ADHD. Importantly, these observations indicate that an animal model of ADHD is not necessary to better understand the neural mechanisms involved in the cognitive/therapeutic effects of low-dose stimulants. This is advantageous given that most animal models of psychopathology involve a high degree of uncertainty regarding the extent to which they model the pathophysiology of a disorder, even when mimicking certain aspects of the behavioral phenotype of that disorder.

Clinically, the therapeutic actions of psychostimulants occur with plasma concentrations in the range of 8 to 40 ng/mL (Swanson and Volkow 2001). Recent work demonstrates that, as with humans, stimulants enhance cognition and calm behavior in monkeys and rodents at doses that produce clinically relevant plasma concentrations (Arnsten and Dudley 2005; Berridge et al. 2006; Devilbiss and Berridge 2008; Kuczenski and Segal 2001, 2002; Zdrale et al. 2008). Combined, these observations demonstrate unambiguously that the cognitive and behavioral effects of low-dose psychostimulants are not unique to ADHD and instead occur in normal humans, monkeys, and rodents.

Neurochemical actions of low-dose psychostimulants

Neurochemically, stimulants inhibit NE and DA reuptake and, depending on the drug and dose, serotonin. Within this drug class, amphetamine also actively stimulates the efflux of DA and NE (Kuczenski and Segal 1994). This latter action is believed to involve amphetamine entry into the catecholamine terminal and the subsequent reverse operation of the transporter (for review see Kuczenski and Segal 1994). In the case of NE, however, this occurs only at relatively high and clinically inappropriate doses associated with pronounced motor activation and stereotypy (Florin et al. 1994). Amphetamine also blocks serotonin reuptake, but this action is limited to high and behaviorally activating doses (Kuczenski et al. 1995). In contrast to amphetamine, methylphenidate acts only as a reuptake blocker for NE and DA, having no impact on serotonin neurotransmission (Kuczenski and Segal 1997). Combined, these observations indicate that the therapeutic/cognition-enhancing actions of low-dose stimulants involve inhibition of NE and/or DA reuptake and are not dependent on inhibition of serotonin reuptake or drug-induced increases in catecholamine release/efflux. A lack of involvement of serotonin in the therapeutic actions of stimulants is consistent with previous observations indicating that selective serotonin reuptake inhibitors are relatively ineffective in the treatment of ADHD (Green 1992).

When administered at relatively high doses associated with hyperactivity or stereotypy, stimulants elicit large increases in extracellular levels of NE and DA widely throughout the brain (Kuczenski and Segal 1992; Kuczenski et al. 1995; Moghaddam et al. 1993). Initially, emphasis was placed on the role of striatal (particularly nucleus accumbens) DA in the locomotor-activating and reinforcing actions of the psychostimulants (Carr and White 1986; Kelley et al. 1989; Kelly et al. 1975; Koob and Bloom 1988; Wise and Bozarth 1987). However, additional work demonstrates a critical role of NE α_1 receptors, particularly within the PFC, in the reinforcing and locomotor-activating effects of these drugs (Blanc et al. 1994; Drouin et al. 2002; Kokkinidis and Anisman 1978). These latter observations indicate that it is inappropriate to view these behavioral effects of stimulants as largely dependent on DA and not NE.

In contrast to behaviorally activating doses of stimulants, low and clinically relevant doses of these drugs produce a qualitatively different pattern of action on brain catecholamine systems. Specifically, clinically relevant doses of methylphenidate preferentially target NE and DA levels in the PFC (Fig. 17.2). Thus, at low and cognition-enhancing doses that produce clinically appropriate peak plasma concentrations, methylphenidate produces a prominent increase in extracellular levels of NE and DA within the PFC while having substantially reduced actions in cortical (somatosensory cortex, hippocampus) and subcortical (accumbens, medial septum) regions outside the PFC (Berridge et al. 2006; Drouin et al. 2006; Kuczenski and Segal 2001, 2002). This preferential sensitivity of PFC NE and DA to low-dose stimulants may involve low DA transporter levels within the PFC combined with an ability of the NE transporter to clear both NE and DA (Carboni et al. 1990; Sesack et al. 1998).

The neurochemical actions of low-dose methylphenidate suggest that the cognition-enhancing/therapeutic actions of low-dose stimulants involve, at least in part, drug-induced increases in rates of NE and DA neurotransmission within the PFC. Consistent with this, recent studies demonstrate that direct infusion of methylphenidate into the medial PFC of the rat improves PFC-dependent function as measured in a delayed-response test of spatial working memory comparable with that seen with systemic administration (Spencer et al. 2011).

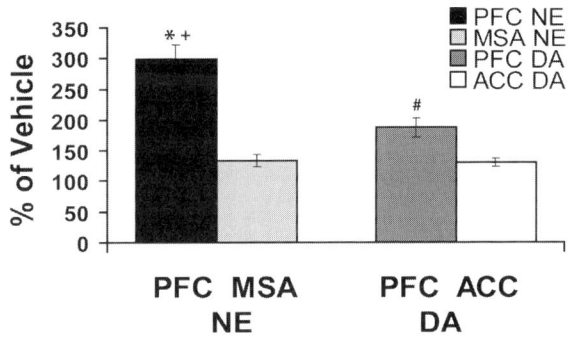

Figure 17.2. Cognition-enhancing doses of methylphenidate (MPH) increase extracellular norepinephrine (NE) and dopamine (DA) preferentially within the prefrontal cortex (PFC). Shown are the effects of a cognition-enhancing dose of MPH that produces clinically relevant peak plasma concentrations (0.5 mg/kg, intraperitoneally) on extracellular levels of NE and DA in the PFC, NE in the medial septal area (MSA), and DA in the nucleus accumbens core (ACC). Data are an average (± SEM) of two 15-minute samples collected 15–45 minutes following drug treatment and are expressed as percent of vehicle treatment. At this dose, MPH produced only a modest (~30%) increase in NE and DA levels outside the PFC. In contrast, within the PFC, this dose of MPH produced a substantially larger increase in NE and DA levels. Moreover, the increase in PFC NE levels (~200%) was significantly larger than that seen for PFC DA (~85%). A similar pattern of effects was observed with oral administration of a cognition-enhancing dose (2.0 mg/kg) of MPH that produced plasma concentrations comparable to those seen with intraperitoneal administration of 0.5 mg/kg MPH. *$P < 0.001$ relative to MSA NE; +$P < 0.001$ relative to PFC DA, #$P < 0.05$ relative to ACC DA. Modified from Berridge et al. (2006).

Effects of low-dose psychostimulants on noradrenergic neuronal discharge

Norepinephrine and DA neurons display both spontaneous and phasic (evoked) discharge, each associated with distinct behavioral processes. In the case of the noradrenergic nucleus, locus ceruleus (LC), tonic/spontaneous discharge is highly state dependent, with higher rates observed with increasing in arousal (for review see Berridge 2008a). Phasic LC discharge is elicited in response to behaviorally relevant sensory stimuli, but only at modest tonic discharge rates corresponding to moderate levels of arousal (for review see Berridge and Waterhouse 2003). Both phasic and tonic discharge have been implicated in higher cognitive processes, including attention and working memory (Arnsten and Li 2005; Clayton et al. 2004; Rajkowski et al. 1994).

High-dose stimulants profoundly suppress LC discharge via activation of somatodendritic α_2 receptors (Curtis et al. 1993; Pitts and Marwah 1987). In contrast, cognition-enhancing doses of methylphenidate produce only a modest suppression of both tonic and phasic discharge (Fig. 17.3; Devilbiss and Berridge 2006). The functional consequence of the decrease in LC tonic discharge is likely negated by drug-induced increases in NE levels in LC terminal fields. Moreover, although these doses of methylphenidate modestly suppress phasic discharge of LC neurons, the signal-to-noise ratio for phasic vs. tonic LC discharge is largely unchanged (Fig. 17.3). Thus, the therapeutic actions of low-dose methylphenidate may not stem directly from alterations in LC discharge firing patterns. However, given the proposed role of phasic LC discharge in higher cognitive function (Clayton et al. 2004; Rajkowski et al. 1994), the ability of low-dose methylphenidate to preserve the ability of LC neurons to respond phasically to sensory events and to relay this signal/information to terminal fields may contribute to the cognition-enhancing actions of low-dose psychostimulants. Alternatively, the robust elevation in NE levels in the PFC seen with cognition-enhancing doses of stimulants may blunt the signal-to-noise ratio for phasic NE release associated with phasic LC discharge, potentially leading to a decrease in sensitivity to distracting/irrelevant stimuli. It seems likely that cognition-enhancing doses of psychostimulants will similarly influence DA neuronal discharge, though this has yet to be determined.

Effects of low-dose psychostimulants on prefrontal cortex neuronal activity

The net effect of drug-induced increases in NE/DA efflux within the PFC combined with modest alterations in discharge rates/patterns of PFC-projecting NE and DA neurons is difficult to predict. To better understand the neuromodulatory actions of low-dose stimulants on PFC neuronal activity, recent studies examined the effects of low-dose methylphenidate on PFC neuronal discharge in awake rats. This work indicates that cognition-enhancing doses of methylphenidate exert minimal effects on spontaneous discharge rates of PFC neurons while increasing the responsiveness of PFC neurons to afferent signals (Fig. 17.4; Devilbiss and Berridge 2008). Across an ensemble of PFC neurons, low-dose methylphenidate increased the dominant representation of afferent input to the PFC

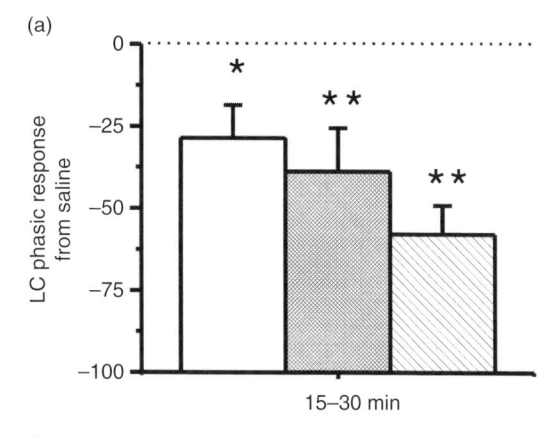

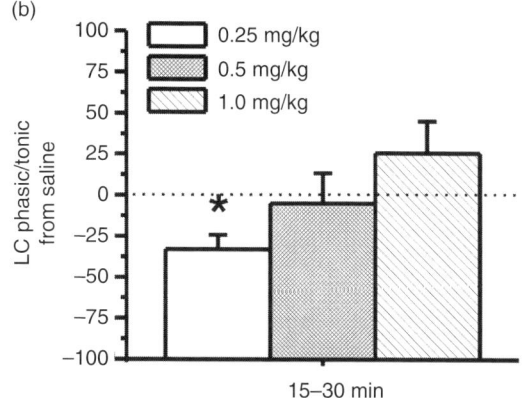

Figure 17.3. Cognition-enhancing doses of methylphenidate exert a modest influence on tonic and phasic locus ceruleus (LC) discharge. Shown are the effects of varying doses of methylphenidate (intraperitoneally) on the magnitude of LC phasic discharge in the halothane-anesthetized rat. Doses examined included the cognition-enhancing dose of 0.5 mg/kg (Devilbiss and Berridge 2008). Evoked discharge was elicited by brief electrical stimulation of the foot (Devilbiss and Berridge 2006). For all treatments, data were normalized by calculating the percent change from predrug conditions and then expressed as the mean change from vehicle (saline, ± SEM). (A) Effects of low-dose methylphenidate on the magnitude of phasic LC discharge, expressed as a change from saline treatment, for a 15-minute period that began 15 minutes following drug treatment ($n = 60$ stimulus presentations). Methylphenidate produced a dose-dependent decrease in phasic discharge that was relatively mild at the 0.5-mg/kg dose. (B) Effects of methylphenidate on the signal-to-noise ratio of phasic responses (relative to tonic discharge). Because methylphenidate-induced suppression of phasic discharge was associated with a similar magnitude suppression of tonic discharge (Devilbiss and Berridge 2006), methylphenidate had minimal effects on the signal-to-noise ratio for phasic discharge, particularly at the 0.5-mg/kg dose. Similar effects were observed with oral methylphenidate administration. *$P < 0.05$, **$P < 0.01$ relative to saline controls. Modified from Devilbiss and Berridge (2006).

while reducing less dominant patterns of activity, actions that were not observed outside the PFC (Devilbiss and Berridge 2008). Modestly higher doses

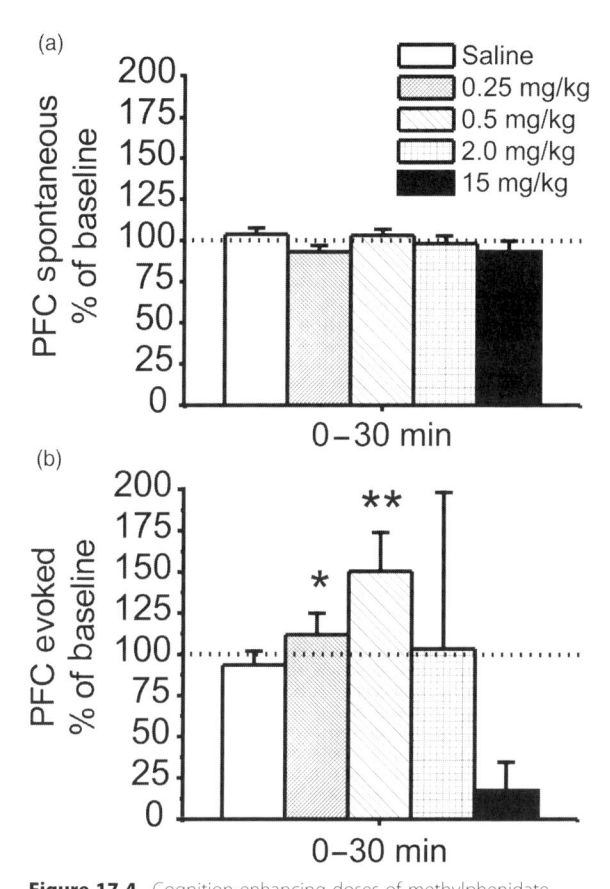

Figure 17.4. Cognition-enhancing doses of methylphenidate (MPH) preferentially increase the responsiveness of prefrontal cortex (PFC) neurons. Shown are the effects of varying doses of methylphenidate on spontaneous discharge and excitatory evoked responses (elicited by brief electrical stimulation of the hippocampus) of PFC neurons in the awake, freely moving rat. Doses examined included the cognition-enhancing dose of 0.5 mg/kg (Devilbiss and Berridge 2008). All data are expressed as the percent change from predrug conditions (± SEM). (A) Spontaneous discharge of PFC neurons was minimally affected by low doses of methylphenidate. (B) Hippocampal stimulus evoked excitatory discharge in PFC neurons exhibited a dose-dependent inverted-U facilitation/suppression. The maximal facilitation of PFC responses to hippocampal input was observed following the 0.5-mg/kg dose. A behaviorally activating dose of MPH (15.0 mg/kg) resulted in a suppression of stimulus evoked activity well below baseline levels. $^*P < 0.05$, $^{**}P < 0.01$ relative to baseline. Modified from Devilbiss and Berridge (2008).

that fail to improve PFC-dependent cognition (2.0 mg/kg) did not increase the responsiveness of PFC neurons, while a high and behaviorally activating dose (15 mg/kg) produced a profound suppression of evoked discharge of PFC neurons (Fig. 17.4; Devilbiss and Berridge 2008). Thus, across a range of doses, only cognition-enhancing doses of psychostimulants facilitate the responsiveness of PFC neurons.

Combined, these observations indicate that the cognitive/therapeutic effects of low-dose psychostimulants involve enhanced signal processing abilities of PFC neurons, potentially biasing neuronal responses to stronger and more salient information. Conversely, the cognitive-impairing effects of high doses of stimulants likely arise from suppressed prefrontal neuronal responsiveness. Consistent with these observations, results from imaging studies demonstrate that cognition-enhancing doses of stimulants increase the efficiency of PFC activity in normal subjects (Mehta et al. 2000). A similar but more pronounced profile is observed in subjects with ADHD (Clark et al. 2007).

Cognition-enhancing actions of low-dose stimulants involve α2 and D1 receptors

Evidence reviewed above indicates that the cognition-enhancing actions of low-dose stimulants involve preferential targeting of PFC catecholamine neurotransmission. α_2 and D_1 receptors located within the PFC facilitate both PFC neural activity and PFC-dependent function (see above). The actions of low-dose methylphenidate on PFC neuronal signal processing are similar to those seen with optimal rates of α_2 and D_1 receptor stimulation. Combined, these observations suggest that cognition-enhancing actions of psychostimulants involve PFC α_2 and/or D_1 receptors. Consistent with this, the cognition-enhancing actions of methylphenidate are prevented by systemic pretreatment with an α_2 antagonist or a D_1 antagonist, at doses that have no impact on baseline cognitive function (Arnsten and Dudley 2005). When combined with information reviewed above, these observations suggest that the cognition-enhancing effects of low-dose methylphenidate are dependent on both α_2 and D_1 receptors located within the PFC.

Summary: neurobiology of low-dose psychostimulants

Low-dose psychostimulants exert cognition-enhancing and behavior-calming actions in both ADHD and normal populations, acting as cognitive enhancers broadly across the population. The ability of low-dose stimulants to improve PFC-dependent function is likely critical for the therapeutic actions of these drugs. Current evidence demonstrates that low and clinically relevant doses of psychostimulants exert neurochemical and behavioral actions that are qualitatively distinct from those of higher doses associated with abuse and addiction. In particular, low-dose psychostimulants preferentially influence PFC catecholamines, PFC neuronal signaling, and PFC-dependent cognition/behavior. Additional evidence suggests that the cognitive and therapeutic effects of low-dose psychostimulants involve enhanced signaling at α_2 and D_1 receptors located within the PFC.

It is important to note that, contrary to the commonly held view, DA is neither the primary target of low-dose stimulants nor the sole participant in the cognitive/behavioral actions of these drugs. Indeed, cognition-enhancing doses of methylphenidate produce larger increases in PFC NE levels than in PFC DA, while blockade of α_2 receptors prevents psychostimulant-induced improvement in cognitive function. Moreover, an involvement of NE in the therapeutic actions of stimulants is entirely consistent with the therapeutic actions of noradrenergic α_2 agonists and selective NE reuptake blockers in ADHD, described below. Of course, cognition-enhancing doses of stimulants also increase PFC DA levels and stimulant-induced improvement in PFC-dependent function is prevented by D_1 receptor blockade. Thus, the available evidence indicates that the cognition-enhancing actions of low-dose psychostimulants involve both NE α_2 and DA D_1 receptors within the PFC.

The fact that PFC catecholamines are strongly implicated in the cognitive/therapeutic actions of low-dose stimulants does not rule out an involvement of catecholamines outside the PFC in these behavioral actions. Nonetheless, the fact that low doses of stimulants produce only modest increases in NE/DA efflux in areas associated with stimulant-induced motor activation (e.g., accumbens) and arousal (medial septum) appears to explain why low doses of these drugs preferentially impact PFC-dependent processes while being devoid of behaviorally activating or arousal-enhancing actions. The fact that low-dose stimulants exert a modest impact on circuitry believed to underlie the abuse liability of these drugs (i.e., accumbens DA) is consistent with evidence indicating that the appropriate use of low-dose stimulants does not increase, and may reduce, the liability for drug abuse in ADHD populations (Biederman 2003; Wilens *et al.* 2003).

Nonstimulant medications
Tricyclic antidepressants and selective norepinephrine reuptake inhibitors

Low-dose methylphenidate and amphetamine largely act as NE and DA reuptake inhibitors. Another class of drugs that blocks catecholamine reuptake is the tricyclic antidepressants. Interestingly, these drugs are also effective in the treatment of ADHD (Green 1992). As a class, these drugs act as monoamine reuptake inhibitors, particularly for NE and serotonin (Baldessarini 1985). However, across the individual members of this class, these compounds display differing selectivity for the different monoamine transporters. Thus, whereas imipramine displays high-affinity binding for both the serotonin and NE transporters, desipramine is highly selective for the NE transporter (Bolden-Watson and Richelson 1993; Wong *et al.* 1982).

The most intensively studied tricyclic for use in ADHD is desipramine, which is effective in treating ADHD in children, adolescents, and adults (Biederman *et al.* 1989; Biederman *et al.* 1986; Gastfriend *et al.* 1984, 1985; Rapoport *et al.* 1985; Spencer *et al.* 1993). Interestingly, for reasons that are poorly understood, desipramine appears effective in a subset of patients who are relatively unresponsive to psychostimulants (Biederman *et al.* 1989). Tricyclic antidepressants also bind to and block a variety of receptors, actions that are typically viewed as contributing to the side-effect profile of these drugs (e.g., anticholinergic, cardiovascular, sedative effects; Baldessarini 1985; Wong *et al.* 1982). Consistent with this view, relative to the other tricyclic antidepressants, desipramine displays a lower affinity for many of these receptors and is associated with a lower side-effect profile, but not reduced efficacy (Biederman *et al.* 1989; Gastfriend *et al.* 1984, 1985; Green 1992).

Atomoxetine, a nontricyclic selective NE reuptake blocker, is also effective in the treatment of ADHD (Michelson *et al.* 2003; Newcorn *et al.* 2008; Spencer *et al.* 1998). Atomoxetine lacks the affinity for neurotransmitter receptors associated with the tricyclic antidepressants and, correspondingly, is largely devoid of tricyclic-like side effects (Wong *et al.* 1982; Zerbe *et al.* 1985). Similar to that seen with the stimulants, atomoxetine improves cognitive function in both normal human subjects and subjects with ADHD (Chamberlain *et al.* 2007; Seu *et al.* 2009).

The neural circuitry underlying the therapeutic actions of desipramine and atomoxetine is not well understood. However, despite the selectivity of these compounds for the NE transporter, they nonetheless increase extracellular levels of both NE and DA in the PFC. Consistent with their primary pharmacological action (i.e., NE reuptake blockade), these drugs have minimal effects on DA levels outside the PFC, at least in regions largely devoid of NE fibers (Bymaster et al. 2002; Carboni et al. 1990). The ability of these drugs to increase both NE and DA levels in the PFC is posited to result from the fact that the NE transporter displays a high affinity for DA (Horn 1973; Raiteri et al. 1977) and plays a prominent role in DA clearance in the PFC due to a limited density of DA transporters in this region (Carboni et al. 1990).

Like desipramine and atomoxetine, the tricyclic nortriptyline displays a high selectivity for the NE transporter and is also effective in the treatment of ADHD (Prince et al. 2000). In contrast, although the tricyclic compound mianserin displays high selectivity for the NE transporter, this compound is ineffective in the treatment of ADHD (Winsberg et al. 1987). An important difference between mianserin and these other NE reuptake blockers is that mianserin displays relatively high affinity for α_2 receptors, where it acts as an antagonist (Baldessarini 1985). Thus, similar to that seen with the stimulants (Arnsten and Dudley 2005), blockade of α_2 receptors appears to eliminate the cognition-enhancing/therapeutic effects of selective NE reuptake blockers. Moreover, preliminary data indicate that atomoxetine-induced improvement in PFC function in animals is dependent on both NE α_2 and DA D_1 receptors (Gamo et al. 2010). Therefore, the ability of stimulants and selective NE reuptake blockers to improve PFC-dependent function is dependent on both α_2 and D_1 receptors, presumably located in the PFC.

α_2 Agonists

The nonselective α_2 agonist clonidine has long been used in the treatment of ADHD (Hunt et al. 1985). The ability of clonidine to decrease extracellular levels of NE is opposite to that observed with the stimulants, tricyclics, and atomoxetine (as well as the monoamine oxidase inhibitors; see section below). This difference between clonidine and other drug classes effective in treating ADHD was initially difficult to reconcile. A significant advance in our understanding of noradrenergic function was the identification of postsynaptic α_2 receptors within the PFC and the demonstration that these receptors promote PFC-dependent cognition (for review see Arnsten et al. 1996; Berridge et al. 1993; Wang et al. 2007). This work suggests that the cognition-enhancing effects of α_2 agonists likely stem from their direct stimulation of postsynaptic α_{2A} receptors.

Consistent with this hypothesis, the α_{2A}-preferring agonist guanfacine is effective in the treatment of ADHD while lacking the potent sedative actions of clonidine (Biederman et al. 2008; Hunt et al. 1995; Scahill et al. 2001). A limiting factor in the use of clonidine in ADHD is its sedative/hypotensive effects (Hunt et al. 1985), which likely involve clonidine-induced suppression of NE release via stimulation of α_2 autoreceptors (for review see Berridge 2008b) and stimulation of brainstem blood pressure–regulating imidazoline I1 receptors (van Zwieten and Chalmers 1994). Guanfacine displays lower sedative/hypotensive effects presumably due to its lower affinity, relative to clonidine, for α_{2B}, α_{2C}, imidazoline I1, and presynaptic α_{2A} receptors (Engberg and Eriksson 1991; van Zwieten and Chalmers 1994). As with the tricyclics and atomoxetine, guanfacine may be beneficial in patients who respond suboptimally to the psychostimulants (Scahill et al. 2001).

Similar to the psychostimulants and atomoxetine, guanfacine improves PFC-dependent behavior in normal human and animal subjects (Franowicz and Arnsten 1998; Jakala et al. 1999). Animal studies demonstrate that guanfacine enhances a wide range of PFC-dependent functions via direct actions within the PFC (Avery et al. 2000; Mao et al. 1999; Steere and Arnsten 1997). Moreover, guanfacine strengthens synaptic inputs to PFC neurons and enhances prefrontal network connectivity, similar to that seen with the psychostimulants (Wang et al. 2007).

Monoamine oxidase inhibitors

Though used less extensively than the other drug classes reviewed, monoamine oxidase inhibitors are also effective in the treatment of ADHD in children and adults (Green 1992; Shenker 1992). By inhibiting the enzyme monoamine oxidase, these drugs interfere with the degradation of NE, DA, and serotonin, resulting in an increase in catecholamine/monoamine neurotransmission. As with the stimulants and tricyclic antidepressants, the impact of the monoamine oxidase inhibitors on NE, DA, and serotonin catabolism varies across individual compounds in this class of drugs. For example, low-dose deprenyl, a monoamine oxidase B inhibitor, is believed to have a reduced impact on NE relative to DA and serotonin (Baldessarini 1985). Interestingly, low-dose deprenyl has been reported to be relatively ineffective in the treatment of ADHD (Green 1992; Rapoport et al. 1985; Shenker 1992; Zametkin and Rapoport 1987). Thus, the therapeutic efficacy of the monoamine oxidase inhibitors appears correlated with their ability to increase NE neurotransmission.

Inhibition of monoamine oxidase has been reported for amphetamine, although this occurs only at relatively high doses inappropriate for clinical use (for review see Kuczenski and Segal 1994). Moreover, methylphenidate does not cross the cell membrane and thus does not gain access to monoamine oxidase. Therefore, despite previous suggestions (Mefford and Potter 1989), the therapeutic actions of stimulants in the treatment of ADHD most likely do not involve inhibition of monoamine oxidase.

Summary: pharmacology of attention deficit hyperactivity disorder

Multiple drug classes have proven effective in the treatment of ADHD. Where examined, the cognition-enhancing actions of these drugs are observed in both normal and ADHD-affected subjects. Across this broad range of pharmacological compounds, all have in common the ability to increase NE, and to a lesser extent DA, neurotransmission within the PFC. In the case of the psychostimulants and the selective NE reuptake inhibitors, evidence indicates that their cognition-enhancing/therapeutic actions are dependent on both α_2 and D_1 receptors. In the case of the α_2 agonists, their therapeutic actions likely involve direct actions at postsynaptic α_{2A} receptors.

Potential use of selective dopamine reuptake inhibitors

Low-dose stimulants block the reuptake of both NE and DA. As reviewed above, several selective NE reuptake inhibitors have proven useful in the treatment of ADHD. In contrast, to date little work has been done with selective DA reuptake inhibitors. The use of DA reuptake inhibitors in the treatment of ADHD has been hampered by both a limited selection of compounds and the stimulant-like abuse potential of these drugs. A series of benztropine analogs was described that display selective and high-affinity binding for the DA transporter (Katz et al. 1999; Newman et al. 1994; Raje et al. 2005). Surprisingly, these compounds do not produce stimulant-like behavioral effects. For example, these drugs lack locomotor-activating properties, do not produce cocaine-like discriminative effects (Katz et al. 1999; Newman et al. 1994), do not maintain cocaine-like rates of responding in self-administration paradigms (Woolverton et al. 2000, 2001), and do not produce a cocaine-like conditioned place-preference (Li et al. 2005). Although the basis for this nonstimulant-like behavioral profile is unknown, contributing factors may include slower onset of action in the brain (Loland et al. 2008).

One well-characterized benztropine analog is AHN 2–005, involving an aryll substitution (Katz et al. 2004). We recently observed that this compound improves performance in a test of spatial working memory, similar to that seen with the psychostimulants (Schmeichel and Berridge 2010). Thus, these compounds may offer a new nonstimulant alternative for pharmacological treatment of ADHD. Given the competitive nature of DA clearance through the NE transporter in the PFC, it is expected that increases in DA levels in this region are likely to result in an increase in NE levels. Limited microdialysis studies appear to confirm this hypothesis (Berridge and Schmeichel, unpublished observations). Future studies will need to compare the broader cognitive actions of these drugs, the degree to which they affect PFC DA and NE, and the degree to which they are effective in the treatment of ADHD.

Pharmacology vs. etiology of attention deficit hyperactivity disorder

The above-reviewed information suggests a prominent role of NE and DA in the pharmacology of ADHD. Researchers have tended to extrapolate from this pharmacology to the underlying biological causes of ADHD, suggesting that NE and/or DA participate in the etiology of the disorder. Although this is possible, it is important to note that treatments can be therapeutic while not targeting the primary/proximal origins of a disorder. As reviewed above, catecholamines act as neuromodulators, modifying the sensitivity of neurons to afferent signals. Available evidence suggests that low-dose stimulants and other cognitive enhancers used to treat ADHD shift neuronal activity within modestly dysregulated PFC circuits (via actions of PFC catecholamine receptors). Theoretically, this action would occur even if a dysregulation of PFC circuitry arises from mechanisms independent of catecholamines. For example, if ADHD symptoms reflect slower maturation of PFC network connections, the facilitation of existing connections through α_{2A} and D1 receptor stimulation would be expected to strengthen PFC regulation of behavior and attention. Thus the fact that stimulants are effective in the treatment of ADHD does not necessarily indicate that ADHD involves dysfunctional catecholamine signaling.

Nonetheless, given that ADHD is highly heritable, there is substantial interest in the degree to which catecholamine-related genes may contribute to this disorder. Numerous studies have identified multiple catecholamine-related gene alleles associated with ADHD, including NE and DA receptors, DA and NE transporters, and dopamine β-hydroxylase, the enzyme required for NE synthesis (Bobb *et al.* 2005; Daly *et al.* 1999; Roman *et al.* 2002). Genetic insults to dopamine β-hydroxylase are particularly interesting, because they reduce NE production and have been associated with weaker sustained attention, impaired PFC executive function, and increased impulsivity (Bellgrove *et al.* 2006; Kieling *et al.* 2008).

Despite these statistically significant genetic associations, in general the variance in the disorder explained by any one of these genes is small (Gizer *et al.* 2009). Evidence also suggests that certain of these genes can act as modifier genes in ADHD, modulating clinical features rather than being responsible for the behavioral phenotype of the disorder (Mill *et al.* 2006). Although these considerations do not rule out an involvement of catecholamine-related genes in ADHD, they suggest that, individually, the majority of these genes are unlikely to play a major role in the etiology of ADHD.

Heterogeneity of attention deficit hyperactivity disorder

The majority of pharmacological studies have focused on patients with the combined subtype of ADHD who have symptoms of both inattention and impulsivity/hyperactivity. It has been proposed that the primarily inattentive form of ADHD involves different neural mechanisms from those associated with ADHD with hyperactivity/impulsivity. Thus, primarily inattentive ADHD is not associated with deficits in behavioral inhibition, a key function of the PFC, whereas the attentional deficits observed in this subtype have been suggested to reflect deficits in more posterior cortical attentional systems (for review see Solanto *et al.* 2007). However, when this possibility was systematically examined, no evidence for a difference in anterior vs. posterior attentional processes was observed across the primarily inattentive and combined hyperactive/inattentive subtype (Solanto *et al.* 2007). Nonetheless, the differences in phenotype across the subtypes of ADHD are likely to reflect differing neural substrates to some extent. Our understanding of the pharmacology and neurobiology of the primarily inattentive subtype of ADHD is extremely limited, representing an important area for future research.

Conclusions

Attention deficit hyperactivity disorder is a serious disorder that affects a sizeable portion of the population. Low-dose psychostimulants and other nonstimulant drugs are remarkably effective in treating ADHD. Importantly, the cognition-enhancing and behavior-calming actions of these drugs occur in both normal individuals and individuals with ADHD. From a drug-discovery perspective, this observation indicates that an animal model of ADHD is not required for identifying novel targets or new compounds with potential for use in the treatment of ADHD.

Over the past 10 years, we have gained significant new insight into the pharmacological mechanisms and neurocircuitry involved in the cognition-enhancing and therapeutic actions of ADHD-related drugs. This work suggests that the therapeutic actions of a broad array of drugs used in the treatment of ADHD involve enhanced DA and/or NE signaling at α_2 and D_1 receptors in the PFC. For example, low-dose psychostimulants and selective NE reuptake inhibitors (desipramine and atomoxetine) increase extracellular levels of *both* NE and DA preferentially in the PFC while having significantly reduced actions outside the PFC. Similarly, clinically relevant doses of methylphenidate preferentially enhance PFC neuronal responsiveness. The electrophysiological and behavioral/

cognitive effects of low-dose stimulants are similar to those observed with direct stimulation of PFC α_2 and D_1 receptors. Moreover, the cognition-enhancing actions of low-dose stimulants, tricyclics, and atomoxetine are prevented by α_2 and D_1 receptor blockade. Combined, these observations indicate a critical role of PFC catecholamines in the therapeutic actions of all drug classes used to treat ADHD. This conclusion is consistent with the pivotal role of the PFC in regulating attention and behavior and evidence indicating PFC dysregulation in ADHD.

These observations suggest that new pharmacological treatments that enhance PFC D_1 and/or α_2 neurotransmission while avoiding excessive stimulation of NE/DA receptors outside the PFC may prove efficacious in the treatment of ADHD. Novel compounds may target NE/DA transporters, receptors, and/or intracellular second messengers to achieve this action. Despite the apparent prominent role of the PFC in the therapeutic actions of ADHD, drug actions outside the PFC may nonetheless be important for maximal therapeutic benefit. For example, all of the drug classes described above influence DA and/or NE neurotransmission outside the PFC, even though the magnitude of these actions may be substantially lower than that seen in the PFC. A better understanding of the neurocircuitry involved in the cognitive/therapeutic effects of psychostimulants and other drugs used in the treatment of ADHD will be an important issue for development of novel treatments for this disorder.

Acknowledgments
This work was supported by PHS grants, MH081843, DA000389, the Wisconsin Institutes of Discovery, and the University of Wisconsin Graduate School.

Disclosure statement
Amy F.T. Arnsten has a license agreement with Shire Pharmaceuticals for the development of guanfacine for the treatment of ADHD. She also performs consulting and speaking engagements with Shire and has received grant money from Shire to examine the mechanism of action of ADHD medications.

References

Abikoff H, Hechtman L, Klein RG et al. 2004. Social functioning in children with ADHD treated with long-term methylphenidate and multimodal psychosocial treatment. *J Am Acad Child Adolesc Psychiatry* **43**:820–829.

Arnsten AF. 2000. Stress impairs prefrontal cortical function in rats and monkeys: role of dopamine D1 and norepinephrine alpha-1 receptor mechanisms. *Prog Brain Res* **126**:183–192.

Arnsten AF. 2007. Catecholamine and second messenger influences on prefrontal cortical networks of "representational knowledge": a rational bridge between genetics and the symptoms of mental illness. *Cereb Cortex* **17** (Suppl. 1):i6–i15.

Arnsten AF, Dudley AG. 2005. Methylphenidate improves prefrontal cortical cognitive function through alpha2 adrenoceptor and dopamine D1 receptor actions: relevance to therapeutic effects in attention deficit hyperactivity disorder. *Behav Brain Funct* **1**:2.

Arnsten AF, Li BM. 2005. Neurobiology of executive functions: catecholamine influences on prefrontal cortical functions. *Biol Psychiatry* **57**:1377–1384.

Arnsten AF, Steere JC, Hunt RD. 1996. The contribution of alpha 2-noradrenergic mechanisms of prefrontal cortical cognitive function. Potential significance for attention-deficit hyperactivity disorder. *Arch Gen Psychiatry* **53**:448–455.

Aron AR, Robbins TW, Poldrack RA. 2004. Inhibition and the right inferior frontal cortex. *Trends Cogn Sci* **8**:170–177.

Avery RA, Franowicz JS, Studholme C, van Dyck CH, Arnsten AF. 2000. The alpha-2A-adrenoceptor agonist, guanfacine, increases regional cerebral blood flow in dorsolateral prefrontal cortex of monkeys performing a spatial working memory task. *Neuropsychopharmacology* **23**:240–249.

Baldessarini RJ. 1985. Antidepressant agents. In *Chemotherapy in Psychiatry*. Cambridge, MA: Harvard University Press, pp. 130–234.

Barkley RA. 2002. Major life activity and health outcomes associated with attention-deficit/hyperactivity disorder. *J Clin Psychiatry* **63** (Suppl. 12): 10–15.

Barkley RA, Fischer M, Smallish L, Fletcher K. 2002a. The persistence of attention-deficit/hyperactivity disorder into young adulthood as a function of reporting source and definition of disorder. *J Abnorm Psychol* **111**:279–289.

Barkley RA, Murphy KR, Dupaul GI, Bush T. 2002b. Driving in young adults with attention deficit hyperactivity disorder: knowledge, performance, adverse outcomes, and the role of executive functioning. *J Int Neuropsychol Soc* **8**:655–672.

Bellgrove MA, Hawi Z, Gill M, Robertson IH. 2006. The cognitive genetics of attention deficit hyperactivity disorder (ADHD): sustained attention as a candidate phenotype. *Cortex* **42**:838–845.

Berridge CW. 2008*a*. The locus coeruleus-noradrenergic system and stress: implications for post-traumatic stress disorder (PTSD). In *Post-Traumatic Stress Disorder: Basic Science and Clinical Practice*. Shiromani PJ, Keane TM, LeDoux JE, eds. New York, NY: Humana/Springer, pp. 213–230.

Berridge CW. 2008*b*. Noradrenergic modulation of arousal. *Brain Res Rev* **58**:1–17.

Berridge CW, Arnsten AF, Foote SL. 1993. Noradrenergic modulation of cognitive function: clinical implications of anatomical, electrophysiological and behavioural studies in animal models [editorial]. *Psychol Med* **23**:557–564.

Berridge CW, Devilbiss DM, Andrzejewski ME *et al*. 2006. Methylphenidate preferentially increases catecholamine neurotransmission within the prefrontal cortex at low doses that enhance cognitive function. *Biol Psychiatry* **60**:1111–1120.

Berridge CW, Stalnaker TA. 2002. Relationship between low-dose amphetamine-induced arousal and extracellular norepinephrine and dopamine levels within prefrontal cortex. *Synapse* **46**:140–149.

Berridge CW, Waterhouse BD. 2003. The locus coeruleus-noradrenergic system: modulation of behavioral state and state-dependent cognitive processes. *Brain Res Brain Res Rev* **42**:33–84.

Biederman J. 2003. Pharmacotherapy for attention-deficit/hyperactivity disorder (ADHD) decreases the risk for substance abuse: findings from a longitudinal follow-up of youths with and without ADHD. *J Clin Psychiatry* **64** (Suppl. 1):3–8.

Biederman J, Baldessarini RJ, Wright V, Knee D, Harmatz JS. 1989. A double-blind placebo controlled study of desipramine in the treatment of ADD: I. Efficacy. *J Am Acad Child Adolesc Psychiatry* **28**:777–784.

Biederman J, Faraone SV, Spencer T *et al*. 1993. Patterns of psychiatric comorbidity, cognition, and psychosocial functioning in adults with attention deficit hyperactivity disorder. *Am J Psychiatry* **150**:1792–1798.

Biederman J, Gastfriend DR, Jellinek MS. 1986. Desipramine in the treatment of children with attention deficit disorder. *J Clin Psychopharmacol* **6**:359–363.

Biederman J, Melmed RD, Patel A *et al*. 2008. A randomized, double-blind, placebo-controlled study of guanfacine extended release in children and adolescents with attention-deficit/hyperactivity disorder. *Pediatrics* **121**:e73–e84.

Birnbaum S, Gobeske KT, Auerbach J, Taylor JR, Arnsten AF. 1999. A role for norepinephrine in stress-induced cognitive deficits: alpha-1-adrenoceptor mediation in the prefrontal cortex. *Biol Psychiatry* **46**:1266–1274.

Birnbaum SG, Yuan PX, Wang M *et al*. 2004. Protein kinase C overactivity impairs prefrontal cortical regulation of working memory. *Science* **306**:882–884.

Blanc G, Trovero F, Vezina P *et al*. 1994. Blockade of prefronto-cortical alpha 1-adrenergic receptors prevents locomotor hyperactivity induced by subcortical D-amphetamine injection. *Eur J Neurosci* **6**:293–298.

Bobb AJ, Addington AM, Sidransky E *et al*. 2005. Support for association between ADHD and two candidate genes: NET1 and DRD1. *Am J Med Genet B Neuropsychiatr Genet* **134B**:67–72.

Bolden-Watson C, Richelson E. 1993. Blockade by newly-developed antidepressants of biogenic amine uptake into rat brain synaptosomes. *Life Sci* **52**:1023–1029.

Brozoski TJ, Brown RM, Rosvold HE, Goldman PS. 1979. Cognitive deficit caused by regional depletion of dopamine in prefrontal cortex of rhesus monkey. *Science* **205**:929–932.

Bunge SA, Ochsner KN, Desmond JE, Glover GH, Gabrieli JD. 2001. Prefrontal regions involved in keeping information in and out of mind. *Brain* **124**:2074–2086.

Bush G, Valera EM, Seidman LJ. 2005. Functional neuroimaging of attention-deficit/hyperactivity disorder: a review and suggested future directions. *Biol Psychiatry* **57**:1273–1284.

Bymaster FP, Katner JS, Nelson DL *et al*. 2002. Atomoxetine increases extracellular levels of norepinephrine and dopamine in prefrontal cortex of rat: a potential mechanism for efficacy in attention deficit/hyperactivity disorder. *Neuropsychopharmacology* **27**:699–711.

Carboni E, Tanda GL, Frau R, Di CG. 1990. Blockade of the noradrenaline carrier increases extracellular dopamine concentrations in the prefrontal cortex: evidence that dopamine is taken up in vivo by noradrenergic terminals. *J Neurochem* **55**:1067–1070.

Carr GD, White NM. 1986. Anatomical disassociation of amphetamine's rewarding and aversive effects: an intracranial microinjection study. *Psychopharmacology (Berl)* **89**:340–346.

Casey BJ, Epstein JN, Buhle J *et al*. 2007. Frontostriatal connectivity and its role in cognitive control in parent–child dyads with ADHD. *Am J Psychiatry* **164**:1729–1736.

Castellanos FX, Lee PP, Sharp W *et al*. 2002. Developmental trajectories of brain volume abnormalities in children and adolescents with attention-deficit/

hyperactivity disorder. *J Am Med Assoc* **288**:1740–1748.

Castellanos FX, Tannock R. 2002. Neuroscience of attention-deficit/hyperactivity disorder: The search for endophenotypes. *Nat Rev Neurosci* **3**:617–628.

Cedarbaum JM, Aghajanian GK. 1977. Catecholamine receptors on locus coeruleus neurons: pharmacological characterization. *Eur J Pharmacol* **44**:375–385.

Chamberlain SR, Del Campo N, Dowson J et al. 2007. Atomoxetine improved response inhibition in adults with attention deficit/hyperactivity disorder. *Biol Psychiatry* **62**:977–984.

Chao LL, Knight RT. 1995. Human prefrontal lesions increase distractibility to irrelevant sensory inputs. *Neuroreport* **6**:1605–1610.

Clark L, Blackwell AD, Aron AR et al. 2007. Association between response inhibition and working memory in adult ADHD: a link to right frontal cortex pathology? *Biol Psychiatry* **61**:1395–1401.

Clayton EC, Rajkowski J, Cohen JD, Aston-Jones G. 2004. Phasic activation of monkey locus ceruleus neurons by simple decisions in a forced-choice task. *J Neurosci* **24**:9914–9920.

Curtis AL, Conti E, Valentino RJ. 1993. Cocaine effects on brain noradrenergic neurons of anesthetized and unanesthetized rats. *Neuropharmacology* **32**:419–428.

Dalley JW, Cardinal RN, Robbins TW. 2004. Prefrontal executive and cognitive functions in rodents: neural and neurochemical substrates. *Neurosci Biobehav Rev* **28**:771–784.

Daly G, Hawi Z, Fitzgerald M, Gill M. 1999. Mapping susceptibility loci in attention deficit hyperactivity disorder: preferential transmission of parental alleles at DAT1, DBH and DRD5 to affected children. *Mol Psychiatry* **4**:192–196.

Devilbiss DM, Berridge CW. 2006. Low-dose methylphenidate actions on tonic and phasic locus coeruleus discharge. *J Pharmacol Exp Ther* **319**:1327–1335.

Devilbiss DM, Berridge CW. 2008. Cognition-enhancing doses of methylphenidate preferentially increase prefrontal cortex neuronal responsiveness. *Biol Psychiatry* **64**:626–635.

Drouin C, Darracq L, Trovero F, et al. 2002. Alpha1b-adrenergic receptors control locomotor and rewarding effects of psychostimulants and opiates. *J Neurosci* **22**:2873–2884.

Drouin C, Page M, Waterhouse B. 2006. Methylphenidate enhances noradrenergic transmission and suppresses mid- and long-latency sensory responses in the primary somatosensory cortex of awake rats. *J Neurophysiol* **96**:622–632.

Engberg G, Eriksson E. 1991. Effects of alpha 2-adrenoceptor agonists on locus coeruleus firing rate and brain noradrenaline turnover in N-ethoxycarbonyl-2-ethoxy-1,2-dihydroquinoline (EEDQ)-treated rats. *Naunyn Schmiedebergs Arch Pharmacol* **343**:472–477.

Florin SM, Kuczenski R, Segal DS. 1994. Regional extracellular norepinephrine responses to amphetamine and cocaine and effects of clonidine pretreatment. *Brain Res* **654**:53–62.

Franowicz JS, Arnsten AF. 1998. The alpha-2a noradrenergic agonist, guanfacine, improves delayed response performance in young adult rhesus monkeys. *Psychopharmacology (Berl)* **136**:8–14.

French GM. 1959. Locomotor effects of regional ablations of frontal cortex in rhesus monkeys. *J Comp Physiol Psychol* **52**:17–24.

Funahashi S, Bruce CJ, Goldman-Rakic PS. 1989. Mnemonic coding of visual space in the monkey's dorsolateral prefrontal cortex. *J Neurophysiol* **61**:331–349.

Fuster JM, Alexander GE. 1971. Neuron activity related to short-term memory. *Science* **173**:652–654.

Gabbott PL, Warner TA, Jays PR, Salway P, Busby SJ. 2005. Prefrontal cortex in the rat: projections to subcortical autonomic, motor, and limbic centers. *J Comp Neurol* **492**:145–177.

Gamo NJ, Wang M, Arnsten AFT. 2010. Methylphenidate and atomoxetine enhance prefrontal function through alpha 2-adrenergic and dopamine D1 receptors.. *J Am Acad Child Adolesc Psychiatry* **49**:1011–1023.

Gastfriend DR, Biederman J, Jellinek MS. 1984. Desipramine in the treatment of adolescents with attention deficit disorder. *Am J Psychiatry* **141**:906–908.

Gastfriend DR, Biederman J, Jellinek MS. 1985. Desipramine in the treatment of attention deficit disorder in adolescents. *Psychopharmacol Bull* **21**:144–145.

Gizer IR, Ficks C, Waldman ID. 2009. Candidate gene studies of ADHD: a meta-analytic review. *Hum Genet* **126**:51–90.

Green WH. 1992. Nonstimulant drugs in the treatment of attention-deficit hyperactivity disorder. *Child Adolesc Psychiatr Clin North Am* **1**:449–465.

Greenhill LL. 2001. Clinical effects of stimulant medication in ADHD. In *Stimulant Drugs and ADHD: Basic and Clinical Neuroscience*. Solanto MV, Arnsten AFT, Castellanos FX, eds. New York, NY: Oxford University Press, pp. 31–71.

Hechtman L, Abikoff H, Klein RG et al. 2004. Academic achievement and emotional status of children with ADHD treated with long-term methylphenidate and multimodal psychosocial treatment. *J Am Acad Child Adolesc Psychiatry* **43**:812–819.

Horn AS. 1973. Structure-activity relations for the inhibition of catecholamine uptake into synaptosomes from noradrenaline and dopaminergic neurones in rat brain homogenates. *Br J Pharmacol* **47**:332–338.

Hunt RD, Arnsten AF, Asbell MD. 1995. An open trial of guanfacine in the treatment of attention-deficit hyperactivity disorder. *J Am Acad Child Adolesc Psychiatry* **34**:50–54.

Hunt RD, Minderaa RB, Cohen DJ. 1985. Clonidine benefits children with attention deficit disorder and hyperactivity: report of a double-blind placebo-crossover therapeutic trial. *J Am Acad Child Psychiatry* **24**:617–629.

Jakala P, Riekkinen M, Sirvio J et al. 1999. Guanfacine, but not clonidine, improves planning and working memory performance in humans. *Neuropsychopharmacology* **20**:460–470.

Jensen PS, Garcia JA, Glied S et al. 2005. Cost-effectiveness of ADHD treatments: findings from the multimodal treatment study of children with ADHD. *Am J Psychiatry* **162**:1628–1636.

Johnson A, van der Meer MA, Redish AD. 2007. Integrating hippocampus and striatum in decision-making. *Curr Opin Neurobiol* **17**:692–697.

Katz JL, Izenwasser S, Kline RH, Allen AC, Newman AH. 1999. Novel 3alpha-diphenylmethoxytropane analogs: selective dopamine uptake inhibitors with behavioral effects distinct from those of cocaine. *J Pharmacol Exp Ther* **288**:302–315.

Katz JL, Kopajtic TA, Agoston GE, Newman AH. 2004. Effects of N-substituted analogs of benztropine: diminished cocaine-like effects in dopamine transporter ligands. *J Pharmacol Exp Ther* **309**:650–660.

Kelley AE, Gauthier AM, Lang CG. 1989. Amphetamine microinjections into distinct striatal subregions cause dissociable effects on motor and ingestive behavior. *Behav Brain Res* **35**:27–39.

Kelly PH, Seviour PW, Iversen SD. 1975. Amphetamine and apomorphine responses in the rat following 6-OHDA lesions of the nucleus accumbens septi and corpus striatum. *Brain Res* **94**:507–522.

Kieling C, Genro JP, Hutz MH, Rohde LA. 2008. The -1021 C/T DBH polymorphism is associated with neuropsychological performance among children and adolescents with ADHD. *Am J Med Genet B Neuropsychiatr Genet* **147B**:485–490.

Kokkinidis L, Anisman H. 1978. Involvement of norepinephrine in startle arousal after acute and chronic d-amphetamine administration. *Psychopharmacology (Berl)* **9**:285–292.

Koob GF, Bloom FE. 1988. Cellular and molecular mechanisms of drug dependence. *Science* **242**:715–723.

Kuczenski R, Segal DS. 1992. Regional norepinephrine response to amphetamine using dialysis: comparison with caudate dopamine. *Synapse* **11**:164–169.

Kuczenski R, Segal DS. 1994. Neurochemistry of amphetamine. In *Amphetamine and Its Analogues: Psychopharmacology, Toxicology and Abuse*. Cho AK, Segal DS, eds. San Diego, CA: Academic Press, pp. 81–113.

Kuczenski R, Segal DS. 1997. Effects of methylphenidate on extracellular dopamine, serotonin, and norepinephrine: comparison with amphetamine. *J Neurochem* **68**:2032–2037.

Kuczenski R, Segal DS. 2001. Locomotor effects of acute and repeated threshold doses of amphetamine and methylphenidate: relative roles of dopamine and norepinephrine. *J Pharmacol Exp Ther* **96**:876–883.

Kuczenski R, Segal DS. 2002. Exposure of adolescent rats to oral methylphenidate: preferential effects on extracellular norepinephrine and absence of sensitization and cross-sensitization to methamphetamine. *J Neurosci* **22**:7264–7271.

Kuczenski R, Segal DS, Cho AK, Melega W. 1995. Hippocampus norepinephrine, caudate dopamine and serotonin, and behavioral responses to the stereoisomers of amphetamine and methamphetamine. *J Neurosci* **15**:1308–1317.

Lewis DA. 2001. The catecholamine innervation of primate cerebral cortex. In *Stimulant Drugs and ADHD: Basic and Clinical Neuroscience*. Solanto MV, Arnsten AFT, Castellanos FX, eds. New York, NY: Oxford University Press, pp. 77–103.

Li SM, Newman AH, Katz JL. 2005. Place conditioning and locomotor effects of N-substituted, 4'¢,4'¢'-difluorobenztropine analogs in rats. *J Pharmacol Exp Ther* **313**:1223–1230.

Loland CJ, Desai RI, Zou MF et al. 2008. Relationship between conformational changes in the dopamine transporter and cocaine-like subjective effects of uptake inhibitors. *Mol Pharmacol* **73**:813–823.

Loo SK, Humphrey LA, Tapio T et al. 2007. Executive functioning among Finnish adolescents with attention-deficit/hyperactivity disorder. *J Am Acad Child Adolesc Psychiatry* **46**:1594–1604.

MacDonald E, Kobilka BK, Scheinin M. 1997. Gene targeting – homing in on alpha 2-adrenoceptor-subtype function. *Trends Pharmacol Sci* **18**:211–219.

Maher B. 2008. Poll results: look who's doping. *Nature* **452**:674–675.

Makris N, Biederman J, Valera EM et al. 2007. Cortical thinning of the attention and executive function networks in adults with attention-deficit/hyperactivity disorder. *Cereb Cortex* **17**:1364–1375.

Mannuzza S, Klein RG, Bessler A, Malloy P, Hynes ME. 1997. Educational and occupational outcome of hyperactive boys grown up. *J Am Acad Child Adolesc Psychiatry* **36**:1222–1227.

Mannuzza S, Klein RG, Bessler A, Malloy P, LaPadula M. 1993. Adult outcome of hyperactive boys. Educational achievement, occupational rank, and psychiatric status. *Arch Gen Psychiatry* **50**:565–576.

Mannuzza S, Klein RG, Bonagura N et al. 1991. Hyperactive boys almost grown up. V. Replication of psychiatric status. *Arch Gen Psychiatry* **48**:77–83.

Mao ZM, Arnsten AF, Li BM. 1999. Local infusion of an alpha-1 adrenergic agonist into the prefrontal cortex impairs spatial working memory performance in monkeys. *Biol Psychiatry* **46**:1259–1265.

McGaughy J, Sarter M. 1995. Behavioral vigilance in rats: task validation and effects of age, amphetamine, and benzodiazepine receptor ligands. *Psychopharmacology (Berl)* **117**:340–357.

Mefford IN, Potter WZ. 1989. A neuroanatomical and biochemical basis for attention deficit disorder with hyperactivity in children: a defect in tonic adrenaline mediated inhibition of locus coeruleus stimulation. *Med Hypotheses* **29**:33–42.

Mehta MA, Owen AM, Sahakian BJ et al. 2000. Methylphenidate enhances working memory by modulating discrete frontal and parietal lobe regions in the human brain. *J Neurosci* **20**:RC65.

Mehta MA, Sahakian BJ, Robbins TW. 2001. Comparative psychopharmacology of methylphenidate and related drugs in human volunteers, patients with ADHD, and experimental animals. In *Stimulant Drugs and ADHD: Basic and Clinical Neuroscience*. Solanto MV, Arnsten AFT, Castellanos FX, eds. New York, NY: Oxford University Press, pp. 303–331.

Michelson D, Adler L, Spencer T et al. 2003. Atomoxetine in adults with ADHD: two randomized, placebo-controlled studies. *Biol Psychiatry* **53**:112–120.

Mill J, Caspi A, Williams BS et al. 2006. Prediction of heterogeneity in intelligence and adult prognosis by genetic polymorphisms in the dopamine system among children with attention-deficit/hyperactivity disorder: evidence from 2 birth cohorts. *Arch Gen Psychiatry* **63**:462–469.

Miller EK, Cohen JD. 2001. An integrative theory of prefrontal cortex function. *Annu Rev Neurosci* **24**:167–202.

Moghaddam B, Berridge CW, Goldman-Rakic PS, Bunney BS, Roth RH. 1993. In vivo assessment of basal and drug-induced dopamine release in cortical and subcortical regions of the anesthetized primate. *Synapse* **13**:215–222.

Newcorn JH, Kratochvil CJ, Allen AJ et al. 2008. Atomoxetine and osmotically released methylphenidate for the treatment of attention deficit hyperactivity disorder: acute comparison and differential response. *Am J Psychiatry* **165**:721–730.

Newman AH, Allen AC, Izenwasser S, Katz JL. 1994. Novel 3 alpha-(diphenylmethoxy)tropane analogs: potent dopamine uptake inhibitors without cocaine-like behavioral profiles. *J Med Chem* **37**:2258–2261.

Paspalas CD, Goldman-Rakic PS. 2004. Microdomains for dopamine volume neurotransmission in primate prefrontal cortex. *J Neurosci* **24**:5292–5300.

Pitts DK, Marwah J. 1987. Electrophysiological actions of cocaine on noradrenergic neurons in rat locus ceruleus. *J Pharmacol Exp Ther* **240**:345–351.

Pratt WE, Mizumori SJ. 2001. Neurons in rat medial prefrontal cortex show anticipatory rate changes to predictable differential rewards in a spatial memory task. *Behav Brain Res* **123**:165–183.

Prince JB, Wilens TE, Biederman J et al. 2000. A controlled study of nortriptyline in children and adolescents with attention deficit hyperactivity disorder. *J Child Adolesc Psychopharmacol* **10**:193–204.

Raiteri M, del Carmine R, Bertollini A, Levi G. 1977. Effect of sympathomimetic amines on the synaptosomal transport of noradrenaline, dopamine and 5-hydroxytryptamine. *Eur J Pharmacol* **41**:133–143.

Raje S, Cornish J, Newman AH et al. 2005. Pharmacodynamic assessment of the benztropine analogues AHN-1055 and AHN-2005 using intracerebral microdialysis to evaluate brain dopamine levels and pharmacokinetic/pharmacodynamic modeling. *Pharm Res* **22**:603–612.

Rajkowski J, Kubiak P, Aston-Jones G. 1994. Locus coeruleus activity in monkey: phasic and tonic changes are associated with altered vigilance. *Brain Res Bull* **35**:607–616.

Rapoport JL, Buchsbaum MS, Weingartner H et al. 1980. Dextroamphetamine – its cognitive and behavioral-effects in normal and hyperactive boys and normal men. *Arch Gen Psychiatry* **37**:933–943.

Rapoport JL, Inoff-Germain G. 2002. Responses to methylphenidate in attention-deficit/hyperactivity disorder and normal children: update 2002. *J Atten Disord* **6**:S57–S60.

Rapoport JL, Zametkin A, Donnelly M, Ismond D. 1985. New drug trials in attention deficit disorder. *Psychopharmacol Bull* **21**:232–236.

Rebec GV, Bashore TR. 1984. Critical issues in assessing the behavioral effects of amphetamine. *Neurosci Biobehav Rev* **8**:153–159.

Roman T, Schmitz M, Polanczyk GV et al. 2002. Further evidence for the association between attention-deficit/hyperactivity disorder and the dopamine-beta-hydroxylase gene. *Am J Med Genet* **114**:154–158.

Rubia K, Overmeyer S, Taylor E et al. 1999. Hypofrontality in attention deficit hyperactivity disorder during higher-order motor control: a study with functional MRI. *Am J Psychiatry* **156**:891–896.

Scahill L, Chappell PB, Kim YS et al. 2001. A placebo-controlled study of guanfacine in the treatment of children with tic disorders and attention deficit hyperactivity disorder. *Am J Psychiatry* **158**:1067–1074.

Scheffler RM, Brown TT, Fulton BD et al. 2009. Positive association between attention-deficit/hyperactivity disorder medication use and academic achievement during elementary school. *Pediatrics* **123**:1273–1279.

Schmeichel BE, Berridge CW. 2010. Selective dopamine reuptake inhibitors improve prefrontal-dependent function and elevate norepinephrine and dopamine levels within the prefrontal cortex: relevance to ADHD. *Soc Neurosci Abstr* **508**:17.

Segal DS. 1975. Behavioral and neurochemical correlates of repeated d-amphetamine administration. *Adv Biochem Psychopharmacol* **13**:247–262.

Seidman LJ, Valera EM, Makris N et al. 2006. Dorsolateral prefrontal and anterior cingulate cortex volumetric abnormalities in adults with attention-deficit/hyperactivity disorder identified by magnetic resonance imaging. *Biol Psychiatry* **60**:1071–1080.

Sesack SR, Hawrylak VA, Matus C, Guido MA, Levey AI. 1998. Dopamine axon varicosities in the prelimbic division of the rat prefrontal cortex exhibit sparse immunoreactivity for the dopamine transporter. *J Neurosci* **18**:2697–2708.

Seu E, Lang A, Rivera RJ, Jentsch JD. 2009. Inhibition of the norepinephrine transporter improves behavioral flexibility in rats and monkeys. *Psychopharmacology (Berl)* **202**:505–519.

Shaw P, Eckstrand K, Sharp W et al. 2007. Attention-deficit/hyperactivity disorder is characterized by a delay in cortical maturation. *Proc Natl Acad Sci USA* **104**:19649–19654.

Shenker A. 1992. The mechanism of action of drugs used to treat attention-deficit hyperactivity disorder: focus on catecholamine receptor pharmacology. *Adv Pediatr* **39**:337–382.

Sheridan MA, Hinshaw S, D'Esposito M. 2007. Efficiency of the prefrontal cortex during working memory in attention-deficit/hyperactivity disorder. *J Am Acad Child Adolesc Psychiatry* **46**:1357–1366.

Smiley JF, Williams SM, Szigeti K, Goldman-Rakic PS. 1992. Light and electron microscopic characterization of dopamine-immunoreactive axons in human cerebral cortex. *J Comp Neurol* **321**:325–335.

Solanto MV. 1998. Neuropsychopharmacological mechanisms of stimulant drug action in attention-deficit hyperactivity disorder: a review and integration. *Behav Brain Res* **94**:127–152.

Solanto MV, Gilbert SN, Raj A et al. 2007. Neurocognitive functioning in AD/HD, predominantly inattentive and combined subtypes. *J Abnorm Child Psychol* **35**:729–744.

Spencer RC, Klein RM, Berridge CW. 2011. Psychostimulant act within the prefrontal cortex to improve cognitive function. *Biol Psychiatry* doi:10.1016/j.bio.psych.2011. 12.002.

Spencer T, Biederman J, Kerman K, Steingard R, Wilens T. 1993. Desipramine treatment of children with attention-deficit hyperactivity disorder and tic disorder or Tourette's syndrome. *J Am Acad Child Adolesc Psychiatry* **32**:354–360.

Spencer T, Biederman J, Wilens T, Faraone SV. 1994. Is attention-deficit hyperactivity disorder in adults a valid disorder? *Harv Rev Psychiatry* **1**:326–335.

Spencer T, Biederman J, Wilens T et al. 1998. Effectiveness and tolerability of atomoxetine in adults with attention deficit hyperactivity disorder. *Am J Psychiatry* **155**:693–695.

Steere JC, Arnsten AF. 1997. The alpha-2A noradrenergic receptor agonist guanfacine improves visual object discrimination reversal performance in aged rhesus monkeys. *Behav Neurosci* **111**:883–891.

Still GF. 1902. Some abnormal psychical conditions in children. *Lancet* **i**:1008–1012.

Swanson J, Volkow N. 2001. *Pharmacokinetic and Pharmacodynamic Properties of Methylphenidate in Humans*. New York, NY: Oxford University Press.

Tannock R, Schachar RJ, Carr RP, Logan GD. 1989. Dose-response effects of methylphenidate on academic performance and overt behavior in hyperactive children. *Pediatrics* **84**:648–657.

U'Prichard DC, Bechtel WD, Rouot BM, Snyder SH. 1979. Multiple apparent alpha-noradrenergic receptor binding sites in rat brain: effect of 6-hydroxydopamine. *Mol Pharmacol* **16**:47–60.

Vaidya CJ, Austin G, Kirkorian G et al. 1998. Selective effects of methylphenidate in attention deficit hyperactivity disorder: a functional magnetic resonance study. *Proc Natl Acad Sci USA* **95**:14494–14499.

Van Tol HH, Bunzow JR, Guan HC et al. 1991. Cloning of the gene for a human dopamine D4 receptor with high affinity for the antipsychotic clozapine. *Nature* **350**:610–614.

van Zwieten PA, Chalmers JP. 1994. Different types of centrally acting antihypertensives and their targets in the central nervous system. *Cardiovasc Drugs Ther* **8**:787–799.

Vertes RP. 2006. Interactions among the medial prefrontal cortex, hippocampus and midline thalamus in emotional and cognitive processing in the rat. *Neuroscience* **142**:1–20.

Vijayraghavan S, Wang M, Birnbaum SG, Williams GV, Arnsten AF. 2007. Inverted-U dopamine D1 receptor actions on prefrontal neurons engaged in working memory. *Nat Neurosci* **10**:376–384.

Visser SN, Lesesne CA, Perou R. 2007. National estimates and factors associated with medication treatment for childhood attention-deficit/hyperactivity disorder. *Pediatrics* **119** (Suppl. 1): S99–S106.

Voorn P, Vanderschuren LJ, Groenewegen HJ, Robbins TW, Pennartz CM. 2004. Putting a spin on the dorsal-ventral divide of the striatum. *Trends Neurosci* **27**:468–474.

Wang M, Ramos BP, Paspalas CD *et al.* 2007. Alpha2A-adrenoceptors strengthen working memory networks by inhibiting cAMP-HCN channel signaling in prefrontal cortex. *Cell* **129**: 397–410.

Weiss G, Hechtman L, Milroy T, Perlman T. 1985. Psychiatric status of hyperactives as adults: a controlled prospective 15-year follow-up of 63 hyperactive children. *J Am Acad Child Psychiatry* **24**:211–220.

Wender PH, Reimherr FW, Wood D, Ward M. 1985. A controlled study of methylphenidate in the treatment of attention deficit disorder, residual type, in adults. *Am J Psychiatry* **142**:547–552.

Wilens TE, Biederman J, Lerner M. 2004. Effects of once-daily osmotic-release methylphenidate on blood pressure and heart rate in children with attention-deficit/hyperactivity disorder: results from a one-year follow-up study. *J Clin Psychopharmacol* **24**:36–41.

Wilens TE, Faraone SV, Biederman J, Gunawardene S. 2003. Does stimulant therapy of attention-deficit/hyperactivity disorder beget later substance abuse? A meta-analytic review of the literature. *Pediatrics* **111**:179–185.

Wilkins AJ, Shallice T, McCarthy R. 1987. Frontal lesions and sustained attention. *Neuropsychologia* **25**:359–365.

Winsberg BG, Camp-Bruno JA, Vink J, Timmer CJ, Sverd J. 1987. Mianserin pharmacokinetics and behavior in hyperkinetic children. *J Clin Psychopharmacol* **7**:143–147.

Wise RA, Bozarth MA. 1987. A psychomotor stimulant theory of addiction. *Psychol Rev* **94**:469–492.

Wong DT, Threlkeld PG, Best KL, Bymaster FP. 1982. A new inhibitor of norepinephrine uptake devoid of affinity for receptors in rat brain. *J Pharmacol Exp Ther* **222**:61–65.

Woolverton WL, Hecht GS, Agoston GE, Katz JL, Newman AH. 2001. Further studies of the reinforcing effects of benztropine analogs in rhesus monkeys. *Psychopharmacology (Berl)* **154**:375–382.

Woolverton WL, Rowlett JK, Wilcox KM *et al.* 2000. 3'- and 4'-chloro-substituted analogs of benztropine: intravenous self-administration and in vitro radioligand binding studies in rhesus monkeys. *Psychopharmacology (Berl)* **147**:426–435.

Zametkin AJ, Rapoport JL. 1987. Neurobiology of attention deficit disorder with hyperactivity: where have we come in 50 years? *J Am Acad Child Adolesc Psychiatry* **26**:676–686.

Zdrale A, Meier TB, Berridge CW, Populin LC. 2008. Effect of methylphenidate on monkey prefrontal cortex-mediated behavior. Presented at the annual meeting of the Society for Neuroscience, Washington, DC, November 15–19. Abstract 388.17.

Zerbe RL, Rowe H, Enas GG *et al.* 1985. Clinical pharmacology of atomoxetine, a potential antidepressant. *J Pharmacol Exp Ther* **232**:139–143.

Chapter 18
Epigenetic mechanisms in central nervous system disorders

Swati Gupta, Ryley Parrish, and Farah D. Lubin

Epigenetic regulation of chromatin structure results in the stable maintenance of gene expression via covalent modifications of the DNA or its associated histone proteins (reviewed in Jiang *et al.* 2008). Within the nucleus the DNA interacts with histone proteins within the nucleosome core. Histones, being positively charged, associate with the negatively charged phosphodiester backbone of DNA to result in a highly compacted nucleosome structure known as chromatin. The unraveling of compacted chromatin is necessary for gene transcription to occur and is subject to environmental influences (Colvis *et al.* 2005; Jiang *et al.* 2008; Levenson and Sweatt 2005; Tsankova *et al.* 2007; Weaver *et al.* 2006).

Chromatin structure regulation or chromatin remodeling is the molecular correlate of the transitioning between densely packed heterochromatin (closed to gene transcription) and loosely packed euchromatin (open to gene transcription). Conversion of heterochromatin to its more open form, euchromatin, involves the unraveling of the chromatin structure and making the DNA accessible to co-activator complexes and the transcriptional machinery. Here we explore the epigenetic manipulating compounds affecting chromatin remodeling and their ability to influence gene transcription. Such compounds offer a novel therapeutic approach for the treatment of altered chromatin structure regulation in CNS disorders.

Brief overview of epigenetic chromatin remodeling mechanisms
Covalent post-translational histone modifications

The histone family of proteins is well classified and consists of histones H1, H2a, H2b, H3, and H4. The H1 class of proteins does not form part of the nucleosomal core but is associated with the spacer DNA connecting the nucleosomal cores. Each nucleosome is composed of 146 base pairs of double-stranded DNA wound around eight histone proteins arranged as homo- or heterodimers (reviewed in Deutsch *et al.* 2008). Histones H3 and H4 form a heterodimer that combines with another heterodimer of histones H3 and H4 to form a tetramer. This tetramer combines with another tetramer composed of two histone H2A and H2B homodimers to form the compact octamer nucleosome core. The histone proteins are rich in basic amino acids such as lysine and arginine. The N-terminal tail of the histone proteins is unstructured, constituted mainly of lysine residues, extends outwardly from the nucleosomal core, and is subject to covalent post-translational modifications (Berger 2007; Jiang *et al.* 2008; Peterson and Laniel 2004).

Epigenetic manipulations of chromatin are achieved by post-translational modifications of the free N-terminal histone tails (Fig. 18.1). To date, five post-translational modifications of N-terminal histone tails have been identified: acetylation, phosphorylation, methylation, sumoylation, and ubiquitinylation (Allis *et al.* 2007; Jenuwein and Allis 2001; Peterson and Laniel 2004). Briefly, histone phosphorylation (H3 ser10) and histone acetylation (H3 lys9, 14, 22, H4 lys5, 8, 12, 16) result in active gene transcription (Strahl and Allis 2000). Histone sumoylation and ubiquitinylation cause repression of gene expression (Berger 2007; Peterson and Laniel 2004) whereas, depending on the residue and number of functional methyl groups added, histone methylation may result in the repression or activation of gene transcription (reviewed in Berger 2007).

The addition of the acetyl group neutralizes the positive charge of the basic histone protein, thus

---

Translational Neuroscience, ed. James E. Barrett, Joseph T. Coyle and Michael Williams. Published by Cambridge University Press. © Cambridge University Press 2012.

Chapter 18: Epigenetic mechanisms in central nervous system disorders

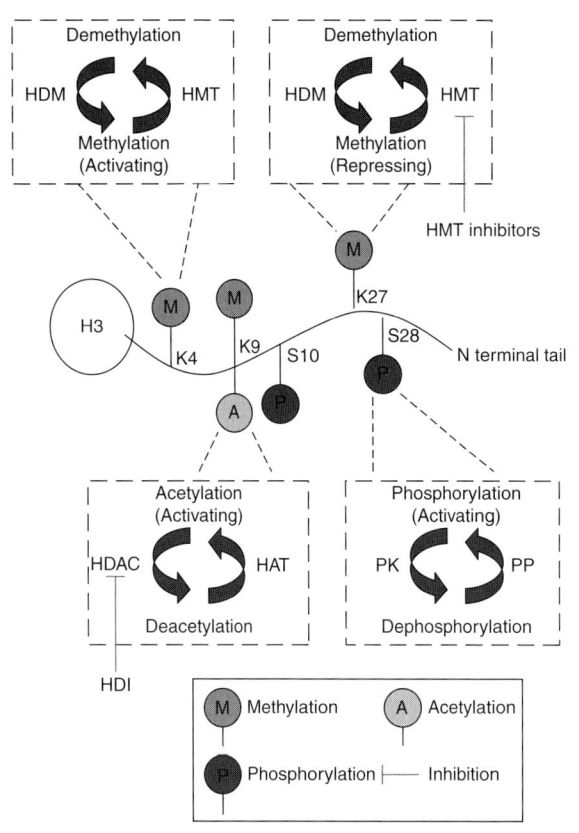

Figure 18.1. Covalent post-translational modifications of histones. Schematic drawing of the covalent histone modifications observed in histone H3, which include acetylation, phosphorylation, and methylation. Lysine methylation is catalyzed by histone methyltransferases (HMT), and the reverse reaction is catalyzed by histone demethylases (HDM). Methylation of lysine residue can result in gene activation or repression. Histone H3 lysine acetylation is catalyzed by histone acetyl transferase (HAT) and deacetylated by histone deacetylases (HDAC). Histone deacetylase inhibitors (HDI) target HDAC resulting in decompaction of chromatin. Serine phosphorylation is catalyzed by protein kinases (PK) and reversed by protein phosphatase (PP). H3, histone-3; K, lysine; S, serine.

relieving chromatin compaction and promoting gene expression (Deutsch et al. 2008). Acetylation and de-acetylation of histone tails have been primarily characterized in the H3 and H4 classes of histone proteins. Specifically, acetylation of histones H3 and H4 has been well characterized in the CNS to mediate memory formation (Alarcon et al. 2004; Barrett and Wood 2008; Bredy et al. 2007; Chwang et al. 2006; Colvis et al. 2005; Fischer et al. 2007; Guan et al. 2002, 2009; Jiang et al. 2008; Kumar et al. 2005; Levenson et al. 2004; Levenson and Sweatt 2005; Lubin et al. 2008; Lubin and Sweatt 2007; Swank and Sweatt 2001; Vecsey et al. 2007; Wood et al. 2006).

The addition of acetyl groups is carried out by a group of enzymes known as histone acetyl transferases (HATs), which transfer the acetyl group of acetyl-coenzyme A to the –NH+ residue of lysine residues (reviewed in Abel and Zukin 2008). A well-known example of a protein with HAT activity is the transcriptional co-activator p300 and cyclic adenosine monophosphate response element binding (CREB) protein-binding protein (CBP), which interacts with the co p300/CBP-associated factor (PCAF). Interestingly, the co-activator p300/CBP/PCAF complex mediates acetylation of the amino terminal ends of all core histone proteins as well as other non-histone targets such as transcription Y-related factors, which results in active transcription (reviewed in Deutsch et al. 2008).

Histone deacetylases (HDACs) catalyze the reversible reaction wherein the removal of the acetyl group causes the cessation of gene expression. The HDAC proteins have been classified into four groups: class I HDAC isoforms (HDAC 1, 2, 3, and 8) are found mainly in the nucleus whereas class II HDAC isoforms (HDAC 4, 5, 6, 7, 9, and 10) shuttle in and out of the nucleus (reviewed in Leipe and Landsman 1997; reviewed in Verdone et al. 2005). Less is understood about the role of class III (sirtuins) and class IV (HDAC 11) HDAC isoforms in the nervous system. Interestingly, other molecular targets exist for HDACs besides histones. Indeed, extensive research using HDAC inhibitors (HDI) has revealed effects on non-histone proteins that are related to acetylation. For example, HDI alter the activity of many transcription factors that are also acetylated by HATs, including ACTR, cMyb, E2F1, EKLF, FEN 1, GATA, HNF-4, HSP90, Ku70, NFκB, PCNA, p53, RB, Runx, SF1 Sp3, STAT, TFIIE, TCF, and YY1 (reviewed in Yang and Seto 2007). This complex interplay makes the exact mechanisms by which HDI alter gene expression unclear and is the focus of ongoing research. Nonetheless, HDI have a long history of use in the treatment of various neurological disorders including psychiatric illnesses, mood disorders, and epilepsy.

Therapeutic applications using HDI require selectivity because acetylation modulates only 2–5% of gene expression, and HDAC isoforms are expressed in a tissue-specific manner. Commonly used HDAC inhibitors include sodium butyrate (SB), sodium phenylbutyrate, trichostatin A, and suberoylanilide hydroxamic acid. These HDI promote enhanced expression of selective genes, arrest cell division, and promote apoptosis of transformed cells (reviewed in Deutsch *et al.* 2008). It is crucial to note that the use of HDI as a potential therapeutic agent will not result in global increases in gene expression but rather in selective gene enhancement in specific cell and tissue types. This selectivity of HDI is being exploited to treat neuropsychiatric disorders that involve altered transcriptional dysregulation. For example, work by the Tsai laboratory shows that systemic injections of SB in their neurodegenerative animal model resulted in dendritic sprouting, an increase in synapse number, reinstated learning behavior, and recovery of long-term memory (Fischer *et al.* 2007). Furthermore, recent work by the same group implicates the HDAC 2 isoform as the principal mediator in enhancement of long-term memory formation with HDI-suberoylanilide hydroxamic acid (Guan *et al.* 2009).

Histone methylation, another well-characterized post-translational modification of histones, was discovered almost 40 years ago (Murray 1964). Unlike histone acetylation and phosphorylation, histone methylation can have different effects on gene transcription based on the amino acid residue of the histone tail being modified within the cell. An additional level of complexity is present, because each lysine residue can add up to three methyl residues, resulting in three states: mono-, di-, and trimethylated. These lysine methylated states can have disparate effects on the transcriptional machinery and are differentially distributed across the chromatin fibers. For example, the trimethylated form of the lysine 4 residue of histone H3 is associated with transcriptional active sites whereas the monomethylated form at the same lysine 4 site is associated with enhancer regions that are at a distance from the transcriptional start sites of the genes (Martin and Zhang 2005; Sims *et al.* 2003). Another noteworthy example of methylation disparity is observed with the monomethylated marks at lysine 9 and 27 of histone H3 and lysine 20 of histone H4 that are associated with active gene transcription whereas the di- and trimethylated forms at these same lysine sites are associated with gene repression (reviewed in Akbarian and Huang 2009).

In general, the addition of the methyl group to the lysine residue preserves its positive charge; this reaction is mediated by a group of enzymes known as histone methyltransferases (HMT). Arginine residues are mono- or dimethylated by the protein arginine methyltransferase (PRMT) (reviews in Akbarian and Huang 2009; Pourreau-Schneider 1975). Families of proteins catalyzing the histone methylation reaction in the brain have been identified, and perturbation of their activity affects normal brain functioning. For example, the H3K9-specific histone methyltransferase, SET domain bifurcated 1 (SETDB1), also known as Erg-associated protein with SET domain (ESET), is present in elevated levels within the striatum of patients with Huntington's disease, resulting in global H3K9 hypertrimethylation and potentially in neuronal dysfunction. The reverse reaction can also occur. For example, histone demethylation is carried out by histone demethylases, which include the lysine-specific demethylase 1 (LSD1) protein. The LSD1 protein demethylates histone H3 lysine 4, resulting in active gene transcription. Novel biguanide and bisguanidine polyamine analogs inhibit LSD1, which was once used as a therapeutic approach to activate gene transcription of silenced genes involved in colorectal cancer. Nonselective monoamine oxidase, a widely used antidepressant, causes LSD1 inhibition (Szyf 2009). Work by Akbarian and colleagues shows decreased trimethylation of histone H3 at lysine 4 of the GAD promoter in the prefrontal cortex of schizophrenic patients. Furthermore, knock-in studies of a truncated form of mixed-lineage leukemia 1 (Mll1), a histone methyltransferase expressed in γ-aminobutyric acid (GABA)-ergic and other cortical neurons, resulted in decreased trimethylation of histone H3 at lysine 4 at GABAergic gene promoters (Akbarian and Huang 2009).

Covalent modifications of DNA

In addition to post-translational modification of histone proteins, DNA can also be epigenetically marked via methylation (Fig. 18.2A). DNA methylation is catalyzed by a group of enzymes called DNA methyltransferases (DNMTs), which transfer the methyl group from the donor S-adenosylmethionine (SAM) to the 5' position of the cytosine pyramidal ring (Fig. 18.2B). In general, cytosines at CpG sites found within a CpG island, defined as a large number of cytosine-guanine dinucleotide sequences linked by phosphodiester bonds, are methylated (see Chen *et al.* 1991; Goldberg *et al.* 2007 for reviews). The methylated CpG dinucleotides are found explicitly in inactive gene promoter

Chapter 18: Epigenetic mechanisms in central nervous system disorders

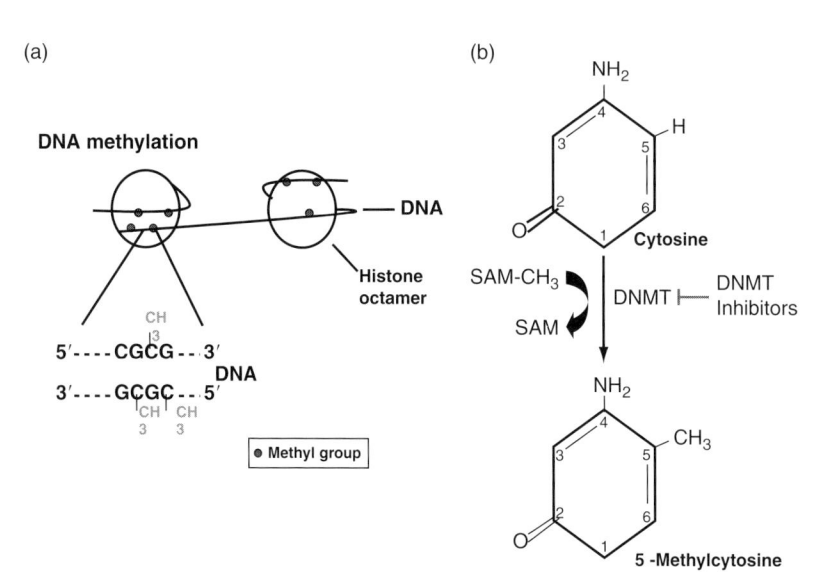

Figure 18.2. Covalent DNA modifications. (A) DNA methylation occurring at cytosine residues of CpG sites renders the DNA inaccessible to transcription. (B) Mechanism of DNA methylation: the enzyme DNA methyltransferase (DNMT) catalyzes the conversion of cytosine to 5-methylcytosine. The methyl group is donated by S-adenosylmethionine (SAM). DNMT inhibitors block DNA methylation.

regions. The CpG dinucleotides are under-represented as would be expected based on probability, yet 70% of them are methylated (Colvis et al. 2005; Jiang et al. 2008; Laird and Jaenisch, 1996; Levenson and Sweatt, 2005).

The methylated CpG residues are docking sites for proteins containing the methyl-binding domain such as methyl CpG binding protein-2 (MeCP2) (reviewed in Deutsch et al. 2008; Szyf 2009). MeCP2 recruits histone-modifying proteins that aid in the formation of the heterochromatin. It is important to note that epigenetic mechanisms are not isolated events; rather they interact and influence each other. Indeed, unmethylated CpG sites at gene promoter regions that are influenced by methyl-binding domain protein activity are dependent on the chromatin microenvironment state, which includes histone modifications. A striking example is the complex interplay between DNA methylation and histone methylation observed with unmethylated histone H3 at lysine 4, which becomes the docking site for DNMTs, resulting in de novo DNA methylation and switching off of gene expression (Szyf 2009). Aberrant DNA methylation levels have been observed at gene promoter sites of patients suffering from schizophrenia and depression (reviewed in Roth et al. 2009). A study of the DNA methylation patterns in neuropsychiatric patients may help shed light on the molecular pathology of these diseases.

Extensive research in the nervous system has supported the idea that epigenetic chromatin structure regulation plays a crucial role in development, cellular differentiation, behavior, and memory formation. It is increasingly apparent that epigenetic mechanisms are responsive to environmental influences and are linked to the cellular machinery. A prototype example is T cells of the mammalian immune system. Numerous epigenetic mechanisms such as histone modifications and DNA methylation modulate gene expression and thus play a role in the commitment of the precursor T cell to its various differentiated states. These processes underlie the formation of persistent immunologic memory cells in response to transient environmental stimuli (Levenson and Sweatt 2005). The epigenetic mechanisms occurring in terminally differentiated neurons are dynamic and transient. Neurodegenerative disorders (Parkinson's and Alzheimer's diseases, epilepsy), neurodevelopmental disorders (fragile X syndrome, autism) and neuropsychiatric disorders (depression, anxiety, substance abuse) all involve cognitive impairment and synaptic disorder, making epigenetic modulators a convincing target for pharmacological intervention. The following sections focus on the molecular mechanisms affecting epigenetic remodeling under physiological and pathological conditions and provide new insights into the possible therapeutic interventions at the level of the epigenome for treatment of neurological and psychiatric disorders.

Neurological disorders

Alzheimer's disease

Alzheimer's disease (AD) is a degenerative brain disorder that results in a progressive decline in one's cognition, memory, and learning. It is estimated that approximately 26 million people worldwide are living with AD, and AD is the most common neurodegenerative disorder. AD is generally characterized by progressive neuronal cell death that affects areas of the brain necessary for cognition and normal brain function. Pathological markers of AD are the accumulation of protein deposits of amyloid-β, resulting in the formation of plaques that build up extracellularly and tangles of a protein called tau that build up intracellularly. Although the effect of plaque and tangle buildup is unclear in the etiology of AD, scientists speculate that they affect gene transcription and neuronal plasticity and can ultimately lead to neuronal cell death. Amyloid-β is produced when amyloid precursor protein (APP) is cleaved abnormally by either β- or γ-secretase. Interestingly, the promoter of the APP gene is rich in CpG dinucleotides, indicating the possibility that APP could be epigenetically regulated and subject to environmental stimuli. It was indeed shown that in the cerebral cortex of the human brain, the APP promoter region between −226 to −101 has 13 potential methylation sites. Methylated cytosines in at least one of these locations were found 26% of the time in people under the age of 70 compared with 8% methylation in individuals over the age of 70 (Tohgi *et al.* 1999). This finding has led to the hypothesis that decreased methylation in the APP promoter with aging may be a risk factor for increased amyloid-β deposits in brain regions.

Amyloid-β buildup can be cleared out of the brain by neprilysin (NEP), an enzyme responsible for amyloid-β degradation. Brains from people with AD and aging people show both a decrease in NEP and global DNA hypomethylation. A recent study reviewed the effects of amyloid-β on global DNA hypomethylation and the DNA methylation state of NEP. Application of amyloid-β in murine cerebral endothelial cell cultures effectively induced global DNA hypomethylation whereas it caused an increase in NEP gene promoter hypermethylation. The increase in methylation in the promoter of the NEP gene was correlated with a decrease in NEP mRNA expression and protein expression (Chen *et al.* 2009). Manipulation of DNA methylation could be a possible approach to treat patients with AD, but much more work is needed to address how certain genes could be targeted while others are left unaffected.

As discussed previously, cognitive deficits are one of the major symptoms of AD. Scientists have investigated innovative ways to alleviate cognitive deficits in AD patients. One such approach has been to look to HDI, the idea being that alterations in post-translational modifications of histone proteins lead to altered gene transcription associated with cognitive disorders in AD. The therapeutic applications of HDI have recently been tested in a well-established mouse model of AD using the HDI sodium 4-phenylbutyrate (4-PBA). Indeed, administration of 4-PBA recovered memory deficits in a mouse model of AD. Furthermore, these transgenic mice had a deficit in histone acetylation that was recovered due to administration of 4-PBA (Ricobaraza *et al.* 2009). Thus, HDI are a promising novel therapeutic approach for potentially reversing memory deficits in patients with AD. Although these studies are promising, additional research is required to rule out possible deleterious effects of HDI on the human brain and body.

Parkinson's disease

Parkinson's disease (PD) is a progressive neurological disease that affects nearly 2% of people over the age of 65. PD is a movement disorder condition that is characterized by tremors, muscle rigidity, bradykinesia, and postural instability. These symptoms are due to a loss of dopaminergic neurons in the substantia nigra, but the underlying etiology of the neuronal cell loss is not well understood. Nevertheless, one clinical sign associated with PD is aggregates of α-synuclein, a normally soluble protein that forms insoluble fibrils called Lewy bodies, which are present in most patients with PD. Much of the current research in PD has focused on α-synuclein and the formation of Lewy bodies in order to shed light on the cause of PD. One reason for this emphasis is that a deficiency in the α-synuclein gene has been shown to be a cause for familial PD. Furthermore, α-synuclein over-expression causes dopaminergic cell loss in animal studies (Lakso *et al.* 2003; Wakamatsu *et al.* 2008).

Recent work indicates that α-synuclein promotes neuronal toxicity (Kontopoulos *et al.* 2006). Interestingly, administration of HDI has been shown to rescue α-synuclein-induced neuronal toxicity. α-synuclein binds directly to histones, reducing acetylated histone H3 levels (Kontopoulos et al. 2006). Further evidence indicates that blocking sirtuin 2 (a specific histone deacetylase) also rescued α-synuclein neuronal toxicity and led to a decrease in dopaminergic cell death (Outeiro et al. 2007). This evidence shows that HDI could have a marquee role in PD treatment, including slowing the progression of the disease. Further studies are warranted to delineate if such treatments might be effective in humans because most of the current work has been performed in cell culture or *Drosophila*.

Epilepsy

Epilepsy is a neurological disorder that affects about 1% of the population and involves recurrent, unprovoked seizures. The molecular processes that underlie epilepsy in patients are still largely unknown; however, treatment through medication for the seizures associated with the disorder has been largely effective at controlling the seizures in most cases. Valproic acid (VPA) has been used to control seizures for decades in epileptic patients. VPA inhibits GABA transaminase, an enzyme that plays a role in the degradation and synthesis of GABA. VPA has now been shown to be a potent inhibitor of class I HDAC isoforms.

The implications of VPA as an HDI in epilepsy have only recently started to be explored. Temporal lobe epilepsy is the most common type of epilepsy in adults. Epileptogenic injuries are believed to induce abnormal sprouting of mossy fibers (granule cell axons) in the dentate gyrus of the hippocampus along with an increase in adult neurogenesis (Bengzon et al. 1997; de Lanerolle et al. 1989; Parent et al. 1997; Reimann et al. 1997). Some data indicate that this process contributes to the development of epilepsy (Buckmaster et al. 2002). VPA blocks neurogenesis and differentiation of hippocampal progenitor cells in vivo along with a correlating increase in histone acetylation (Hsieh et al. 2004). Furthermore, the action of VPA is believed to be responsible for blockade of the aberrant neurogenesis induced by seizure activity, which is believed to be blocked by the action of VPA as an HDI (Jessberger et al. 2007). Cognitive deficits are also experienced among patients with epilepsy. In addition to blocking aberrant neurogenesis, VPA reverses cognitive impairments in a rodent model of epilepsy, presumably due to blocking HDACs (Jessberger et al. 2007).

Seizures induce many changes in gene expression, including changes in glutamate receptor 2 (an AMPA receptor subunit), which shows a seizure-induced downregulation in gene expression. Seizures also alter brain-derived neurotrophic factor (*bdnf*) gene expression, which is upregulated due to seizures. Changes in gene expression at *glutamate receptor-2* and *bdnf* have been shown to correlate with changes in histone acetylation at the promoter regions of the two genes (Huang et al. 2002). A decrease in histone acetylation at the *glutamate receptor-2* promoter was reversed by administration of HDI (Huang et al. 2002). The role of epigenetics in the etiology of epilepsy is just beginning to be understood. As this picture becomes clearer, different HDI will play a role in the treatment and possible prevention of symptoms associated with epilepsy, such as reversal of cognitive deficits in epileptic patients.

Neurodevelopmental and neuropsychiatric disorders

Anxiety disorders

Early life experiences have a strong, lasting effect on stress- and anxiety-mediated behavioral responses in an organism. In rodents, experiments show that maternal care influences an offspring's ability to combat stress and anxiety by altering the development of the endocrine and behavioral responses (Szyf et al. 2007). The maternal effects are mediated through modulation of the glucocorticoid epigenome of the hippocampus. Stress triggers the activation of the hypothalamus-pituitary-adrenal axis (HPA), resulting in the production of glucocorticoid steroid hormone by the adrenals (Lupien et al. 2009). Glucocorticoid receptors (GR) are present throughout the brain. Activated GR receptors can act as transcription factors and regulate gene expression. In rodents, a high degree of maternal care results in enhanced GR expression and a more modest HPA response to stress. Alternatively, decreased maternal care results in lowered GR expression and an elevated HPA response to stress. Blockage of the difference in hippocampal GR levels results in elimination of the effect of maternal care on individual HPA responses to stress. Specifically, the nerve growth factor-inducible protein A (NGFI-A), which is a transcription factor that binds to the brain-specific GR promoter site, is subject to DNA methylation and histone acetylation.

Enhanced maternal care results in DNA demethylation and histone acetylation at the NGFI-A promoter. Thus, strengthening NGFI-A binding culminates in increased hippocampal GR expression.

Interestingly, central infusion of the HDAC blocker trichostatin A abolishes the low maternal care effects on histone acetylation, DNA methylation, GR expression, and HPA responses of the offspring. However, infusion with L-methionine, a precursor of S-adenosylmethionine that serves as the donor for the methyl groups required during DNA methylation, resulted in increased methylation of the NGFI-A GR promoter binding site, decreased GR expression, and enhanced HPA responses to stress (Weaver et al. 2006). Thus, manipulation of epigenetics at a latter age can counter the behavioral alterations established by early life experiences. These experiments epitomize the use of epigenetic tools as therapeutic agents to combat stress- and anxiety-related disorders. Epigenetic remodeling as established by the experiments described previously can prove to be beneficial in treating patients with post-traumatic stress disorder such as war veterans.

Depression

Major depressive disorder is the most common disorder of the brain, with a lifetime risk of 16.2% in the USA (reviewed in Abel and Zukin 2008). The symptoms include depressed mood, anhedonia (reduced ability to experience pleasure from natural rewards), irritability, difficulties in concentrating, and abnormalities in appetite and sleep (neurovegetative symptoms) (Tsankova et al. 2006). Depression mainly occurs idiopathically and may be associated with risk factors such as stressful experiences, cancer, and endocrine abnormalities. The hippocampus is one of the primary brain regions implicated in the pathophysiology of depression. Reduced volumes of hippocampus have been observed in depressed human patients. Antidepressant agents developed so far act by increasing the synaptic levels of neurotrophins such as serotonin and norepinephrine and do so over a span of 2–4 weeks. This delayed response between administration of the drugs and alleviation of symptoms suggests that the neurotransmitters may affect other mechanisms that are responsible for the therapeutic effect (Nelson et al. 1989).

A possible mechanism for the slow stable changes following treatment with antidepressant agents is epigenetic remodeling. For example, increased histone H3 acetylation levels at *bdnf* promoters 4 and 6 (referred to as promoters 3 and 4 in the old *bdnf* nomenclature, respectively) correlate with increased total *bdnf* mRNA transcripts (Tsankova et al. 2004), which is hypothesized to be the therapeutic effect of electroconvulsive shock therapy used to treat depression. Antidepressant treatment has resulted in elevated levels of *bdnf* gene expression, which in turn can modulate neural activity and behavior. Specifically, chronic imipramine treatment induces histone H3 lysine acetylation as well as histone H3 lysine 4 methylation at the *bdnf* promoter site. It has been established that imipramine is acting via HDAC 5 by downregulating the latter. HDAC 5 overexpression results in neutralizing the effects of imipramine (Tsankova et al. 2006). Interestingly, imipramine affects the *bdnf* levels of depressed animals and not the control animals, hence making it suitable for therapeutic treatment. Systemic injection of SB, a nonselective HDI, has antidepressive effects. SB acts to increase *bdnf* expression within the hippocampus. This finding would suggest that HDI might function as an antidepressant or effectively enhance the action of existing antidepressants.

Chronic defeat stress, a behavioral learning paradigm commonly used to study depression, results in dimethylation of H3 lysine-27 at the *bdnf* promoter, culminating in repression of gene transcription (Deutsch et al. 2008). Studies investigating the role of SB as a single drug compared with a combined uptake with the selective serotonin reuptake inhibitor (SSRI) fluoxetine for alleviating depression in mice have been carried out (Deutsch et al. 2008; Schroeder et al. 2007). The behavioral test results show that indeed combining the antidepressant fluoxetine with SB is more efficacious than a single dosage of fluoxetine. Thus, the combination of brain region-selective HDI SB together with a SSRI might eventually be a promising novel antidepressant treatment strategy that warrants further exploration in experimental animal models.

Schizophrenia

Schizophrenia is a chronic, debilitating neuropsychiatric disorder. It affects about 1.1% of the US population, age 18 and above. It is characterized by three categories of symptoms: (1) positive symptoms – hallucinations, delusions, and thought disorder;

(2) negative symptoms – apathy, inappropriate mood, and poverty of speech; and (3) cognitive dysfunction defined by impaired working memory and conceptual disorganization (reviewed in Roth et al. 2009). Antipsychotic drugs used thus far for treatment act only to alleviate the symptoms. Thus, a better understanding of the pathophysiology of schizophrenia is required to generate more efficacious drugs.

Although nongenetic risk factors including winter birth and obstetric birth have been identified as potential causative agents, it is the genetic factors that seem to have a much stronger impact. Studies have been carried out in twins to identify the degree of genetic influence on the etiology of the disease (reviewed in Roth et al. 2009). Previous studies revealed that risk of schizophrenia is substantially higher for monozygotic (53%) compared with dizygotic twins (15%) (reviewed in Roth et al. 2009). In addition, several studies concluded an overall heritability estimate of 68% for the underlying liability of schizophrenia (reviewed in Roth et al. 2009).

Biochemical analyses of postmortem samples from patients with schizophrenia demonstrate a downregulation of the *reelin* and *glutamic acid decarboxylase-1* (*GAD1*) genes specifically in the hippocampus and cortical brain regions. The *reelin* gene encodes an extracellular matrix protein that is important for development and synaptic integrity and is a chief player in long-term potentiation, the molecular correlate of learning. *Reelin* is expressed predominantly in GABAergic neurons. GABAergic neurons also express the *GAD1* gene that encodes GAD67, the enzyme that synthesizes the neurotransmitter GABA from glutamate (Huang et al. 2007). Extensive studies show that hypermethylation at the two gene promoters parallels a decrease in the respective mRNA levels. A genome-wide epigenetic approach reveals 100 loci with altered CpG methylation in patients with schizophrenia, affirming the role of epigenetic dysregulation in the disorder. Altered DNA methylation has been observed at gene promoters pivotal for the normal functioning of the dopaminergic and serotonergic pathways. Use of specific DNMT blockers to return the hypermethylated gene promoters to their normal states may serve as a possible remedy.

Not surprisingly, altered histone modifications are also observed in patients with schizophrenia. An upregulation of the HDAC isoform, HDAC1, is observed in the prefrontal cortex of patients, making HDI a potential avenue for further investigation as a treatment. Huang and colleagues further implicated Mll1 (histone methyltransferase) in the pathophysiology of schizophrenia (Huang et al. 2007). They observed decreased histone H3 lysine 4 trimethylation (active gene transcription mark) and Mll1 occupancy at the *GAD1* promoter. Treatment with clozapine, an antipsychotic drug commonly used in schizophrenia, acts via increase in histone H3 lysine 4 tri-methylation and Mll1 occupancy at the *GAD1* promoter (Huang et al. 2007). However, further research focusing on the possible interplay between histone H3 lysine 4 hypomethylation, enhanced HDAC activity, and hyper DNA methylation at the *GAD1* promoter is yet to be done. Furthermore, although beneficial effects of HDAC and DNMT inhibition have been observed in rodent models for cognitive deficits, their efficiency in humans has not been tested.

Fragile X syndrome

Fragile X syndrome is one of the most recognizable forms of inherited mental retardation. The disease is caused as a result of transcriptional silencing of the fragile X mental retardation 1 (*FMR1*) gene. Amplification of the CGG repeats has been observed in the 5' untranslated region of the gene. Patients with fragile X syndrome exhibit more than 200 CGG repeats together with methylation of most of the cytosine of the CGG repeat (O'Donnell and Warren 2002). Hypermethylation of the promoter region becomes amenable to MECP2 binding. MECP2 in turn recruits HDAC isoforms, which bring about chromatin condensation by removal of acetyl groups, making the DNA inaccessible to the transcriptional machinery (Chiurazzi et al. 1998). Thus, hypermethylation of the DNA culminates in gene silencing and loss of the protein product, the fragile X mental retardation protein. The latter is an RNA binding protein that associates with translating polyribosomes as part of a large messenger ribonucleoprotein and modulates the translation of its RNA ligands. In vitro and in vivo neuronal studies have implicated fragile X mental retardation protein in the formation of synapses, and the loss of the protein affects synaptic plasticity.

CGG hypermethylation has been strongly implicated as the underlying cause of fragile X syndrome in experiments in which 5-azadeoxycytidine, a DNA demethylating drug, has been used to counter the extensive methylation (Chiurazzi et al. 1998). These studies concluded that using 5-azadeoxycytidine results in resumption of FMR1 gene transcription, as shown by restoration of the specific mRNA and protein product. This process is accompanied by extensive demethylation at the promoter region. The studies also infer that hypermethylation is the root cause of gene silencing and not the extensive amplification of CGG. These experiments underscore the importance of epigenetic manipulation for therapeutic intervention in treating cognitive impairment associated with fragile X syndrome. More rigorous studies of the efficiency of treatment with 5-azadeoxycytidine in mouse models of fragile X syndrome are required.

Autism

Autism is a prevalent developmental disorder that is categorized along with Asperger syndrome, Rett syndrome, and childhood disintegrative disorder to form a group called autism spectrum disorders (reviewed in Abel et al. 1997). Autistic patients are characterized by problems with verbal and nonverbal communication, impaired social interaction, and unusual, repetitive, or severely limited activities and interests. Brain tissue recovered from autistic patients exhibits reduced levels of the *reelin* gene transcript (Fatemi et al. 2005). The *reelin* gene has previously been implicated in Asperger syndrome (Fatemi et al. 2005). Children suffering from autism have decreased levels of SAM/SAH (S-adenosylhomocysteine) in their plasma, suggesting the possibility of abnormal methylation profiles (James et al. 2004). Brain tissue analysis reveals a lower expression of *MeCP2*, again implicating impaired DNA methylation (Hendriksen et al. 2001). Additionally, autism has been observed in conjunction with an incidence of prenatal exposure to HDI-VPA (Christianson et al. 1994). Together, these findings demonstrate that chromatin modifications play a role in autism spectrum disorders. Thus, the use of HDI to reverse the reduced levels of important genes associated in autism, such as *reelin* and *MeCP2*, is a plausible therapeutic approach.

Substance abuse

Drug addiction is a psychiatric disorder that involves a continuation of drug use and the subsequent development of drug-seeking behavior despite the consequences. Drug addiction is a curable disorder: former addicts can live normal productive lives; nevertheless, relapse occurs in many cases. Due to the addictive nature of drug use and the propensity of addicts to relapse, scientists have focused on understanding the mechanisms behind drug addiction. Drug use affects the mesolimbic system, which includes alterations in gene transcription in the ventral tegmental area, the nucleus accumbens, the prefrontal cortex, and the basolateral amygdala (Koob and Kreek 2007; Nelson et al. 1989). Furthermore, drug use has also been shown to cause changes in chromatin structure that correlate with the altered gene transcription associated with drug use (Jiang et al. 2008).

Cocaine is a stimulant that increases dopamine levels in brain regions involved in the mesolimbic system (Nelson et al. 1989). Acute cocaine exposure causes activation of immediate early genes *c-fos* and *fosb* in the nucleus accumbens; this process correlates with an increase in histone H4 acetylation in the promoter regions of the genes (Kumar et al. 2005). Chronic cocaine exposure showed no changes in c-fos or fosb hyperacetylation; however, H3 acetylation was observed at the *bdnf* and *Cdk5* promoters (Kumar et al. 2005). Moreover, stable changes in histone acetylation have been observed even 2 weeks after withdrawal from cocaine in the prefrontal cortex, along with changes in gene expression associated with the histone acetylation changes (Jiang et al. 2008). Furthermore, histone phosphorylation and methylation changes have also been observed due to cocaine exposure (Jiang et al. 2008). Interestingly, administration of HDI directly into the nucleus accumbens greatly enhances the rewarding effects of cocaine (Kumar et al. 2005).

Stimulants such as cocaine are not the only drugs that cause changes in histone modification. Ethanol, one of the most commonly abused drugs, is a central nervous system depressant, and epigenetic mechanisms are also altered due to ethanol use. Acute exposure to alcohol caused decreases in HDAC activity while causing hyperacetylation in histones H3 and H4 in the amygdala of a rodent model (Pandey et al. 2008). However, alcohol withdrawal after chronic exposure correlated with an increase in HDAC activity and a decrease in acetylation of histones H3 and H4 while also being associated with anxiety, a common symptom of

Chapter 18: Epigenetic mechanisms in central nervous system disorders

Table 18.1. Candidate epigenetic modifications as potential therapeutic targets associated with central nervous system disorders.

Associated disorder	Epigenetic modification	Associated gene	HDI/ DNA demethylating agents	Reference
Alzheimer's disease	Histone acetylation DNA methylation	NEP↓ APP↑	Sodium 4-phenylbutyrate 5-Azadeoxycytidine?	(Chen et al. 2009; Ricobaraza et al. 2009; Tohgi et al. 1999)
Anxiety	Histone acetylation DNA methylation	GR↓ NGFI-A↑	Trichostatin-A L-methionine	(Lupien et al. 2009; Weaver et al. 2006)
Autism	Histone acetylation	Reelin↓ MeCP2	Valproic acid Trichostatin-A	(Hendriksen et al. 2001)
Depression	Histone acetylation	BDNF↓	Sodium butyrate	(Schroeder et al. 2007; Tsankova et al. 2006)
Epilepsy	Histone acetylation	BDNF↓ GluR2; GRIA2	Valproic acid	(Hsieh et al. 2004; Huang et al. 2002; Jessberger et al. 2007)
Fragile X syndrome	DNA methylation	FMR1↑	5-Azadeoxycytidine	(Chiurazzi et al. 1998; Chiurazzi et al. 1999)
Parkinson's disease	Histone acetylation	α-synuclein↓	Sirtuin 2 Sodium butyrate SAHA	(Kontopoulos et al. 2006; Outeiro et al. 2007)
Schizophrenia	DNA methylation Histone acetylation	Reelin↑ GAD1↓	5-Azadeoxycytidine? Zebularine	(Chen et al. 2002; Huang and Akbarian 2007; Huang et al. 2007; Roth et al. 2009)
Substance abuse	Histone acetylation	c-Fos↓ BDNF Cdk5	Sodium sutyrate	(Kumar et al. 2005; Pandey et al. 2008)

alcohol withdrawal. The anxiety associated with alcohol withdrawal, along with the deficits in acetylation of histones H3 and H4, was alleviated by the administration of HDI (Pandey et al. 2008). The evidence points toward epigenetics playing a role in drug-induced gene transcription and in the underlying behavior associated with drug use. Although additional studies are needed, several potential therapeutic benefits through epigenetic manipulation show promise. As has been demonstrated, HDI may decrease anxiety associated with withdrawal from ethanol use.

Future directions and conclusions

A common theme that emerges from the disorders mentioned above is that they share several phenotypes such as cognitive deficits. This principal feature may share common molecular players encoded by inter-related genes. Indeed, aberrant gene expression is a common feature of most of these disorders, which may arise through several avenues including altered HAT, HDAC, HMT, and DNMT activity. It is conceivable that functional interaction and extensive cross-talk occurs between the various histone modifications and DNA methylation. For example, binding of the transcription factor II D to the histone H3 lysine 4 residue is greatly enhanced if the proximal lysine 9 and 14 residues are acetylated. Treatment with SB-HDI results not only in hyperacetylation but also in an increase in histone H3 lysine 4 methylation at specific gene promoter sites (Akbarian and Huang 2009; Szyf 2009). Thus, as epigenetic mechanisms continue to be linked to cognitive dysfunctions, we need a better understanding of the complex molecular interaction and regulation of these processes.

Alterations in covalent modifications of histones and associated DNA modulate gene expression, to yield altered gene expression patterns, which may ultimately contribute to the phenotypic manifestation of neurological disorders. These modifications impinge directly on the transcriptional machinery and accessory proteins that are recruited to the DNA for gene silencing or gene activation. Using compounds that can inhibit the covalent modifications and that function to restore normal transcriptional equilibrium poses new therapeutic avenues for the treatment of several brain disorders (Table 18.1). For example, neurodevelopmental disorders that commence at an early stage can be treated with these chromatin-altering compounds at a later developmental stage to modulate DNA transcription. Another salient feature of epigenetic modulators is that they exert their effects in a cell-specific and gene-specific manner, rendering the drugs more precise and efficacious in countering the underlying transcriptional dysregulation. Although still in its elementary stages, further investigation of chromatin-modifying drugs as a therapeutic approach for neuropsychiatric, neurodevelopmental, and neurological disorders may produce positive results.

Acknowledgments

This work was supported by the National Institute of Health grant MH82106 and the Evelyn F. McKnight Brain Research Foundation. The authors declare no conflicting financial interests.

References

Abel T, Nguyen PV, Barad M et al. 1997. Genetic demonstration of a role for PKA in the late phase of LTP and in hippocampus-based long-term memory. *Cell* **88**:615–626.

Abel T, Zukin RS. 2008. Epigenetic targets of HDAC inhibition in neurodegenerative and psychiatric disorders. *Curr Opin Pharmacol* **8**:57–64.

Akbarian S, Huang HS. 2009. Epigenetic regulation in human brain-focus on histone lysine methylation. *Biol Psychiatry* **65**:198–203.

Alarcon JM, Malleret G, Touzani K et al. 2004. Chromatin acetylation, memory, and LTP are impaired in CBP+/-mice: a model for the cognitive deficit in Rubinstein–Taybi syndrome and its amelioration. *Neuron* **42**:947–959.

Allis CD, Berger SL, Cote J et al. 2007. New nomenclature for chromatin-modifying enzymes. *Cell* **131**:633–636.

Barrett RM, Wood MA. 2008. Beyond transcription factors: the role of chromatin modifying enzymes in regulating transcription required for memory. *Learn Mem* **15**:460–467.

Bengzon J, Kokaia Z, Elmer E et al. 1997. Apoptosis and proliferation of dentate gyrus neurons after single and intermittent limbic seizures. *Proc Natl Acad Sci USA* **94**:10432–10437.

Berger SL. 2007. The complex language of chromatin regulation during transcription. *Nature* **447**:407–412.

Bredy TW, Wu H, Crego C et al. 2007. Histone modifications around individual BDNF gene promoters in prefrontal cortex are associated with extinction of conditioned fear. *Learn Mem* **14**:268–276.

Buckmaster PS, Zhang GF, Yamawaki R. 2002. Axon sprouting in a model of temporal lobe epilepsy creates a predominantly excitatory feedback circuit. *J Neurosci* **22**:6650–6658.

Chen KL, Wang SS, Yang YY et al. 2009. The epigenetic effects of amyloid-beta (1–40) on global DNA and neprilysin genes in murine cerebral endothelial cells. *Biochem Biophys Res Commun* **378**:57–61.

Chen L, MacMillan AM, Chang W et al. 1991. Direct identification of the active-site nucleophile in a DNA (cytosine-5)-methyltransferase. *Biochemistry* **30**:11018–11025.

Chen Y, Sharma RP, Costa RH, Costa E, Grayson DR. 2002. On the epigenetic regulation of the human reelin promoter. *Nucleic Acids Res* **30**:2930–2939.

Chiurazzi P, Pomponi MG, Pietrobono R et al. 1999. Synergistic effect of histone hyperacetylation and DNA demethylation in the reactivation of the FMR1 gene. *Hum Mol Genet* **8**:2317–2323.

Chiurazzi P, Pomponi MG, Willemsen R, Oostra BA, Neri G. 1998. In vitro reactivation of the FMR1 gene involved in fragile X syndrome. *Hum Mol Genet* **7**:109–113.

Christianson AL, Chesler N, Kromberg JG. 1994. Fetal valproate syndrome: clinical and neuro-developmental features in two sibling pairs. *Dev Med Child Neurol* **36**:361–369.

Chwang WB, O'Riordan KJ, Levenson JM, Sweatt JD. 2006. ERK/MAPK regulates hippocampal histone phosphorylation following contextual fear conditioning. *Learn Mem* **13**:322–328.

Colvis CM, Pollock JD, Goodman RH et al. 2005. Epigenetic mechanisms and gene networks in the nervous system. *J Neurosci* **25**:10379–10389.

de Lanerolle NC, Kim JH, Robbins RJ, Spencer DD. 1989. Hippocampal interneuron loss and plasticity in human temporal lobe epilepsy. *Brain Res* **495**:387–395.

Deutsch SI, Rosse RB, Mastropaolo J, Long KD, Gaskins BL. 2008. Epigenetic therapeutic strategies for the treatment of neuropsychiatric disorders: ready for prime time? *Clin Neuropharmacol* **31**:104–119.

Fatemi SH, Snow AV, Stary JM et al. 2005. Reelin signaling is impaired in autism. *Biol Psychiatry* **57**:777–787.

Fischer A, Sananbenesi F, Wang X, Dobbin M, Tsai LH. 2007. Recovery of learning and memory is associated with chromatin remodelling. *Nature* **447**:178–182.

Goldberg AD, Allis CD, Bernstein E. 2007. Epigenetics: a landscape takes shape. *Cell* **128**:635–638.

Guan JS, Haggarty SJ, Giacometti E et al. 2009. HDAC2 negatively regulates memory formation and synaptic plasticity. *Nature* **459**:55–60.

Guan Z, Giustetto M, Lomvardas S et al. 2002. Integration of long-term-memory-related synaptic plasticity involves bidirectional regulation of gene expression and chromatin structure. *Cell* **111**:483–493.

Hendriksen H, Datson NA, Ghijsen WE et al. 2001. Altered hippocampal gene expression prior to the onset of spontaneous seizures in the rat post-status epilepticus model. *Eur J Neurosci* **14**:1475–1484.

Hsieh J, Nakashima K, Kuwabara T, Mejia E, Gage FH. 2004. Histone deacetylase inhibition-mediated neuronal differentiation of multipotent adult neural progenitor cells. *Proc Natl Acad Sci USA* **101**:16659–16664.

Huang HS, Akbarian S. 2007. GAD1 mRNA expression and DNA methylation in prefrontal cortex of subjects with schizophrenia. *PLoS One* **2**: e809.

Huang HS, Matevossian A, Whittle C et al. 2007. Prefrontal dysfunction in schizophrenia involves mixed-lineage leukemia 1-regulated histone methylation at GABAergic gene promoters. *J Neurosci* **27**:11254–11262.

Huang Y, Doherty JJ, Dingledine R. 2002. Altered histone acetylation at glutamate receptor 2 and brain-derived neurotrophic factor genes is an early event triggered by status epilepticus. *J Neurosci* **22**:8422–8428.

James SJ, Cutler P, Melnyk S et al. 2004. Metabolic biomarkers of increased oxidative stress and impaired methylation capacity in children with autism. *Am J Clin Nutr* **80**:1611–1617.

Jenuwein T, Allis CD. 2001. Translating the histone code. *Science* **293**:1074–1080.

Jessberger S, Nakashima K, Clemenson GD Jr et al. 2007. Epigenetic modulation of seizure-induced neurogenesis and cognitive decline. *J Neurosci* **27**:5967–5975.

Jiang Y, Langley B, Lubin FD, Renthal W et al. 2008. Epigenetics in the nervous system. *J Neurosci* **28**:11753–11759.

Kontopoulos E, Parvin JD, Feany MB. 2006. Alpha-synuclein acts in the nucleus to inhibit histone acetylation and promote neurotoxicity. *Hum Mol Genet* **15**:3012–3023.

Koob G, Kreek MJ. 2007. Stress, dysregulation of drug reward pathways, and the transition to drug dependence. *Am J Psychiatry* **164**:1149–1159.

Kumar A, Choi KH, Renthal W et al. 2005. Chromatin remodeling is a key mechanism underlying cocaine-induced plasticity in striatum. *Neuron* **48**:303–314.

Laird PW, Jaenisch R. 1996. The role of DNA methylation in cancer genetics and epigenetics. *Annu Rev Genet* **30**:441–464.

Lakso M, Vartiainen S, Moilanen AM et al. 2003. Dopaminergic neuronal loss and motor deficits in *Caenorhabditis elegans* overexpressing human alpha-synuclein. *J Neurochem* **86**:165–172.

Leipe DD, Landsman D. 1997. Histone deacetylases, acetoin utilization proteins and acetylpolyamine amidohydrolases are members of an ancient protein superfamily. *Nucleic Acids Res* **25**:3693–3697.

Levenson JM, Riordan KJ, Brown KD. et al. 2004. Regulation of histone acetylation during memory formation in the hippocampus. *J Biol Chem* **279**:40545–40559.

Levenson JM, Sweatt JD. 2005. Epigenetic mechanisms in memory formation. *Nat Rev Neurosci* **6**:108–118.

Lubin FD, Roth TL, Sweatt JD. 2008. Epigenetic regulation of BDNF gene transcription in the consolidation of fear memory. *J Neurosci* **28**:10576–10586.

Lubin FD, Sweatt JD. 2007. The IkappaB kinase regulates chromatin structure during reconsolidation of conditioned fear memories. *Neuron* **55**:942–957.

Lupien SJ, McEwen BS, Gunnar MR, Heim C. 2009. Effects of stress throughout the lifespan on the brain, behaviour and cognition. *Nat Rev Neurosci* **10**:434–445.

Martin C, Zhang Y. 2005. The diverse functions of histone lysine methylation. *Nat Rev Mol Cell Biol* **6**:838–849.

Murray K. 1964. The occurrence of epsilon-N-methyl lysine in histones. *Biochemistry* **3**:10–15.

Nelson RB, Linden DJ, Hyman C, Pfenninger KH, Routtenberg A. 1989. The two major phosphoproteins in growth cones are probably identical to two protein kinase C substrates correlated with persistence of long-term potentiation. *J Neurosci* **9**:381–389.

O'Donnell WT, Warren ST. 2002. A decade of molecular studies of fragile X syndrome. *Annu Rev Neurosci* **25**:315–338.

Outeiro TF, Kontopoulos E, Altmann SM et al. 2007. Sirtuin 2 inhibitors rescue alpha-synuclein-mediated toxicity in models of Parkinson's disease. *Science* **317**:516–519.

Pandey SC, Ugale R, Zhang H, Tang L, Prakash A. 2008. Brain chromatin remodeling: a novel mechanism of alcoholism. *J Neurosci* **28**:3729–3737.

Parent JM, Yu TW, Leibowitz RT et al. 1997. Dentate granule cell neurogenesis is increased by seizures and contributes to aberrant network reorganization in the adult rat hippocampus. *J Neurosci* **17**:3727–3738.

Peterson CL, Laniel MA. 2004. Histones and histone modifications. *Curr Biol* **14**:R546–551.

Pourreau-Schneider N. 1975. In vitro growth promotion of rat leukemia L5222 cells in the presence of 2-mercaptoethanol. *J Natl Cancer Inst* **55**:1467–1470.

Reimann T, Hempel U, Krautwald S et al. 1997. Transforming growth factor-beta1 induces activation of Ras, Raf-1, MEK and MAPK in rat hepatic stellate cells. *FEBS Lett* **403**:57–60.

Ricobaraza A, Cuadrado-Tejedor M, Perez-Mediavilla A et al. 2009. Phenylbutyrate ameliorates cognitive deficit and reduces tau pathology in an Alzheimer's disease mouse model. *Neuropsychopharmacology* **34**:1721–1732.

Roth TL, Lubin FD, Sodhi M, Kleinman JE. 2009. Epigenetic mechanisms in schizophrenia. *Biochim Biophys Acta* **1790**:869–877.

Schroeder FA, Lin CL, Crusio WE, Akbarian S. 2007. Antidepressant-like effects of the histone deacetylase inhibitor, sodium butyrate, in the mouse. *Biol Psychiatry* **62**:55–64.

Sims RJIII, Nishioka K, Reinberg D. 2003. Histone lysine methylation: a signature for chromatin function. *Trends Genet* **19**:629–639.

Strahl BD, Allis CD. 2000. The language of covalent histone modifications. *Nature* **403**:41–45.

Swank MW, Sweatt JD. 2001. Increased histone acetyltransferase and lysine acetyltransferase activity and biphasic activation of the ERK/RSK cascade in insular cortex during novel taste learning. *J Neurosci* **21**:3383–3391.

Szyf M. 2009. Epigenetics, DNA methylation, and chromatin modifying drugs. *Annu Rev Pharmacol Toxicol* **49**:243–263.

Szyf M, Weaver I, Meaney M. 2007. Maternal care, the epigenome and phenotypic differences in behavior. *Reprod Toxicol* **24**:9–19.

Tohgi H, Utsugisawa K, Nagane Y et al. 1999. Reduction with age in methylcytosine in the promoter region-224 approximately-101 of the amyloid precursor protein gene in autopsy human cortex. *Brain Res Mol Brain Res* **70**:288–292.

Tsankova N, Renthal W, Kumar A, Nestler EJ. 2007. Epigenetic regulation in psychiatric disorders. *Nat Rev Neurosci* **8**:355–367.

Tsankova NM, Berton O, Renthal W et al. 2006. Sustained hippocampal chromatin regulation in a mouse model of depression and antidepressant action. *Nat Neurosci* **9**:519–525.

Tsankova NM, Kumar A, Nestler EJ. 2004. Histone modifications at gene promoter regions in rat hippocampus after acute and chronic electroconvulsive seizures. *J Neurosci* **24**:5603–5610.

Vecsey CG, Hawk JD, Lattal KM et al. 2007. Histone deacetylase inhibitors enhance memory and synaptic plasticity via CREB: CBP-dependent transcriptional activation. *J Neurosci* **27**:6128–6140.

Verdone L, Caserta M, Di Mauro E. 2005. Role of histone acetylation in the control of gene expression. *Biochem Cell Biol* **83**:344–353.

Wakamatsu M, Ishii A, Iwata S et al. 2008. Selective loss of nigral dopamine neurons induced by overexpression of truncated human alpha-synuclein in mice. *Neurobiol Aging* **29**:574–585.

Weaver IC, Meaney MJ, Szyf M. 2006. Maternal care effects on the hippocampal transcriptome and anxiety-mediated behaviors in the offspring that are reversible in adulthood. *Proc Natl Acad Sci USA* **103**:3480–3485.

Wood MA, Attner MA, Oliveira AM, Brindle PK, Abel T. 2006. A transcription factor-binding domain of the coactivator CBP is essential for long-term memory and the expression of specific target genes. *Learn Mem* **13**:609–617.

Yang XJ, Seto E. 2007. HATs and HDACs: from structure, function and regulation to novel strategies for therapy and prevention. *Oncogene* **26**:5310–5318.

Chapter 19

Section summary and perspectives: Neurodevelopmental disorders and regulation of epigenetic changes

James E. Barrett and Joseph T. Coyle

The broad scope of the discipline of neuroscience is emphasized in the final section of this book, which focuses on neurodevelopmental disorders and epigenetic regulation. Autism spectrum disorders (ASD), fragile X syndrome (FXS), and attention deficit hyperactivity disorder (ADHD) are among the topics covered in the preceding chapters. These topics are integrated into and expanded upon in the final chapter of this section on epigenetics, which addresses these conditions and many of the other neurological and psychiatric disorders covered in previous sections of this book. As such, this summary and perspective is a review of these important, active areas of neurodevelopmental research and a forecast, as much as possible, of the direction further research is likely to take. Many of these directions have only recently emerged but offer the potential for accelerating further progress in these areas. Although there have been major advances in the treatment of ADHD, as reviewed in Chapter 15 by Stigler et al., Berridge et al. note in Chapter 17 that we are at the beginning stages of developing effective therapeutics for ASD and FXS and for other neurodevelopmental disorders not specifically addressed in these sections (e.g., Rett syndrome and Down syndrome).

In some respects, the neurodevelopmental disorders present many of the same challenges as the neurological and psychiatric disorders discussed in previous sections of this volume. For example, as is true with neurodegenerative disorders such as Alzheimer's disease and Parkinson's disease, ASD, Rett syndrome, and other neurodevelopmental disorders are progressive; early diagnosis and treatment are likely critical for effective intervention. Where are the appropriate windows for intervention? Is it the case that the requirements for effective treatment differ at various developmental stages? Is it possible to block the onset or progression of these disorders by early intervention with appropriate therapeutics? Where are the appropriate windows for timely intervention? As is the case with both neurological and psychiatric disorders, there are multiple distinct symptomatic components to neurodevelopmental disorders. For example, Roberts et al. (2011) point out that ASD is characterized by impairments in social reciprocity and language and communication and by stereotypic and repetitive behaviors. It would seem unlikely that a drug directed toward a single target symptom would be able to address these vastly different symptom domains, again speaking to the possible need to develop combination or multitarget drugs to treat effectively the totality of ASD symptoms. An additional challenge is that not all of these symptoms are uniformly present (or absent) in all individuals who have ASD and, once appropriate therapeutics are identified for each of the symptoms associated with this disorder, it may be necessary to adjust dosages to target only those symptoms that are most problematic. Despite the wide variety of medications that have been evaluated in the attempts to treat ASD and FXS, which have included antidepressants, antipsychotics, anticonvulsants, and psychomotor stimulants, none has proved effective in either disorder; several, namely the antipsychotic medications that have been used to treat self-injury, aggression, and behavioral disturbances in ASD, cause serious side effects, such as akathesia and weight gain (Dölen et al. 2010; Rossignol 2009).

Despite these difficulties and complexities, there has recently been progress in our understanding of the pathogenesis of FXS, yielding clear possibilities for potential treatments for this disorder as well as for ASD, which shares symptomatic features with FXS. In many respects, FXS is regarded as a potential

---

Translational Neuroscience, ed. James E. Barrett, Joseph T. Coyle and Michael Williams. Published by Cambridge University Press. © Cambridge University Press 2012.

"molecular doorway" to a better understanding of and treatment approaches to other neurodevelopmental disorders (Berry-Kravis et al. 2011). A major difference between research on several of the neurodevelopmental disorders, particularly FXS, and that on the adult-onset neuropsychiatric disorders is the fact that the neurodevelopmental disorders have clear genetic etiologies. Elucidating the genetic causes has permitted the development of genetic animal models with face validity. These gene-based models have been extensively characterized, ultimately leading to the clinic with mechanistically based compounds that followed the extensive preclinical research. Because FXS is a Mendelian single-gene disorder, it has been somewhat easier to probe the molecular pathophysiology associated with this disease and to generate genetic animal models that have been characterized both molecularly and behaviorally. Indeed, the joint approaches of genetics and molecular biology have converged with parallel developments in neurobiology and pharmacology to generate a testable hypothesis of the role of the metabotropic glutamate 5 (mGluR5) antagonist in treating individuals with FXS, resulting in several clinical trials that are now under way (Krueger and Bear 2011).

Understanding the molecular mechanisms causing a disorder and then proceeding from basic research to clinical evaluation is in many respects *the* model for translational neuroscience. We can expect that there will also be "reverse translation" as the clinical findings from ongoing trials then feed back to basic research and to the model systems and targets currently being employed. The translational approach taken with FSX also provides a perspective on the time required to arrive at a stage ripe for therapeutic intervention based on rational hypotheses and experimental evidence. As indicated in Chapters 15 and 16 and as documented in Krueger and Bear (2011), FXS, originally known as the Martin–Bell syndrome, was first described in 1943 as an X-linked form of inherited mental retardation. It took another 26 years before the constriction on the X-chromosome that was diagnostic for this condition was identified. This discovery led to the identification of the gene in 1991, followed by the description of the protein in 1993, and, in 1994, by the generation of a knockout mouse. This mouse model has been extensively characterized during the intervening years, connecting the dendritic pathology to the mechanism of action of the fragile X mental retardation protein,

FMRP (Dölen et al. 2010). Thus, this timeline, starting in 1943 with the description of the disorder and culminating in the initiation of clinical trials with a proof of concept compound, spans nearly 60 years. During the intervening 60-year period, progress in molecular biology, genetics, neurobiology, and pharmacology resulted in enabling steps in generating insight into the disorder, into the potential role of mGluRs in neurobiology and behavior, and into the integration of the information from these diverse disciplines to permit clinical assessment. Translating basic research into clinical benefit is a lengthy process that requires tremendous synthetic efforts and interdisciplinary research. One would hope that, given the present state of knowledge in molecular biology and neuroscience, the timeline from disorder identification to testable therapeutics might now be greatly abbreviated.

As is the case with several of the disorders covered in this book, there are a number of challenges in pursuing clinical trials and in the development of clinical trial designs of compounds for treating FXS, ASD, and other neurodevelopmental disorders. Many of these are summarized by Berry-Kravis et al. (2011) and include (i) how best to assess side effects in cognitively impaired individuals who may not be able to accurately report symptoms; (ii) how to determine the most appropriate age at which to initiate treatment; e.g., clinical trials with adults pose fewer issues but it may be best to assess the efficacy of a compound earlier in the developmental cycle; (iii) the problem surrounding the lack of validated and sensitive outcome measures for behavior, especially cognition; and (iv) the lack of any validated biomarkers that are known to correlate with functional improvement. These issues of the appropriate developmental window for therapeutic intervention, the discovery of validated biomarkers, and the question of whether advances in the pharmacotherapy of FXS may inform possible treatment avenues for other neurodevelopmental disorders may have to await validation of clinical efficacy against one or more components of these disorders.

Despite the concerns about the reversibility of the symptoms of neurodevelopmental disorders, recent findings offer the hope that the window of intervention may be open wider than we think. For example, male mice with the Rett's gene knocked out die at about 60 days of age with severe respiratory and motoric symptoms. Cobb et al. (2010) engineered a mouse in which MeCP2 was knocked out but which possessed another copy of the MeCP2 gene that could be conditionally expressed. When the male mice that were within days of death were treated so that MeCP2 was again expressed, the phenotype was rapidly reversed and the mice survived. Down syndrome is the consequence of the disordered expression of the genes on an entire chromosome, HAS 21, although a small subset of these genes plays a dominant role in the phenotype. Das and Reeves (2011) exploited a mouse in which this subset of critical genes is triplicated, resulting in many of the phenotypic features of Down syndrome including cognitive impairments. Behavioral and electrophysiological studies linked the cognitive impairments in the adult Down syndrome mouse to GABAergic dysfunction in the hippocampus. A GABA receptor modulator that has successfully reversed these cognitive symptoms is now entering a clinical trial. Thus, we have two recent encouraging examples whereby adult intervention may have remarkable therapeutic effects in severe neurodevelopmental disorders. The fact that there appear to be clear points of pharmacological intervention based on a heightened understanding of the molecular and pathophysiological aspects of these disorders, coupled with the identification of pharmacological agents that address these deficits in model systems, is a significant step toward the successful treatment of these disabilities.

Epigenetics

The developmental biologist Conrad Waddington coined the term epigenetics in 1940 to describe "the interaction of genes with their environment, which bring the phenotype into being" (Waddington 1940). This definition was extended somewhat later by Waddington with the following statement: "It is possible that an adaptive response can be fixed without waiting for the occurrence of a mutation" (Waddington 1942). As Gräff et al. (2011) pointed out, these two statements framed two key aspects of epigenetic processes, namely their plasticity and their potential heritability, which, as a consequence, carries the implication that there may well be long-term stability associated with the epigenetic changes. Since the original formulation of the term, epigenetics has had many definitions and meanings but generally, the term refers to heritable traits in cells and organisms that do not involve changes in the underlying DNA sequence (Russo et al. 1996). According to Gräff et al. (2011), "epigenetic mechanisms provide an organism with the molecular means to promptly react to environmental contingencies with stable alterations in gene expression." Alterations in DNA methylation and modifications in chromatin, as examples of epigenetic regulation, can persist throughout an organism's life and even for multiple generations, despite the lack of change in the underlying DNA sequence (Csoka and Szyf 2009). The conditions for inducing such alterations and the precise mechanisms contributing to those alterations, along with an exploration of the potential means of intervention, represent one of the most vigorous areas of research in contemporary molecular biology and have captured the attention of many investigators in the area of neuroscience.

Epigenetics and neurodevelopmental disorders

There is increasing recognition that many CNS disorders, including those involving neurodevelopment, may represent disorders of epigenetic regulation (Mehler 2008). With epigenetic regulation appearing to be so fundamental in CNS development, it is not surprising that dysregulation of epigenetic mechanisms can play an important role in contributing to these disorders. Chapter 18 by Gupta et al. covers a wide range of psychiatric, neurological, and neurodevelopmental disorders, which share common phenotypes including, among others, cognitive deficits. Indeed, one of the first demonstrations that a common form of epigenetic modification, histone acetylation, could be modified in the CNS was shown to occur during memory formation (Levenson et al. 2004). As this rapidly expanding field develops and as new avenues yield insight into mechanisms underlying dysfunction in epigenetic mechanisms, new treatment opportunities for these disorders will become available. Already, early preclinical studies have suggested a role for histone deacetylase inhibitors in reversing some of the symptoms in a mouse model of Rett syndrome (Guy et al. 2007), and additional histone deacetylase inhibitors are being evaluated in clinical trials for other neurological disorders (Sananbenesi and Fischer 2009). Although this area of research is still evolving and many questions remain, there is considerable enthusiasm about potential applications and about the ability to utilize these mechanisms in the development of new therapeutic approaches and as biomarkers. Indeed, Csoka and Szyf (2009) have suggested that many commonly used drugs can produce epigenetic changes that can be manifested in adverse events. Thus, they have proposed the creation of the field of "pharmacoepigenomics," which could ultimately have more impact than that of pharmacogenetics.

Micro RNAs and neurodevelopmental regulation

Recently, a new level of epigenetic regulation by small noncoding RNAs, termed microRNAs (miRNAs), has been discovered that regulates gene expression at different levels. MiRNAs are a class of small noncoding RNAs 18 to 25 nucleotides long that are generated through a series of cleavage steps from long precursor RNA transcripts. The binding of miRNAs to mRNAs silences chromatin, degrades mRNA, and blocks translation. Evidence is mounting that miRNAs play an important role in a variety of human diseases, including CNS disorders in which modifications of DNA methylation and of chromatin appear to be important targets for the development of novel therapeutics (Szyf 2009). At the present time, miRNAs have been found to play an important role in synapse development (Schratt 2009), with implications for a significant role for miRNAs in a number of neurodegenerative and neurodevelopmental disorders (Eacker *et al.* 2009). miRNAs can be regulated by neuronal activity, suggesting that they respond to experience-related events, and can remodel neuronal circuits with enduring effects on behavior. The ability of miRNAs to fine-tune the activity of biological pathways may underlie some of the difficulties associated with linking psychiatric disorders to specific causative genes and may contribute to the heterogeneity of CNS disorders. As Xu *et al.* (2010) have pointed out, it appears that miRNAs are key components not only of the genetic architecture of complex CNS disorders but are also integral parts of the biological pathways that mediate the effects of the primary genetic deficits. It is early in our assessment of the involvement of miRNAs in CNS disorders but there is optimism that more detailed knowledge of the dysregulation of miRNAs in CNS disorders may provide a better understanding of the molecular mechanisms in these disorders and may also provide avenues for progress in biomarker development and in the introduction of new therapeutics.

Conclusions

The further study of epigenetic mechanisms in CNS disorders, including the rapidly emerging role of miRNAs, is an exciting and relatively new endeavor for neuroscience. The field of epigenetics may be an important approach to breaking the bottleneck in the understanding and treatment of neuropsychiatric disorders, providing new insight into the means by which adaptation to the environment results in enduring changes in behavior and stable changes in gene expression. Unlike the DNA sequence, epigenetic changes are reversible, providing opportunities to affect those changes that occur though dysregulation and opening up new opportunities for the treatment of CNS disorders. Understanding how the patterns of DNA methylation change during neuronal differentiation and maturation, how both genetic and environmental factors may result in alterations to these epigenetic pathways during development and into adulthood, and how the resulting insights then generate alternative approaches to therapeutic treatments are all critical aspects of the excitement surrounding this area of research. These studies are expected to be of critical importance for the eventual treatment and prevention of autism and other complex genetic disorders. In addition, as progress in these areas unfolds, it is increasingly likely that there will be heightened attention to the development of epigenomics with the capability of identifying epigenetic biomarkers that may be of greater utility and importance than biomarkers based on genomics. As such, the widespread importance of epigenetic modification to the neurosciences may herald a new era both in our understanding of the pathophysiology of these disorders and in the ability to develop new therapeutics to treat them.

References

Berry-Kravis E, Knox A, Hervey C. 2011. Targeted treatments for fragile X syndrome. *J Neurodevelop Disord* **3**:193–210.

Cobb S, Guy J, Bird A. 2010. Reversibility of functional deficits in experimental models of Rett syndrome. *Biochem Soc Trans* **38**:498–506.

Csoka AB, Szyf M. 2009. Epigenetic side-effects of common pharmaceuticals: a potential new field in medicine and pharmacology. *Med Hypotheses* **73**:770–780.

Das I, Reeves RH. The use of mouse models to understand and improve cognitive deficits in Down syndrome. *Dis Model Mech* 2011 4:596–606.

Dölen G, Carpenter RL, Ocain TD, Bear MF. 2010. Mechanism-based approaches to treating fragile X. *Pharmacol Ther* 127:78–93.

Eacker SM, Dawson TM, Dawson VL. 2009. Understanding microRNAs in neurodegeneration. *Nat Rev Neurosci* 10:837–841.

Gräff J, Kim D, Dobbin, MM, Tsai L-H. 2011. Epigenetic regulation of gene expression in physiological and brain processes. *Physiol Rev* 91:603–649.

Guy J, Gan J, Selfridge J, Cobb S, Bird A. 2007. Reversal of neurological defects in a mouse model of Rett syndrome. *Science* 315:1143–1147.

Krueger DD, Bear MF. 2011. Toward fulfilling the promise of molecular medicine in fragile X syndrome. *Annu Rev Med* 62:411–429.

Levenson JM, O'Riordan KJ, Brown KD *et al.* 2004. Regulation of histone acetylation during memory formation in the hippocampus. *J Biol Chem* 279:40545–40559.

Mehler MF. 2008. Epigenetic principles and mechanisms underlying nervous system functions in health and disease. *Prog Neurobiol* 86:305–341.

Rossignol DA. 2009. Novel and emerging treatments for autism spectrum disorders: a systematic review. *Ann Clin Psychiat* 21:213–236.

Russo VEA, Martienssen RA, Riggs AD, eds. 1996. *Epigenetic Mechanisms of Gene Regulation*. Plainview, NY: Cold Spring Harbor Laboratory Press.

Sananbenesi F, Fischer A. 2009. The epigenetic bottleneck of neurodegenerative and psychiatric diseases. *Biol Chem* 390:1145–1153.

Schratt G. 2009. microRNAs at the synapse. *Nat Rev Neurosci* 10:842–849.

Szyf M. 2009. Epigenetics, DNA methylation, and chromatin modifying drugs. *Annu Rev Pharmacol Toxicol* 49:243–263.

Waddington CH. 1940. *Organizers and Genes*. Cambridge: Cambridge University Press.

Waddington CH. 1942. Canalization of development and the inheritance of acquired characters. *Nature* 150:563–565.

Xu B, Karayiorgou M, Gogos JA. 2010. MicroRNAs in psychiatric and neurodevelopmental disorders. *Brain Res* 1338:78–88.

Chapter 20

Promises and challenges of translational research in neuropsychiatry

David L. Braff

This book is well organized into three sections: psychiatric disorders, neurological disorders, and neurodevelopmental disorders. Each chapter itself represents a domain (e.g., neuropharmacology) or disorder (mood, schizophrenia, autism) that could be, and has been, the subject of *many* books. These scholarly chapters are well balanced and reflect one of the first comprehensive views of neuropsychiatric translational research, with its amazing array of mammalian biological tools that are advancing our understanding of, and possible "bench-to-bedside" (T1) treatment innovations of, a wide array of neuropsychiatric disorders. It is extremely timely from both scientific and broad social perspectives and reflects a scholarly balance of innovative ideas and appropriately cautious optimism for the future.

So what binds these chapters together? The answer is the amazing explosion of knowledge about the complexity of the human brain, with its intricate mammalian biological processes. These processes range from gene expression to brain circuit function and to "mistakes" of Mother Nature (e.g., mutations) that result in neuropsychiatric disorders and can be understood and even potentially ameliorated as we expand our neuroscience "tool kit" of methods to understand and even alter the mammalian neurobiological functions that underlie neuropsychiatric disorders. In general, translational neuroscience uses techniques grounded in genomics, animal models, and cognitive science to advance our understanding and treatment of these disorders.

The dysfunctions and disorders described in this book range from simple, punctate Mendelizing errors in the genome's instruction manual for the human brain to complex circuit-based disorders (Insel *et al.* 2010). These disorders sometimes occur very early in life (at conception) but may be expressed early (fragile X syndrome, autism) or later (Huntington's disease [HD], Parkinson's disease [PD]) in the life cycle, often after a seemingly normal period of brain function. This volume does *not* generally include the brain disorders resulting from a profound and strong environmental (E) insult such as stroke, cancer, or traumatic brain injury, except for a few disorders such as post-traumatic stress disorder. Rather, the book focuses largely on the profoundly diverse array of brain disorders in motor, cognitive, and mood domains that results from the complex interaction of genetically programmed neural circuit miswiring with environmental events (gene × environment [G×E]) (Zammit *et al.* 2010). The results of these "errors" in brain function are as complex as the organ of interest: They include disorders of motor function and nociception (discussed in Chapters 9, 10, 11, 12, and 13), cognition (Chapters 4, 8, and 17), and mood (Chapters 2 and 3) that profoundly disrupt how humans navigate through our socially and physically complex world.

Thus, some disorders, such as HD (Shoulson and Young 2011), have simple "instruction manual" genomic deficits with their detailed and orderly but sad unfolding of genetically mediated influence on the onset of and progressive motor, cognitive, and mood decline of those who lose the Mendelian lottery. Other disorders are more episodic, less well understood, and highly polygenic and complex, such as bipolar affective disorder (see Chapter 3 by Quiroz *et al.*), in which, despite some relatively good interepisode functioning, there is evidence that each manic episode may leave an indelible footprint of progressive neurological dysfunction (Post 2007). Still, many patients with bipolar affective disorder are amazingly *resilient* compared with "equally" psychotic patients with schizophrenia. The field of the neurobiology of resilience and protective factors is relatively new to translational

---

Translational Neuroscience, ed. James E. Barrett, Joseph T. Coyle and Michael Williams. Published by Cambridge University Press. © Cambridge University Press 2012.

neuroscience but is of great importance as we strive to understand the brain disorders and processes described in Chapters 1 through 19. But even some patients with schizophrenia, who are not viewed as a particularly resilient group, show amazing recovery of vocational, social, and symptom functions in the natural course of events. Emil Kraepelin in 1919 (reprinted in Kraepelin 1971) noted that up to almost 15% of patients with schizophrenia, diagnosed with the ominous sounding "dementia praecox," seemed usually to suffer only a single episode and return to fairly good function. This observation is also reflected in Eugene Bleuler's insightful, heterogeneous term, "the group of schizophrenias" (Bleuler 1911). Academicians tend to study the more chronic and disabling forms of neuropsychiatric disorders in people who volunteer for research. This "willing to volunteer but quite ill" stratification is not just true of neuropsychiatry, because some major biomedical and even Nobel prize-winning scientists have studied fairly severe forms of familial disorders such as hypercholesterolemia (Goldstein and Brown 2008), often using the most severe forms of the disorder to gain an initial intellectual foothold on the shifting, murky sands of complex human diseases.

One way of looking at the array of disorders represented in this book, given the 2003 premise of 30,000 or so human genes, the 16,000 genes expressed in the human brain, and the 6,000 to 8,000 genes found *only* in the human brain (Insel and Collins 2003), is to stand back in amazement that so many people do *not* have major motor, cognitive, and mood problems despite the myriad of possible disorders that could occur. Perhaps the plasticity and resilience of the human brain are hallmarks of its evolutionary success, such as it is.

Definition and promises of translational neuropsychiatric research

"Translational research" has been a buzzword for several years. One of the goals of the National Institutes of Health Roadmap for Medical Research along with the Clinical and Translational Research Awards, which funds the Center for Clinical and Translational Sciences, is to make translational research an integral part of biomedical research (National Center for Research Resources 2011). The first Request for Applications for the Clinical and Translational Research Award program defined translational research as follows: "Translational research includes two areas of translation. One is the process of applying discoveries generated during research in the laboratory, and in preclinical studies, to the development of trials and studies in humans. The second area of translational research concerns research aimed at enhancing the adoption of best practices in the community." The first area of translation, from laboratory findings to clinical practice, is labeled T1. The second area of translation, to the community and back, is called T2 translation (Helfand *et al.* 2011).

This book illustrates the promises and challenges facing translational research in neuropsychiatry, neurology, and neurodevelopmental disorders. The promises can be summarized as the potential to wisely apply an explosion of laboratory science to real-world clinical challenges: the so-called T1 translational research paradigm of the bench-to-bedside transformation of treatment informed by our rapidly expanding basic science informatics base. T1 research is augmented by T2 research or the initial dissemination of the bench-to-bedside advances in knowledge to patients' healthcare delivery in order to create robust and widely implemented critical pathways of care. I would add that now there is T3, T4, and "full spectrum" translational research (Selker 2010; Selker and Califf 2011), defined by the expanding roles of the widespread, cost-effective, and feasible application of T1 and T2 concepts, but I would include them as part of stage 3 translational research (see below). For breast cancer, T1 is relatively advanced with the identification of the *BRCA-1* gene (King *et al.* 2001) followed by the creation of risk algorithms of breast cancer and then by genotype-guided therapeutics as a beginning T2 (second stage) advance in therapeutics. In contrast to breast cancer and simpler oncological dilemmas, personalized medicine in neuropsychiatry involves the brain as the organ of interest. The brain is encapsulated in a relatively inaccessible osseous vault and is infinitely more complex than the more accessible, homogeneous, and uniform breast and liver tissues explored in "successful" T1 oncology research. In addition, even if we could easily and safely access brain tissue for biopsy, many of our most trenchant neuropsychiatric disorders are not characterized by simple Mendelizing genomic processes. It is unclear *where* and *when* in the life cycle we would biopsy or harvest accessible tissue (lymphocytes) for many of the disorders represented in this book. In addition, genomic abnormalities in many psychiatric disorders reside in the complex dysregulation of far-ranging, complex neural circuits (Insel *et al.* 2010). Translational neuropsychiatry research is a "young" science (Nestler and Hyman 2010), and many of the mental disorders are attributable to circuit-based rather than punctate lesions or dysfunctions (Swerdlow 2010). T1 translational research in neuropsychiatry is in an exciting but challenging early stage of development. It also appears likely that many complex neural circuit imbalances and dysfunctions may well be "settled" at birth (Swerdlow 2011) and subsequently unfold over time. So, as indicated in the summaries of the sections on neurology and neurodevelopmental conditions (Chapters 6, 14, and 19), neither biological nor pharmacological interventions may be effective later in life, which raises profound ethical dilemmas for efficacious implementation in the earliest stages of life.

Thus, serious neuropsychiatric disorders mostly include a complex tapestry of tangled and dysregulated neural circuits and cellular dysfunctions that occur in a dauntingly hard to quantify matrix of genetic risk, augmented by gene–gene, epistatic, and environmental factors. Relatively well understood exceptions do exist, in that fragile X syndrome and HD (Shoulson and Young 2011) are genomically simpler disorders, and HD has autosomal dominant Mendelizing heritability patterns, but they are the exception rather than the rule. In addition, as Williams and Coyle (Chapter 7) and Williams and Barrett (Chapter 1) point out, many therapeutic advances in psychiatry accrue not from careful incremental research or even from a brainstorm of insight but rather from serendipitous findings (see also Preskorn 2010). This type of chance finding is illustrated by the initial astute but serendipitous discovery of the efficacy of antidepressant and antipsychotic medications. For example, the use of antipsychotics sprang from a relatively rare sequence of events, probably unlikely to recur in the twenty-first century (Klein 2008): (1) A surgeon in the French Navy noted the sedative and related antihistaminic properties of chlorpromazine; (2) he suggested its use in schizophrenia to his colleagues; (3) chlorpromazine's antipsychotic and dopamine antagonist properties led to (4) the dopamine hypothesis of schizophrenia, a Nobel prize-winning accomplishment by Arvid Carlsson, Paul Greengard, and Eric R. Kandel, who were awarded the prize in 2000 for their contributions to neuroscience and psychiatric medicine. This observation of an unlikely recurrence is especially true in the context of today's healthcare delivery system, in which time for reflection, collegial discussion, and subsequent serendipity is not reimbursed via codable conditions or encouraged by health insurance industry policies.

So although the *Book of Life* (the Human Genome Project) trumpeted the accomplishment of sequencing the human genome, the challenges we face in the postsequencing epoch after 2000 remain profound but relatively underacknowledged, despite the clear caveat of Insel and Collins (2003), stated soon after we entered the genomics era in 2003, that "from a discovery perspective we are just entering the genomic era." We must temper our excitement, borne of amazing basic science progress, with hubris borne of the recognition that a 10- to 15-year bench-to-bedside T1 translational period for the interval of basic science findings to the initial delivery of therapeutic agents via clinical trials (e.g., oncology at its best) may be much longer in common but complex neuropsychiatric disorders. The amazing advances in the face of these challenges are the object of most of the scholarly discussions in this book, but even completion of the exciting initial T1 advances still largely await us. One useful metric is to divide translational research into three stages:

Stage 1: *initial laboratory discovery*: no or few applications.
Stage 2: *middle stage*: beginning of success to moderate success in disseminating basic science insights to the bedside of some patients.
Stage 3: *late stage*: feasible, wide implementation of advances via healthcare systems.

In this context, one might estimate that neuropsychiatry is in the middle of stage 1 and oncology is in the beginning of stage 2. We must face the possibility that neuropsychiatry, especially for more complex problems, may not complete the third stage for the next 50–60 years or more.

How is the term translational research actually used?

At the most fundamental level, translational research is a widely used term that is often not clearly defined. Perhaps the T1–T2 parsing is of the greatest utility. Still, a recent (June 2011) PubMed Search of the first 20 citations of "translational research" in neuropsychiatry (see Table 20.1) illustrates a net so broad that it appears dauntingly complex and multidisciplinary.

Chapter 20: Promises and challenges of translational research in neuropsychiatry

Table 20.1. Wide-ranging topics represented by a PUBMED search "translational research in psychiatry" from SNPs and alleles to service users. Is translational science now all of science from genome to social science?

Author	Title	Journal Information
1. Tao J et al.	Deletion of astroglial Dicer causes non-cell-autonomous neuronal dysfunction and degeneration.	J Neurosci 2011;**31**:8306–8319.
2. Callard F et al.	Close to the bench as well as at the bedside: involving service users in all phases of translational research.	Health Expect 2011; May 25. doi: 10.1111/ j.1369–7625.2011.00681.x.
3. Pincus HA.	Academic health centers and comparative effectiveness research: baggage, buckets, basics, and bottles.	Acad Med 2011;**86**:659–660.
4. Paul SM.	Therapeutic antibodies for brain disorders.	Sci Transl Med 2011;**3**:84ps20.
5. Eickhoff SB et al.	Co-activation patterns distinguish cortical modules, their connectivity and functional differentiation.	Neuroimage 2011;**57**:938–949.
6. Teipel SJ et al.	Development of Alzheimer-disease neuroimaging-biomarkers using mouse models with amyloid-precursor protein-transgene expression.	Prog Neurobiol 2011; May 12. [Epub ahead of print].
7. Bloom J et al.	The contribution of common CYP2A6 alleles to variation in nicotine metabolism among European-Americans.	Pharmacogenet Genomics 2011;**21**:403–416.
8. Granger BB and Bosworth HB.	Medication adherence: emerging use of technology.	Curr Opin Cardiol 2011;**26**:279–287.
9. Freathy RM et al.	Genetic variation at CHRNA5-CHRNA3-CHRNB4 interacts with smoking status to influence body mass index.	Int J Epidemiol 2011; May 18. [Epub ahead of print].
10. Siegel SJ.	What can we expect from long-acting formulations for schizophrenia?	Curr Psychiatry Rep 2011;**13**:243–244.
11. Ray R et al.	Human Mu Opioid Receptor (OPRM1 A118G) polymorphism is associated with brain mu-opioid receptor binding potential in smokers.	Proc Natl Acad Sci USA 2011; **108**:9268–9273.
12. Scherma M et al.	The anandamide transport inhibitor AM404 reduces the rewarding effects of nicotine and nicotine-induced dopamine elevations in the nucleus accumbens shell in rats.	Br J Pharmacol 2011; May 9. doi: 10.1111/j.1476–5381.2011. 01467.x [Epub ahead of print].
13. Quednow BB et al.	The schizophrenia risk allele C of the TCF4 rs9960767 polymorphism disrupts sensorimotor gating in schizophrenia spectrum and healthy volunteers.	J Neurosci 2011;**31**:6684–6691.
14. Parr LA.	The evolution of face processing in primates.	Trans R Soc Lond B Biol Sci 2011;**366**:1764–1777.
15. Sim K et al.	Integrated genetic and genomic approach in the Singapore translational and clinical research in psychosis study: an overview.	Early Interv Psychiatry 2011;**5**:91–99.
16. Carter CS et al.	Cognitive neuroscience treatment research to improve cognition in schizophrenia II: developing imaging biomarkers to enhance treatment development for schizophrenia and related disorders.	Biol Psychiatry 2011;**70**:7–12.

Table 20.1. (cont.)

Author	Title	Journal Information
17. Gamaleddin et al.	Cannabinoid receptor stimulation increases motivation for nicotine and nicotine seeking.	Addict Biol 2011; Apr 26. doi:10.1111/ j.1369–1600.2011.00314.x. [Epub ahead of print].
18. Loughead J et al.	Brain activity and emotional processing in smokers treated with varenicline.	Addict Biol 2011; Apr 20. doi: 10.1111/ j.1369–1600.
19. Gamaleddin I et al.	The selective anandamide transport inhibitor VDM11 attenuates reinstatement of nicotine seeking induced by nicotine associated cues and nicotine priming, but does not affect nicotine-intake.	Br J Pharmacol 2011; Apr 18. doi:10.1111/ j.1476–5381.2011.01440.x. [Epub ahead of print].
20. Blondeau K et al.	Increasing body weight enhances prevalence and proximal extent of reflux in GERD patients "on" and "off" PPI therapy.	Neurogastroenterol Motil 2011;23:724-e327.

Table 20.1 reflects the fact that neuropsychiatric translational research now commonly includes health services (Callard et al. 2011), face processing in primates (Parr 2011), therapeutic antibodies for brain disorders (Paul 2011), medication adherence (Granger and Bosworth 2011), genetic variation (Freathy et al. 2011), developing biomarkers (Teipel et al. 2011), opioid receptor polymorphisms (Ray et al. 2011), how genetic variation influences the prepulse inhibition (PPI) biomarker and endophenotype (Quednow et al. 2011). Table 20.1 also illustrates a pitfall for PubMed searches: PPI also refers to protein pump inhibitors. Indeed, Table 20.1 represents a staggering array of research areas and knowledge, and much of it is far from bench-to-bedside research (medication adherence) or T1 bedside implementation. In fact, Weissman makes a valid case for extending translational research to the realm of epidemiology (Weissman et al. 2011).

Thus, the T1 bench-to-bedside mantra of translational research progress may be one of the most appealing but challenging concepts in all of neuropsychiatric science. The term *basic science* – science in a pure, unapplied but knowledge-enhancing form – is an intellectually challenging, essential endeavor. Such true basic exploration of mammalian biology with no explicit ties to any pathophysiology is, of course, important in order to create a foundation from which to support clinically relevant bench-to-bedside experiments. Yet, the concept of nonapplied basic research has a lack of funding and real-world appeal and sometimes seems to be strangely disarticulated from the real world of disease and human suffering compared with, say, problems of a lack of a clean supply of water, of vaccinations, or of the availability of basic antibiotics. So scientists invested in the T1 concept of bench-to-bedside research must be careful to be explicit and clear about expectations and about the course of the T1 and T2 cycles of research goals. That is why the 19 scholarly chapters in this book, with their wise balance of basic and applied science, make such a novel and meaningful contribution to our field, as outlined in the introduction and the summaries of each of the three areas of disorder-defined research on disorders.

We can examine some general examples of T1 research to point out strengths and challenges of this approach. For example, in neuropsychiatric genomics research, the discovery of single-nucleotide polymorphism (SNP) coding errors has led to remarkable discoveries, but none of them have direct, viable bedside application at the current time. That is understandable because translational research takes time, sometimes a lot of time. The HD locus was discovered in 1983, spurred on by the dedication of Nancy Wexler and others, and the gene itself was characterized 10 years later in 1993, a 10-year "locus to gene identification" period for a simple disorder. Then we found that trinucleotide CAG repeats (and corresponding metabolic polyamine toxicity) of base-pair language had an amazingly informative relationship to the age of onset (and morbidity) of HD. It is an amazing scientific finding, but as yet there is no practical treatment for this simple autosomal dominant Mendelizing disease. So along with the realistic short- (less than 25 years) and long-term (greater, perhaps much greater, than 25 years) goals of translational

343

Chapter 20: Promises and challenges of translational research in neuropsychiatry

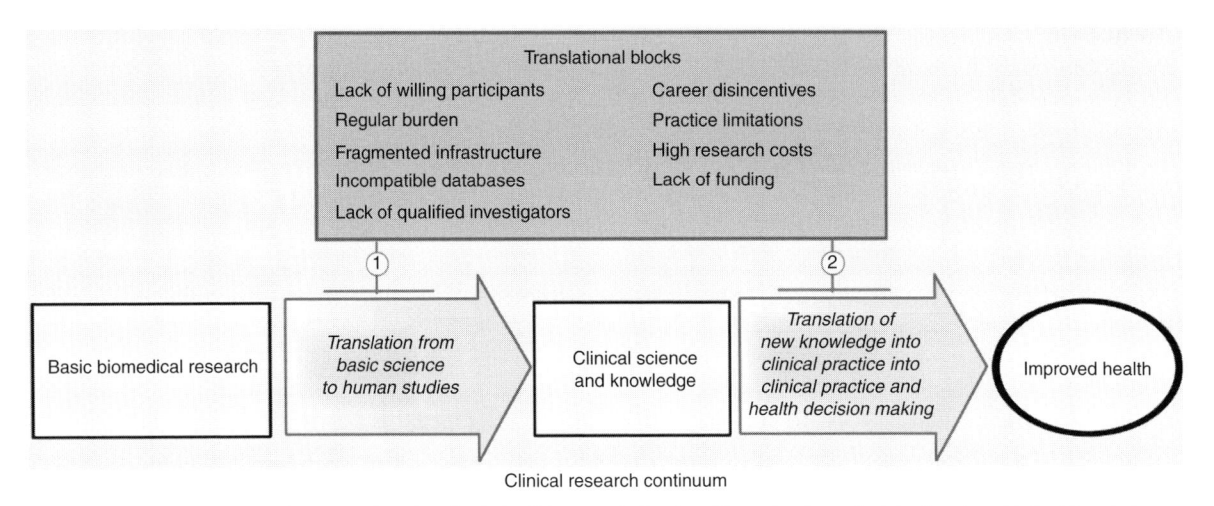

Figure 20.1. Structural impediments to bench-to-bedside (T1) research. Reprinted from the *Journal of the American Medical Association*, Vol. 289, Sung NS, Crowley WF Jr, Genel M *et al.*, Central challenges facing the national clinical research enterprise, pp. 1278–1287, copyright 2003, with permission from the American Medical Association. All rights reserved.

neuropsychiatric research, we must maintain a scholarly view that the explosion of facts (knowledge) we are seeing may take a relatively long time to reach T1 implementation as we try to integrate facts with actual treatment advances. In addition, as discussed below, gene funding for "simple" diseases such as HD may or *may not* lead to efficacious treatments, and some rodent T1 research may not be translatable to *Homo sapiens*.

What are the first steps and first blocks in bench-to-bedside T1 research?

At the most basic level, if we parse our research enterprise into T1 and T2 research endeavors as outlined above, our challenges are many. Some of the structural problems are clearly discussed and summarized by Sung *et al.* (2003) in Fig. 20.1. Other barriers and challenges are discussed below. These blocks (Sung *et al.* 2003) are what could be termed:

Type A: structural and social translational research barriers.

Type B: largely scientific and methodological barriers such as the winner's curse in genetics research (Nakaoka and Inoue 2009).

In this broader framework, a number of issues seem to pop out. Despite the T1 bench-to-bedside phrase, in reality, the first step in translational research is often taking the signs and symptoms of our patients with various neuropsychiatric disorders at the bedside and, via strong inference (Platt 1964),

good hunches, or luck, creating falsifiable hypotheses that can be brought to the basic science laboratory for confirmation. So the T1 "bench-to-bedside" mantra as well as the geneticists' DNA-to-RNA-to-protein mantra is infinitely more complex than it first appears. For example, in schizophrenia research, a corpus of knowledge about clinically observed inhibitory failures in patients and their neural and genomic substrates (e.g., Braff *et al.* 2001; Geyer *et al.* 2001; Swerdlow *et al.* 2001) has been explored in the laboratories of many scientists. This line of research started with the clear descriptions by Bleuler (1911), Kraepelin (1971), and McGhie and Chapman (1961) of patients and their self-described experiences, a subjective starting point. This world is full of inhibitory failures leading to sensory and cognitive gating failures and sensory and cognitive overload, leading in turn to disorganization of navigation through our complex, stimulus-laden world (Braff *et al.* 2007*a*, 2007*b*). Then basic science was used to test falsifiable hypotheses about gating failures via electroencephalography (Grillon *et al.* 1990), animal models (Geyer *et al.* 2001; Swerdlow *et al.* 2001), neurocognition (Gur *et al.* 2001), brain imaging (Hazlett *et al.* 2001), and cellular inhibitory function deficits (Adler *et al.* 1993) in patients with schizophrenia. These studies identified neuroanatomic regions of interest with their specific distributed neural circuit dysfunctions via animal models and brain imaging techniques. So in reality the apparent T1 inhibitory dysfunction approach really started at the bedside with the clinical observations of Bleuler, Kraepelin, and McGhie and Chapman.

Thus, the field went from clinical observation back to the T1 start point of applied basic science and then to clinical science. Such an orderly progression is of value and even possible in other disorders. Still, the "aha!" moment in drug discovery (as noted repeatedly in the 19 preceding chapters) has often been from serendipity rather than from well-planned research programs. Will serendipity be possible for new drug discovery as clinicians spend less and less time with their (under- or noninsured) patients? This outcome seems less likely (Klein 2008). Does our present healthcare delivery system negate this crucial pathway for drug discovery? These are vexing social and medical economics problems. "We still lack the requisite information to create genetic tests for psychiatric risk, diagnosis, and treatment that are robust enough to use responsibly and in a valid manner in psychiatric practice" (Braff and Freedman 2008).

A second largely implicit T1 type B block is the simple but misguided assumption that *knowledge (facts)* = *wisdom (informed use of facts)*, which seems often to be accepted without clear critical appraisal. Although our basic science-based build-up of technology and facts is a great accomplishment, it is but the first step in successful bench-to-bedside research, which can easily be seen as extending 50–100 years for complex disorders (cf. Insel and Collins 2003). How will we integrate genetic and neurobiological knowledge into effective early identification, understanding, and treatment of neuropsychiatric disorders? Several challenging examples of the problems as well as the benefits of basic science T1 discovery are illustrated below.

Scientific conundrums and blocks

> Editors and readers of elite basic science journals such as *Nature*, *Cell*, and *Science* would have difficulty comprehending the importance of studying fat accumulation in smooth muscle cells and hepatocytes. These articles are relevant to medical science because they address important diseases . . ." (Goldstein and Brown 2008).

As these Nobel laureates (and prominent translational researchers) discuss their work on hypercholesterolemia, there is often a "disconnect" between basic science research and real-world, clinically useful implementation. For example, a VIPR-2 mutation was found that is ten times more prevalent in patients with schizophrenia (0.3%) than in controls (0.03%) (Vacic *et al.* 2011). But unless the gene's location is in a crucial neurobiological pathway related to schizophrenia, its "direct effect" might apply to a group of only 0.3% of schizophrenia patients who have the mutation. The authors also concluded that the work may lead to "druggable" targets, but this path to treatment is elusive (cf. Nestler and Hyman 2010; Swerdlow 2011). It is also stated that schizophrenia is not unitary, but Bleuler came to that conclusion over a century ago when he coined the term *the group of schizophrenias*. We still struggle with subtyping issues in schizophrenia. So why is the finding statistically significant? Because if one examines about 8,000 subjects per group (schizophrenia and controls), such a large N will produce a significant P value even though the effect size of the genetic finding is extremely small. So *et al.* (2011) pointed out that, across ten complex diseases, the median of variance explained genomically was only 9.81% "while the variance explained per associated SNP was around 0.25%"! With these and many other similar findings, it is clear that prime basic science journals avidly and understandably publish excellent within-the-box translational (see below) genomic work where effect sizes are very small. This "large N, small effect size, highly significant P value conundrum" (Braff *et al.* 2008) is illustrated by other examples in the highly heritable, mammalian biological realm of height and body mass index (BMI) (e.g., Yang *et al.* 2010) relating to genes in common diseases (Hansen *et al.* 2011). With tens of thousands of subjects examined, the headline-grabbing news was that genes for height and BMI were identified. On closer inspection, however, these "new" genes accounted for only a tiny percentage of the variance in height or BMI (cf. So *et al.* 2011, for a scholarly discussion of this issue in common human diseases). Clearly, careful examination of gene–gene interactions will yield better models for these highly polygenic disorders (Moskvina *et al.* 2011).

The elegant basic science article "Modelling schizophrenia using human induced pluripotent stem cells" (Brennard *et al.* 2011) raises related issues. In Gage's laboratory, Brennard *et al.* "directly reprogrammed fibroblasts from SCZD [schizophrenia] patients into human induced pluripotent stem cells (hiPSCs) and subsequently differentiated these disorder-specific hiPSCs into neurons." These neurons showed diminished neuronal connectivity in

345

Chapter 20: Promises and challenges of translational research in neuropsychiatry

conjunction with decreased neurite number, PSD95-protein levels, and glutamate receptor expression. Many cyclic AMP and WNT signaling pathways showed altered gene expression. Only the little used antipsychotic, loxapine (among other drugs), seemed to reverse some of these findings. This differential drug effect may (or may not) have been due to dosage levels of the drugs (Brennard, personal communication). Thus the authors concluded that "we now report hiPSC neuronal phenotypes and gene expression changes associated with SCZD, a complex genetic psychiatric disorder." But are all the measures (e.g., decreased neurite number) associated with schizophrenia? If so, where in the brain does this occur and when in the life cycle? Three of four of the patients were "Jewish Caucasian" from the Coriell collection and all had multiply affected relatives. The paper itself makes *no* claims regarding therapeutic applications. Interestingly, Brennard and Gage *et al.* are illustrating "translational wisdom" by pursuing a strategy of using biological manipulations to create pluripotential-derived "hippocampal" and dopamine-rich cells and other candidate cells of primary regions of interest in the brains of patients with schizophrenia. This approach is a fascinating, long-term translational strategy.

The main challenge for neuropsychiatric translational research is to establish models of central nervous system (CNS) disease states using induced pluripotent stem cell technology (Pedrosa *et al.* 2011). Animal models are useful for many medical diseases, but for uniquely human disease domains, the use of stem cell technology is far more challenging. First, patient-specific pluripotential stem cells must be created (Durnaoglu *et al.* 2011; Pedrosa *et al.* 2011). Second, these cells must be biologically morphed into functionally relevant or disease model-specific cells (Durnaoglu *et al.* 2011). For neurotransmitter or specific locus disorders like PD, early point mutations may be within reach (Soldner *et al.* 2011). For complex distributed circuit-based disorders and those involving novel targets (Ibrahim and Tamminga 2011) such as schizophrenia or mood disorders, this task is much harder. A complex tapestry of genes, endophenotypes, clinical phenotypes, and domains of function and outcome must all be integrated (Fig. 20.2), a daunting task that is now productively beginning (Cannon and Keller 2006; Gottesman and Gould 2003; Greenwood *et al.* 2011).

I strongly recommend that all basic/translational studies include explicit statements regarding the

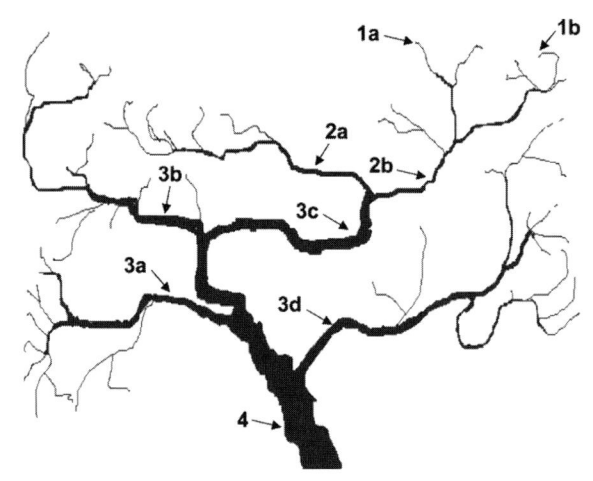

Figure 20.2. Watershed model of the pathway between upstream genes and downstream phenotypes. Specific genes (1a, 1b) contribute variation to narrowly defined endophenotypes such as dopaminergic regulation in the prefrontal cortex (2b). This and other narrowly defined endophenotypes affect more broadly defined endophenotypes, such as working memory (3c). Working memory in conjunction with several other endophenotypes (3a, 3b, 3d) affects phenotypically observable phenotypes, such as symptoms of schizophrenia (4). Reprinted from the *Annual Review of Clinical Psychology*, Vol. 2, Cannon TD, Keller MC, Endophenotypes in the genetic analyses of mental disorders, pp. 267–290, copyright 2006, with permission from Annual Reviews.

practical implications of the work, the (likely) immediacy of results application in the world of the clinic, and the estimated time frame to efficacious and effective clinical implementation, say clearly designating (1) now; (2) within 5 years; (3) perhaps in 10 years; (4) probably 10 years or more; (5) totally unknown. We must remember that the HD linkage result occurred in 1983. It is a simple autosomal dominant disorder, yet almost 30 years later there is no dramatic bench-to-bedside treatment, although treatments are evolving (Shoulson and Young 2011). Unfortunately, for most genomic findings in neuropsychiatry, the answer to "when will this basic science finding lead to specific and significant help for my relative?" lies somewhere in the vast period between 10 years and unknown (or never).

Two other vignettes illustrate the profound scientific and guardian-of-the-public trust mantle issues that neuropsychiatry must address in the context of premature genetic testing for (neuropsychiatry) disorders.

1. Francis Collins paid to have his DNA genotyped for disease risk by three large commercial interests (Collins 2009). The three medical disease risk profiles were highly divergent, reflecting the fact

that in all of medicine (except for some diseases like HD and breast cancer), practical genetic risk testing is not nearly ready for practical implementation even though the premature marketing of these tests goes on largely unregulated.

2. Some tests are marketed directly to consumers, and the results are sent to unsuspecting primary-care doctors (Braff and Freedman 2008). In contrast, anticoagulation therapy with its narrow therapeutic range is amenable for creating drug-dosing algorithms for warfarin (Wu *et al.* 2008), and oncology has dramatically begun to use genomic testing for treatment decisions (e.g., Pander *et al.* 2007). In contrast, direct-to-consumer genetic tests for, say, bipolar disorder (Braff and Freedman 2008) have a computed 90% false negative rate and very poor sensitivity of only 10% versus the desired 95%. Of course, the underlying fact that a specific GRK mutation is three times more likely in bipolar patients than controls is true but practically speaking it is misleading.

"Responsible genetic testing in modern medicine has to take into account not only the promise but also the consequences of offering information to patients" (Braff and Freedman 2008), especially with decisionally impaired patients and their desperate families. We must be much more careful with exactly how we present medical and neuropsychiatric T1 claims to the public lest we overpromise and then have to deal with the inevitable disappointment and even loss of confidence in translational scientists and their work that may be engendered as we have seen, to some degree, in high-throughput oncology translational research (Kolata 2011; Tuma 2010).

Translational neuropsychiatry: from a simple disorder (HD) to a very complex disorder (schizophrenia)

Huntington's disease

One might see HD as one of the simplest genetic disorders in neuropsychiatry (Ho *et al.* 2001; Shoulson and Young 2011). The extensive knowledge we have regarding the etiology and pathogenesis of HD is still impressive. But the lack of any meaningful highly efficacious personalized genomic treatment illustrates the bifurcation of knowledge (facts) and wisdom (what to do with facts) that faces us in T1 research. The majority of various medically "at-risk" patients resist genetic testing; those who do get tested (e.g., for lung cancer susceptibility) often do not perform low-tech behavioral interventions to minimize the risk of developing the disorder (e.g., stop smoking) (Braff and Freedman 2008). This behavior may be due to human nature and demand or to a lack of proper rigorous behavioral medicine educational interventions or both. In HD, 95% of at-risk individuals refuse genetic testing. Why? Perhaps they refuse because there is no known genomic-based treatment, even almost 30 years after the discovery of the HD locus. The only option is to genotype embryos for the mutation and then implant unaffected embryos, an ethical slippery slope indeed.

Our expanding biological knowledge of HD is indeed impressive. The genomic region of interest for HD was found via linkage studies in 1983. Ten years later, the Mendelizing gene that accounts for HD was discovered at 4p16.3, containing a trinucleotide repeat of CAG coding for glutamine calling for cytoplasmic protein limitations in the polyglutamate tracts and regions. In addition, an orderly relationship between the trinucleotide CAG repeat number from generation to generation has been noted. With fewer than 25 to 35 CAG repeats, an individual is not at much risk for developing HD, and age at onset occurs later. Risk increases in an orderly fashion with 36 and 40 repeats to about 100% with many repeats, with juvenile onset occurring in about 7–8% of very dense, repetitive HD CAG carriers in an absolutely orderly and rational manner. This unveiling of levels of risk represents an amazing accomplishment of bench science, but it still awaits the technology and advances to definitively apply to bedside T1 treatment interventions to reduce or preempt tonic polyamine accumulation.

HD is the prototypical "low-hanging fruit" poster child of genetically (but not necessarily biologically) well understood neuropsychiatric disorders (Feigin 1998; Ho *et al.* 2001; Reglodi *et al.* 2011). But, there is just a leading edge of (palliative) therapies (Shoulson and Young 2011). This fact gives us both hope and cause for modesty: hope that we can translate our detailed knowledge of HD into cures and modesty that with a heritable disorder like HD there is a known autosomal Mendelizing heritability single gene. But, after almost 30 years of locus-to-therapy time and many advances in our neuropsychiatric "fact" base, our therapeutic armamentarium is sadly devoid of a practical, ethically acceptable cure or prevention for HD. Another example of a simple disorder that offers challenges is autism (see Chapter 16), with its heartbreaking (and family shattering) consequences. Insel and Collins (2003) noted that autism is a highly genetic disorder, but recent reports of monozygotic twins show that profound in utero environmental risk factors (Hallmayer *et al.* 2011) impact this disorder.

If we apply this type of analysis to bipolar affective disorder (see Chapter 15), anxiety disorder (see Chapter 2), or schizophrenia (see Chapter 4), with their highly polygenic and G×E etiologies, we can only imagine how long it may take to translate basic (and social) science knowledge into efficacious bedside interactions. Plus, even when we have efficacious treatments, they will undoubtedly face ethical, regulatory, practical, cost, side-effect, and compliance barriers. There is a lot of work to do in our still "early stage" science.

Schizophrenia: a complex disorder

Schizophrenia is much more complex than HD, especially from a genetic standpoint: despite 80% heritability, its gene–gene and polygenic G×E interactions are extremely challenging problems or scientific type B blocks to advancing knowledge and treatment. As translational schizophrenia genomic research has progressed, a debate has occurred between adherents of common variant/low penetrance (genome-wide association study [GWAS]-based) versus rare variant/high penetrance (copy number variant [CNV]) modelers. This debate accrues from GWAS adherents' reliance on their widespread search for many common risk variants of mild penetrance (small effect size) versus CNV-based approaches for rare CNVs of large effect size. It is notable that new risk genes and phenes are being discovered for many disorders at a dramatic rate outside of the GWAS platform. Still, there is a profound "missing heritability" problem with schizophrenia and many other neuropsychiatric disorders, perhaps occurring from epistatic, gene–gene interactions (Chou *et al.* 2011). So schizophrenia, an extremely complex disorder, stands in stark contrast to HD.

Owen *et al.* (2010; Visscher *et al.* 2011) eloquently pointed out that the GWAS versus CNV debate may be illusory. They state that "until recently, genome-wide scans for disease risk variants were based on linkage analysis, an approach that can detect only those alleles that confer relatively large effects. The main alternative was the candidate gene association study, which, although better powered than linkage for weak genetic effects, is problematic for phenotypes where pathogenesis is largely unknown. However, systematic searches across the genome for risk alleles of small effect are now possible thanks to the development of array platforms allowing hundreds of thousands of ... SNPs to be assayed." Rather than restate their elegant argument, I refer the interested reader to their manuscripts (cf. Owen *et al.* 2010; Visscher *et al.* 2011). Also, we must remember that the whole area of protective gene and environmental factors is crucial and is quite understudied in complex disorders. Undoubtedly, this area of research will expand rapidly in coming years.

Thus, it is clear that both rare (e.g., *de novo*) mutations and more common vertically transmitted mutations occur and that we are dealing with an admixture of common and rare contributions from disorder to disorder based on the neurobiological pathways that are affected (GAIN Collaborative Research Group *et al.* 2007; Owen *et al.* 2010; Visscher *et al.* 2011). Translating this knowledge from the bench to the bedside *will* be a daunting task after we have determined the relative contributions to these two "bins" of rare and common genetic variations on the relevant mammalian biological pathways for disorders such as schizophrenia. Plus, although rare variants are commonly thought of as highly penetrant (Walsh *et al.* 2008) and GWAS may have hidden heritability in many small effect sizes and gene–gene interactions (Gibson 2010), this story is still evolving. It is possible that even some rare and *de novo* events may have small effect sizes comparable with those identified in GWAS studies, but this issue remains unclear.

Animal models

Modeling of human neuropsychiatric disorders in animals is extremely challenging given the subjective nature of many symptoms, the lack of biomarkers and objective diagnostic tests, and the early state of the relevant neurobiology and genetics (Nestler and Hyman 2010).

Cross-species translational animal models for neuropsychiatric disorders abound, including those for schizophrenic, bipolar, addictive, eating, major depression, anxiety, and many other disorders. As reflected in this book, the major advantage of animal models is the ability of the investigators to directly manipulate the neural and genomic substrates relevant to a particular disorder. Also, social manipulations such as maternal deprivation and isolation rearing allow for dramatic environmental manipulations that are ethically impermissible in human subjects (Geyer et al. 2001). The downside of animal models is the danger of going "a bridge too far" by, for example, anthropomorphizing rodents. For isomorphic measures like PPI, animal models make sense. But then PPI, not schizophrenia, is being modeled. For modeling higher level brain functions such as social cognition, one need only look at the thin, friable cortex of a mouse and observe the primitive but orderly social structures and wonder if rodents can experience phenomena, such as social cognition, which are similar to, if not isomorphic with, phenomena experienced by humans. Can a rodent model account for affective states like depression or just social isolation and withdrawal? I'm not a mouse so I really have no idea what a mouse "feels" or "thinks." For nontalking primates (e.g., rhesus monkeys), the anaclitic depression model seems to have more robust face validity (e.g., McKinney 1984). So choosing the species and life-cycle point of intervention as well as the behavioral and biological targets is crucial in animal model research.

Nestler and Hyman (2010) point out that animal models of neuropsychiatric disorders face many challenges; their views are summarized and extended below.

1. Despite the profoundly negative effects of these disorders on public health, progress in understanding their pathophysiology has been frustratingly slow and the discovery of new therapeutic neuropsychiatric mechanisms is at a near standstill. Big Pharma is therefore exiting from the CNS stage with all of its complexities and is betting on fields such as oncology with its (apparently) simpler models and putatively faster bench-to-bedside applications.
2. Given the limitations in human research, it is hard to imagine substantial progress in understanding pathophysiology or developing therapeutics without good animal models. Unfortunately, current animal models have substantial and often unstated limitations, ranging from weak face and construct validity to poor predictive power for drug efficacy in human disease (Markou et al. 2009).
3. The explosion of infrahuman animal models has not fully addressed the obstacles of modeling dimensions of these disorders that are uniquely human in nature. As discussed above on "modeling schizophrenia," it is difficult to see how invertebrate and cellular preparations of pluripotential stem cells will comprehensively model complex neuropsychiatric disorders, although with 40 or 50 years of detailed work, such modeling may be more feasible. In addition, the availability of mouse knockout technology (vs. rat knockout technology until recently) may have forced murine animal models into the mouse versus rat species-specific arena. This development may represent another type B scientific block: sometimes the availability of technology rather than robust falsifiable hypotheses dictates research endeavors. Nestler and Hyman (2010) pointed out that many of the symptoms used to establish psychiatric diagnoses in humans (hallucinations, delusions, sadness, and guilt) cannot be convincingly modeled in Petri dishes, rodents, or even our nontalking primate "cousins" who share 99% of the human genome. These are indeed significant problems but with effort, wisdom, and time, they may well be overcome or subject to scientifically robust work-arounds.

A vexing issue is how to parse G (gene) from E (environment) and $G \times E$ interactions in animal models of endophenotypes related to neuropsychiatric disorders. In this context, Gottesman and Gould (2003) defined endophenotypes as being (1) quantitative, laboratory-based measures not detected by the naked eye; (2) patients who have quantitative deficits versus normal controls; (3) family members of patients who have intermediate values between patients and normal individuals, and (4) endophenotypes that co-segregate with the disorder. Braff et al. (2007a, 2007b, 2008) describe endophenotypes as filling in the "gene-to-phene gap." Endophenotype research in animal model experiments offers unique advantages. For example, Francis et al. (2003) used an imaginative strategy to answer the relative contributions of genes (Mother Nature) versus environment (Mother Nuture) to schizophrenia-linked endophenotype defects. They took two mouse strains (B-6 and BALB) with different endophenotype behavioral signatures on four quantitative phenotypes. Then they took strain B-6 embryos and implanted them into BALB dams and cross-fostered the resulting pups into rearing by B-6 and BALB dams. Many iterations of this strategy were used (e.g., BALB embryos implanted into B-6 dams and raised by B-6 or BALB dams). Across four quantitative endophenotypes, PPI was the most genetically determined behavior. A B-6 embryo showed B-6 related levels of PPI even when implanted into BALB dams and the resulting pups were reared by BALB dams. This process parsed Mother Nature from Mother Nuture and allowed us to assess the relative G and E as well as G×E determinants of different genetically and environmentally mediated endophenotypic behaviors. This strategy is promising for detecting the genetic versus environmental determinants of endophenotypes of a neuropsychiatric disorder but does not model the entire syndrome. Still, endophenotypes such as PPI are relevant because PPI relies on a well-known modulatory circuit in mammals (Swerdlow and Koob 1987) and, in schizophrenia patients, is both heritable (Greenwood *et al.* 2007) and related to real-world function (Swerdlow *et al.* 2006).

In conclusion, Nestler and Hyman (2010) made reasonable, detailed recommendations for animal model researchers as follows:

1. State the goal. Is this a neurobiological tool or a disease model?
2. State the hypothesis to be tested.
3. List the specific aspects of the illness meant to be modeled.
4. State the type(s) of validators (for example, construct, face, and predictive) applied to the model.
5. State the evidence for and against the validity of the modeling of the context of the validator(s) used.

I would add:

1. State the time frame before the implementation of T1 basic science advances may be likely. This task is difficult but one that will avoid overexuberant (or false) claims and reactive public disappointment (Kolata 2011).
2. State the distance between the species being used and humans on the basis of the biology of the measure being examined. Clearly mice are closer to humans than are zebra fish for most domains. But are mice or rats closer to humans genetically and neural circuit-wise for a specific measure being examined? Also, it would be helpful if scientists included the species being examined in the title and abstracts of articles.

Translating psychosocial and behavioral interventions to their neurobiological substrates: a novel and underutilized translational strategy

Without some fundamental paradigmatic change, it is implausible that pharmacology will, in the foreseeable future, be able to reach backwards two decades [of a patient's life] through a variable web of absent and misguided neural connections, replace missing and improper ones with healthy ones, and thereby disentangle schizophrenia from the self (Swerdlow 2011).

We all wish that we could accelerate our basic understanding of the relationship of CNS dysfunction in neuropsychiatric disorders into more efficacious and effective treatments for our patients and their families. Unfortunately, it must be acknowledged that dramatic basic science discoveries in our field across anxiety (see Chapter 2), addictive (see Chapter 5), mood (see Chapter 3), and psychotic (see Chapter 4) disorders, have not led to dramatic advances in the treatment arena. It is especially noteworthy that, despite the fact that psychosocial therapies account for up to 50% or more of the variance in outcome in, say, depression (Weissman 2007), "treatment" as used in psychiatric jargon often means *only* antidepressant medications. Unlike statin direct-to-consumer advertisements – which advise "diet and exercise" in addition to medications – antidepressant direct-to-consumer advertising seems almost never to advise counseling, relaxation therapy, or diet and exercise, all of which can add therapeutic gains to antidepressant drug response. We have not fully capitalized on translating biological and psychosocial research into a range of full treatment options (Selker and Califf 2011). Despite that void, we now understand that psychosocial interventions (e.g., cognitive behavior therapy and other behavioral interventions) can lead to profound brain reorganization and to the engagement of both impaired and complementary healthy brain circuits to augment comprehensive treatment in disorders such as obsessive-compulsive disorder and depression (Saxena *et al.* 2009; Schwartz *et al.* 1996).

Efficacious treatment strategies consist of psychosocial therapies designed to engage healthy circuits to act as surrogates to aid the functions of terminally damaged circuits and the use of medications that target circuit-based dimensions of pathology such as procognitive drugs for disorders with prominent cognitive deficits from Alzheimer's disease to some depressive disorders to schizophrenia, the prototypical thought disorder. Cognitive disturbances, which are characteristic of depression, were identified as early as 1974 (Braff and Beck 1974) and led to the birth of cognitive–behavioral therapy, as developed by Tim Beck and Arnold Lazarus among others. These effective behavioral medicine interventions earned Aaron Beck the coveted Lasker Prize in 2006. This view of the salience of psychosocial therapies is supported by Myrna Weissman (2007) and others who parsed the outcome from the treatment of depression into roughly equivalent "silos" of medication and behavioral treatment benefits. We should take advantage of both biological and psychosocial treatment domains and interventions. A third domain in treatment is the use of drugs that target specific exacerbations in convergent circuit parts within neural circuits and facilitate the efficacy of the other two interventions. It is also important to note that current treatments may also prevent the neurobiological and psychosocial deterioration that may result from repeated symptomatic exacerbations (Post 2007). This model of treatment is particularly relevant to bipolar affective disorder, schizophrenia, depression, eating, and other disorders, but it may also apply parsimoniously even to motor-dominated disorders such as HD and PD.

One key point is that we widely stress that neuropsychiatric disorders are "biopsychosocial" disorders but then often ignore the fact that psychosocial interventions can reshape brain structure and function alone or in conjunction with biological treatments. This observation is true even if the etiology of a disorder is purely or largely biological. Thus prepulse inhibition (PPI) of the startle response is a useful biomarker (Braff 2010; Braff *et al.* 2001; Geyer *et al.* 2001; Swerdlow *et al.* 2001) and heritable endophenotype (Greenwood *et al.* 2007) of schizophrenia involving many genes and gene pathways (e.g., Greenwood *et al.* 2011). But Dawson and others have shown that PPI can be influenced by simple attentional instructions (Thorne *et al.* 2005). Kumari (personal communication, article in submission) has shown that this highly neurobiological marker of schizophrenia (and other gating disorders) can be normalized with cognitive–behavioral therapies. That is a striking finding, perhaps reflecting a combination of strengthening related, intact neural circuits or increasing the efficiency of the impaired cortico-striato-pallido-thalamic and related cortico-striato-pallido-pontine modulatory circuits that regulate PPI.

A key but too often ignored point of the translational revolution in neuropsychiatry may reside in the power of psychosocial interventions, which, when efficacious, may provide for a more accessible, readily available, cheaper, and low-risk path to moving the brain to normalcy in seriously mentally ill patients. This area of translational, brain-changing social and cognitive interventions is also widely applied across learning and other disorders (Gaab *et al.* 2007; Popov *et al.* 2011). Certainly, pursuing this area of brain-changing psychosocial treatments appears to be as potentially rewarding as many complementary high-tech genomic and medication strategies, which are fraught with challenges regarding how to develop new compounds and unknown and unintended consequences (e.g., will the introduction of pluripotential stem cells into the striatum of patients with HD lead to neural overgrowth, increased tangles, and miswiring?). In addition, some classes of nanotechnology tools (e.g., contact lenses to measure intraocular pressure in glaucoma patients) may never be feasible as direct readouts of biomarker signals in the brain regions implicated in neuropsychiatric disorders. Both biological and psychosocial domains of treatment need to be pursued, often in concert with each other.

Anatomy of the translational neuropsychiatric revolution

> It should not escape our notice" [50 years after Watson and Crick's paper] . . . that we have an opportunity to revolutionize the diagnosis and treatment of mental disorders" (Insel and Collins 2003).

In Crane Britton's seminal, highly revered book, *Anatomy of Revolution* (Britton 1938), the early English (pre-1800), American, French, and Russian revolutions are examined for developmental similarities. One theme that emerged, which applies to our translational research and genomic revolutions in neuropsychiatry, is that a period of initial settled, incremental events is followed by intense (over) enthusiasm for change, often propelled by small numbers of avid adherents (Jacobeans), which is followed by subsequent reflective moderation (The Thermidorian Reaction). In this context, the thoughtful, deep, careful work of Mendel, Darwin, and Watson and Crick (1953) represents a balanced presage that was followed by the current period of sometimes overexuberant claims. Fortunately, the carefully crafted chapters of this book do not suffer from overstatement; as a first volume of neuropsychiatric translational research, this book is a good model of a balanced approach.

Look at the modest text of Watson and Crick's paper, "We wish to suggest a structure for the salt of deoxyribose nucleic acid (D.N.A.). This structure has novel features which are of considerable biological interest." Contrast it with the 24-hour news cycle-driven, often inaccurate, shortcut promotion of biomedical and genomic research findings. Advertisements such as "Get your mouse model started when you're away" are particular favorites of mine. It is now time to leaven the enthusiasm borne of the initial but still limited success of the translational and genomic revolution with careful Thermidorian reflection. In reality, the sequencing of the 3,000,000,000 base pairs of the human genome with its trinucleotide codes was a watershed turn-of-the-millennium event (2000), highly publicized, and an amazing accomplishment. In Britton's parlance, the publicity surrounding the year 2000 opening of "The Book of Life" can be viewed as the somewhat overly enthusiastic centerpiece of the early phase of the genomic revolution in which we are still immersed as we recognize that nuclear DNA is the tip of the clinically relevant genomic iceberg. In fact, over the past decade, questions regarding the sequencing of the human genome have been replaced by a new set of issues. Are gene deserts really biologically inert? Exactly how do epigenetic events change gene expression (see Chapter 18)? How does all of this new information fit into our neuropsychiatric disease models? A lot of intellectually challenging territory remains to be covered. The rapid but still early "evolution" of genomic science – to areas such as gene expression, epigenetics, the transcriptome, and a host of other advances – is setting the table for what is still largely an initial stage 1 phase of careful reflection that is beginning to replace revolutionary zeal. In biomedical research, one might view the decade following the completion of the Human Genome Project (2000–2010), with the development of genomic-guided breast cancer therapies, as the beginning of a stage 2 of downregulated claims and careful assessment of emerging early identification and intervention strategies. Unfortunately, even in the middle of stage 2 in the field of oncology, overpromises and financial and academic incentives have resulted in claims that have failed and that have engendered public outrage (Kolata 2011). This emerging reflection and rise of a transitional Thermidorian period may last 20 or more years for some disorders and longer for other, more complex disorders such as many of those involving the brain, although any such projection is difficult to make. Still, it is notable that we are devising strategies that deal with large numbers of comparisons of gene effects (e.g., Greenwood *et al.* 2011; Lazzeroni and Ray 2010; Ott and Wang 2011).

It is interesting to note that Bill and Melinda Gates (and Warren Buffett) via the Gates Foundation gives $800,000,000 per year for global health, which approaches the annual budget of the United Nations World Health Organization (193 nations). The Gates Foundation is heavily invested in vaccination, eradication of polio, immunization, health services education, and, to a lesser extent, HIV research. Thus, only a small percentage of these charitable donations are directed to T1 research endeavors. Why would such smart people (Bill and Melinda Gates, Warren Buffet) decide to allocate resources to these "low-tech" areas? Perhaps they did so because T1 research is still in its early phases, whereas vaccination or clean drinking water programs have an immediate payoff that is high impact and palpable. Although T1 research has great appeal and promise, it must be noted that researchers should be very clear about (1) *how* their research will impact the "real world" and (2) *when* that impact is likely to occur. We can and must do a better job of educating the public about the great strengths and realistic timelines of neuropsychiatric research.

Pretense of wisdom syndrome

In the paper, "Macroeconomics after the Crisis: Time to Deal with the Pretense-of-Knowledge Syndrome" (Caballero 2010), Ricardo J. Caballero argues that macroeconomics, with its current core of the so-called dynamic stochastic general equilibrium approach "has become so mesmerized with its own internal logic that it has begun to confuse the precision it has achieved about its own world with the precision that it has about the real one."

I would argue that psychiatric translational and genetics research with its emphasis on "facts" and dazzling technology and its relative underemphasis on generating falsifiable general, integrative hypotheses is also in danger of prematurely entering the fine-tuning mode, when we should be in the broad-exploration mode. This broad-exploration mode includes the integration of psychosocial therapies into creating advanced pathways for neuropsychiatric disorders. This mode could be termed a "pretense of wisdom syndrome." We are also too far from the absolute truth about medications and cures for neuropsychiatric disorders to make the overconfident claims that can emerge from the impressive but larger internal logic of the fine-tuning mode at the current core of emerging but still stage 1 neuropsychiatric knowledge. We face many pitfalls that must be overcome as we train a new generation of translational neuroscientists (e.g., Licinio and Wong 2004).

This book does much to advance translational research in the neurosciences. The carefully crafted, scholarly chapters are data driven and well researched and relate well to the broad themes of translational research. This approach is appropriate since So et al. (2011), in reviewing ten complex diseases from Crohn's and types I and II diabetes to AD, bipolar disorder, and schizophrenia point out that "a substantial proportion of heritability remains unexplained." They indicate that "the median *total* variance explained across the 10 diseases was 9.81%" despite the very large Ns utilized and that the most powerful individual SNPs accounted for only 0.25% of the variance of disorders. This missing heritability issue is indeed vexing and may accrue from multiple small gene effects, gene–gene interactions, or as yet unknown factors. So larger and larger Ns are often gathered in a brute force and blunt dissection effort, but, despite these efforts, careful, comprehensive explanations still elude us for many disorders. We must remain open to new paradigms and as-yet undreamed of explanations that our students and their students are yet to develop. Reciprocally, we must be sure not to become so mesmerized by our technology that we allow it, rather than our knowledge of cells, circuits, genes, and outcome (Braff 2011), to drive our neuropsychiatric research programs.

Summary and conclusions

To borrow (and modify) Charles Dickens' famous opening line from *A Tale of Two Cities*, "It is the best of times; it is the most challenging of times."

It is the best of times because translational research in neuroscience has now evolved to a point where our fact base and new techniques offer us and the next few generations of researchers a wonderful opportunity to advance our knowledge of neuropsychiatric disorders and neural circuit-based domains of function (Insel et al. 2010) in the service of better understanding and treating trenchant, complex neuropsychiatric, neurological, and neurodevelopmental problems. The content of this book reflects this veritable explosion of information.

Our main challenges remain how to integrate huge amounts of new facts (knowledge) into comprehensive and realistic translational models and derivative interventions for these disorders (wisdom). This book and the carefully referenced scholarship herein go far in facilitating our goals to advance translational neuropsychiatric research. Indeed, it is an exciting time to be conducting careful translational research in neuroscience. We must recognize that despite an extensive armamentarium of new facts we are in the relatively early stages of a promising translational research revolution. Given the expected important, time-consuming nature of the work, some solvable problems may entail several decades to close the T1 bench-to-beside loop. Other problems may be even more difficult to resolve, even using both neurobiological and psychosocial interventions. Translational research and treatment of the disorders covered in this book are promising, but many of the solutions are long term. Progress will ultimately help our patients and their families cope with the terrible burden of "no fault" clinical disorders as our translational science advances.

These challenges will, in many cases, take decades to resolve and will rely on the robust and exciting science foundation that is currently being constructed. In this context, a number of points are critical to remember:

1. Right now our knowledge (facts) and technology far outpace our ability to wisely integrate the wealth of information being discovered. The T1 and T2 research categorizations are helpful in guiding our ongoing research, but there is now a knowledge-wisdom gap particularly in neuropsychiatric translational research.
2. We should be careful not to allow new technologies to define problems or unnecessarily accelerate claims regarding the problems we are attempting to understand.

3. The time course of many of the more vexing T1 bench-to-bedside challenges can reasonably be expected to be measured in decades, not years. Even a "simple" Mendelizing autosomal dominant disorder (HD) has no genomic informed treatment 30 years after its locus was clearly identified.
4. The "blocks" we face to progress in translational neuroscience research consist of two "bins": type A blocks, which are practical (e.g., enriching the pipeline of well-trained investigators) and involve social and economic resource allocation, and type B blocks, which are conceptual and technical scientific challenges. First, how do we best handle large datasets? For example, the most informative SNPs may account for only 0.25% of the variance in many complex medical disorders. How can we best integrate therapeutic and side-effect information across complicated data sets? Can traditional DSM-based diagnoses and novel intermediate endophenotypes be used in a complementary strategy in order to best complement each other (Braff et al. 2007a, 2007b)? The buildup of new technology will facilitate but hopefully not direct our research endeavors over the next 50 years.
5. The neuropsychiatric translational revolution can be parsed into the following stages:

   Stage 1: early discovery.
   Stage 2: first efficacious interventions and the identification of genomic predictors of dosage and side effects.
   Stage 3: widespread effective applications.

Oncology is probably early in stage 2, neuropsychiatry in the middle of stage 1.

1. We should not allow the "pretense-of-wisdom syndrome" to prematurely facilitate overstating accomplishments that are impressive but only preliminary. We must maintain "realistic expectations" for our science (Swerdlow et al. 2008).
2. Animal and basic science modeling often models functions and endophenotypes rather than disorders. The great utility and limitations of animal models are discussed in this chapter and throughout this book. Caveats are summarized by Nestler and Hyman (2010), Millan (2008) and in this chapter.
3. Genomics (postsequencing genetic science) is an incredibly powerful discipline in its early stages (Insel and Collins 2003). Although "the history of psychiatric genetics is largely a story of unreplicated discoveries and unrealized expectations," this book reinforces the idea that "a new chapter of discovery is about to begin" (Insel and Lehner 2007). We have built much on the foundation laid down by Mendel, Darwin, and Watson and Crick. Early optimism for quick fixes is fading as a reflective Thermidorian (to use Crane Britton's historical parlance) reaction is occurring. Both common and rare genomic events must be incorporated into comprehensive disorder models (Owen et al. 2010). In addition, we must determine the level of knowledge that can be explained based on single gene versus gene network analyses. Then, complementary issues of gene expression, epigenetics, and other emerging disciplines will undoubtedly add to a comprehensive picture of understanding neuropsychiatric disorders.
4. Along with enthusiasm, we face a time fraught with challenges and problems. We should be clear that techniques such as pluripotential stem cell research methods *may* offer initial treatments in the near (10–20 years) future for spinal cord injury and even HD and the neurodegenerative disorders discussed in this book. More complex neuropsychiatric disorders may remain even longer in the scientific queue until significant "high-tech"-mediated enhancements, not to mention "cures," are available. Premature "Gold Rush" (Kolata 2011) claims and commercialization may cause profound social problems. Even in the relatively simple field of oncology, "initial highly publicized breakthroughs turned out to be wrong ... gene-based tests proved worthless ... based on bad science" (Kolata 2011). We must carefully advance our translational science while avoiding headline-grabbing, overreaching claims, especially since many neuropsychiatric patients are decisionally impaired and vulnerable to unwarranted claims. Our science is too good to sacrifice it at the altar of overenthusiastic claims. Modesty is needed to leaven our understandable excitement regarding translational research advances.
5. Translational research in the neurosciences, particularly in neuropsychiatry, must take full advantage of the neural circuit and

brain-reorganizing potential of psychosocial interventions in both animal models and human research. It is not necessary that a complex biological clinical problem has a complex biological treatment (e.g., Weissman, 2007). It is striking that nonbiological psychosocial interventions such as cognitive–behavior therapy and cognitive training and remediation can "reorganize the brain" as assessed by brain imaging and biomarkers (cf. Gaab et al. 2007; Popov et al. 2011; Saxena et al. 2009; Schwartz et al. 1996; Swerdlow 2011). Our circuit- and domain-based understanding (Insel et al. 2010) and treatment of neuropsychiatric disorders must include the integration of both biological and psychosocial tools (Braff 2011). We must resist the common perception that in the neuropsychiatric world "treatment = drugs." It is profoundly self-defeating and untrue. Our complementary biological and cognitive treatment modalities are both needed to develop novel and effective neuropsychiatric treatment strategies.

Given all these challenges, it remains clear that our neuropsychiatric translational science is an incredible foundational resource. As we move forward with a new understanding of the brain's vulnerabilities and resilience, drug therapeutics and side effects, there are a myriad of opportunities documented in this book to advance ways to end the suffering of patients via translational research. Although future advances in these endeavors will probably be slower than we and our patients and their families would like, the amazing advances of the past 20–30 years in the translational research of disorders within the scope of neuroscience are a cause for great hope: hope that we have gained a crucial intellectual and scientific foothold in advancing the comprehensive understanding and treatment of these unique neuropsychiatric "no fault" clinical brain disorders.

Acknowledgments

Supported by NIH grants: MH065571, MH042228, MH085265, MH084071, MH089984, MH07977, MH091350; Department of Veteran's Affairs VISN-22 Mental Illness Research, Education, and Clinical Center (MIRECC), and the Niederhofer Family Foundation.

References

Adler LE, Hoffer LD, Wiser A, Freedman R. 1993. Normalization of auditory physiology by cigarette smoking in schizophrenic patients. *Am J Psychiatry* **150**:1856–1861.

Bleuler E. 1911. *Dementia praecox, oder Gruppe der Schizophrenien*. Leipzig: F. Deuticke.

Blondeau K, Boecxstaens V, Van Oudenhove L et al. 2011. Increasing body weight enhances prevalence and proximal extent of reflux in GERD patients 'on' and 'off' PPI therapy. *Neurogastroenterol Motil* **23**:724–e327.

Bloom J, Hinrichs AL, Wang JC. 2011. The contribution of common CYP2A6 alleles to variation in nicotine metabolism among European-Americans. *Pharmacogenet Genomics* **21**:403–416.

Braff DL. 2010. Prepulse inhibition of the startle reflex: a window on the brain in schizophrenia. *Curr Top Behav Neurosci* **4**:349–371.

Braff DL. 2011. Gating in schizophrenia: from genes to cognition (to real world function?). *Biol Psychiatry* **69**:395–396.

Braff DL, Beck AT. 1974. Thinking disorder in depression. *Arch Gen Psychiatry* **31**:456–459.

Braff DL, Freedman R. 2008. Clinically responsible genetic testing in neuropsychiatric patients: a bridge too far and too soon. *Am J Psychiatry* **165**:952–955.

Braff DL, Freedman R, Schork NJ, Gottesman II. 2007a. Deconstructing schizophrenia: an overview of the use of endophenotypes in order to understand a complex disorder. *Schizophr Bull* **33**:21–32.

Braff DL, Geyer MA, Swerdlow NR. 2001. Human studies of prepulse inhibition of startle: Normal subjects, patient groups, and pharmacological studies. *Psychopharmacology* **156**:234–258.

Braff DL, Greenwood TA, Swerdlow NR et al. 2008. Advances in endophenotyping schizophrenia. *World Psychiatry* **7**:11–18.

Braff DL, Schork NJ, Gottesman II. 2007b. Endophenotyping schizophrenia. *Am J Psychiatry* **164**:705–707.

Brennard KJ, Simone A, Jou J et al. 2011. Modelling schizophrenia using human induced pluripotent stem cells. *Nature* **473**:221–225.

Britton C. 1938. *The Anatomy of Revolution*. New York, NY: Random House.

Caballero RJ. 2010. Macroeconomics after the crisis: time to deal with the pretense-of-knowledge syndrome. *J Econ Perspectives* **24**:85–102.

Callard F, Rose D, Wykes T. 2011. Close to the bench as well as at the bedside: involving service users in all phases of translational research. *Health Expect* May 25. doi: 10.1111/j.1369-7625.2011.00681.x. [Epub ahead of print].

Cannon TD, Keller MC. 2006. Endophenotypes in the genetic

analyses of mental disorders. *Annu Rev Clin Psychol* **2**:267–290.

Carter CS, Barch DM, Bullmore E *et al.* 2011. Cognitive neuroscience treatment research to improve cognition in schizophrenia II: developing imaging biomarkers to enhance treatment development for schizophrenia and related disorders. *Biol Psychiatry* **70**:7–12.

Chou HH, Chiu HC, Delaney NF, Segre D, Marx CJ. 2011. Diminishing returns epistasis among beneficial mutations decelerates adaptation. *Science* **333**:1190–1192.

Collins FS. 2009. *The Language of Life: DNA and the Revolution in Personalized Medicine*. New York, NY: Harper Collins Publishers.

Durnaoglu S, Genc S, Genc K. 2011. Patient-specific pluripotent stem cells in neurological diseases. *Stem Cells Int* **2011**:212487. Epub 2011 Jul 3.

Eickhoff SB, Bzdok D, Laird AR. 2011. Co-activation patterns distinguish cortical modules, their connectivity and functional differentiation. *Neuroimage* **57**:938–949.

Feigin A. 1998. Advances in Huntington's disease: implications for experimental therapeutics. *Curr Opin Neurol* **11**:357–362.

Francis DD, Szegda K, Campbell G, Martin WD, Insel TR. 2003. Epigenetic sources of behavioral differences in mice. *Nat Neurosci* **6**:445–446.

Freathy RM, Kazeem GR, Morris RW *et al.* 2011. Genetic variation at CHRNA5-CHRNA3-CHRNB4 interacts with smoking status to influence body mass index. *Int J Epidemiol* [Epub ahead of print, May 18].

Gaab N, Gabrieli JD, Deutsch GK, Tallal P, Temple E. 2007. Neural correlates of rapid auditory processing are disrupted in children with developmental dyslexia and ameliorated with training: an fMRI study. *Restor Neurol Neurosci* **25**:295–310.

GAIN Collaborative Research Group, Manolio TA, Rodriguez LL *et al.* 2007. New models of collaboration in genome-wide association studies: the Genetic Association Information Network. *Nat Genet* **39**:1045–1051.

Gamaleddin I, Wertheim C, Zhu AZ *et al.* 2011. Cannabinoid receptor stimulation increases motivation for nicotine and nicotine seeking. *Addict Biol* Apr 26. doi:10.1111/j.1369-1600.2011.00314.x. [Epub ahead of print].

Gamaleddin I, Guranda M, Goldberg SR, Lefoll B. 2011. The selective anandamide transport inhibitor VDM11 attenuates reinstatement of nicotine seeking induced by nicotine associated cues and nicotine priming, but does not affect nicotine-intake. *Br J Pharmacol* Apr 18. doi:10.1111/j.1476-5381.2011.01440.x. [Epub ahead of print].

Geyer MA, Krebs-Thomson K, Braff DL, Swerdlow NR. 2001. Pharmacological studies of prepulse inhibition models of sensorimotor gating deficits in schizophrenia: a decade in review. *Psychopharmacology (Berl)* **156**:117–154.

Gibson G. 2010. Hints of hidden heritability in GWAS. *Nat Genet* **42**:558–560.

Goldstein JL, Brown MS. 2008. From fatty streak to fatty liver: 33 years of joint publications in the JCI. *J Clin Invest* **118**:1220–1222.

Gottesman II, Gould TD. 2003. The endophenotype concept in psychiatry: etymology and strategic intentions. *Am J Psychiatry* **160**:636–645.

Granger BB, Bosworth HB. 2011. Medication adherence: emerging use of technology. *Curr Opin Cardiol* **26**:279–287.

Greenwood TA, Braff DL, Light GA *et al.* 2007. Initial heritability analyses of endophenotypic measures for schizophrenia: the consortium on the genetics of schizophrenia. *Arch Gen Psychiatry* **64**:1242–1250.

Greenwood TA, Lazzeroni LC, Murray SS *et al.* 2011. Analysis of 94 candidate genes and 12 endophenotypes for schizophrenia from the Consortium on the Genetics of Schizophrenia. *Am J Psychiatry* [Epub ahead of print, Apr 15].

Grillon C, Courchesne E, Ameli R, Geyer MA, Braff DL. 1990. Increased distractibility in schizophrenic patients. Electrophysiologic and behavioral evidence. *Arch Gen Psychiatry* **47**:171–179.

Gur RC, Ragland JD, Moberg PJ *et al.* 2001. Computerized neurocognitive scanning: II. The profile of schizophrenia. *Neuropsychopharmacology* **25**:777–788.

Hallmayer J, Cleveland S, Torres A *et al.* 2011. Genetic heritability and shared environmental factors among twin pairs with autism. *Arch Gen Psychiatry* [Epub ahead of print, Jul 4].

Hansen T, Ingason A, Djurovic S *et al.* 2011. At-risk variant in TCF7L2 for type II diabetes increases risk of schizophrenia. *Biol Psychiatry* **70**:59–63.

Hazlett EA, Buchsbaum MS, Tang CY *et al.* 2001. Thalamic activation during an attention-to-prepulse startle modification paradigm: a functional MRI study. *Biol Psychiatry* **50**:281–291.

Helfand M, Tunis S, Whitlock EP *et al.* 2011. A CTSA agenda to advance methods for comparative effectiveness research. *Clin Transl Sci* **4**:188–198.

Ho LW, Carmichael J, Swartz J *et al.* 2001. The molecular biology of Huntington's disease. *Psychol Med* **31**:3–14.

Ibrahim HM, Tamminga CA. 2011. Schizophrenia: treatment targets beyond monoamine systems. *Annu Rev Pharmacol Toxicol* **51**:189–209.

Insel TR, Collins FS. 2003. Psychiatry in the genomics era. *Am J Psychiatry* **160**:616–620.

Insel T, Cuthbert B, Gravey M *et al.* 2010. Research domain criteria (RDoC): toward a new classification framework for research on mental disorders. *Am J Psychiatry* **167**:748–751.

Insel TR, Lehner T. 2007. A new era in psychiatric genetics? *Biol Psychiatry* **61**:1017–1018.

King MC, Weiand S, Hale K *et al.* 2001. Tamoxifen and breast cancer incidence among women with inherited mutations in BRCA1 and BRCA2: National Surgical Adjuvant Breast and Bowel Project (NSABP-P1) Breast Cancer Prevention Trial. *J Am Med Assoc* **286**:2251–2256.

Klein DF. 2008. The loss of serendipity in psychopharmacology. *J Am Med Assoc* **299**:1063–1065.

Kolata G. 2011. How bright promise in cancer testing fell apart. *New York Times*, July 7.

Kraepelin E. 1971. *Dementia Praecox and Paraphrenia*. Huntington, NY: RE Krieger Publishing Company.

Lazzeroni LC, Ray A. 2010. The cost of large numbers of hypothesis tests on power, effect size and sample size. *Mol Psychiatry* [Epub ahead of print, Nov. 9].

Licinio J, Wong ML. 2004. Translational research in psychiatry: pitfalls and opportunities for career development. *Mol Psychiatry* **9**:117.

Loughead J, Ray R, Wileyto EP *et al.* 2011. Brain activity and emotional processing in smokers treated with varenicline. *Addict Biol* Apr 20. doi: 10.1111/j.1369-1600. [Epub ahead of print].

Markou A, Chiamulera C, Geyer MA, Tricklebank M, Steckler, T. 2009. Removing obstacles in neuroscience drug discovery: the future path for animal models. *Neuropsychopharmacol Rev* **34**: 74–89.

McGhie A, Chapman J. 1961. Disorders of attention and perception in early schizophrenia. *Br J Med Psychol* **34**:103–116.

McKinney WT. 1984. Animal models of depression: an overview. *Psychiatr Dev* **2**:77–96.

Moskvina V, Cradock N, Muller-Myhsok B *et al.* 2011. An examination of single nucleotide polymorphism selection prioritization strategies for tests of gene–gene interaction. *Biol Psychiatry* **70**:198–203.

Nakaoka H, Inoue I. 2009. Meta-analysis of genetic association studies: methodologies, between-study heterogeneity and winner's curse. *J Hum Genet* **54**:615–623.

National Center for Research Resources. 2011. *NCRR Fact Sheet. Clinical and Translational Science Awards*. Bethesda, MD: National Center for Research Resources. Available at: http://www.ctsaweb.org/docs/CTSA_FactSheet.pdf. [Accessed September 7, 2011].

Nestler EJ, Hyman SE. 2010. Animal models of neuropsychiatric disorders. *Nat Neurosci* **13**:1161–1169.

Ott J, Wang J. 2011. Multiple phenotypes in genome-wide genetic mapping studies. *Protein Cell* **2**:519–522.

Owen MJ, Craddock N, O'Donovan MC. 2010. Suggestion of roles for both common and rare risk variants in genome-wide studies of schizophrenia. *Arch Gen Psychiatry* **67**:667–673.

Pander J, Gelderblom H, Guchelaar HJ. 2007. Insights into the role of heritable genetic variation in the pharmacokinetics and pharmacodynamics of anticancer drugs. *Expert Opin Pharmacother* **8**:1197–1210.

Parr LA. 2011. The evolution of face processing in primates. *Trans R Soc Lond B Biol Sci* **366**:1764–77.

Paul SM. 2011. Therapeutic antibodies for brain disorders. *Sci Transl Med* **3**:84ps20.

Pedrosa E, Sandler V, Shah A *et al.* 2011. Development of patient-specific neurons in schizophrenia using induced pluripotent stem cells. *J Neurogenet* [Epub ahead of print, July 29].

Pincus HA. 2011. Academic health centers and comparative effectiveness research: baggage, buckets, basics, and bottles. *Acad Med* **86**:659–660.

Platt JR. 1964. Strong inference: certain systematic methods of scientific thinking may produce much more rapid progress than others. *Science* **146**:347–353.

Popov T, Jordanov T, Rockstroh B *et al.* 2011. Specific cognitive training normalizes auditory sensory gating in schizophrenia randomized trial. *Biol Psychiatry* **69**:465–471.

Post RM. 2007. Kindling and sensitization as models for affective episode recurrence, cyclicity, and tolerance phenomena. *Neurosci Biobehav Rev* **31**:858–873.

Preskorn SH. 2010. CNS drug development: Part I: The early period of CNS drugs. *J Psychiatr Res* **16**:334–339.

Quednow BB, Ettinger U, Mössner R *et al.* 2011. The schizophrenia risk allele C of the TCF4 rs9960767 polymorphism disrupts sensorimotor gating in schizophrenia spectrum and healthy volunteers. *J Neurosci* **31**:6684–6691.

Ray R, Ruparel K, Newberg A *et al.* 2011. Human Mu Opioid Receptor (OPRM1 A118G) polymorphism is associated with brain mu-opioid receptor binding potential in smokers. *Proc Natl Acad Sci USA* **108**:9268–9273.

Reglodi D, Kiss P, Lubics A, Tamas A. 2011. Review on the protective effects of PACAP in models of neurodegenerative diseases in vitro and in vivo. *Curr Pharm Des* **17**:962–972.

Saxena S, Gorbis E, O'Neill J *et al.* 2009. Rapid effects of brief intensive cognitive-behavioral therapy on brain glucose metabolism in obsessive-compulsive disorder. *Mol Psychiatry* **14**:197–205.

Scherma M, Justinová Z, Zanettini C *et al.* 2011. The anandamide transport inhibitor AM404 reduces the rewarding effects of nicotine and nicotine-induced dopamine elevations in the nucleus accumbens shell in rats. *Br J Pharmacol* May 9. doi: 10.1111/j.1476-5381.2011.01467.x. [Epub ahead of print].

Schwartz JM, Stoessel PW, Baxter Jr, LR, Martin KM, Phelps ME. 1996. Systematic changes in cerebral glucose metabolic rate after successful behavior modification treatment of obsessive–compulsive disorder. *Arch Gen Psychiatry* **53**:109–113.

Selker HP. 2010. Beyond translational research from T1 to T4: Beyond "separate but equal" to integration (Ti). *Clin Transl Sci* **3**:270–271.

Selker HP, Califf RM. 2011. The need for academic leadership in full-spectrum translational research. *Clin Transl Sci* **4**:78–79.

Shoulson I, Young AB. 2011. Milestones in Huntington disease. *Mov Disord* **26**:1127–1133.

Siegel SJ. 2011. What can we expect from long-acting formulations for schizophrenia? *Curr Psychiatry Rep* **13**:243–244.

Sim K, Lee J, Subramaniam M et al. 2011. Integrated genetic and genomic approach in the Singapore Translational and Clinical Research in Psychosis Study: an overview. *Early Interv Psychiatry* **5**:91–99.

So H-C, Gui AHS, Cherny SS, Sham PC. 2011. Evaluating the heritability explained by known susceptibility variants: a survey of ten complex diseases. *Gen Epidemiol* **35**:310–317.

Soldner F, Laganiere J, Cheng AW et al. 2011. Generation of isogenic pluripotent stem cells differing exclusively at two early onset Parkinson point mutations. *Cell* **146**:318–331.

Sung NS, Crowley WF Jr, Genel M et al. 2003. Central challenges facing the national clinical research enterprise. *J Am Med Assoc* **289**:1278–1287.

Swerdlow NR. 2010. Integrative circuit models and their implications for the pathophysiologies and treatments of the schizophrenias. *Curr Top Behav Neurosci* **4**:555–583.

Swerdlow NR. 2011. Are we studying and treating schizophrenia correctly? *Schizophr Res* **130**:1–10.

Swerdlow NR, Geyer MA, Braff DL. 2001. Neural circuit regulation of prepulse inhibition of startle in the rat: current knowledge and future challenges. *Psychopharmacology (Berl)* **156**:194–215.

Swerdlow NR, Koob GF. 1987. Lesions of the dorsomedial nucleus of the thalamus, medial prefrontal cortex and pedunculopontine nucleus: effects on locomotor activity mediated by nucleus accumbens-ventral pallidal circuitry. *Brain Res* **412**:233–243.

Swerdlow NR, Light GA, Cadenhead KC et al. 2006. Startle gating deficits in a large cohort of patients with schizophrenia: relations, medications, symptoms, neurocognition, and level of function. *Arch Gen Psychiatry* **63**:1325–1335.

Swerdlow NR, Weber M, Qu Y, Light GA, Braff DL. 2008. Realistic expectations of prepulse inhibition in translational models for schizophrenia research. *Psychopharmacology (Berl)* **199**:331–388.

Teipel SJ, Buchert R, Thome J, Hampel H, Pahnke J. 2011. Development of Alzheimer-disease neuroimaging-biomarkers using mouse models with amyloid-precursor protein-transgene expression. *Prog Neurobiol* [Epub ahead of print, May 12].

Thorne GL, Dawson ME, Schell AM. 2005. Attention and prepulse inhibition: the effects of task-relevant, irrelevant, and no-task conditions. *Int J Psychophysiol* **56**:121–128.

Tao J, Wu H, Lin Q et al. 2011. Deletion of astroglial Dicer causes non-cell-autonomous neuronal dysfunction and degeneration. *J Neurosci* **31**:8306–8319.

Tuma RS. 2010. Duke scandal shines light on systemic problems in high-throughput experiments. *Oncology Times* **32**:13–15.

Vacic V, McCarthy S, Malhotra D et al. 2011. Duplications of the neuropeptide receptor gene VIPR2 confer significant risk for schizophrenia. *Nature* **471**:499–503.

Visscher PM, Goddard ME, Derks EM, Wray NR. 2011. Evidence-based psychiatric genetics, AKA the false dichotomy between common and rare variant hypotheses. *Mol Psychiatry* June 14. doi: 10.1038/mp.2011.65. [Epub ahead of print].

Walsh T, McClellan JM, McCarthy SE et al. 2008. Rare structural variants disrupt multiple genes in neurodevelopmental pathways in schizophrenia. *Science* **320**:539–543.

Watson JD, Crick FHC. 1953. Molecular structure of nucleic acids: a structure for deoxyribose nucleic acid. *Nature* **171**:737–738.

Weissman MM. 2007. Cognitive therapy and interpersonal psychotherapy: 30 years later. *Am J Psychiatry* **164**:693–696.

Weissman MM, Brown AS, Talati A. 2011. Translational epidemiology in psychiatry: linking population to clinical and basic sciences. *Arch Gen Psychiatry* **68**:600–608.

Wu AH, Wang P, Smith A et al. 2008. Dosing algorithm for warfarin using CYP2C9 and VKORC1 genotyping from a multi-ethnic population: comparison with other equations. *Pharmacogenomics* **9**:169–178.

Yang J, Benyamin B, McEvoy BP et al. 2010. Common SNPs explain a large proportion of the heritability for human height. *Nat Genet* **42**:565–569.

Zammit S, Owen MJ, Lewis G. 2010. Misconceptions about gene–environment interactions in psychiatry. *Evid Based Ment Health* **13**:65–68.

Index

locators in **bold** refer to figures/tables

ACC (anterior cingulate cortex) 56–59
acetylation, histone proteins 336. *See also* epigenetics
acid sensing ion channels **233**
acute pain 168, 169, 170. *See also* pain therapeutics
addictive disorders 107–108, 115, 122–123
   cross-tolerance 109–110
   genetics 113–114, 123
   inhibitory systems 114
   medication-assisted treatment strategies 109
   new strategies 112–114
   nicotine 111–112
   partial agonists 111
   plasticity, cellular/synaptic 107, 115, 123
   receptor antagonists 110–111
adenosine A2 antagonists 204–205
adenylyl cyclase 29–32
ADHD (attention-deficit hyperactivity disorder) 267–269, 303, 309–310, 313–314
   catecholamines 304–305
   clonidine/guanfacine 311
   dopamine reuptake inhibitors 312
   etiology 312–313
   genetics 313
   heterogeneity 313
   monoamine oxidase inhibitors 311–312
   pharmacological treatment, basic principles 305, 312
   prefrontal cortex 303–304, 308–309
   psychostimulants 303, 306–310
   tricyclic antidepressants 269, 310–311
adrenocorticotropic hormone (ACTH) 178
AEDs. *See* antiepileptic drugs
AFFIRM (Natalizumab Safety and Efficacy in Relapsing-Remitting Multiple Sclerosis) study 189
agranulocytosis 3

AHN 2-005 312
AKTi gene 86–87, 90
alcohol use 329–330
αβ integrins 184
α-synuclein 199, 255, 325–326
ALS. *See* amyotrophic lateral sclerosis
ALS2 gene 216–217
ALS4 gene 217
Alzheimer's disease 149–150, 162. *See also* tau hypothesis
   amyloid precursor-like proteins 153–154
   anti-inflammatory drugs 135–136
   biomarkers 131–132, 254–255
   clinical features/neuropathy/ biochemistry 151–153
   clinical trials 137
   combination therapies 161–162
   current treatments 130, 153
   early pathology 131
   environmental factors 130
   epigenetics 325, **330–331**
   and epilepsy 228
   experimental manipulations/ therapeutic strategies 159–162
   gene-based drug discovery 139–140
   genetics 132, **133**, 155
   immunotherapy 160–161
   metabolic syndrome 136
   mild cognitive impairment 150–151
   transgenic models 156–159
   translational neuroscience 253
AMPA receptors 41–42, 45, 46–48
amphetamine 303, 304
amygdala **16**, 18–19, 48–49, 57, 58
amyloid hypothesis, Alzheimer's disease. *See* tau hypothesis
amyloid precursor-like proteins (APLPs) 153–154
amyotrophic lateral sclerosis 224
   animal models 215
   biomarkers 215–216, 255
   cell-specific drug intervention targets 217–218
   clinical trials 218–220, **221**
   current treatments 131
   environmental factors 130
   gene therapy 221–222
   genetics 134, **135**, 216–217

   heterogeneity 214–215
   interfering RNA/antisense oligonucleotides 223–224
   stem cell therapy 222–223
   traditional drug targets 220–221
   translational neuroscience 214–216, 218
Anatomy of Revolution (Britton) 351
anesthetics, and neuropathic pain 169
angiogenesis, and epilepsy 229–230
angiogenin 217
animal models 253, 255–257. *See also* endophenotypes, transgenic models, translational neuroscience
   addictive disorders 108–109
   ADHD 306
   AMPA receptors 46–48
   amyotrophic lateral sclerosis 215
   approach–avoidance behaviors 18–19, **284**
   autism spectrum disorders 275, 277–278, 280–287, **289**, **291**
   biomarkers 254
   epilepsy 236, 238
   epileptogenesis 236–237
   methylphenidate **309**
   mood disorders 31–32, 35, 39–41, 59–60
   multiple sclerosis 186–187
   neurobiology of fear 14–15, **16**
   neurological disorders 138
   pain therapeutics 170–172
   Parkinson's disease 206
   psychiatric disorders 1, 7
   schizophrenia 88–91
anisomycin 20
anterior cingulate cortex 56–59
antidepressant drugs 4–6, 118
   ADHD 269, 310–311
   autism 264, 292
   epigenetics 327
   neuropathic pain 169
antiepileptic drugs 230–232, **233**
   combination therapies 239
   comparative data 243–244
   development of new 240–241

359

Index

antiepileptic drugs (cont.)
  dose prediction 243
  drug resistance 238–239
  mechanism of action 231, **232**
  for nonepileptic conditions 169, 242, 243
  preclinical screening 232–242
  side effects 239–240
anti-inflammatory drugs
  Alzheimer's disease 135–136
  multiple sclerosis 178
antipsychotic drugs 3–4, 118
antisense oligonucleotides 223–224
anxiety disorders 4, 14, 22, 120.
    See also benzodiazepines
  epigenetics 326–327, **330–331**
  extinction-based treatment 16–18
  extinction–reconsolidation combined approaches 22
  memory consolidation/reconsolidation 18–22
  neurobiology of fear 14–15, **16**
  plasticity, cellular/synaptic 123
Aph-1 gene 159
APLPs (amyloid precursor-like proteins) 153–154
apolipoprotein (*APP*) gene 155
apoptosis 94–95, 132, 206
applied science 343
approach–avoidance behaviors, animal models 18–19, **284**
aquaporin-4 181
ARPs (AMPA receptor potentiators) 46–48
ASD. *See* autism spectrum disorders
ASTIN stroke study 257
atomexitine 310
attention-deficit hyperactivity disorder. *See* ADHD
auditory evoked related potentials 83–84
auditory evoked responses 289–290
autism spectrum disorders 261–264, 273–274, 293
  animal models 275, 277–278, 280–287
  cognitive endophenotypes 287
  comorbidity 286–287
  diffusion tensor imaging 275–276
  drug development 291–293, 334
  environmental factors 282
  epigenetics 329, **330–331**
  genetics 280–281
  magnetic resonance spectroscopy 275–276
  magnetoencephalography 274–276, 277–278, 289
  model specificity assessment 287

molecular endophenotypes 288
neuroanatomy 288
neuroimaging, basic principles 289–291
neurophysiological endophenotypes 288–289
resting state magnetoencephalography 275
translational neuroscience 276–280, 287–291, 348
validation criteria, preclinical models 279–280
autoimmune hypotheses
  autism spectrum disorders 282
  multiple sclerosis 180–182
avoidance paradigms, animal models 18–19, **284**
AVP (plasma arginine vasopressin) 49
axonal damage
  epilepsy 229–230
  multiple sclerosis 182

BACE1/2 genes 154, 158, 159
baclofen 114
B-cell lymphoma 2 31
Bcl-2 gene 35–38
BDNF (brain-derived neurotrophic factor)
  amyotrophic lateral sclerosis **219**
  autism spectrum disorders 288, 292
  epigenetics 50, 327
  mood disorders 5, 31, 33–35, **36**, 121
  schizophrenia 87, 94
  substance abuse 329–330
behavioral interventions 350–351, 354–355
behavioral phenotypes.
    See endophenotypes
bench-to-bedside perspective ix, 339, 340–341, **344**
benzodiazepines 2, 4, 17
benztropine analogs 312
β-blockers 282. *See also* propranolol
biochemical endophenotypes, autism 288
biogenic amine hypothesis 4
biomarkers 253, 254–255
  Alzheimer's disease 131–132, 254–255
  amyotrophic lateral sclerosis 215–216, 255
  animal models 254
  autism spectrum disorders 273–274, 277–278, 290–291
  definitions 254
  epilepsy 247–248
  multiple sclerosis 186, 187–188, 255
  neurological disorders 131–132, 139
  Parkinson's disease 203–204, 206

bipolar disorder 339
  neurogenesis **30**
  protein kinase C inhibition 33
  translational neuroscience 348
blood–brain barrier 135, 234
body mass index (BMI) 345
BPD. *See* bipolar disorder, mood disorders
breast cancer 340
buprenorphine 111
bupropion 111–112

caffeine 136, 199, 205
cAMP response element binding protein (CREB) 29–33, 49, 121
cancer pain, animal models 172
cannabis use 88
capsaicin model of pain therapeutics 173
CART (cocaine-and-amphetamine-regulated transcript) 31
catecholamines 304–305
catechol-O-methyltransferase (*COMT*) genotype 88
causality. *See also* environmental factors
  ADHD 312–313
  autism 276, 282
  epilepsy 228
  neurological disorders 129, 130, 138
  psychiatric disorders 1, 48–50
celecoxib **219**, 220
cell replacement therapy 136
chance, role in drug discovery 341, 345
childhood abuse 48–50
chlordiazepoxide 2
chlorpromazine 2, 80
chlorpyrifos 282
cholinesterase inhibitors 130
CHRNA4/CHRNAB2 genes 238
chromatin 321–324.
    See also epigenetics
chronic defeat 327
chronic fatigue 42
chronic pain 168–169. *See also* pain therapeutics
cigarette smoking 111–112, 136, 199
clinical trials 253. *See also* AFFIRM, CONSIST, IMPACT, SENTINEL, STAR*D
  Alzheimer's disease 161
  amyotrophic lateral sclerosis 218–220, **221**
  design 257
  epilepsy 246–248
  multiple sclerosis 179, 191
  neurodevelopmental disorders 335
  neurological disorders 137, 257
  Parkinson's disease 204–205, 206
  psychiatric disorders 7–8, 19–20

Index

CLOCK gene 122
clonidine 311
clozapine 3, 80, 92
CNV-based models (copy number variants) 90–91, 124, 348
cocaine 329–330
cocaine-and-amphetamine-regulated transcript (CART) 31
coenzyme Q$_{10}$ **219**, **221**
cognitive–behavioral therapy 61, 351
cognitive functioning
    ADHD 306, 309–310
    Alzheimer's disease 150–151, 325
    autism spectrum disorders 287
    schizophrenia 84
coherence analysis 278
combination therapies 254, 258–259
    Alzheimer's disease 161–162
    epilepsy 239
communicative functioning, autism 284–286
compensatory heterogeneity 276
component symptom complex approach 7
COMT (catechol-O-methyltransferase) gene 88
conditioned responses (CR) 14–15, 107, 120
CONSIST trial 92
constipation 198
construct validity
    autism spectrum disorders 279, 282
    seizure tests/epilepsy models 234
copy number variants (CNV) 90–91, 124, 348
corticosteroids 178.
    See also gluticocorticoids
covalent modifications.
    See also epigenetics
    DNA 323–324
    histone 321–323
craving 122. See also addictive disorders
CREB (cAMP response element binding protein) 29–33, 49, 121
cross-tolerance 109–110
cyclic adenosine monophosphate pathway (cAMP) 29–32
cyclophosphamide **219**
cyclosporine **219**
cysteine 92, 115
cytokines, neuroactive 41–42, 88–89.
    See also inflammatory cytokines

DAT imaging 203
DATATOP study 206
d-cycloserine (DCS) 16–18, 93
declarative memory 18
deep brain stimulation (DBS) 54, 136, 201–202
default mode network (DMN) 151
definitions
    biomarkers 254
    epigenetics 336
    seizure tests/epilepsy models 233
    translational neuroscience ix, 340–343
degenerative disorders.
    See neurodegenerative disorders
deltaFosB transcription factor 32–33
dementia, amyotrophic lateral sclerosis 215. See also Alzheimer's disease
demyelination, multiple sclerosis 181–182
dendritic spine remodeling 53
depression. See also antidepressants
    5-HT hypothesis 5
    epigenetics 327, **330–331**
    NMDA receptor antagonists 5
desipramine 310
detoxification 109
developmental disorders.
    See neurodevelopmental disorders
Devic's disease 181
dextromethorphan **219**
diabetes
    Alzheimer's disease 136
    transgenic models 256
diagnostic issues
    autism spectrum disorders 273
    neurodevelopmental disorders 334
    neurological disorders 139
    Parkinson's disease 203
Diagnostic and Statistical Manual of Mental Disorders (DSM) 8, 123–124
diazepam **231**
diet, ketogenic 241–242
diffusion tensor imaging (DTI) 275–276
DiGeorge syndrome 90–91
DISC1 gene
    autism spectrum disorders 292
    schizophrenia 85, 90
DJ-1 gene 200
DNA, covalent modifications 323–324.
    See also epigenetics
dopamine
    ADHD 267–268, 304–305, 312
    Parkinson's disease 130, 197, 201
    psychostimulants 306–310
    schizophrenia 3, 80, 82, 91
    tricyclic antidepressants 311
Down syndrome 336

DSM (*Diagnostic and Statistical Manual of Mental Disorders*) 8, 123–124
DTI (diffusion tensor imaging) 275–276
dysbindin gene 86, 90
dyskinesia 201

EAE model, multiple sclerosis 186–187
early intervention 334
early life events 48–50, 326–327
ECT (electroconvulsive therapy) 327
EDSS (Expanded Disability Status Scale) 189, **190**
EEG (electroencephalography) 83–84, 277–278
electrical kindling **235**, 236
electrophysiological measures, schizophrenia 83–84
endogenous opioid system 112–114, 123
endophenotypes 349–350, 354
    autism 283–287, 288–289, **291**, **346**
environmental factors
    autism spectrum disorders 282
    multiple sclerosis 130
    neurological disorders 130
    Parkinson's disease 198–199
enzymes 233
epigenetics 321, 336, 337.
    See also genetics
    chromatin remodeling mechanisms 321–324
    future directions **330–331**
    neurodevelopmental disorders 328–329, 336–337
    neurological disorders 325–326
    neuropsychological disorders 125, 326–328
    substance abuse 329–330, **330–331**
epilepsy 228–232, 248.
    See also antiepileptic drugs
    epigenetics 326, **330–331**
    future directions 246–248
    genetics 228, 238
    models 233
    nonpharmacological approaches 241–242
    preclinical screening 234–242
    proof-of-concept studies 242–244
    regulatory pathways **231**, 245–246
    and traumatic brain injury **237**, 246–247
epileptogenesis 229–230, 236–237
Epstein–Barr virus (EBV) 180
ErbB4 gene 90
escape deficits 32–33, 35
etanercept 42

361

Index

ethics, memory consolidation disruption 18
etiology. *See* causality
European regulation of AEDs 245–246
Expanded Disability Status Scale (EDSS) 189, **190**
exposure therapy, anxiety disorders 17–18
extinction-based treatment, anxiety 15, 16–18, 22

face validity
　autism spectrum disorders 279
　seizure tests/epilepsy models 234
FAD gene 155, 156–159
fatigue states 42
fear, neurobiology of 14–15, **16**. *See also* anxiety disorders
fibromyalgia **170**. *See also* neuropathic pain
fine-tuning 352–353
5-HT hypothesis 3, 4, 49
　autism 261–264, 288
　depression 5
FMR1 gene 264, 281, 290–291, 292, 328–329. *See also* fragile X syndrome
fMRI (functional magnetic resonance imaging), pain 174
folic acid 265–266
Food and Drug Administration (FDA), US **231**, 245–246
forced swim test 31–32, 33–34
fragile X syndrome 264–267, 280, 281, 290–291, 292
　epigenetics 328–329, **330–331**
　metabotropic glutamate receptors 334–335
　translational neuroscience 335
fused in sarcoma (*FUS*) gene 217

G protein-coupled receptors 233
GABA functioning
　addictive disorders 114
　autism spectrum disorders 275–276, 293
　epilepsy 240, 326
　magnetoencephalography **276**
　mood disorders 59
　schizophrenia 82–83, 93, 118–119
gabapentin **219**, 231
GAD1 (glutamic acid decarboxylase-1) gene 328
gain-of-function mutations 199–200
γ-aminobutyric acid. *See* GABA functioning
gamma neural synchrony 290–291
γ-secretase 154, 160
gap junctions **233**

GAPDH (glyceraldehyde phosphate dehydrogenase) 206
Gates Foundation 352
gene-based drug discovery 139–140
gene silencing 223–224
gene therapy
　amyotrophic lateral sclerosis 221–222
　neurological disorders 139
　Parkinson's disease 136
genetic testing 346–347
genetics. *See also* epigenetics
　addictive disorders 113–114, 123
　ADHD 313
　Alzheimer's disease 155
　amyotrophic lateral sclerosis 216–217
　autism spectrum disorders 280–281
　epilepsy 228, 238
　fragile X syndrome 335
　Huntington's disease 347
　mood disorders 28, 56–57
　multiple sclerosis 185
　neurological disorders 132–137
　Parkinson's disease **133–134**, 199–200
　psychiatry, translational medicine 118
　schizophrenia 85, 90–91, 119–120, 327–328
genome-wide association studies 132
　Parkinson's disease 200
　psychiatry 124
　schizophrenia 4, 85, 348
genomics 354
glatiramer acetate 178, 186, **187**
glial cells 59, 94–95
glucocorticoids 20, 21–22, 49–51
glutamate. *See also* NMDA receptors
　addictive disorders 115
　amyotrophic lateral sclerosis 215
　anxiety disorders 16–18
　autism spectrum disorders 292
　epilepsy 326
　mood disorders 5, 36, 42–48, 59
　schizophrenia 3–4, 83, 91–93, 118–119
glutamine 59
glutathione **219**
glyceraldehyde phosphate dehydrogenase (GAPDH) 206
glycine 16–18, 92
glycogen synthase kinase 3 (*GSK-3*) 29–32, 38–39, **40**
gray matter
　animal models 59–60
　lithium 37, **38**
　multiple sclerosis 182

neurophysiological imaging 57–58
　schizophrenia 94–95
　structural neuroimaging 56–57
growth factors, neural 33–35. *See also* BDNF
GSK-3 (glycogen-synthase kinase-3) inhibitors 6
guanfacine 311
GWAS. *See* genome-wide association studies

haloperidol 80
HATs (histone acetyl transferases) 322
HDAC (histone deacetylase) inhibitors (HIDs)
　Alzheimer's disease 322–323, 325
　anxiety disorders 327
　depression 327
　epilepsy 326
　schizophrenia 328
　substance abuse 329–330
head size, autism spectrum disorders 288
heavy metals 282
height, and body mass index (BMI) 345
hemispheric lateralization, language functioning 290
herbicides 198–199
HIDS. *See* HDAC inhibitors
hippocampus 48–49, 57, 121, 327
hiPSCs (human induced pluripotent stem cells) 125, 345–346
histone acetyl transferases (HATs) 322
histone deacetylases. *See* HDAC inhibitors
histone proteins
　acetylation 336
　covalent posttranslational modifications 321–323
　methylation 322
historical perspectives
　ADHD 267
　fragile X syndrome 265–266
　multiple sclerosis 178–180
　neurodevelopmental disorders 261
　neurological disorders 129–130
　psychiatric disorders 1
human induced pluripotent stem cells (hiPSCs) 125, 345–346
Huntington's disease 339, 343–344
　causality 130
　current treatments 131
　genetics 134, **135**
　translational neuroscience barriers/ obstacles 347–348
hyperserotonemia 261–263
hypothalamic-pituitary-adrenal axis 48–49, 57, 326–327

IGF1 (insulin-like growth factor 1) **219**
imipramine 310
immune system, autism spectrum disorders 288
immunotherapy
  Alzheimer's disease 160–161
  multiple sclerosis 180
IMPACT (International MS Secondary Progressive Avonex Controlled Trial) 189, **190**
imprinting 125
in vitro to *in vivo* applications. *See* translational research
incomplete transgenic models 255
individualized medicine 123, 186
infection 119
  and autism 282
  and multiple sclerosis 178, 180
inflammation
  epilepsy 229–230, 242, 247–248
  pain 168, 169, 170–171. *See also* pain therapeutics
  Parkinson's disease 199
inflammatory cytokines
  biomarkers 132
  mood disorders 121–122
  plasticity, cellular/synaptic **43**
  schizophrenia 88–89, 95
influenza infection 119
inhibitory systems 114. *See also* GABA functioning
insecticides 198–199, 282
insulin resistance 136
insulin-like growth factor 1 (IGF1) **219**
integration, knowledge 352–353
integrins 184
interfering RNA (RNAi) 223–224
interferon 178, 183, 186, **187**
interleukin-2 gene 185
intermediate phenotypes 83–85
International MS Secondary Progressive Avonex Controlled Trial (IMPACT) 189, **190**
intervention, early 334
ion channels, acid sensing **233**
iproniazid 2
istradefylline 204–205

ketamine 5, 46, 118–119
ketogenic diet 241–242
kinases 206
kindling 229–230, **235**, 236, **237**, 238
knowledge
  integration 352–353
  pretense-of-wisdom syndrome 352–353, 354
kynurenine 121–122

lamotrigine 93, **219**, **231**, 236, 238, 239
language functioning, autism 284–286, 290
latent inhibition 84
lateralization, language functioning 290
L-dopa 197, 201, 202
learned helplessness paradigm 32–34, 35, 53
learning. *See also* memory
  addictive disorders 107
  schizophrenia 93
levetiracetam **231**, 238–239
Lewy bodies 198, 199
LFPs (local field potentials) 278, **279**
life expectancy
  epilepsy 228
  Parkinson's disease 202
life events, early 48–50, 326–327
ligand-gated ion channels **233**
literature search, PUBMED **342**
lithium 36–37, 122
  glycogen synthase kinase 3 38–39, **40**
  gray matter 37, **38**
  historical perspective 2
local field potentials (LFPs) 278, **279**
loss-of-function mutations 200
LRRK2 gene 200

M100 274–276, 289
magnetic mismatch field 274–276, 290
magnetic resonance imaging. *See* MRI
magnetic resonance spectroscopy (MRS) 275–276
magnetoencephalography (MEG) 274–276, 277–278, 289
maintenance treatment, addictive disorders 109–110
major depressive disorder (MDD). *See* depression, mood disorders
major histocompatibility complex 120, 133, 180, 185
major tranquilizers 3–4, 118
mania. *See* bipolar disorder, mood disorders
maternal care 48–50, 326–327
maximal electroshock (MES) test 235–236
MDD (major depressive disorder). *See* depression, mood disorders
MeCP2 gene 281, 292
medial prefrontal cortex 54–57
MEG (magnetoencephalography) 274–276, 277–278, 289
melatonin 5
memory formation/consolidation 18–22, 93, 336
MES (maximal electroshock) test 235–236

metabolic syndrome 136
metabolomics, Parkinson's disease 203–204
metabotropic glutamate receptors (nGluRs) 48, 266, 334–335
methadone 109–110
methylation. *See also* epigenetics
  DNA 323–324
  fragile X syndrome 328–329
  histone proteins **322**, 323
methylphenidate 292, 303
  ADHD 304
  animal models **309**
  cognitive functioning 306, 309
  psychostimulants 307–308
mianserin 311
microglia 160
microRNAs 124–125, 337
mild cognitive impairment (MCI) 150–151. *See also* cognitive functioning
minocycline **219**
mismatch negativity 274–276, 290
mitochondrial function
  Alzheimer's disease 134, 139
  Parkinson's disease 200
mitoxantrone 186, **187**
molecular endophenotypes, autism 288
monoamine oxidase inhibitors 311–312
monoaminergic neurotransmitters 27, 28–29
mood disorders 27–29, 30, 61–62, 121–122. *See also* anxiety disorders, bipolar disorder, depression, neurocircuitry of mood disorders
  animal models 31–32, 35, 59–60
  Bcl-2 family proteins 35–38
  BDNF 5, 31, 33–35, **36**, 121
  cyclic adenosine monophosphate pathway 29–32
  dendritic spine remodeling 53
  early life events 48–50
  epigenetics 326–327, **330–331**
  glucocorticoid receptors 49–51
  glutamate/glutamine/GABA 42–48, 59
  glycogen synthase kinase 3 38–39, **40**
  growth factors/neurotrophins 33–35
  neuroactive cytokines 41–42
  neurocircuitry 53–57, 60–61
  neurogenesis 51–53, 121
  neuropathology 59
  neurophysiological imaging 57–59

363

Index

mood disorders (cont.)
  NMDA receptors 36, 45–46, 121–122
  p11 39–41
  plasticity, cellular/synaptic 123
  protein kinase C inhibition 33
  stress models 121
  structural neuroimaging 56–57
  transcription factors 32–33
mortality rates
  epilepsy 228
  Parkinson's disease 202
motor neurone diseases.
  See amyotrophic lateral sclerosis
motor symptoms, Parkinson's disease 197–198
mouse screens, autism 282–283.
  See also animal models
MRI (magnetic resonance imaging)
  multiple sclerosis 179–180, 187–188
  pain therapeutics 174
MRS (magnetic resonance spectroscopy) 275–276
MS. *See* multiple sclerosis
MTP (mitochondrial transition pore) function 134
mTOR cascade 247–248, 292
multiple sclerosis 120, 178, 191
  animal models 186–187
  biomarkers 255
  current treatments 131
  drug targets 183–186
  environmental factors 130
  future directions 190–191
  genetics 133, **135**, 185
  historical perspective 178–180
  neuroimaging 187–188
  outcome measures/scales 188–190
  pathogenesis 180–182, **184**
  pharmacodynamic markers 186
  translational neuroscience 183
Multiple Sclerosis Functional Composite (MSFC) measure 189–190
mutations
  autism spectrum disorders 280–281
  gain-of-function 199–200
  loss-of-function 200
  superoxide dismutase gene 215

N-acetyl-L-cysteine **219**
naloxone/naltrexone 110–111, 112–114, 123
natalizumab 183, **184**, 186, **187**
Natalizumab Safety and Efficacy in Relapsing-Remitting Multiple Sclerosis (AFFIRM) study 189
National Institutes of Health (NIH) Clinical Center ix

Research Domain Criteria Project 123–124
roadmap ix
Nav1.7 gene 170
NCT (nicastrin) transgenic models 159
negative predictive value 242–243
neprilysin 325
nerve growth factor-inducible protein A (NGFI-A) 326–327
neural synchrony, autism 290–291
neuregulin 1 gene (*NRG1*) 86
neuroactive cytokines 41–42, 88–89.
  See also inflammatory cytokines
neuroanatomy, autism 288
neurobiological substrates, behavioral interventions 350–351
neurodegenerative diseases 36–37.
  See also Alzheimer's disease, amyotrophic lateral sclerosis, multiple sclerosis, Parkinson's disease
neurodevelopmental disorders 261, 269, 334–336. *See also* ADHD, autism, fragile X syndrome
  clinical trials 335
  epigenetics 328–329, 336–337
  historical perspectives 261
  schizophrenia model 88–89
neurodevelopmental regulation, microRNAs 337
neurogenesis 29, **30**
  epilepsy 229–230
  mood disorders 51–53, 121
neuroimaging. *See also* DTI, EEG, fMRI, MRI, MRS, PET
  autism spectrum disorders 289–291
  mood disorders 56–59
  multiple sclerosis 187–188
  pain therapeutics 173–174
neuroinflammation. *See* inflammation
neurological disorders 129–130, 140.
  See also Alzheimer's disease, amyotrophic lateral sclerosis, multiple sclerosis, epilepsy, Parkinson's disease
  animal models 255–257
  biomarkers 131–132, 139, 254–255
  causality 129, 130, 138
  challenge of finding new treatments 131–132
  clinical trials 137, 257
  combination therapies 258–259
  common themes 138–139, **138–140**
  current treatments 130–131
  gene-based drug discovery 139–140
  genetics 132–137, **133–134**
neuropathic pain 168–169, **170**, 171–172. *See also* pain therapeutics

neurophysiological endophenotypes, autism 288–289
neuroplasticity. *See* plasticity
neuropsychiatric disorders. *See* psychiatry
Neuro-QOL project 190
neurotoxins. *See* environmental factors
neurotransmitters. *See also* dopamine; 5-HT, norepinephrine
  ADHD 304–305
  monoaminergic 27, 28–29
  psychostimulants 306–307
  transporters **233**
neurotrophins 33–35, 288.
  See also BDNF
NF1 gene 292
nicotine 111–112, 136, 199
nicotinic acetylcholine receptors 93
NIH. *See* National Institutes of Health
NLGN3 gene 290–291
NMDA receptors. *See also* glutamate
  anxiety disorders 16–18, 21, 120
  autism spectrum disorders 292
  mood disorders 5, 36, 45–46, 121–122
  schizophrenia 3–4, 87–88, 90, 91–93, 118–119
nociceptive pain 168, 169, 170.
  See also pain therapeutics
norepinephrine (noradrenaline) 4
  ADHD 268–269, 304–305
  psychostimulants 306–310
  tricyclic antidepressants 311
nortryptyline 311
Notch processing 135
NR2B gene 46. *See also* NMDA
NRG1-ErbB4 (neuregulin) gene 90
NSAID (non-steroidal anti-inflammatory drugs)
  Alzheimer's disease 135–136
  inflammatory pain 169
  nociceptive pain 169
  Parkinson's disease 136, 199

'oddball' experimental designs 274–276, 290
olfactory dysfunction 198
opioid system, endogenous 112–114, 123
orbital prefrontal cortex, 54–57
organophosphate insecticides 198–199, 282
oscillatory deficits, schizophrenia 84
oxidative stress 92, 95, 132

364

Index

p11 gene 39–41
Paced Auditory Serial Addition Test (PASAT) 189
pain therapeutics 168–169, 174
 animal models 170–172
 experimental human models 173
 neuroimaging 173–174
 pharmacological treatment 169, **170**
 R & D 169–170
 translational neuroscience 172–173
paradoxical effects, psychostimulants 306
paraquat 198
Parkinson's disease 197, 207
 adenosine A2A antagonists 204–205
 apoptosis pathway 206
 biomarkers 203–204, 206
 clinical trials 137
 current treatments 130, 200–202
 early pathology 131
 environmental factors 130, 198–199
 epigenetics 325–326, **330–331**
 genetics **133–134**, 199–200
 mortality rates/life expectancy 202
 motor symptoms 197–198
 neurodegeneration 202
 new treatment strategies 136–137
 non-motor symptoms 198
 treatment complications 202
 unmet needs of current therapies 202–203
PASAT (Paced Auditory Serial Addition Test) 189
pentoxifylline **219**
personalized medicine 123, 186
pesticides 198–199, 282
PET (positron emission tomography) 174
pharmacodynamic markers. *See* biomarkers
pharmacoepigenomics 337
phenotypes
 behavioral. *See* endophenotypes
 intermediate 83–85
 screening 256–257
phenytoin **231**, 238
phosphodiesterase (PDE) 31–32
PINK1 gene 200
placebo effect
 amyotrophic lateral sclerosis 220
 epilepsy 245
 multiple sclerosis 191
 psychiatric disorders 7–8
plasticity, cellular/synaptic 123
 addictive disorders 107, 115
 autism spectrum disorders 292
 cytokines, neuroactive 41–42
 epilepsy 229–230
 inflammatory cytokines 43

mood disorders 29, 34, **52**, 61
 schizophrenia 89
POC. *See* proof-of-concept studies
positive predictive value 242
positron emission tomography (PET) 174
posttraumatic stress disorder (PTSD) 14, **15**, 18–22
PPI (prepulse inhibition) 84, 288, 351
pramipexole 37–38
predictive validity
 autism spectrum disorders 279
 seizure tests/epilepsy models 234
predictive value, negative/positive 242–243
prefrontal cortex
 ADHD 303–304, 308–309
 catecholamines 304–305
 mood disorders 53–54
 psychostimulants 309–310
 stress 48–49
prepulse inhibition 84, 288, 351
pretence-of-wisdom syndrome 352–353, 354
proconvulsant drugs 241
promiscuous drugs 258
proof-of-concept (POC) studies
 epilepsy 242–244
 multiple sclerosis 191
propionic acid 282
propranolol 19–20, 21–22
protein kinase A 29–32
protein kinase C 33
protein misfolding 129, 139. *See also* tau hypothesis
proteomics, Parkinson's disease 203–204
PS1/2 gene 155, 158
pseudo-placebo effect 245
psychiatric disorders 1–2, 8–9. *See also* specific disorders
 animal models 7
 clinical trials 7–8
 diagnosis 8
 epigenetics 326–327
 future directions 123–125
 historical perspectives 1
 plasticity, cellular/synaptic 123
 translational neuroscience 6–7, 118, 125, 351–352
psychosocial interventions 350–351, 354–355
psychostimulants 303, 304, 306–310
 and cognitive functioning 306, 309–310
PTEN gene 292
PTSD (posttraumatic stress disorder) 14, **15**, 18–22
PTZ (pentylenetetrazol) test 235–236

publication bias 257
PUBMED literature search **342**

quinolinic acid 121–122

R & D. *See also* clinical trials
 neurological disorders 139
 pain therapeutics 169–170
 psychiatric disorders ix–x
radioligand binding 2
rapamycin 247–248, 292
rapid-eye movement behavior disorder (RBD) 198
rasagiline 206
reelin gene 328, 329
refractoriness creep 245
regeneration, neural 35. *See also* plasticity
regulation, legal 245–246
repetitive behaviors 286
Research Domain Criteria Project 123–124
resilience, cellular 29
 resting state magnetoencephalography 275
Rett syndrome 120, 280, 281, 335
reward systems 108–109
riluzole 45, 131, 218, **219**
risperidone 291
rituximab 183
RNAi (interfering RNA) 223–224
rotenone 199

S100A10 gene 39–41
saccadic eye-movement 288–289
S-adenosylhomocysteine (SAM) 329
SARs (structure-activity relationships) 2
SB (drug) 327
schizophrenia 81, 95–96, 118–120, 339. *See also* antipsychotic drugs
 animal models 88–91
 apoptosis 94–95
 BDNF 87, 94
 dopaminergic activity 3, 82, 91
 epigenetics 327–328, **330–331**
 GABA receptors 82–83, 93, 118–119
 genetics 85, 90–91, 119–120, 327–328
 genome-wide association studies 4
 glutamate function 3–4, 83, 91–93, 118–119
 historical perspective 80–81
 intermediate phenotypes 83–85
 NMDA receptors 3–4, 87–88, 90, 118–119
 novel therapeutic targets 91–95
 plasticity, cellular/synaptic 123
 synaptic connectivity 81–82

365

Index

schizophrenia (cont.)
  translational neuroscience barriers/obstacles 345–346, 348
SCN1A gene 238, 241
secretase 154, 160
seizure tests 233
senataxin (*ALS4*) gene 217
SENTINEL (Safety and Efficacy of Natalizumab in Combination with Interferon in Patients with Relapsing-Remitting Multiple Sclerosis) study 189
serendipity, roll in drug discovery 341, 345
serotonin. *See* 5-HT, SSRIs
signaling pathways
  mood disorders 29, 35, 38–39, **40**, 61
  NRG1-ErbB4 90
signatures, electrophysiological 273–274, 277–278. *See also* biomarkers
single nucleotide polymorphisms (SNPs) 85, 343
6-Hz seizure test **235**, 238–239
SMN gene 217
smoking 111–112, 136, 199
social behavior
  autism spectrum disorders 283–284
  schizophrenia 84–85
social defeat 32, 33
social isolation 32
SOD1 gene 214, 215, 216, 223–224
sodium ion channel 170
sodium phenylbutyrate **219**
spike-wave discharges **235**, 236
SSRIs (selective serotonin reuptake inhibitors) 5, 264, 292
STAR*D (Sequenced Treatment Alternatives to Relieve Depression) trial 8
startle response 84, 288, 351
status epilepticus model 237
stem cell therapy
  amyotrophic lateral sclerosis 222–223
  neurological disorders 139
  Parkinson's disease 136
stress 48–49, 59–60, 121, 326–327. *See also* posttraumatic stress disorder
structure–activity relationships (SARs) 2
subcutaneous pentylenetetrazol (PTZ) test 235–236
subgenual ACC (anterior cingulate cortex) 56–59

substance abuse. *See* addictive disorders
superoxide dismutase (*SOD1*) gene 214, 215, 216, 223–224
survival of motor neuron (*SMN*) gene 217
synaptic connectivity, schizophrenia 81–82
synaptic vesicle protein (SV2A) 240

tail suspension test 31–32
tamoxifen 33, 120
TARDNA-binding protein (TDP-43) 217
target-based drug screening 256–257
tau hypothesis 132, 134–135, 149, 151–153
  biomarkers 132
  epigenetics 325
  immunotherapy 160–161
  transgenic models 156–158
TBI (traumatic brain injury) **237**, 246–247
temporal lobe epilepsy 326
tetrabenazine 131
therapeutic index, AEDs 239
therapeutic window, AEDs 235
thimerosal 282
time to *n*th seizure study design 244
timelines, proof-of-concept trials 243
timolol 21
TNF (tumor necrosis factor) receptor-1 35, 41
TNFα chimeric antibodies 135–136
topiramate **219**, **231**, 239
transcranial magnetic stimulation 136, 244
transcriptomics 29–33, 203–204
transferin receptors 135
transgenic models 7. *See also* animal models
  Alzheimer's disease 156–159
  amyotrophic lateral sclerosis 215
  α-synuclein 255
translational neuroscience, general references
  barriers/obstacles 344–347, 348–350, 354
  definitions ix, 340–343
  stages 340–345, 354
translocation in liposarcoma gene 217
trauma. *See* life events, posttraumatic stress disorder, stress
traumatic brain injury (TBI) **237**, 246–247
tricyclic antidepressants 269, 310–311

tryptophan 262, 263–264. *See also* 5-HT hypothesis
TSC1/2 genes 247, 281, 292
tuberous sclerosis 247–248, 280, 281, 290–291
tumor necrosis factor (TNF) receptor-1 35, 41
tyrosine kinase B receptors 33

ubiquitin proteasome system (UPS) 200
UCH-L1 gene 200
ultraviolet model, pain therapeutics 173
unbridged gap, translational research paradigm 6
US Food and Drug Administration (FDA) **231**, 245–246

vaccination, and autism 282
validation criteria, preclinical models of autism 279–280
validity. *See also* construct/face/predictive validity
  animal models 7, 108–109
  DSM 123–124
  seizure tests/epilepsy models 233–234
valley of death translational research paradigm 6
valproate/valproic acid
  autism 122, **231**, 282, 290, 292
  epilepsy 326
  mood disorders 39, 45
varenicline 111–112
vascular endothelial growth factor (VEGF) 34–35, 221
velocardiofacial syndrome 90–91
verapamil **219**
vesicle-associated protein (*VAPB*) gene 217
vitamin E **219**
voltage-gated ion channels **233**
vulnerability factors, addictive disorders 108

watershed model, endophenotypes **346**
websites
  clinical trials 221
  cytokines, neuroactive 42
white matter 61, 304
wisdom, pretense of 352–353, 354
withdrawal symptoms 109

xaliproden **219**